*Editor*

# JOHN MARQUIS CONVERSE, M.D.

Lawrence D. Bell Professor of Plastic Surgery,
New York University School of Medicine

*Assistant Editor*

## JOSEPH G. McCARTHY, M.D.

Associate Professor of Surgery (Plastic Surgery),
New York University School of Medicine

*Editor, section on The Hand*

## J. WILLIAM LITTLER, M.D.

Chief of Plastic and Reconstructive Surgery,
The Roosevelt Hospital, New York City

SECOND EDITION

# RECONSTRUCTIVE PLASTIC SURGERY

*Principles and Procedures
in Correction, Reconstruction
and Transplantation*

## VOLUME SEVEN
## THE LOWER EXTREMITY
## THE TRUNK
## THE GENITOURINARY TRACT

W. B. SAUNDERS COMPANY
Philadelphia • London • Toronto
Mexico City • Rio de Janeiro • Sydney • Tokyo

W. B. Saunders Company: West Washington Square
Philadelphia, PA 19105

1 St. Anne's Road
Eastbourne, East Sussex BN21 3UN, England

1 Goldthorne Avenue
Toronto, Ontario M8Z 5T9, Canada

Apartado 26370—Cedro 512
Mexico 4, D.F., Mexico

Rua Coronel Cabrita, 8
Sao Cristovao Caixa Postal 21176
Rio de Janeiro, Brazil

9 Waltham Street
Artarmon, N.S.W. 2064, Australia

Ichibancho, Central Bldg., 22-1 Ichibancho
Chiyoda-Ku, Tokyo 102, Japan

| Complete Set | 0-7216-2691-2 |
| Volume 1 | 0-7216-2680-7 |
| Volume 2 | 0-7216-2681-5 |
| Volume 3 | 0-7216-2682-3 |
| Volume 4 | 0-7216-2683-1 |
| Volume 5 | 0-7216-2684-X |
| Volume 6 | 0-7216-2685-8 |
| Volume 7 | 0-7216-2686-6 |

Reconstructive Plastic Surgery

Last digit is the print number:   9   8   7   6   5

# CONTRIBUTORS

## TO VOLUME SEVEN

VINKO ARNERI, M.D.

Professor of Plastic Surgery and Specialist in General Surgery, Military Medical Academy, Belgrade. Director, Klinika za Plasticku Hirurgiju, V.M.A., Belgrade, Yugoslavia.

SHERRELL J. ASTON, M.D.

Assistant Professor of Surgery (Plastic Surgery), New York University School of Medicine. Assistant Attending Surgeon, Institute of Reconstructive Plastic Surgery, New York University Medical Center. Chief, Plastic Surgery Service, Veterans Administration Hospital, New York; Associate Attending Surgeon, Manhattan Eye, Ear and Throat Hospital, New York.

EARL Z. BROWNE, JR., M.D.

Assistant Professor, Division of Plastic Surgery, University of Utah College of Medicine. Surgeon, University Medical Center, Salt Lake City, Utah.

ROSS M. CAMPBELL, M.D.

Formerly Associate Professor of Clinical Surgery (Plastic Surgery), New York University School of Medicine, and Attending Surgeon in Plastic Surgery, Institute of Reconstructive Plastic Surgery, New York University Medical Center, New York.

BRADFORD CANNON, M.D.

Clinical Professor of Surgery (Emeritus), Harvard Medical School. Senior Consulting Staff, Massachusetts General Hospital, Boston, Massachusetts.

JOHN MARQUIS CONVERSE, M.D.

Lawrence D. Bell Professor of Plastic Surgery, New York University School of Medicine; Director, Institute of Reconstructive Plastic Surgery, New York University Medical Center; Director of Plastic Surgery Service, Bellevue Hospital; Consultant in Plastic Surgery, Manhattan Eye, Ear and Throat Hospital and Veterans Administration Hospital, New York.

DOUGLAS S. DAHL, M.D.

Assistant Professor of Surgery, University of Utah College of Medicine. Active Staff, University Medical Center, Salt Lake City, Utah.

JOSÉ DELGADO, M.D.

Clinical Associate Professor of Surgery (Plastic Surgery), New York University School of Medicine. Associate Attending Surgeon, Institute of Reconstructive Plastic Surgery, New York University Medical Center, Bellevue Hospital, and Manhattan Eye, Ear and Throat Hospital, New York.

### WALLACE M. DENNISON, M.D., F.R.C.S.(Ed.), F.R.C.S.(Glasg.)

Formerly Barclay Lecturer in Surgery of Childhood, University of Glasgow; Senior Surgeon and Chairman of the Division of Surgery, Royal Hospital for Sick Children and Surgical Paediatric Unit, Stobhill Hospital, Glasgow; Paediatric Surgeon, Royal Maternity Hospital, Glasgow, Scotland.

### CHARLES J. DEVINE, JR., M.D.

Professor and Chairman, Department of Urology, Eastern Virginia Medical School. Chief, Department of Urology, Medical Center Hospitals, Inc. and DePaul Hospital; Active Staff, Children's Hospital of the King's Daughters, General Hospital of Virginia Beach, Bayside Hospital, and Chesapeake General Hospital, Norfolk, Virginia.

### PATRICK C. DEVINE, M.D.

Professor, Department of Urology, Eastern Virginia Medical School. Director, Urology Residency Program, Medical Center Hospitals, Inc. and DePaul Hospital; Active Staff, Children's Hospital of the King's Daughters, Norfolk, Virginia; Consultant, U.S. Naval Hospital, Portsmouth, and Veterans Administration Center, Hampton, Virginia.

### LEONARD T. FURLOW, M.D.

Clinical Associate Professor of Plastic Surgery, University of Florida School of Medicine. Attending Plastic Surgeon, Alachua General Hospital and North Florida Regional Hospital; Consultant in Plastic Surgery, Veterans Administration Hospital, Gainesville, Florida.

### RALPH GER, M.D.

Professor of Surgery and Professor of Anatomy, Albert Einstein College of Medicine. Director of Surgery, Hospital of the Albert Einstein College of Medicine, Bronx, New York.

### JOSEPH W. HAYHURST, M.D.

Clinical Assistant Professor of Plastic Surgery, University of Oklahoma College of Medicine. Director of the Microsurgery Unit, Presbyterian Hospital, Oklahoma City, Oklahoma.

### HERBERT HÖHLER, M.D.

Chief of the Department of Plastic and Reconstructive Surgery, St. Markus Krankenhaus, Frankfurt am Main, Germany.

### CHARLES E. HORTON, M.D.

Professor and Chairman, Department of Plastic Surgery, Eastern Virginia Medical School. Chief of Plastic Surgery, Medical Center Hospitals, Inc.; Consultant, DePaul Hospital and Children's Hospital of the King's Daughters, Norfolk, Virginia.

### STEPHEN R. LEWIS, M.D.

Professor of Surgery and Chief, Division of Plastic Surgery, The University of Texas Medical Branch. Consultant, St. Mary's Infirmary and Galveston County Memorial Hospital, Galveston, Texas.

### JOSEPH G. McCARTHY, M.D.

Associate Professor of Surgery (Plastic Surgery), New York University School of Medicine. Associate Director, Institute of Reconstructive Plastic Surgery, New York

University Medical Center. Attending Surgeon, University Hospital, Bellevue Hospital, Manhattan Eye, Ear and Throat Hospital, and Veterans Administration Hospital, New York.

## JOHN B. McCRAW, M.D.

Associate Clinical Professor of Plastic Surgery, Eastern Virginia Medical School. Attending Surgeon, Medical Center Hospitals, Inc., Norfolk, Virginia; Consultant to Public Health and U.S. Naval Hospitals, Portsmouth, Virginia, and Bethesda, Maryland.

## FRED M. MASSEY, M.D.

Chief, Gynecologic Oncology, Wilford Hall U.S.A.F. Medical Center, Lackland Air Force Base, Texas.

## JOHN CLARKE MUSTARDÉ, M.B., Ch.B., D.O.M.S., F.R.C.S., F.R.C.S.(Glasg.)

Clinical Lecturer in Plastic Surgery, University of Glasgow. Consultant Plastic Surgeon, West of Scotland Plastic Surgery Unit, Canniesburn Hospital, Glasgow; Royal Hospital for Sick Children, Glasgow; Ballochmyle Hospital, Ayrshire; and Seafield Sick Children's Hospital, Ayr, Scotland.

## KENNETH L. PICKRELL, M.D.

Professor of Plastic and Reconstructive Surgery, Duke University Medical Center. Consultant Plastic Surgeon, Veterans Administration Hospitals, Durham and Fayetteville, and Memorial Hospital, Greensboro, North Carolina.

## IVO PITANGUY, M.D.

Professor of Plastic and Reconstructive Surgery, Catholic University of Rio de Janeiro. Chief, Plastic Reconstructive Unit, Santa Casa do Rio de Janeiro General Hospital, Rio de Janeiro, Brazil.

## THOMAS D. REES, M.D.

Clinical Professor of Surgery (Plastic Surgery), New York University School of Medicine. Attending Surgeon, Institute of Reconstructive Plastic Surgery, New York University Medical Center. Visiting Surgeon, Bellevue Hospital; Chairman, Department of Plastic Surgery, Manhattan Eye, Ear and Throat Hospital, New York.

## CLIFFORD C. SNYDER, M.D.

Professor and Chairman, Division of Plastic Surgery, University of Utah College of Medicine. Chief, Surgical Services, Veterans Administration Hospital; Chief, Plastic Surgery Service, Shriners Hospital for Crippled Children, Salt Lake City, Utah.

## RICHARD BOIES STARK, M.D.

Professor of Clinical Surgery, Columbia University College of Physicians and Surgeons. Attending Surgeon in Charge of Plastic Surgery, St. Luke's Hospital, New York.

## DONALD WOOD-SMITH, M.B., F.R.C.S.E.

Associate Professor of Surgery (Plastic Surgery), New York University School of Medicine. Surgeon Director, Department of Plastic Surgery, Manhattan Eye, Ear and Throat Hospital; Attending Surgeon, Institute of Reconstructive Plastic Surgery, New York University Medical Center; Visiting Surgeon in Plastic Surgery, Bellevue Hospital; Attending Surgeon, Veterans Administration Hospital; Consultant, New York Eye and Ear Infirmary, New York.

# CONTENTS

ix

## *Part Six. The Genitourinary System*

*Part Four*

# THE LOWER
# EXTREMITY

# CHAPTER 86

# RECONSTRUCTIVE SURGERY OF THE LOWER EXTREMITY

BRADFORD CANNON, M.D.,
JOHN D. CONSTABLE, M.D.,
LEONARD T. FURLOW, M.D.,
J. W. HAYHURST, M.D.,
JOSEPH G. MCCARTHY, M.D.,
AND JOHN B. MCCRAW, M.D.

Closure of Defects of the Lower
Extremity by Muscle Flaps
*Ralph Ger, M.D.*

Closure of Defects of the Lower
Extremity by Myocutaneous Flaps
*John B. McCraw, M.D.*

The methods and principles of reconstructive surgery of the lower extremity are similar to those of reconstructive procedures elsewhere in the body. There are, however, certain unique anatomical characteristics of the lower extremities which may alter the standard reconstructive techniques. The anterior aspect of the tibia is covered only by a layer of skin with minimal subcutaneous tissue. Consequently a cutaneous defect of the pretibial area usually involves bone and does not provide a suitable bed for skin grafting. Another anatomical characteristic is the pattern of vascular anastomoses around the knee which makes possible the use of undelayed direct retrograde flaps in this area. However, the absence of such anastomoses below the knee endangers the vascularization of local flaps in this area. Furthermore, arteriosclerotic changes in the elderly and diabetic angiopathic changes complicate lower extremity reconstructive procedures in these patients.

The lack of readily accessible sources of flap donor tissue requires special methods of transfer, such as cross-leg, muscle, or microvascular free flaps. Newer reconstructive techniques have decreased the need for cross-leg fixation.

Another unique anatomical characteristic is the irreplaceable weight-bearing skin of the sole of the foot, which calls for special consideration in choosing tissue for repair.

Because of the dependent position of the legs, they require a longer period of protection and support for the healing tissues, a period considerably longer than that required in other parts of the body. Adjunctive measures such as leg elevation and wraparound dressings promote venous and lymphatic return. These special characteristics are but a few of those which must be considered when one is undertaking reconstructive procedures in the lower extremity.

The chapter is divided into two major sections: (1) reconstructive problems of the lower extremity, and (2) reconstructive procedures used in resurfacing cutaneous defects of the lower extremity.

## RECONSTRUCTIVE PROBLEMS OF THE LOWER EXTREMITY

Reconstructive problems of the lower extremity can be divided into several categories which will be considered separately. Plastic surgical techniques frequently prove invaluable in dealing with many of the pathologic conditions involving the lower extremity.

1. Problems following *acute trauma* are the commonest and perhaps the most frequently overlooked. Trauma may produce damage or destruction to skin only (burn, avulsion, crush), may involve the skin and underlying soft tissues (deep burn, laceration, crush), or may involve soft tissues and bone with or without a break in the skin (deep burn, fracture, severe crush). *The restoration of an intact cutaneous covering is the primary surgical requisite following trauma of the lower extremity because deep healing can be no better than the surface covering.* Restoration of the surface as soon as possible after injury is essential to prevent further contamination, to avoid the development of infection and suppuration, and to lessen fibrosis and interference with local blood supply. Tension and hematoma formation jeopardize healing in a primarily closed wound. If an acceptable primary repair is impossible, delayed primary closure or skin transplantation by a graft or a flap may be required. Hueston and Gunther (1967) advocated the primary use of a cross-leg flap to achieve cutaneous coverage following trauma, especially when

there is associated major skeletal injury and loss of the tendo Achilles. Surgical methods of resurfacing traumatic defects are discussed later in the chapter.

2. Circulatory insufficiency (arterial, venous, and lymphatic) may result in chronic ulceration, edema, and other disabilities of the dependent lower extremities. These problems challenge the skills of the reconstructive surgeon.

3. Tumors of the lower extremities may be either benign or malignant. They present problems in reconstruction because of their location, because of associated involvement of osseous structures, and because of spread through the lymphatics to the regional lymph nodes. The types of tumors encountered include carcinoma, melanoma, lymphangioma, and hemangioma.

4. Osteomyelitis, either post-traumatic or hematogenous in origin, is often associated with extensive loss of the overlying soft tissue. Resurfacing the defect with a skin flap, in addition to curettage of the involved bone, is often required.

5. Congenital anomalies, such as supernumerary toes and syndactyly, require careful evaluation before reshaping of the foot in order to simplify the fitting of shoes and to prevent problems in walking. In patients with constricting bands, excision and revision of the scar are required to improve the circulation in the distal portion of the extremity.

6. Finally, there is a miscellaneous group of disabilities of the lower extremity which at one time or another require surgical reconstruction. These include the plantar wart, plantar callus, keratosis plantaris, neurotrophic ulcers, the ingrown toenail, and the sequelae of irradiation for benign or malignant disease.

### Trauma

Trauma to the lower extremity may be of little consequence or may be of such magnitude that the healing of the deep tissues is temporarily or permanently impaired. The soft tissue repair must be constantly kept in mind and not treated lightly despite what may appear to be a minor injury. Failure of primary wound healing not only occurs in compound injuries with or without loss of skin but also complicates the open reduction of simple fractures if closure is attempted in the presence of significant subcutaneous or subfascial edema. Spontaneous rupture of the unbroken skin occurs occasionally if its circulation is impaired by tension.

Wounds of the lower extremity must be managed like soft tissue wounds elsewhere on the body. There are no exceptions to the principles of debridement and closure of the wound.

A special type of lower extremity trauma is the avulsion injury in which a flap of skin and subcutaneous tissue is raised, usually in the pretibial region. The surgeon must resist the temptation to resuture the flap, as the major portion is destined to necrosis because of extensive soft tissue injury and intravascular sludging.

The safest course is to resect the major portion of the avulsed flap and apply split-thickness skin grafts to the defect (either immediately or after 24 to 72 hours), provided the recipient bed is suitable for skin grafting. Connelly (1973) proposed the following test to determine the viability of the avulsed flap:

1. Elevate the leg for one minute.
2. Inflate a tourniquet around the thigh.
3. Lower the leg.
4. Deflate the tourniquet.
5. The point to which the circulation (pink color) returns correlates with the future line of demarcation. The avulsed flap should be debrided to this line.

The treatment of acute thermal burns is discussed in Chapter 18. It should be reemphasized, however, that in circumferential full-thickness burns of the lower extremity, radical fasciotomy may be required to prevent circulatory embarrassment, and separate incisions of the individual compartments are necessary.

The management of frostbite is discussed in Chapter 19, and the techniques available for reconstruction of the cold-injured foot follow later in the chapter.

**Bone Cavities.** A deep cavity in bone is fortunately seen less commonly in civilian practice than in the military. The missile that penetrates the tibia below the knee joint and the bumper fracture, usually compounded in the upper portion of the tibia, are common causes. Throughout the full length of the tibia, however, there is a minimum of soft tissue available anteriorly for primary coverage, and if there is a loss of bone substance as well, additional tissue for filling the cavity may be difficult to secure. Many concave surfaces of the lower leg are temporarily closed by lining the bone cavity with skin grafts applied to the thinly granulating surfaces. The temporary skin dressing of the wound may suffice permanently if a sufficiently strong surrounding bony framework remains to ensure adequate bony strength for normal use. If minimal bone remains or if there is nonunion, bone grafting is indicated.

If an adequate local flap is available for the covering tissue, autogenous cancellous iliac bone chips may be used to fill the cavity. The temporary lining skin graft must be removed with care to eliminate every bit of epithelial tissue; residual epithelium may become a source of infection and destroy the transplanted tissue or may form a cyst, which becomes the site of recurring local infection. The completely denuded cavity is filled with the bone grafts and is finally covered with a skin flap as discussed later in the chapter.

## Circulatory Disabilities

In the treatment of surface defects or cutaneous ulcers associated with venous, arterial, or lymphatic disease, correction of the underlying vascular disorder must be part of the therapeutic regimen.

**Venous Disease.** The commonest manifestation of circulatory disease with which the plastic surgeon is likely to be concerned is that of "varicose," "postphlebitic," "post-thrombotic," or "stasis" ulcers. These latter terms are used to distinguish more accurately the individual etiologies of similar lesions. Varicose ulcer is the oldest term, but it is incomplete, since only about 25 per cent of these lesions are due solely to the pathology of the varicose veins. Many ulcers have a definite history of antecedent deep thrombophlebitis and are therefore properly termed postphlebitic or post-thrombotic; this is not always the case, since ulceration may be due to incompetence of the deep veins or to varicose veins.

The essential factor in the development of these ulcers, regardless of whether the specific cause is varicose veins, deep thrombophlebitis, or silent venous thrombosis, is venous hypertension secondary to mechanical failure of the venous valves to support the venous blood returning from the extremity. It is now recognized that the critical factor in the return of venous blood to the heart from the legs, while dependent, is the pumping action of the muscles of the leg, which propels the blood of the deep venous system. The pumping action, however, is entirely dependent upon the integrity of the valves in the veins, and if these are destroyed, there is a retrograde backing up of blood in the superficial system, with relative local venous hypertension. If the incompetency of the valves is restricted to the superficial system (as in varicose veins), the deep veins will be unaffected. However, if there is destruction in the perforating veins that connect the deep and superficial systems, there will be reversal of the usual flow in these vessels, and the "muscle pump" will add more blood to the already distended superficial veins rather than pushing it upward out of the limb.

Once the process of relative venous hypertension has been established, there are progressive secondary changes in the limb, including increased capillary permeability, local extravascular extravasation of red cells with consequent hemosiderin deposition, irritation of the subcutaneous tissues, and the formation of dense scar tissue over which the skin becomes at first atrophic, tender, and erythematous, then exceedingly thin and fragile, and finally ulcerated. The site of ulceration will be determined by the area of maximal venous insufficiency but is characteristically near or over the medial malleolus. As long as the basic venous abnormality is not corrected or controlled, the ulcers will usually persist, and even if they heal occasionally, they are subject to frequent recurrence.

TREATMENT OF THE CUTANEOUS DEFECT. Since the skin ulcers are the most obvious and distressing evidence of venous disease, therapy must be aimed at closure of these lesions. In most cases treatment of the venous insufficiency will result in a rapid spontaneous healing of the ulcers. External support in the form of elastic bandages or elastic stockings is generally sufficient to promote healing of the ulcer. Although surgical treatment of the incompetent veins can be accomplished in the presence of open ulcerations, it is preferable to delay definitive vein surgery until the ulcers are healed. The location of the ulcers, as well as the scarring and induration around them, usually prevents the successful treatment by excision and direct closure.

A split-thickness skin graft is the treatment of choice, in some cases, for a large unhealed ulcer after the area has been sufficiently prepared. Frequent dressing changes will generally provide sufficient preparation, and local chemotherapy, antibiotics, or enzymatic debriding agents are unnecessary.

If skin grafting is feasible, healing will be of a better quality than when the wound is allowed to heal spontaneously; the graft heals with a cushion of underlying dermis, in contrast to the thin, atrophic, and unstable scar epithelium that grows in from the edges of the wound and is always vulnerable to minimal trauma.

A thin skin graft is preferable, since the ulcer bed tends to be densely scarred and the potential for vascularization of the graft is often less than

ideal. Local or distant skin flaps are rarely indicated in venous disease of the leg, since satisfactory healing can usually be obtained without these more complicated methods.

Thompson and Ell (1974) have advocated the dermal overgrafting technique in covering venous ulcers (Fig. 86–1). They have stated that serial application of skin grafts on a venous ulcer bed will yield a firm and resilient cover (see Chapter 6).

Any form of skin grafting requires complete bed rest for at least two weeks, with continuous elevation of the leg, and may eliminate the possibility of treating the ulcer on an ambulatory basis with adequate support.

Nearly all venous ulcers heal spontaneously if the underlying venous insufficiency is corrected by elevation or external elastic support or both. If the underlying venous insufficiency is not corrected, vascularized grafts fail to heal or break down as soon as the patient starts to ambulate.

DEFINITIVE SURGERY. In the very aged or poor risk patient, the healing of the ulcer with subsequent careful elastic support may represent the definitive treatment of the venous disease. In the majority of patients, however, closure of the ulcer—whether by elevation and bed rest, ambulatory treatment with firm support, or grafting—is only a preparation to more definitive surgery to correct the venous hypertension.

In patients with varicose veins alone, careful ligation and stripping of the long and short saphenous venous systems is generally sufficient. However, in those patients with incompetent perforating veins between the deep and superficial venous systems, it is also essential that these be divided (Linton, 1953; Cockett, 1955), if necessary, by designing a large skin flap and elevating the fascia over the muscles of the medial half of the lower leg to identify and ligate the connecting perforating veins. Occasionally such an extensive flap heals with some areas of necrosis. If the venous disease has been controlled, the skin flap heals satisfactorily, even if preoperatively it looks incapable of survival. It is important that the perforating vein or veins located characteristically directly under the site of ulceration be divided, and the surgeon should not hesitate to incise or dissect below the newly healed graft if necessary; otherwise, recurrence of the ulceration is almost certain.

Skin grafts placed over the dense scar of an old ulcer without further vein surgery do not remain healed; they do remain healed if the ulcer and scar are initially excised widely. Presumably, this is because incompetent veins are interrupted during the excision. Skin grafts placed

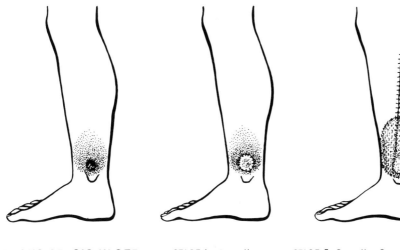

**VENOUS STASIS ULCER**

A

STAGE 1. Operation.
Skin graft to ulcer.

STAGE 2. Operation 3 weeks later.
Strip varicose veins.
Dermal overlay graft (extensive).
Ligation venous perforators of gaiter area.

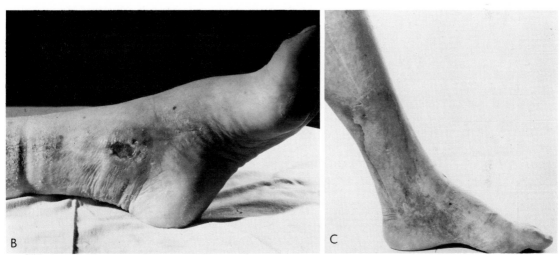

**FIGURE 86–1.** *A,* Technique of dermal overgrafting of a venous ulcer. *B,* Preoperative appearance of a varicose ulcer present for seven years. *C,* Appearance ten years after two dermal overgrafts, stripping of the varicose veins, and ligation of the perforating veins of the lower leg. (From Thompson, N., and Ell, P. J.: Dermal overgrafting in the treatment of venous stasis ulcers. Plast. Reconstr. Surg., *54*:290, 1974. Copyright © 1974, The Williams & Wilkins Company, Baltimore.)

over densely scarred ulcers survive indefinitely, provided that the underlying venous disease is controlled.

**Arterial Disease.** The causes of inadequate arterial circulation to the skin or to the extremities may be neurologic (exemplified by Raynaud's disease), obliterative, or obstructive. In most cases the sequelae of arterial insufficiency are not as well localized as in peripheral venous disease. Arterial disease is characterized by a progression from functional limitation of the extremity without pain (intermittent claudication) to pain at rest, atrophic skin changes, and finally superficial ulceration and gangrene.

These changes generally progress most rapidly at the most distant portion of the extremities. Diabetic arterial disease is peculiar in that there is extensive obliterative disease of the small end arteries without obligatory involvement of the major peripheral vessels. Consequently, gangrenous changes may be apparent in the presence of adequate pulses.

The distinction between ulcers due to venous insufficiency and those due to arterial inadequacy can usually be easily made, but both may occasionally be present at the same time. Ulcers caused by arterial insufficiency are usually accompanied by changes in the arterial supply elsewhere in the limb. They are generally located peripherally and are characteristically painful (but not in diabetics with neuropathy). They often appear rather dry and shallow, and they lack the thick, indurated, moist edges of most venous ulcers.

TREATMENT. As in venous disease, considerations of the care of the local lesion for which grafting or plastic surgical closure is considered are secondary to the diagnosis and treatment of the underlying vascular disease. Unless this is subject to significant surgical or medical control, conservative and local methods of treatment of an ischemic lesion are much less likely to be successful. Whereas nearly all venous ulcers can be healed relatively quickly by conservative measures alone, the majority of ulcers caused by arterial insufficiency do not respond similarly. While venous hypertension can be eliminated by elevation of the limb, there is no equally good way of increasing local arterial circulation; in most cases in which the arterial blood supply has become insufficient to maintain the viability of the skin or of a digit, it will also not be adequate to support the healing of an incision or the vascularization of a skin graft.

Therapy aimed at improving arterial blood supply depends upon the etiology of the insufficiency. In cases of neurovascular disease or Raynaud's disease, medical treatment with a sympathetic block or sympathectomy may provide temporary relief of the arterial spasm and allow the skin lesions or amputation sites to heal spontaneously or be satisfactorily grafted.

In occlusive disease of the arterial system of the lower extremity, appropriate physical examination with or without arteriography or the Doppler flow meter generally shows whether the obstruction is proximal to the popliteal bifurcation. If the obstruction is in the small vessels of the arterial "runoff," surgical improvement of the arterial blood supply is more difficult. The latter situation is characteristic of diabetic arterial disease, in which the toes may become gangrenous in the presence of a palpable pedal pulse.

Depending on the site of the block in the arterial tree, various vascular reconstructive techniques, such as vein grafts or plastic prostheses and endarterectomy are available. When arterial circulation to the area showing insufficiency, gangrene, or ulceration is restored, healing will commence spontaneously and may be accelerated by split-thickness skin grafting of the ulcers. In many cases surgical improvement in circulation can be considered only as temporary. It may be important to lose no time in closing extensive ulcers with a graft or in performing a transmetatarsal or even higher amputation

while sufficient circulation is still present to allow surgery to be done safely and the wound to heal satisfactorily.

In many diabetics or other patients in whom the local arterial circulation cannot be improved by surgery, the use of Buerger's exercises, bed rest with the legs flat or slightly downward, and meticulous cleansing and debridement will improve the local situation to the extent that a thin skin graft may accelerate the healing of the lesion.

Inadequate arterial circulation in the remainder of the limb generally precludes the use of skin flaps in these patients. An attempt to effect surgical closure of an amputation stump that has failed to heal because of irremediable arterial insufficiency generally results only in further necrosis of previously viable tissue, and a higher level of amputation is usually required.

In patients in whom concomitant severe venous and arterial disease is present in a limb, a combination of treatments is indicated. Caution must be exercised in surgery of the lower leg for the control of venous disease if there is, concomitantly, inadequate arterial blood supply to support adequate wound healing.

**Lymphatic Disease.** The etiology and treatment of lymphatic disease and lymphedema of the lower extremity are discussed in Chapter 87.

### Tumors of the Lower Extremity

Tumors of the lower extremity are benign (hemangioma, lymphangioma) or malignant (malignant melanoma, squamous cell carcinoma). Sclerosing hemangiomas are small, firm, subcutaneous nodules which are peculiar to the pretibial area. Lymphangiomas may involve the lower extremity and have been associated with constricting bands (Kitlowski, 1957). The treatment of hemangiomas and lymphangiomas is discussed in Chapter 65.

While wide and deep excision of melanomas has become the accepted therapy, the role of regional node dissection has generated considerable controversy (see Chapter 65). The bed of the resulting cutaneous defect is usually a muscle, which provides a suitable site for the application of a split-thickness skin graft.

### Osteomyelitis

Osteomyelitis may be either acute or chronic and either post-traumatic or hematogenous in origin.

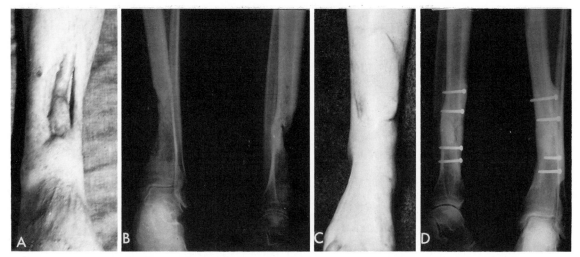

**FIGURE 86–2.** A closed, comminuted, spiral fracture of the tibia treated by open reduction and plating. When the wound broke open, there was considerable necrosis of skin, sequestration of much of the anterior portion of the tibia, and severe infection in the local tissues (*A*). The granulating areas surrounding the exposed bone were covered by skin grafts, and after the sequestra were removed, the viable bone was also covered with skin grafts. With the elimination of infection by wound closure, bone union progressed to a solid but weak bone bridge in the tibia (*B*). A cross-leg flap (*C*) from the opposite thigh was used to replace the skin grafts and provide a well-vascularized and flexible cover of normal skin over the damaged tibia. Finally, the tibia was strengthened by a bone graft inserted beneath the flap (*D*). (From Cannon, B.: Soft-tissue repairs. *In* Fractures and Other Injuries, by members of the Fracture Clinic, Massachusetts General Hospital. Chicago, Year Book Medical Publishers, 1958.)

In the patient with osteomyelitis, a draining sinus, and a surrounding area of scar tissue, initial treatment consists of excision of the scar and sinus tract and curettage of the involved bone. Crikelair and Symonds (1966) have demonstrated the value of immediate coverage with a cross-leg flap at the time of debridement of a chronic osteomyelitis ulcer.

In the face of active infection, bone grafting of an osseous defect should be deferred (Fig. 86–2). However, autogenous bone grafting is feasible in conjunction with a flap transfer in the same operative session, provided that the wound is clean and vascularization of the bone graft is ensured by the skin flap, which should overlap the involved area for better blood supply. Coverage by an appropriate antibiotic is indicated.

The development of free vascularized bone grafts (Taylor, Miller, and Ham, 1975) offers a new technique of replacing lower extremity osseous defects.

### Congenital Anomalies

Congenital anomalies of the lower extremity include constricting bands, supernumerary toes, and syndactylism.

**Congenital Constricting Bands.** Congenital constricting bands are seen in the fingers and toes in one of every 2000 to 2500 births (Blackfield and Hause, 1951). They are less frequently seen proximal to the wrist or ankle. The presence of distal edema is variable. Kitlowski (1957) reported a massive lymphangioma of the leg associated with a constricting band.

Blackfield and Hause (1951) devised the following classification:

1. Shallow grooves which are only slightly noticeable.

2. Deeper grooves encroaching into the subcutaneous tissue and muscles.

3. An extremely deep groove which encircles the bone and causes lymph stasis distal to the band.

Sarnat and Kagan (1971) added two additional categories in which there was pseudoarthrosis under the constricting band.

In some patients other members of the family have similar constricting bands, and the lesions are felt to be hereditary in nature. Other bands have been attributed to amniotic bands (Kohler, 1962), such as postinflammatory adhesions between the amnion and fetus or holes in the membrane that had been pierced by the affected extremity.

Treatment consists of excision of the band and Z-plasty elongation. Reconstruction should be done in two stages, half of the circumference being corrected at each surgical procedure (Fig. 86–3).

**Supernumerary Toes.** Supernumerary toes

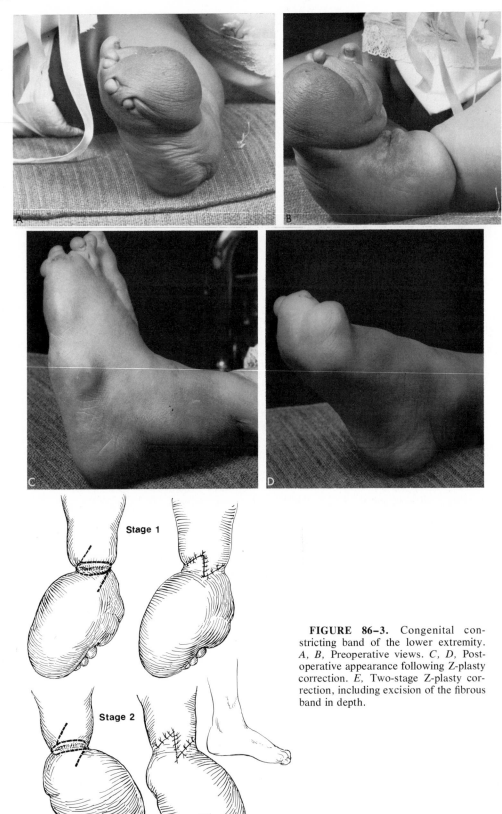

**FIGURE 86–3.** Congenital constricting band of the lower extremity. *A, B,* Preoperative views. *C, D,* Postoperative appearance following Z-plasty correction. *E,* Two-stage Z-plasty correction, including excision of the fibrous band in depth.

are usually located laterally and may or may not contain osseous elements. Amputation is usually advised, but the incision should be confined to the dorsal and lateral aspect of the foot to avoid any problems with weight-bearing.

**Syndactylism.** Syndactylism does not pose the problem that it does in the upper extremity (see Chapter 79). If correction is sought, the same Z-plasty techniques can be applied.

### Miscellaneous

Miscellaneous problems unique to the lower extremity are plantar wart, plantar callus, keratosis plantaris, neurotrophic ulcer, and ingrown toenail.

**Plantar Wart.** The plantar wart, insignificant though it may appear, is a disabling lesion for the patient and presents a therapeutic dilemma for the physician. A multiplicity of therapeutic methods ranging from psychotherapy to surgical excision have been recommended and used.

The plantar wart is similar to warts occurring elsewhere in the body except that it is flattened by the pressure of weight-bearing. The responsible virus is filterable, and from the filtrate the wart can be reproduced. The wart virus is a papovavirus with a diameter of approximately 38 m$\mu$ (Fitzpatrick, 1971). The wart can be transmitted, and seeding or dissemination is promoted by moisture of the skin of the foot. The wart is surrounded by a thick callus which conceals its papillomatous surface. After the callus is shaved off, the wart appears as a soft white or brownish tuft of tissue, often exquisitely tender to pressure. Pain is the usual complaint for which treatment is sought. On microscopic examination, the wart can be identified by elongated rete pegs which bend inward at the margins to assume a spherical shape. Vacuolated cells in the upper malpighian layer of the epidermis are characteristic.

The lesion is a purely epidermal one, and the treatment need be concentrated only in the epidermal layer of the skin. In the foot the wart may seem to be deeper than the epidermis because of the thick overlying callus which conceals it. Nevertheless, microscopic examination shows that only the epidermal layer is involved.

TREATMENT. In the absence of pain, the wart is a benign process and should be left alone. No treatment should be considered which will risk any permanent changes in the skin of the sole of the foot. Treatment is indicated only if the wart is painful or interferes with walking.

Methods of treatment vary according to the severity of the lesion. Relief of pressure by means of commercially available adherent soft plastic rings is a conservative form of treatment. Destruction of the lesion, however, may be indicated.

The first step is to expose the wart by paring away the callus. Opinions diverge concerning the appropriate method. The technique most generally used is the topical application of one of a large number of chemical agents from fuming nitric acid to formalin soaks. The chemical agents also include concentrated trichloroacetic acid combined with a medicated (salicylic acid, 40 per cent) corn plaster, salicylic acid (5 per cent) in collodion, dichloracetic acid, silver nitrate stick, podophyllin, and glacial acetic acid. Cryotherapy in the form of liquid nitrogen or carbon dioxide snow for a few seconds produces an inflammatory reaction which can destroy the wart. Destructive heat in the form of carefully limited desiccation combined with curettage is effectively used by many dermatologists. Local anesthetic agents, usually with epinephrine added, eliminate the pain and, on occasion, the wart. Other recommended solutions are thrombosing agents or bismuth salts.

Full-thickness surgical excision, which may require the rotation of a local flap, is a last resort because the resulting scar may be painful with weight-bearing.

Radiation in any form, much used in the past, is contraindicated. The irreversible late consequences of irradiation—atrophy, scarring, pain, and ulceration—prohibit the use of this dangerous method of treatment of a benign process such as a plantar wart. If a radiation ulcer develops following such therapy, excision and coverage by a flap raised from the non–weight-bearing portion of the foot are indicated (see Fig. 86–10).

Plantar warts have often been confused with plantar calluses. The two lesions must be differentiated, as the treatment of each is different.

**Plantar Callus.** The plantar callus is usually located over the metatarsal head and rarely appears in crops. Roentgen study usually shows a misplaced metatarsal head.

Treatment consists of replacing the metatarsal head by a transfer of the extensor digitorum longus tendon to the metatarsal shaft, as recommended by Kiehn, Earle, and Des Prez (1973).

**Keratosis Plantaris.** Keratosis plantaris is a hereditary disease characterized by excessive keratin production on the sole of the foot. The lesion should be excised with preservation of sufficient subcutaneous tissue in order to support a skin graft (Kisner and Hendrix, 1973).

**Neurotrophic Ulcers.** Plantar neurotrophic ulcers are usually secondary to diabetes, while a smaller number are associated with leprosy. They are often located over the plantar metatarsal head, usually of the great toe.

Neurovascular island flaps have been recommended to resurface the defect with innervated skin (Snyder and Edgerton, 1965; Kaplan, 1969).

**Ingrown Toenail.** The term "ingrown toenail" is generally used for hypertrophic, painful, inflammatory, and often extremely disabling changes surrounding the toenail of the first toe and occasionally the other toes. The term is probably a misnomer, because there is seldom an abnormality of the nail. More frequently, inflammatory or hypertrophic changes occur at the nail margin along the nail groove. DuVries (1959) has suggested "hypertrophy of the ungual labia" as a more precise descriptive diagnosis.

The compressive effect of shoes that narrow the space between the nail and the adjacent soft tissues of the nail groove and the nail lip is probably the primary etiologic factor, which produces chronic irritation, hypertrophy of surrounding tissues, and occasionally acute suppurative inflammation.

Three common causes have been described. First, a normally growing nail, improperly trimmed, may have a marginal spur which projects into the nail groove and produces local pain and inflammation. Second, an abnormal distortion of one or both of the lateral margins of the nail may cause it to grow inward toward the soft tissues along the marginal groove. Finally, a normally developing nail may, because of a tight shoe, cause hypertrophic changes in the surrounding soft tissues. Such hypertrophy, which is occasionally the result of a congenital overgrowth, narrows the nail groove and causes the lateral margins of the normal nail to "dig into" the unyielding adjacent tissues.

TREATMENT. A number of surgical procedures have been recommended for correction of this annoying disability. Preventive measures are desirable and effective but often overlooked. Shoes of sufficient size to permit free mobility of the toes will decrease the likelihood of the ingrown toenail. If there is a tendency for the toenail to grow into the soft tissues at the distal end of the nail groove, the nail should be guided over the soft tissues to project to the end of the toe. A small wisp of cotton inserted beneath the sharp edge of the ingrowing nail will minimize the incising pressure on the soft tissues. Careful trimming of the margins of the nail as it grows along the nail groove will avoid the development of spurs which may be the precursors of acute inflammation.

In the presence of acute suppuration in the nail groove, it is essential that the side of the nail be excised to its origin. The removal of the offending "foreign body" parallel to the nail groove is essential so that no fragment remains beneath the eponychium to cut into the soft tissue.

When hypertrophic changes take place in the soft tissues adjacent to the nail groove, a number of operative procedures have been suggested either for reducing the hypertrophic tissues or for reconstructing the soft tissues around the growing nail. The simplest of these procedures consists of the excision of a wedge of hypertrophic tissue along the side of the toe adjacent to the nail groove to permit a rotation of the superficial tissue away from a position overlapping the edge of the nail.

A more complicated procedure, essentially a reconstruction of the nail grooves, has been suggested by DuVries (1959). Through an incision along one or both sides of the nail, the hypertrophic tissue is excised. The nail margins are then elevated and detached from the bed, and the incised skin edges are tucked beneath the nail and secured by sutures passed through the nail itself. This reconstructive procedure effectively restores a normal relationship between the nail and its adjacent soft tissues.

## RECONSTRUCTIVE PROCEDURES USED IN RESURFACING CUTANEOUS DEFECTS OF THE LOWER EXTREMITY

### Closure by Primary Approximation

Many traumatic wounds can be closed by primary approximation, provided that there is no extensive loss of skin. In fact, the vast majority of leg lacerations can be closed using the techniques discussed in Chapter 1.

Attempts to close wounds of the lower leg with significant loss of substance by primary closure after extensive undermining of the wound margins are usually unsuccessful because of excessive tension and resulting tissue ischemia. In the thigh, the looser tissue allows closure of larger defects.

Delayed primary closure as practiced in military surgery is often indicated in severely contused wounds with edema or other evidence of disturbed local circulation. In the interval, the wound can be covered by commercially available porcine xenografts or cadaver allografts. Delayed primary closure is accomplished between the fifth and seventh days. By that time much of the edema has subsided, and contamination from the exposed surface has not yet developed into clinically evident infection. The usefulness of the method is unquestioned.

### Closure by Skin Grafting

Skin grafting is a useful alternative method of wound closure when primary suture cannot be employed or delayed primary suture is inappropriate. Most wounds with significant skin loss can be closed by a skin graft applied directly on subcutaneous tissues, muscles (Fig. 86–4), or even cancellous bone. Skin grafts are usually used following release of burn contractures of the popliteal space (Fig. 86–5).

Delayed skin grafting (see Chapter 6) is indicated if hemostasis in the recipient bed is incomplete. When there is reason for delay, a graft applied two to five days later will have every prospect for success. Whether the skin graft will provide definitive covering is immaterial, since its main purpose is to restore an intact covering so that healing can progress

unhampered. Final determination of the permanent usefulness of the skin graft can be made at a later date.

The concept of dermal overgrafting was introduced by Webster (1958) in the treatment of unstable scars of the leg. Its application has subsequently been expanded by Hynes (1959) and Thompson (1960; Thompson and Ell, 1974). The technique is particularly suited to resurfacing defects of the lower extremity, since it is simple and obviates the need for more complex multistaged procedures. Thompson and Ell (1974) reported a decrease in the use of cross-leg flaps in the treatment of acute leg injuries from 1 in 170 emergency admissions during the five-year period ending in 1962 to 1 in 800 patients during the five-year period ending in 1972. As mentioned earlier in the chapter, the technique finds particular application in the treatment of venous stasis ulcers and cutaneous defects of weight-bearing surfaces (Fig. 86–6).

The surface epithelium, if present, can be removed by dermabrasion or a freehand knife. The split-thickness skin graft to be applied should be cut as thick as possible, so that in the serial application of the grafts, a thick laminated layer of dermis can be built up. A second skin graft can be applied three weeks later. The details of the technique are discussed in Chapter 6.

### Closure by Skin Flaps

A skin flap is indicated when neither primary or delayed primary closure nor skin grafting of

**FIGURE 86–4.** *A,* Extensive avulsion of the posterior surface of the thigh. *B,* Despite the fact that the defect extended as far as the muscle bellies of the thigh, a skin graft applied to the raw surface proved effective in providing permanent coverage. Weight-bearing was well tolerated, because sufficient soft tissue provided by the massive muscle bellies of the posterior thigh served as a cushion between the thin skin graft and the underlying bony structures.

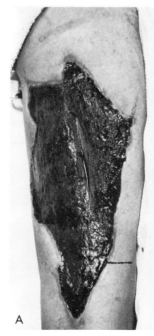

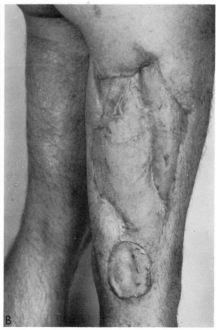

A    B

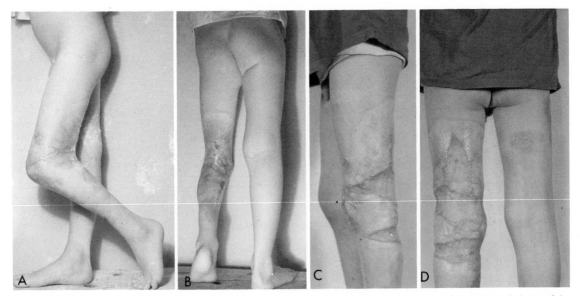

**FIGURE 86–5.** *A, B,* A burn contracture of the leg which significantly limits extension of the knee. *C, D,* Release of the contracture required horizontal relaxing incisions above and below the knee. Each incision extended halfway around the extremity. The vertical incision in the thigh was needed to diminish the circumferential constriction. Repair was done with split-thickness grafts removed from the opposite thigh.

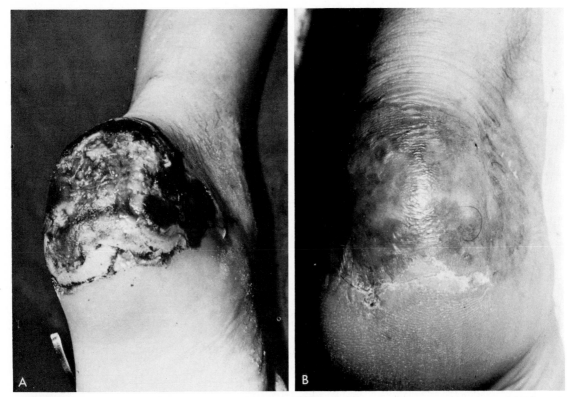

**FIGURE 86–6.** Dermal overgrafting of a calcaneal defect. *A,* Preoperative appearance. *B,* Following serial skin grafting. Sufficient dermis was provided so that weight-bearing was well tolerated. (From Thompson, N., and Ell, P. J.: Dermal overgrafting in the treatment of venous stasis ulcers. Plast. Reconstr. Surg., *54*:290, 1974.)

the acute wound is possible. Replacement of scar tissue or a skin graft in a healed wound with a skin flap is often required at a later date as a preliminary step to definitive reconstructive surgery. The indications are legion: in the acute wound, a flap transferred over bare bone devoid of periosteum may make the difference between viability or sequestration of the bone; the unprotected fracture site without adequate covering may become a focus of infection and nonunion, whereas union may be accelerated with the added blood supply of a transferred skin flap; tendons, nerves, or joints exposed as a result of acute trauma must be covered by a flap if the procedure is at all possible.

The skin flap is used in late repair to replace scar tissue or furnish improved blood supply in poorly vascularized areas. An area of bony nonunion often heals spontaneously merely by virtue of the improved local blood supply when the overlying scar tissue is replaced by a well-vascularized skin flap. Joints, areas of functional stress, and weight-bearing surfaces require the additional cushioning effect of subcutaneous tissue between the deep tissues and the skin. A flap of skin and subcutaneous tissue is often an essential preliminary to definitive reconstructive surgery involving the tendon, bone, or nerve.

**Types of Skin Flaps.** Skin flaps may be shifted from local or from distant areas. Especially in the foot, local tissue is often preferable to remote tissue because there are significant differences between the skin of the sole of the foot and the type of skin in areas from which distant flaps are removed. Where this is impossible, the choice must be made between a muscle flap covered by a skin graft, a flap from the opposite leg (a cross-leg flap), a flap from the groin as a microvascular free flap, a flap from the abdominal wall carried on the arm as an intermediate host (a jump flap), and a delayed tube flap. The transfer of distant flaps is an ordeal for the patient, and its use is less frequent since the development of newer techniques, such as microvascular free flaps, myocutaneous flaps, and muscle flaps, to be discussed later in the chapter.

The judicious, forward-looking planning of a flap, whether from a local or distant area, whether direct or delayed, is essential to the achievement of a successful result. The defect to be covered must be carefully mapped on the donor area with an allowance of at least 25 per cent excess to compensate for the normal shrinkage of the skin after transfer. This is especially true in flaps that are prepared or transferred in multiple stages. The location from which the flap is taken must be suitable; that is, it should not be from a weight-bearing area or an area exposed to trauma; neither should it be from an area where an unsightly donor scar would be conspicuous; and it is desirable, if possible, to transplant skin of the same thickness and texture as that which originally occupied the recipient defect.

The flap must be planned so that it will reach the full extent of the defect to be covered without excessive tension, while causing minimal patient discomfort and involving the least complicated problems of immobilization. An important point in technique, particularly when a flap is being transplanted over a defect which is poorly vascularized, is to design the flap so that it is of adequate size to overlap the defect into the adjacent well-vascularized tissues. Thus some of the tissue adjacent to the defect must be sacrificed to provide a hospitable recipient site for the flap.

The flap must be planned so that the transfer can be accomplished as expeditiously as possible. It should also be planned so that it can be positioned without kinking and without tension. Finally, the donor site of the flap should be covered by skin grafts, if it cannot be closed primarily.

LOCAL FLAPS. The direct undelayed flap, completely mobilized at the time of transfer without any preliminary preparation, is useful in the lower extremity. Its survival depends on an adequate blood supply through a sufficiently broad pedicle. The surgical adage that a flap can be twice as long as the width of its pedicle is especially inapplicable in the extremities, par-

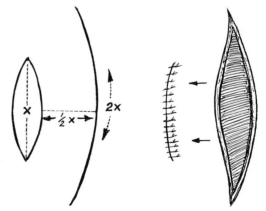

**FIGURE 86–7.** Bipedicle flap for elliptical defects. The incision parallel to the primary defect is a relaxing incision. To be adequate, the length of this incision should be twice that of the primary defect. The width of the flap should be at least half the length of the primary defect. The lateral incision should parallel the curve of the primary defect. A flap prepared with these dimensions can be moved easily into the new position. The donor site is closed with a split-thickness skin graft.

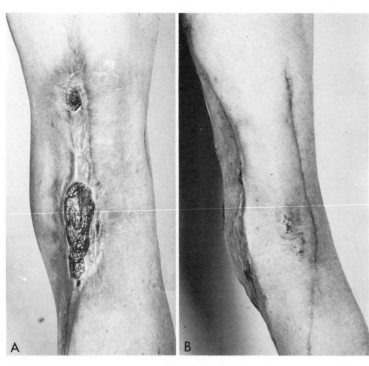

FIGURE 86–8. *A,* Deeply penetrating chronic wound of the leg. This
type of wound can be successfully
closed only by a flap which carries its
own blood supply and furnishes nutrition to the damaged tissues. *B,* A bipedicle flap from behind the knee was
used in the repair in order to employ
skin in the neighborhood of the defect.
The flap was delayed in several stages
because of its excessive length in relation to width. The choice of local tissue
obviated the more complex repair by a
distant flap.

ticularly in older patients. Various types of undelayed direct flaps are satisfactory when
removed from areas where sufficient blood
supply can be ensured.

Crawford (1957) has emphasized the role of
local flaps in covering cutaneous defects of the
lower extremities. Delays are often indicated,
and he advocated bipedicle flaps (Figs. 86–7
and 86–8). If a bipedicle flap is used, the flap
must be designed so that it is twice the width
of the defect. Local flaps are especially suitable
in the knee region (Fig. 86–9) because of the
abundant circulation in the genicular vessels
(White, Dupertuis, Gaisford, and Musgrave,
1957).

A local flap can be raised from the non–
weight-bearing surface of the sole of the foot
and used to cover defects secondary to the
treatment of plantar warts (Fig. 86–10). Because
of its broad pedicle, delay is not indicated. The
flap is contraindicated in older individuals with
arterial insufficiency.

Amputation of the toe at the metatarsal level
and filleting of the skin have been advocated to
cover defects in the area of the metatarsal head
(Fig. 86–11).

DISTANT FLAPS

*The cross-leg flap.* One of the most frequently performed flap techniques of the lower
extremity is the cross-leg flap, which was initially described by Hamilton in 1854. Because of
the subcutaneous position of the tibia and the
frequency of compound fractures of the tibia and
fibula, flap repair in this area is often necessary.
It is usually accepted that a calf-leg flap is preferable to a thigh-leg flap, which places the patient in a less comfortable position and which is
principally indicated for female patients who
wish to avoid a visible secondary defect of the
leg. The thigh-leg flap is also more suitable for
closing larger defects and in patients in whom
the opposite calf cannot be used because of
scars or other injuries.

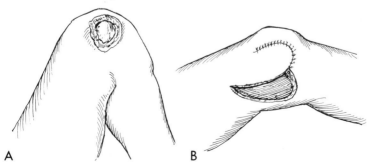

FIGURE 86–9. *A,* Ulceration over
the lateral aspect of the knee with
penetration into the knee joint. *B,* Repair by a local flap which was rotated
to cover the defect; a skin graft was
used to cover the donor area of the
flap.

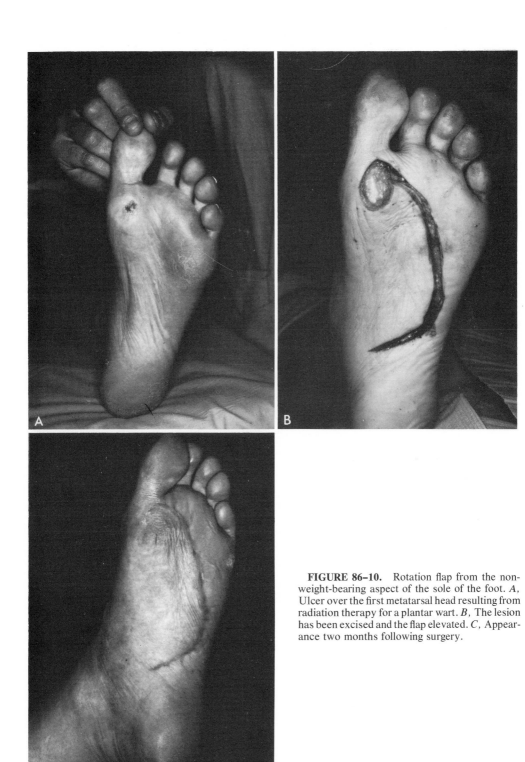

**FIGURE 86–10.** Rotation flap from the non-weight-bearing aspect of the sole of the foot. *A*, Ulcer over the first metatarsal head resulting from radiation therapy for a plantar wart. *B*, The lesion has been excised and the flap elevated. *C*, Appearance two months following surgery.

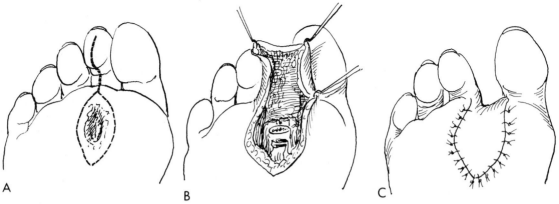

A        B        C

**FIGURE 86–11.**    Amputation of the toe with filleting of the soft tissue to resurface a defect of the plantar surface of the metatarsal head.

The flap is planned with the patient on the operating table, a pattern of the defect being used as the imaginary pedicle (for details, see Chapter 6, p. 199). The flap should be planned to be of a generous size in order to overlap the defect in every direction and allow insertion of the flap into healthy, well-vascularized tissues. Whenever possible, the flap should be designed in such a way that its lymphatics will be directed in the same direction as the lymphatics of the region, in order to restore lymphatic drainage rapidly from the distal portion of the extremity. Delay is indicated if the length-width ratio exceeds 1½ to 1. The cross-leg flap should not undergo the slightest degree of tension lest the circulation be impaired.

A raw area is usually present between the donor and recipient sites on the undersurface of the flap. This raw area may be closed by the hinge-flap technique (Fig. 86–12) or by a split-thickness skin graft. The hinge-flap technique has the advantage that it increases the surface of contact between the recipient site and the flap and also provides additional tissue which facilitates the insetting of the flap after the pedicle has been severed.

In terms of flap donor sites, the best blood supply is in the medial aspect of the calf and the anterior aspect of the lower one-third of the thigh; the poorest blood supply is situated in the posterior calf and posterior thigh (Stark, 1952).

The most favorable area for a donor site is the anteromedial aspect of the calf for resurfacing defects of the dorsum and sole of the foot, medial malleolus, and anterior tibial surface. Alternate donor sites include the anterior thigh (proximal base) to the medial malleolus (Fig. 86–13, *A*); anterior thigh (distal base) to the pretibial area (Fig. 86–13, *B*); posteromedial calf to the posterolateral leg (Fig. 86–13, *C*); and cross-foot flaps from the contralateral plantar arch to re-

surface heel defects (Fig. 86–13, *D*) (Mir y Mir, 1954).

The flap is raised from the deep fascia and the legs are approximated either in a parallel position one to the other or in a cross-leg position. After excision of all scar tissue, bone sequestra, and granulation tissue, the flap is applied over the defect and its edges sutured to the defect. Ideally, 75 per cent of the flap (and not less than 30 per cent) is embedded at the time of transfer.

Fixation has been traditionally obtained by plaster. Most surgeons prefer to apply the plaster after completion of the cross-leg flap proce-

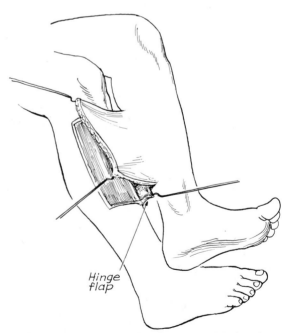

*Hinge flap*

**FIGURE 86–12.**    Cross-leg flap. The flap has been raised from the posteromedial aspect of the leg with an anterior pedicle. Note the hinge flap to cover the raw surface of the pedicle. (From Converse, J. M.: Plastic repair of the extremities by non-tubulated pedicle skin flaps. J. Bone Joint Surg., *30*:1, 1948.)

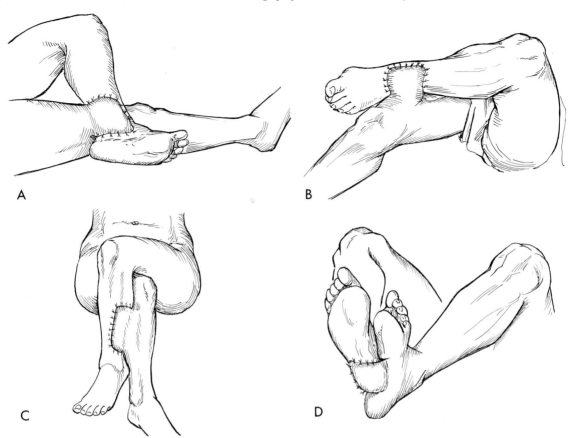

**FIGURE 86–13.** Alternative donor sites for cross-leg flap. *A,* Anterior thigh flap to medial malleolar area. *B,* Anterior thigh flap to lower pretibial region. *C,* Cross-leg flap to anterolateral defect. *D,* Cross-foot flap (Mir y Mir).

dure. The application of the plaster is facilitated by performing the operation on a Hawley type of orthopedic table. Other surgeons prefer to apply the casts prior to the operation, cutting a window in the respective casts at the site of the defect and at the donor site.

Transosseous pin fixation has recently been employed (Constant and Grabb, 1968; Adams and associates, 1969; Stern, 1972) and offers several advantages, such as increased patient comfort and exposure of the operative site for frequent examination. It is important to maintain flexion of the knees of both extremities in order to avoid an uncomfortable position in extension, which may lead to considerable postoperative stiffness, particularly in older patients. Elevation of both legs during the postoperative period assists venous return and lymphatic drainage of the extremities. The pedicle can be either totally or serially severed at two to three weeks and the proximal end of the flap sutured into the defect.

Because of thromboembolic phenomena associated with cross-leg flaps, Letterman, Schur-

ter, and Prandoni (1961) recommended prophylactic anticoagulation. They also felt that dividing and insetting the flap could be accomplished in older patients while the patient was anticoagulated.

In patients over 40 years of age undergoing cross-leg flaps, a high percentage manifest some type of thromboembolic disease; in addition, older patients have peripheral arterial disease. For these reasons the use of cross-leg flaps has been discouraged in this age group. However, Hayes (1962) reported 24 patients over 50 years of age undergoing the cross-leg flap procedure. There were only three failures, and there was no incidence of permanent joint damage, acute thromboembolism, or chronic intermittent claudication. Stark and Kaplan (1972) reported only two complications (thrombophlebitis and pressure sore) in nine elderly patients following cross-leg flap procedures. The authors felt age per se should not be a contraindication to the use of a cross-leg flap, provided the peripheral circulation is adequate.

On the other end of the age spectrum, Argamaso and associates (1973) reported three patients under 15 years of age who tolerated the cross-leg position.

In a review of 114 cross-leg flaps, White, Dupertuis, Gaisford and Musgrave (1957) reported a 19 per cent failure rate. In this study it was concluded that thigh-based cross-leg flaps were preferable to calf flaps, as they were associated with fewer failures and delays. In addition, in this site longer flaps were possible, and fixation and care were less complex.

*The tube flap.* When a microvascular free flap or a cross-leg flap is unfeasible, a distant tube flap may be indicated to resurface a lower extremity defect (Fig. 86–14).

The tube flap is usually removed from the anterolateral aspect of the abdomen and transferred via the wrist or occasionally by the caterpillar technique. The main indication for this technique is the repair of a defect of the leg in a young female patient who cannot tolerate the position of transfer and in whom the cross-leg flap is contraindicated because of the secondary disfigurement resulting from the cross-leg flap technique or because of absence of part of the limb from amputation.

Several shortcomings in the use of tube flaps deserve mention. The tube flap may be almost unlimited in its length, but its width is dependent on sufficient looseness of the tissues to permit formation of a tube. A tube flap with a large circumference may be so bulky and inflexible

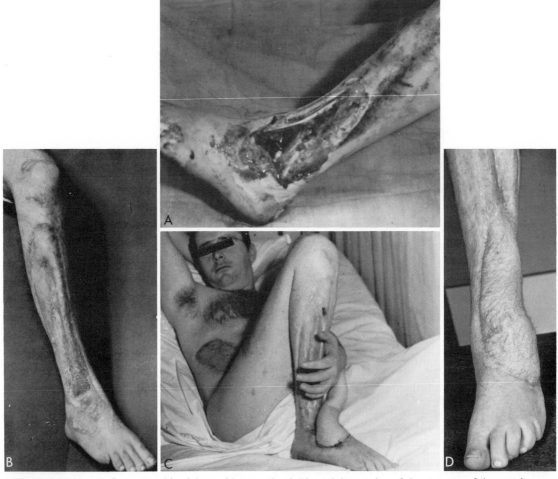

**FIGURE 86–14.** *A,* Severe crushing injury with necrosis of skin and destruction of the contents of the anterior compartment of the lower leg. *B,* Operative debridement of all devitalized tissue was done within 24 hours, and the wound was closed with a skin graft from the opposite thigh. The skin graft proved stable except over the ankle joint, where it lay directly on the joint surfaces. A tube flap from the abdominal wall, with the wrist as the intermediate carrier (*C*) was transferred in multiple stages to replace the skin graft in the lower half of the leg and to provide a cushion over the ankle joint. *D,* When the patient began to move the ankle, the flap separated from the bone at this level. Better anchorage for the flap was secured by drilling multiple holes in the thick bony cortex of the tibia and the talus. (From Cannon, B.: Soft-tissue repairs. *In* Fractures and Other Injuries, by members of the Fracture Clinic of the Massachusetts General Hospital. Chicago, Year Book Medical Publishers, 1958.)

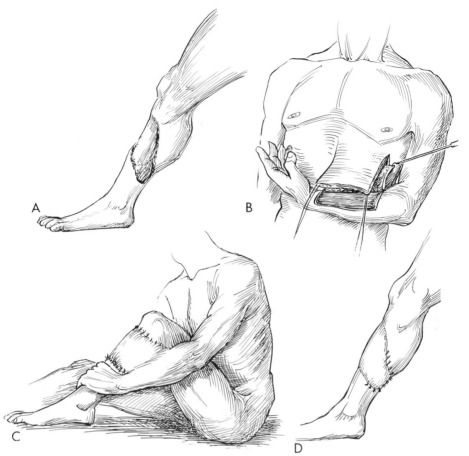

**FIGURE 86–15.** Typical steps in the preparation and transfer of an open jump flap to the lower leg. (From Cannon, B.: The use of open jump flaps in lower extremity repairs. Plast. Reconstr. Surg., 2:336, 1947. Copyright © 1947, The Williams & Wilkins Company, Baltimore.)

that it cannot be easily transferred from one attachment to another. A tube flap, in common with all flaps, shrinks. Shrinkage in the long axis is limited by the attachments at either end. Circumferential shrinkage is limited by the amount of fat within the tube. An excess of fat may constrict circulation and delay healing; a minimum of fat allows shrinkage.

The main disadvantages of the tube flap technique are that multiple procedures are required, and reconstruction entails a considerable amount of time (see Chapter 6). The development of muscle flaps, myocutaneous flaps, and microvascular free flaps has decreased the need for tube flaps.

*The jump flap.* Extensive surface defects of the lower extremity can seldom be covered by a flap from the opposite leg. Neither can the leg be readily and adequately resurfaced by a tube flap because of the limitations in the dimensions of the tube. The jump flap from the abdominal or chest walls carried on the ulnar or radial aspect of the forearm as an intermediary host is a

method of dealing with such large defects (Fig. 86–15). The technique also provides for the most rapid transfer of distant flaps.

Converse (1948) reported the transfer of a jump flap raised from the anterolateral aspect of the thorax and abdomen to cover a defect extending over an area (30 × 42 cm) on the lower anterior aspect of the thigh, knee, and midportion of the leg. The presence of chronic osteomyelitis of 12 years' duration, draining sinuses, and sequestrating bone required the excision of the scarred soft tissues and the sequestrating bone; the flap was transferred in the same operative session. The flap, which was considerably larger than the defect, was planned to overlap into the adjacent well-vascularized tissues.

The success of the jump flap from the abdominal wall depends on the maintenance of a short, broad pedicle throughout all stages of the transfer. Sufficient mobility of the leg, shoulder, and body is essential to permit the shifting of the carrier arm in juxtaposition with the lower leg or foot. Selection of the ipsilateral or contralateral arm depends on which will accomplish the transfer with minimal discomfort to the patient in the compromised position. The method should be restricted to children and young adults, as older patients do not tolerate the long period of immobilization and the position of transfer. As in all flaps, an excess of at least one-third in the size of the flap is necessary to compensate for shrinkage. The main advantage of the jump flap is that an adequate amount of tissue can be secured.

## AXIAL PATTERN FLAPS IN THE LOWER EXTREMITY

A significant advance in lower extremity reconstruction has been the introduction of axial pattern flap principles (see Chapter 6). McGregor and Morgan (1973) made the distinction between random pattern flaps and those flaps having an independent and functionally self-contained arteriovenous system (axial pattern flaps).

Development of cutaneous axial flaps in the lower extremity has lagged behind other areas, probably as a result of an incomplete understanding of the anatomy and an underestimation of the local vascular capacity to support flaps of high length-width ratio. Furthermore, the reliability of certain lower extremity random pattern flaps has been emphasized. Nonetheless, reliable axial pattern flaps have been defined, one supplied by the plantar artery and the other by the dorsalis pedis artery.

Lower extremity axial pattern flaps were first suggested by Moberg (1964), who described an island flap of volar great toe skin supplied by the deep branch of the dorsalis pedis artery. Subsequently, Snyder and Edgerton (1965) used island flaps consisting of the skin of the second and third toes and metatarsal pad based on the lateral plantar vessels; and Kaplan (1969) transferred the skin of the volar aspect of the great toe supplied by the medial plantar vessels. All of these small island flaps were used to resurface neurotrophic heel ulcers, and they established the feasibility of local arterialized and sensory-innervated foot flaps.

**The Dorsalis Pedis Flap.**    The first large axial flap in the lower extremity was reported by McCraw and Furlow (1975). This flap is based on the dorsalis pedis artery and the dorsal venous arch and has been used successfully to resurface defects of the dorsum of the foot, both malleoli, and the heel. The dorsalis pedis flap is a true axial pattern flap, with predictable axial and random components. Flap survival, whether the flap is an "island" or is attached by a skin pedicle, is equally good and should allow the flap to be used for Achilles tendon and pretibial area defects.

DESIGN OF THE DORSALIS PEDIS FLAP.    The large dorsalis pedis flap extends from the medial aspect of the first metatarsal to the lateral aspect of the fifth metatarsal, distally to the metatarsal necks, and proximally to the midportion of the extensor retinaculum (see Fig. 86–16). The flap includes the dorsal venous arch, the dorsalis pedis artery and vein, and the terminal sensory branches of the peroneal nerve.

The largest dorsalis pedis flap comprised the entire dorsal foot skin and measured approximately 12 cm in width and 14 cm in length in the adult foot. The distal 2 cm of this flap is a "random" area, particularly if the flap is carried distally to the web spaces of the toes (see Chapter 6). Delay is advisable if such a large flap is employed.

Smaller flaps, centralized on the dorsalis pedis vessels, can be raised without delay if a portion of the dorsal venous arch is included.

"Island" flaps are practical but cannot be extended proximal to the midportion of the extensor retinaculum, where the dorsalis pedis vessels enter the flap. Delay is required only when a large "random" area is transferred. Because the flap is a "self-contained vascular territory" (Smith, 1973), the width of the flap base is relatively unimportant. This allows one to narrow the flap base by back-cutting to increase flap mobility, incorporating "island" flap principles in pedicle flap applications.

RAISING THE FLAP.    Using the pneumatic tourniquet, a skin incision is made medial to the extensor hallucis longus tendon. Dissection is carried lateral to this tendon, where the dense extensor hallucis longus fascia is divided longitudinally. The deep underlying muscular fascia is divided, the surface of the second dorsal interosseous muscle being exposed. The muscle is penetrated by the deep branch of the dorsalis pedis artery approximately 3 cm above the great toe web space (Figs. 86–16 and 86–17). *One must identify the distal and proximal parts of the dorsalis artery prior to ligation and division of the deep branch of the dorsalis pedis artery.* The dorsalis pedis artery is adherent to the undersurface of the flap, and its delicate vascular attachments must not be separated from the flap. The dorsalis pedis artery is carefully dissected away from the tarsal bones and elevated with the upper flap, after the vessel beneath the extensor hallucis longus fascia has been exposed and the

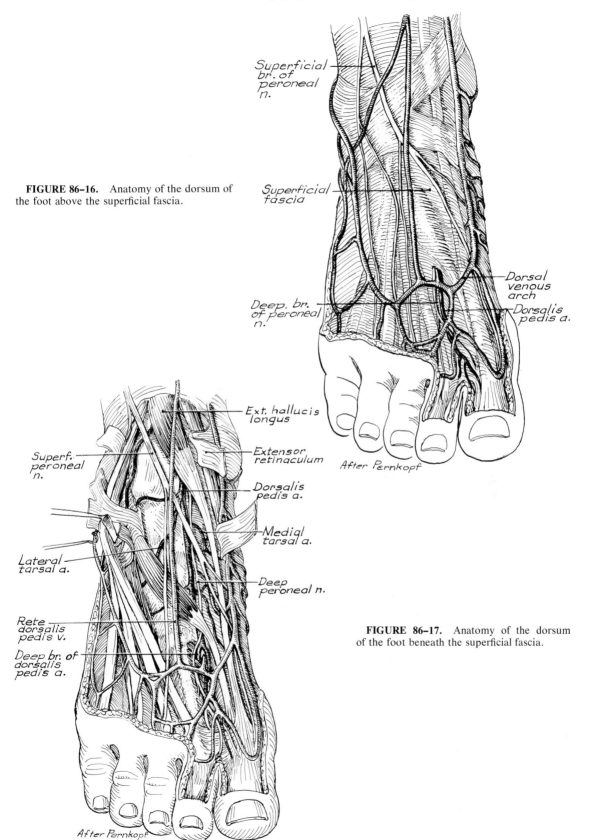

**FIGURE 86–16.** Anatomy of the dorsum of the foot above the superficial fascia.

Superficial br. of peroneal n.

Superficial fascia

Deep. br. of peroneal n.

Dorsal venous arch

Dorsalis pedis a.

After Pernkopf

Ext. hallucis longus

Extensor retinaculum

Superf. peroneal n.

Dorsalis pedis a.

Medial tarsal a.

Lateral tarsal a.

Deep peroneal n.

Rete dorsalis pedis v.

Deep br. of dorsalis pedis a.

After Pernkopf

**FIGURE 86–17.** Anatomy of the dorsum of the foot beneath the superficial fascia.

extensor hallucis brevis tendon divided. The remaining elevation is uncomplicated and consists of distal division of the neurovascular structures at the web spaces and elevation of the flap from the paratenon of the long and short toe extensors. Following this maneuver, flap mobility is gained by incising the extensor retinaculum, the skin, and the fatty attachments of the vascular pedicle to the ankle joint. All but the upper centimeter of the extensor retinaculum can be divided without causing "bowstring" of the extensor tendons.

APPLICATIONS OF THE DORSALIS PEDIS FLAP. A dorsalis pedis flap was used in a 20 year old male who sustained an avulsion injury in a motorcycle accident, losing the skin and all extensor tendons to the lateral four toes; the injury was complicated by osteomyelitis of the cuboid bone (Fig. 86–18).

The osteomyelitic bone was excised, four joint spaces being exposed. The area was immediately covered with a small central dorsalis pedis flap.

Another case is that of a 21 year old male who was involved in a motorcycle accident in which he sustained knee and ankle fractures in the same extremity. Full-thickness resurfacing of the medial ankle skin was deemed necessary to permit ankle fusion (Fig. 86–19). A large dorsalis pedis flap was raised. When viability was assured, the defect was excised, and the flap was immediately inset. After two weeks, the dorsalis pedis artery and vein were divided, and at three weeks the remaining unused flap was returned to its donor site. Healing was uncomplicated. The patient subsequently underwent ankle fusion.

Local arterialized flap coverage, without immobilization, is desirable and expeditious when one is dealing with lower extremity defects. The dorsalis pedis flap has been successfully used to provide coverage of both malleoli, the dorsum of the foot, the midsole, and portions of the heel. Cadaver dissections and other "island" dorsalis pedis flap applications suggest that the flap may be useful to resurface the Achilles tendon or pretibial areas.

The use of the dorsalis pedis flap requires that the donor site be skin-grafted. Skin grafts are successfully vascularized on normal paratenon and have proved to be durable if minimal preventive measures against local trauma are followed.

## MICROVASCULAR FREE FLAPS OF THE LOWER EXTREMITY

The goal of rapid full-thickness cutaneous coverage of large defects of the lower extremity

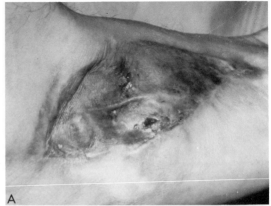

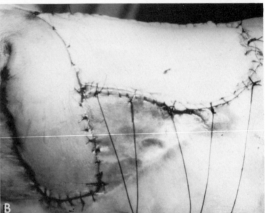

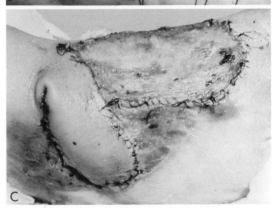

**FIGURE 86–18.** A dorsalis pedis flap used to resurface a defect over the lateral aspect of the dorsum of the foot. *A,* Osteomyelitic ulcers in a skin grafted area of the lateral aspect of the dorsum of the foot. *B,* Immediate dorsalis pedis flap inset. *C,* Healed flap and donor site graft at two weeks.

has been facilitated by the development of microvascular surgery, which permits immediate transfer and revascularization of large composites of tissue. The principles of microvascular flaps are discussed in Chapter 14 and replantation techniques in Chapter 77.

**Indications for Use of Microvascular Free Flaps.** It is axiomatic that a flap should not be

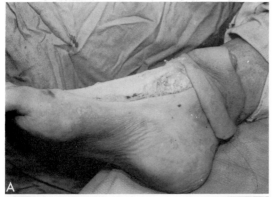

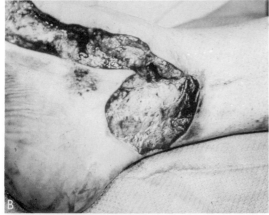

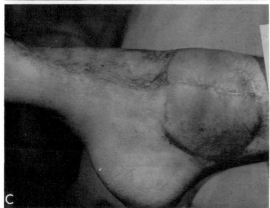

**FIGURE 86–19.** Dorsalis pedis flap used to resurface a defect over the medial malleolus. *A,* Flap excursion and viability determined prior to excision of the medial malleolar ulcer. *B,* Ulcer and unstable scar excised. *C,* Dorsalis pedis flap covering the medial malleolus after the remaining flap is returned to the anterior aspect of the ankle.

used if a skin graft will suffice. The simplest procedure that will achieve a satisfactory result should be used in resurfacing defects of the lower extremity. Only when a simpler procedure will not suffice should a distant flap be considered.

**Preoperative Evaluation**

COVERAGE.    The size, thickness, durability, texture, and cosmetic requirements of the area

to be covered should be evaluated. The flap need not always be as large as the defect. It is frequently possible to cover only a portion of the defect with the flap and the remainder with a split-thickness skin graft (see Fig. 86–24). The thickness and durability needs for the flap may vary from one portion of the defect to the other, for example, when the defect extends to the weight-bearing surfaces of the foot. The texture and cosmetic appearance of flaps of the lower extremity may be important considerations, especially in young women.

RECIPIENT SITE.    The location, availability, accessibility, size, and length of the recipient vessels is confirmed prior to creating the recipient defect or raising the donor flap. The anterior tibial artery and its venae comitantes are excellent recipient vessels and can be brought to virtually any area in the lower leg. If the pedicle of the donor vessels from the flap is sufficiently long, the anastomoses can be placed well away from the recipient defect, a technique which is desirable when an irradiated area or a recipient defect with residual infection is being covered.

Ideally the recipient site should be free of infection and covered with a healed split-thickness skin graft. This is not always possible, and, fortunately, the microvascular flap has some capacity to clear residual infection of the soft tissues and/or bone. However, every effort should be made to place the microvascular anastomoses outside the area of infection. At least one flap may have been lost because of late infection at the site of the vascular anastomoses (Vasconez, 1974).

DONOR SITE.    The selection of the donor site will depend upon the previous evaluation of coverage requirements of the recipient site and upon the character of the recipient vessels.

The groin flap (see Chapter 6) is versatile and readily available and can be designed in very large dimensions (McGregor and Jackson, 1972). The texture and quality of skin are excellent, particularly in thin patients. The donor site can usually be closed primarily, and the residual defect is easily concealed (see Fig. 86–22). In obese patients the excessive thickness of the flap and the technical problems related to its insetting may make it unsuitable for some defects.

The dorsum of the foot offers a thinner alternative in the dorsalis pedis flap with a pedicle of donor vessels which can be made quite long (Fig. 86–20). The flap can include most of the dorsum of the foot, an area frequently measuring 10 cm × 10 cm.

**Operative Technique.**    Total operative time is

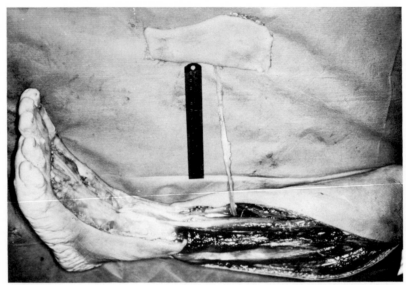

**FIGURE 86–20.**   A dorsalis pedis island flap with a pedicle in excess of 20 cm in length.

shortened by the use of two operative teams, one to prepare the recipient site, the other to raise the flap and close the donor site. A microvascular surgeon is useful on each team to prevent inadvertent trauma to the donor or recipient vessels. As an initial step, the location, size, and length of the donor and recipient vessels are confirmed. The flap is not raised until the recipient and donor vessels have been delineated. If satisfactory vessels are not found, the donor site and/or recipient vessels can be changed. The anterior tibial vessels may be approached anywhere along their course to the dorsalis pedis flap, depending upon the length of the donor pedicle which is required. The vessels supplying the groin flap are approached through an incision over the femoral vessels along the medial border of the flap (O'Brien, MacLeod, Hayhurst, and Morrison, 1973).

The donor flap is usually made 10 to 20 per cent larger than the proposed recipient defect to allow for some margin of error and to facilitate closure. However, experimental evidence has shown that microvascular flaps can tolerate normal or greater than normal tension without difficulty (Hayhurst, Mladick, and Adamson, 1974). A pattern taken from the recipient defect is useful in determining the size and shape of the flap. The flap is left attached to its feeder vessels until immediately prior to the actual anastomosis to the recipient vessels in order to minimize ischemia time.

Preparation of the recipient defect includes undermining of the skin edges, meticulous hemostasis, and dissection of the recipient vessels.

The donor artery of the flap is divided and tagged with a suture or small hemoclip. The end of the artery is allowed to remain open for escape of blood from the flap, and the veins are likewise ligated, divided, and tagged. Blood is allowed to drain freely from the flap, but perfusion of the flap is not practiced. Experimental and clinical evidence (Hayhurst, Mladick, and Adamson, 1974) has shown that perfusion is not necessary, and recent studies done in the reimplantation of hind limbs in rats by Harashina (1974) suggest that perfusion may actually decrease the chances of a successful replant. The flap is moved to the recipient area, and immediate preparations are made for the microvascular repairs. The techniques of microvascular repair are discussed in Chapter 14.

**Use of Microvascular Free Flaps in Resurfacing Defects of the Lower Extremity.**   The technique of microvascular free flap coverage of lower extremity defects can be demonstrated by illustrative case histories.

CASE HISTORY NUMBER 1.   A 15 year old girl was admitted to the hospital shortly after the onset of an acute toxic febrile illness. There were extensive purpuric lesions over both extremities, especially the lower legs (Fig. 86–21, *A*); the trunk and head and neck were spared.

The history revealed a bout of infectious mononucleosis approximately six weeks prior to admission from which she had apparently recovered and resumed normal activity and health. A decreased fibrinogen level was noted, and a diagnosis of purpura fulminans with disseminated intravascular coagulation was made.

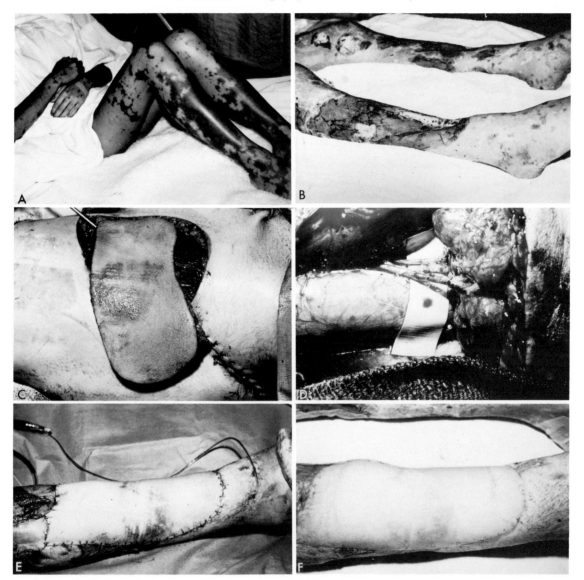

**FIGURE 86–21.** Lower extremity purpuric lesions which progressed to full-thickness skin defects. *A,* Early appearance. *B,* All lesions were covered with skin grafts except a small area of the left tibia and a larger area of the right tibia. Multiple drill holes failed to produce granulations. *C,* Microvascular free groin flap. The partially raised groin flap remains attached to its feeder vessels. The central dark area on the flap is the site of a previously harvested split-thickness skin graft. Note beginning closure of the donor defect. *D,* Anastomosis of the tibial vessels to the flap vessels. *E,* Note the relatively pale color of the flap immediately after transfer. *F,* Two weeks postoperatively.

The patient was treated with cortisone and heparin, to which she responded.

The ecchymotic lesions progressed to full-thickness sloughs of skin at the site of most of the purpuritic lesions, and in the anterior aspect of the lower leg, there was deeper involvement with loss of the fascia and muscle mass, particularly involving both anterior tibial compartments. The lesions were treated with Sulfamylon, frequent dressing changes, debridement, and eventual skin grafting of all areas but the exposed portions of both lower tibias. Multiple

drill holes failed to produce any granulation tissue, and roentgenograms showed early osteomyelitis (Fig. 86–21, *B*). It was felt that early flap coverage was indicated.

A suitable donor area was not available on the opposite lower extremity, and the joint stiffness and arthritic symptoms produced by the systemic illness suggested the inadvisability of a distant skin flap.

The decision was therefore made to perform a microvascular free flap. A large flap was removed from the left groin (Fig. 86–21, *C*), and

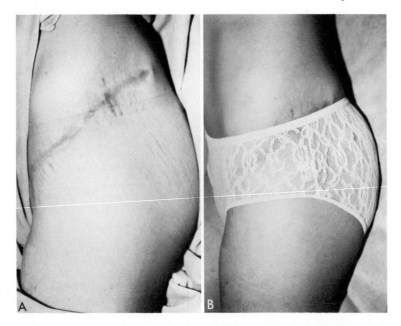

**FIGURE 86–22.** The donor site in the groin. *A,* Six months postoperatively. *B,* The donor site is easily concealed.

the superficial circumflex iliac artery and vein were sutured end-to-end to the anterior tibial artery and one of its venae comitantes (Fig. 86–21, *D*). The second vena comitans of the anterior tibial artery was sutured to a deep vein in the flap. The flap healed primarily (Fig. 86–21, *E, F*), and the donor site was easily concealed (Fig. 86–22).

CASE HISTORY NUMBER 2. A 13 year old boy became entangled in the power take-off of a tractor and suffered a compound fracture of both bones of the right lower leg with avulsion of skin and 12.5 cm of the lower third of the fibula; a distal 4-cm segment of the fibula was left attached at the ankle. The initial treatment by debridement of the soft tissues and internal fixation of the tibia was followed 10 days later by further debridement and application of a split-thickness skin graft (Fig. 86–23, *A*).

A small portion of exposed bone in the center of the wound continued to drain purulent material and was treated with frequent dressing changes and gentamicin cream. At one month postoperatively there was persistent drainage around a small fragment of exposed bone in the wound. The fragment of bone was removed (Fig. 86–23, *B*), followed by the transfer of a microvascular free flap from the left groin to the right lower leg. The anterior tibial artery and its two venae comitantes were anastomosed to the superficial circumflex iliac artery and its venae comitantes and a more superficial skin vein from the groin flap (Fig. 86–23, *C, D*).

Postoperatively the patient was placed on intravenous antibiotics, oral aspirin, and Persantine. The flap healed primarily without incident.

CASE HISTORY NUMBER 3.* A 17 year old boy suffered an accidental shotgun wound of his right foot and ankle (Fig. 86–24, *A*). After extensive debridement and frequent dressing changes, the granulating wound appeared to be relatively clean and ready for application of a split-thickness skin graft except for exposure of the talus in the central portion of the wound (Fig. 86–24, *B*). A femoral angiogram showed that the anterior tibial artery was interrupted by the injury but was patent to approximately 10 cm above the ankle.

Twelve days after the original injury, a flap was transferred from the left groin to the defect at the ankle, and the superficial circumflex iliac vessels were anastomosed to the tibial vessels. The first arterial anastomosis was unsatisfactory and was revised at the initial operation. Flap circulation remained satisfactory until approximately six hours postoperatively, when there was slowing of the capillary refill time, and the color of the flap changed from pale pink to a dusky blue.

Removal of some of the sutures from the flap seemed to provide a temporary improvement in circulation, but reoperation was required approximately 24 hours postoperatively. At reoperation, a thrombosis of the lower end of the anterior tibial artery was noted. After resection of the anastomosis, careful examination under the microscope showed additional unrecognized damage to the distal anterior tibial artery. After adequate resection of the distal end of the an-

---

*From O'Brien, MacLeod, Hayhurst, and Morrison, 1973.

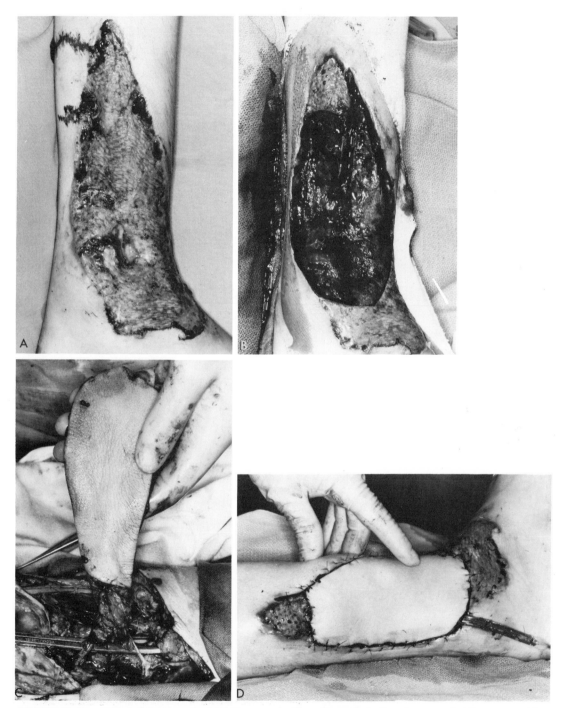

**FIGURE 86–23.** Defect of the lower leg initially covered with a skin graft. *A*, Bone is exposed at the upper and lower ends of the defect. *B*, The recipient defect is prepared and the necrotic bone excised. *C*, Flap raised and left attached to artery and vein. *D*, Completed microvascular free flap. Note the suction drain and skin graft of the residual defect.

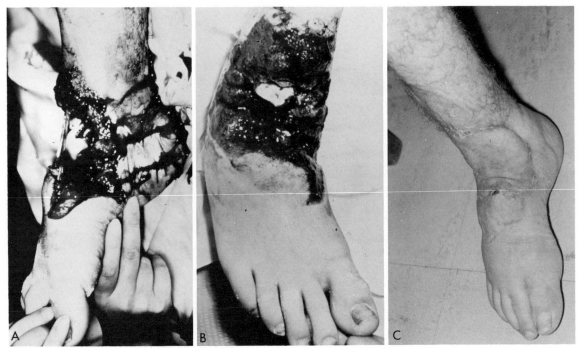

**FIGURE 86–24.** Shotgun wound of the ankle. *A*, Initial appearance. Note the exposed talus. *B*, Granulating wound with exposed talus in the center. *C*, Healed microvascular free groin flap with skin grafts at the edges.

terior tibial artery, its length was insufficient to reach the flap vessels. A vein graft was used to bridge the gap between the anterior tibial artery and the flap.

There was an immediate return of circulation to the flap with bleeding from the edges. Most of the bluish discoloration of the flap resolved slowly over a period of several days. Split-

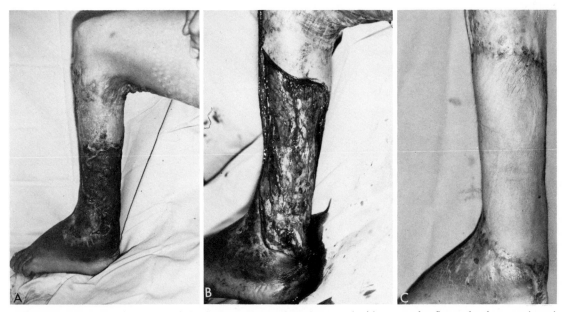

**FIGURE 86–25.** Persistent ulcer following attempts to close the wound with a cross-leg flap and a thoracoepigastric tube flap. *A*, Initial appearance. *B*, Debridement of the ulcer and scar with exposure of bone and tendon. *C*, Five weeks postoperatively, showing satisfactory healing of a large microvascular free groin flap.

thickness skin grafts were required at the edges of the flap, and the flap healed without further difficulties (Fig. 86–24, *C*).

CASE HISTORY NUMBER 4.* A 26 year old man had a large ulcer on his left leg at the site of a previous fracture (Fig. 86–25, *A*). There was exposure of the fibula with osteomyelitis. Two previous attempts to treat the lesion with a cross-leg flap and a thoracoepigastric tube flap had failed. Following wide debridement of the leg (Fig. 86–25, *B*), a microvascular flap from the left groin was applied to the defect with anastomosis of the superficial circumflex iliac vessels to the anterior tibial vessels. At four weeks the flap was well-healed, and the patient was exercising without difficulty (Fig. 86–25, *C*).

## Closure of Defects of the Lower Extremity by Muscle Flaps

### RALPH GER, M.D.

The closure of tissue defects by the transplantation of mobilized muscle bellies with their intact neurovascular bundles offers the following benefits:

1. A rigid-walled, deep cavity, resisting closure by any other means, can be obliterated, e.g., a bony cavity or a chronic cavity lined by thick fibrous or fibrocalcific walls.

2. The vascularity of the area is increased. On the arterial side, this may promote or accelerate healing. On the venous and lymphatic sides, it is possible that drainage is improved.

3. Adherence of skin to underlying rigid structures (e.g., bone) is prevented.

4. A skin graft, split- or full-thickness, or a skin flap can be applied to the transferred muscle, which is an ideal recipient site.

5. Muscle is, in most instances, freely and locally available for immediate and prompt use in the closure of a defect.

6. The implantation of muscle may, either by itself or acting as a vehicle for chemotherapeutic agents, aid in controlling a persistent infection.

7. Closure of a large cavity by a muscle flap stops the leakage of protein-rich exudate, leading to improvement of the patient's general condition.

**Principles of the Technique.** The incision, which obviously varies according to the involved area, is, in general, longitudinal in design in order to avoid severing of the cutaneous nerves. It does not cross skin creases and may diverge to enclose the ulcerated area itself.

The primary lesion is excised with as much of the associated scar as possible, consistent with the likely possibility of obtaining adequate skin cover. The most easily available muscle is dissected and sufficiently mobilized, with its neurovascular supply intact, to fill the defect. During mobilization, it is useful to retain the aponeurotic sheath, which serves as an anchor for stabilizing sutures. The muscle is secured to the surrounding skin, subcutaneous tissue, fascia, or periosteum by chromic catgut (3–0) sutures. The skin is approximated on either side of the muscle, and drainage is provided as necessary.

Skin grafting may be performed by three different methods: (1) a skin graft may be placed on the muscle at the end of the operation; (2) the graft may be taken at this time and stored for delayed application; or (3) the graft can be taken and applied five to seven days later. All three methods have been used.

The disadvantage of primary grafting is that the muscle may ooze excessively, and there may subsequently be small areas of necrosis. The disadvantage of delayed application of stored skin is that accurate suturing of the graft cannot be performed without anesthesia, except in paraplegics.

**Defects in the Region of the Hip.** Large deep wounds in the region of the hip joint commonly follow resection of the femoral head and neck for septic arthritis and decubitus ulcers. Such a defect, lined by thick fibrous walls containing contaminated material, cannot usually be closed by a rotation flap, which covers only the superficial part of the lesion. The problem is such that closure by a distant skin flap and disarticulation combined with closure of the defect by thigh flaps in one or two stages are often the only alternatives (Conway and associates, 1951; Georgiade, Pickrell, and Maguire, 1956; Steiger and Curtiss, 1968).

The muscle selected depends on the depth and extent of the defect. For a trochanteric ulcer, the sartorius is used if the lesion is superficial, and the rectus femoris is employed for a larger and deeper defect. For an even larger lesion, both muscles may be utilized, or the vastus lateralis may be the muscle of choice (Ger, 1971; Ger and Adar, 1973).

TECHNIQUE. The patient is placed in a supine position with the pelvis tilted to the side opposite to the lesion. The incision encircles the lesion and is extended inferiorly down along the

---

*Courtesy of Dr. Kiyonori Harii, Tokyo, Japan.

long axis of the thigh, overlying the muscle selected for transposition. The muscle is exposed, divided inferiorly, and mobilized proximally until sufficient length has been gained to allow it to fill the defect free of any tension (Fig. 86–26). The walls of the lesion are excised and any necrotic material removed. The belly is turned on itself and placed into the defect, making sure that it reaches the bottom of the cavity (Fig. 86–27). To date, 16 trochanteric defects have been corrected by the author using the following muscles: sartorius, 4; rectus femoris, 9; and vastus lateralis, 3.

**Defects Involving the Knee.** Lesions in the region of the knee may lead to serious complications, as the bony components of the joint lie largely in a subcutaneous location. On the medial side, one muscle, the sartorius, crosses the posterior aspect of the joint, the other muscles represented only by well-formed tendons. On the lateral side there are no muscles crossing the joint, and posteriorly both heads of the gastrocnemius cover the joint capsule. Exposure of bone or cartilage at the bottom of a deep wound does not lend itself to resurfacing by any kind of skin cover. Awaiting closure by granulation tissue followed by skin cover may be successful, but failure carries severe penalties: septic arthritis, osteomyelitis, and destruction of the epiphyseal plate.

Four patients with lesions in which skin loss caused exposure of the joint were seen by the author. Three cases followed deep burns; two involved the femoral condyle and distal diaphysis, and one involved the tibial condyle. The femoral condyle and distal diaphysis were covered by the transposed lower end of the sartorius muscle (Fig. 86–28) and the tibial condyle by the transposed medial head of the gastrocnemius. In the fourth patient, the head of the fibula with its tibiofibular articulation was exposed as the result of an ill-fitting plaster cast. This lesion was covered by the lateral head of the gastrocnemius (Fig. 86–29).

**Defects of the Leg.** Ulcerative lesions of the leg present special difficulties in their management, mainly because of the unique anatomical features of the part. Over the medial aspect of the tibia and over the fibula, the periosteum is covered only by a thin layer of subcutaneous tissue and immobile skin. Arterial studies show a relatively poor supply, especially in the lower

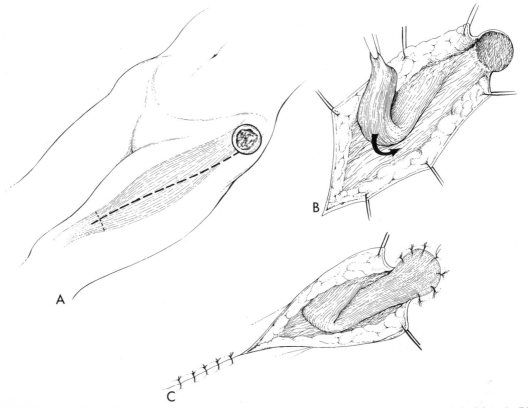

**FIGURE 86–26.**   Closure of a trochanteric defect with a rectus femoris muscle flap. *A,* Lines of skin incision. *B,* Division and rotation of the mobilized muscle. *C,* Muscle implanted into and sutured to the edge of the defect.

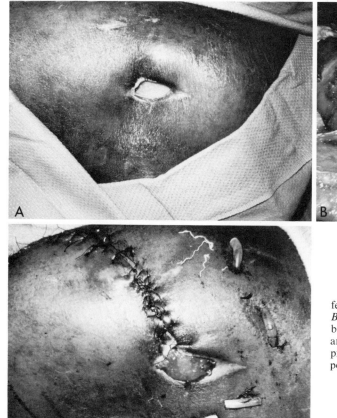

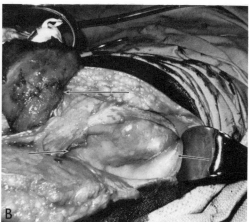

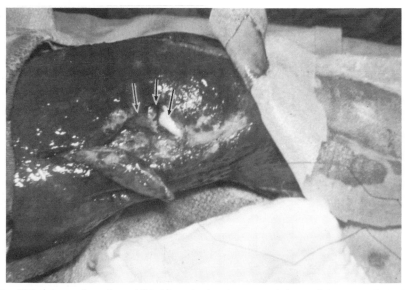

**FIGURE 86–27.** Trochanteric cutaneous defect in a paraplegic patient. *A,* Initial appearance. *B,* Actual size of the defect (13 × 8 cm) indicated by arrows. The mobilized rectus femoris (upper arrow) prior to mobilization. *C,* The muscle occupies the entire defect. Rubber booties indicate the peripheral attachment of the muscle.

**FIGURE 86–28.** Third degree burn in a child. Note the involvement of the medial aspect of the femoral diaphysis (upper arrow), epiphyseal disc (middle arrow), and articular cartilage of the femoral condyle (lower arrow). The sartorius muscle has been mobilized prior to transposition into the defect.

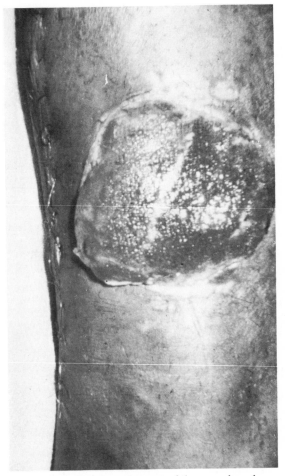

**FIGURE 86–29.** Lateral aspect of the upper leg, showing the lateral head of the gastrocnemius transposed to cover an ulcer exposing the fibular head, superior tibiofibular articulation, and the common peroneal nerve. The line of the incision is seen posteriorly.

leg (Dodd and Cockett, 1956). The superficial venous return, unaided by muscular action and hampered by gravity, is partly dependent on a system of valved communicating veins, commonly the site of pathologic processes. Skin loss over the tibia or upper and lower fibula from trauma, with or without fracture, surgery, or chronic ulceration results in a lesion based on bone.

The indications (Ger, 1972) for closure of leg defects by muscle transposition and skin graft include:

1. Acute traumatic lesions with skin loss and damage to the underlying structures.

2. Acute infections with skin loss and exposure of the underlying structures.

3. Chronic ulcerative lesions. The procedure may be indicated in the treatment of the following conditions: stasis ulceration, chronic os-teomyelitis, postexcisional defects, and ulcers resulting from unstable scars.

SKIN LOSS WITH DAMAGE TO DEEPER STRUCTURES. When tendons are exposed or fractures have occurred, some form of cover is necessary. Traditional methods were discussed earlier in the chapter, but another approach to the treatment of open fractures was introduced as a result of wartime experiences (Converse, 1941, 1942; Dehne and associates, 1961a, b, Witschi and Omer, 1970). These authors advocated initial debridement, long-leg plaster immobilization, and delayed skin grafts. An unacceptable incidence of osteomyelitis and an adherent thin scar in an easily injured superficial position, possible antecedents to recurrent osteomyelitis and ulceration respectively, remain the main criticisms of this approach.

Closure by muscle transposition has the following disadvantages: the destruction of available muscle may invalidate the procedure, and operative manipulation may theoretically spread existing contamination. However, in traumatic cases the wound is left open for drainage for five to seven days before skin grafts are applied. The operation does have complications and sequelae, which will be described later. On the other hand, in addition to the previously described advantages, loss of tendons through exposure is prevented, and granulation tissue is covered with less chance for the development of fibrous tissue.

In a series of 23 defects of the leg, 15 involved the tibia (11 of the middle third of the shaft, 1 the upper third, and 3 the lower third); 3 involved the fibula; and in 5 patients both bones have been involved. The results have been satisfactory, primary healing occurring without the development of osteomyelitis or nonunion. A clinical example is shown in Figure 86–31.

ACUTE INFECTIONS WITH SOFT TISSUE LOSS. Primary infections of the leg leading to destruction of the deeper structures occur not uncommonly in diabetic patients. There may be resulting exposure of the tendons, particularly the tendo calcaneus, and exposure of the underlying bones and ankle joint. Special efforts should be made to protect these structures, as their involvement may progress to loss of the limb. The tendo calcaneus can be protected by dissecting out the attached soleus muscle and covering its surface with a skin graft; the ankle joint has been covered by the peroneus brevis and flexor hallucis longus muscles (Ger, 1972).

CHRONIC STASIS ULCERATION. While control of the underlying venous hypertension is necessary, the fibrous tissue, at times calcified or ossified, with its covering of atrophic skin

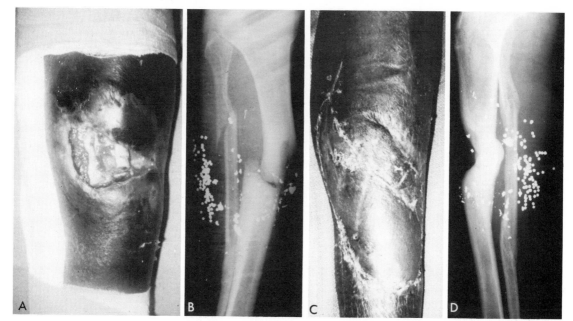

**FIGURE 86–30.** Chronic osteomyelitis of the middle tibia shaft and overlying cutaneous defect. *A,* Initial appearance. *B,* Roentgenogram showing the residual shots from the original gunshot injury. Note the pathologic fracture at the site of the chronic osteomyelitis. *C,* Healed wound following transposition of the soleus and flexor digitorum muscle flaps and application of split-thickness skin grafts. *D,* Roentgenogram showing healing at the fracture sites.

constitutes an irreversible state unaffected by the relief of the hypertension and shows a persistent tendency to ulcerate. Ideally, as with any other unstable scar tissue, such tissues should be excised. The steps in the operative treatment are as follows:

1. Excision of the ulcer and as much surrounding pathologic tissue as can be removed, consistent with the likely possibility of obtaining adequate skin cover.

2. Ligation and division of the exposed perforating veins.

3. Mobilization of a muscle belly to fill the defect and fixation of the muscle.

4. Immediate or delayed skin graft application.

ULCERS ASSOCIATED WITH CHRONIC OSTEOMYELITIS. Several types of ulcers associated with chronic osteomyelitis warrant application of the muscle flap technique:

1. Nonhealing superficial ulcer: the osteomyelitis has been controlled, the problem being inadequate covering of the sclerosed bone by a thin epithelial layer. Traditional methods, including cross-leg flaps, have their disadvantages, and coverage by muscle transposition after excision of the excess bone is a suitable approach.

2. Deep bone-based ulcer: the main difficulty is obliteration of a rigid-walled cavity. This is an ideal indication for the use of a muscle flap, which obliterates the defect, improves the blood supply, and allows suitable skin cover.

3. Multiple sinuses with inflammatory changes of the surrounding soft tissue. Extensive debridement results in a large uncovered bony cavity, the filling of which by a muscle flap followed by skin grafting is an acceptable solution.

4. Multiple skin-lined sinuses leading to the implantation of keratinizing squamous epithelium with resultant inflammatory reaction. The epithelium may show a typical pseudoepitheliomatous hyperplasia, which, on occasion, may proceed to frank carcinoma.

A clinical example of a chronic ulcer associated with osteomyelitis is illustrated in Figure 86–30.

### Surgical Technique of Mobilization of Specific Muscles

GASTROCNEMIUS MUSCLE (Fig. 86–32). The medial head of the gastrocnemius muscle can be used to cover the upper medial aspect of the tibia and a portion of the knee joint, depending on its size. The lateral head can be employed to resurface the superior tibiofibular joint, the upper fibula, and a part of the knee joint. Either head can be exposed by a vertical incision passing from the crease of the popliteal fossa inferiorly in the midline to a point just proximal to the lower limit of the bulge produced

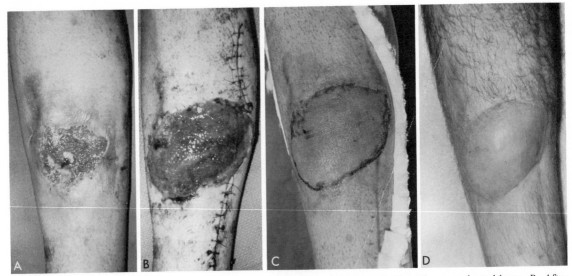

**FIGURE 86–31.** Open fracture of the midtibia. *A,* Appearance of the wound. Note the comminuted bone. *B,* After debridement and transposition of a soleus muscle flap. *C,* Twelve days following debridement and closure of the defect and one week after application of split-thickness skin graft on the muscle bed. *D,* Eight months after reconstruction.

by the gastrocnemius; the incision curves medially or laterally, depending on which muscle is to be mobilized. The short saphenous vein and the sural nerve are respectively located before and after division of the deep fascia. The two heads are easily separated and the selected head is mobilized by sharp dissection at the musculotendinous junction and by proceeding proximally as far as the main neurovascular bundle opposite the tibial condyles. Finger dissection between the muscle and the deep fascia in an anterior direction establishes a tunnel through which the muscle belly, deep surface uppermost, is passed. Compression of the muscle by the skin bridge is prevented by excising the underlying deep fascia.

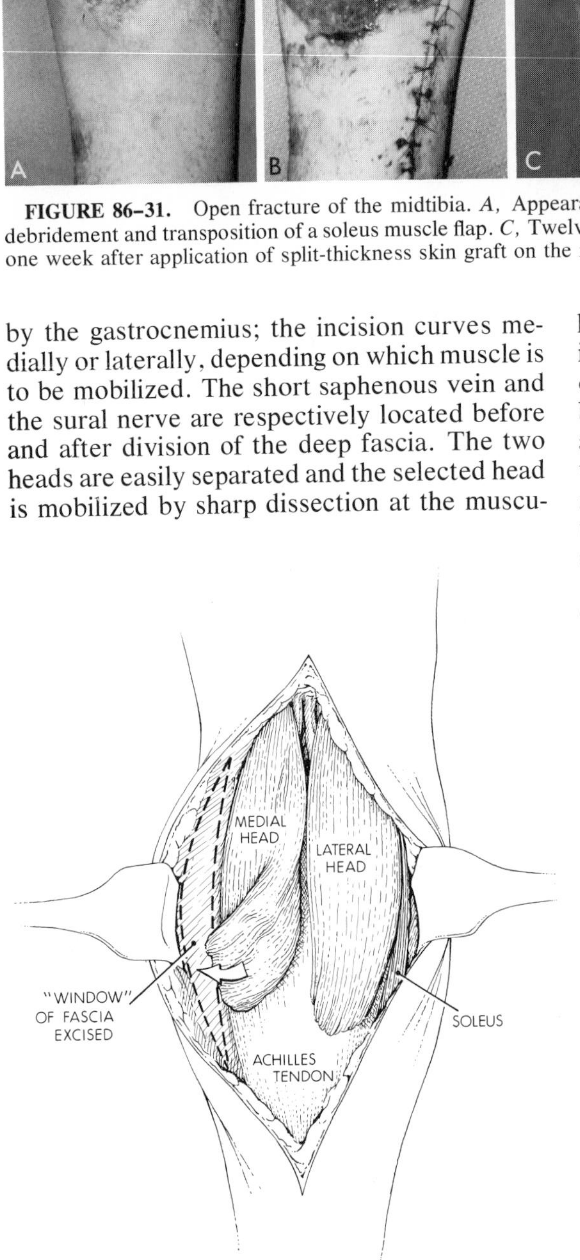

SOLEUS, FLEXOR DIGITORUM LONGUS, AND THE MEDIAL PART OF THE FLEXOR HALLUCIS LONGUS MUSCLES (Fig. 86–33). A vertical incision midway between the tibia and the tendo calcaneus from a point 2.5 cm above the middle of the leg to a point 1.25 cm above the medial malleolus affords adequate exposure of the soleus, flexor digitorum longus, and the medial portion of the flexor hallucis longus.

*Soleus muscle.* After division of the deep fascia, the medial border of the tendo calcaneus is identified (Fig. 86–34), with the plantaris tendon lying in close attendance. Traction on three or four stay sutures placed in the medial border of the tendo calcaneus facilitates separation of the soleal fibers. The separation is easily commenced 5 cm above the lowest fibers, carried across the whole width of the tendon, and then dissected distally until the lowermost fibers are divided. A stay suture is placed in the lower end of the muscle. The anterior border of the muscle is defined and easily separated from the fascial septum covering the neurovascular bundle and the deep muscles. Several soleal veins passing deeply and superficially require division and ligation as the mobilization proceeds up to the

"WINDOW" OF FASCIA EXCISED

MEDIAL HEAD

LATERAL HEAD

SOLEUS

ACHILLES TENDON

**FIGURE 86–32.** Mobilization of the medial head of the gastrocnemius muscle.

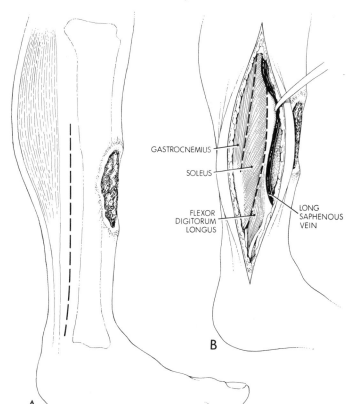

**FIGURE 86–33.** The line of incision (*A*) and the planes of dissection (*B*) for exposing and mobilizing the soleus muscle.

GASTROCNEMIUS

SOLEUS

FLEXOR DIGITORUM LONGUS

LONG SAPHENOUS VEIN

A

B

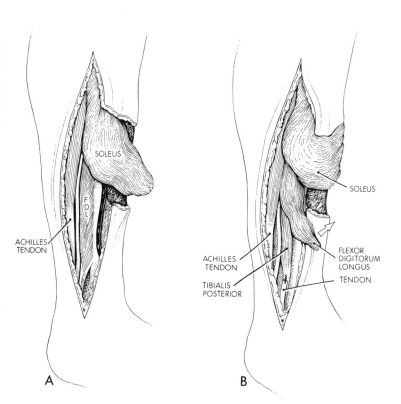

SOLEUS

F D L

ACHILLES TENDON

A

SOLEUS

ACHILLES TENDON

TIBIALIS POSTERIOR

FLEXOR DIGITORUM LONGUS

TENDON

B

**FIGURE 86–34.** The soleus muscle alone (*A*) transposed to cover an anterior defect or in combination with the flexor digitorum longus (*B*) for a larger defect.

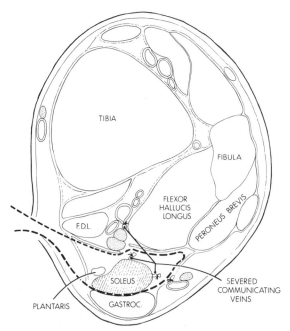

**FIGURE 86–35.** Planes of dissection to mobilize the soleus muscle. Communicating veins are divided and ligated.

distal tibial attachment (Fig. 86–35). The fibers are separated from their tendinous insertion, traction on the soleal stay suture and counter-traction via those in the tendo calcaneus facilitat-

ing this division. As the dissection proceeds proximally, branches draining laterally into the short saphenous vein may require attention. Sufficient muscle is mobilized to cover the defect, maximal liberation being gained by detaching the muscle from its tibial origin. It should be mentioned that at times the large bulk of a well-developed soleus muscle is more than is required to cover the defect. In this situation, the muscle can be split along a central line of division, and the medial component only can be used. In general, the whole soleus can cover the middle two quarters of the tibial shaft.

*Flexor digitorum longus muscle.* This muscle may be mobilized to cover a small defect. It may also be used to supplement the soleus (see Fig. 86–34) in covering a superior defect or to supplement the abductor hallucis in a lower defect.

It is usual to commence the mobilization inferiorly, where the tendon must be differentiated from that of the closely related tibialis posterior. The flexor digitorum longus is divided at its origin by sharp dissection and by blunt dissection from its fascial attachment. After division of the tendon, its lower end is sutured to that of the tibialis posterior. It may be elected to dissect the muscle belly off the tendon, leaving the latter more functionally intact.

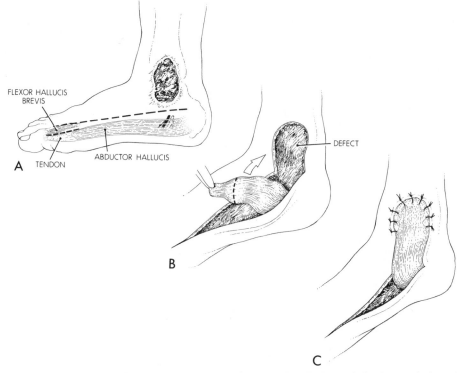

**FIGURE 86–36.** Abductor hallucis muscle flap. *A,* Skin incision. *B,* Muscle mobilized posteriorly and its tendon excised. *C,* Muscle rotated superiorly and sutured into the medial malleolar defect.

*Flexor hallucis longus muscle.* This muscle is the bulkiest of all the extrinsic foot muscles at the level of the ankle joint, being aptly described as the "beef of the heel" (Last, 1972). However, full advantage cannot be taken of its size, as it is difficult to transpose. This difficulty stems from its position, arising deeply from the lower two-thirds of the posterior fibular surface, with the large peroneal artery in intimate relationship to its origin. Mobilization does not permit easy transposition in either a medial or lateral direction. It has been used on occasion to cover the posterior aspect of the ankle joint and to cover the posteroinferior surface of the medial malleolus.

ABDUCTOR HALLUCIS MUSCLE (Fig. 86–36). This muscle may be used to cover the medial aspect of the heel, ankle joint, and tibial malleolus. The slightly convex incision passes just above the medial border of the foot from the medial surface of the calcaneus to the medial surface of the first metatarsophalangeal joint. The tendon is divided, separated sharply from the flexor hallucis brevis, and mobilized posteriorly until the main neurovascular supply is encountered about 1 cm anterior to its calcaneal origin. The muscle is rotated superiorly across the medial aspect of the ankle joint.

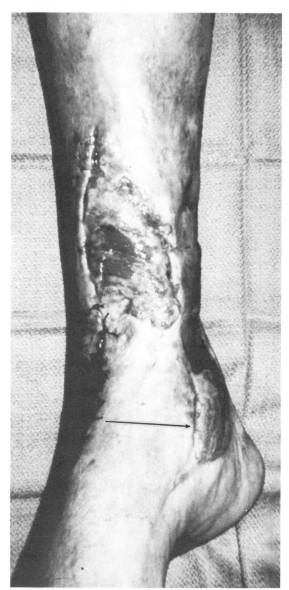

**FIGURE 86–38.** Anterior leg ulcer resurfaced by the extensor digitorum longus muscle. A full-thickness skin graft applied on a previously transposed abductor hallucis muscle is indicated by the arrow.

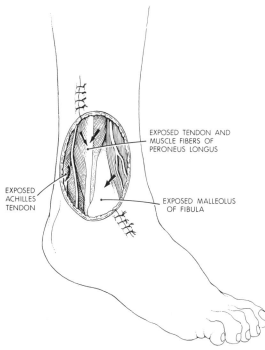

EXPOSED TENDON AND
MUSCLE FIBERS OF
PERONEUS LONGUS

EXPOSED
ACHILLES
TENDON

EXPOSED MALLEOLUS
OF FIBULA

**FIGURE 86–37.** Defect of the lower lateral side of the leg, with exposure of the fibular malleolus, peroneus longus tendon, and tendo calcaneus. These are covered by the peroneus tertius, peroneus brevis, and the lower fibers of the soleus muscles, respectively.

**Defects of the Lower Lateral Third of the Leg** (Fig. 86–37). Loss of skin in this area results in a wound exposing the fibular malleolus and the tendons of the peroneus longus and tendo calcaneus muscles. These structures may be covered by mobilization of the peroneus tertius, peroneus brevis, and soleus muscles, respectively.

Generally, the cutaneous defect does not provide adequate exposure for this procedure and requires enlargement by a vertical incision extended superiorly to expose the soleus muscle, and inferiorly to expose the peroneus tertius.

The superficial peroneal and sural nerves are preserved.

The peroneus tertius muscle is mobilized by dividing its tendon and separating it sharply from the extensor digitorum longus along a line medial to its tendon. After its fibular origin is divided, it is transposed to cover the fibular malleolus. On occasion, the peroneus tertius is absent, in which case the peroneus brevis muscle is used. The peroneus longus tendon is easily covered by burying the tendon in the underlying peroneus brevis by tying interrupted 3–0 chromic catgut sutures placed in the muscle on either side of the tendon. The tendo calcaneus can be covered by dissecting the soleus muscle off the tendon and rotating it laterally.

**Defects of the Lower Part of the Lateral Leg and Ankle Joint.** The muscles just discussed cannot cover a defect at or below the lower part of the lateral malleolus. The abductor digiti minimi muscle is well situated for this purpose. A slightly convex incision is designed just above the lateral border of the foot. After the tendon is divided, it is dissected free from the flexor digiti minimi brevis and mobilized proximally until the neurovascular bundle is reached. The muscle can then be rotated superiorly to cover a defect at or below the lower part of the lateral malleolus.

**Defects of the Anterior Aspect of the Leg.** The extensor digitorum longus and extensor hallucis longus are, in general, not substantial muscles and have been used mainly to supplement other muscles; on occasion, however, they have been utilized singly (Fig. 86–38).

**Defects of the Sole of the Foot.** While small defects of the sole of the foot can be closed by rotation flaps from the non–weight-bearing surface (see Fig. 86–10), larger defects may require cross-leg or distant flaps (Converse, 1964; Grabb and Smith, 1968; May, 1971). Ulcers of the hindfoot may be managed by excision of the defect, transposition of either the abductor hallucis or abductor digiti minimi, depending on the side of the defect, and coverage by a local rotation flap or thick split-thickness skin graft. The choice is dependent on the site of the lesion relative to weight-bearing. The operative technique is diagrammatically illustrated in Figure 86–39; patients thus treated are shown in Figures 86–40 and 86–41.

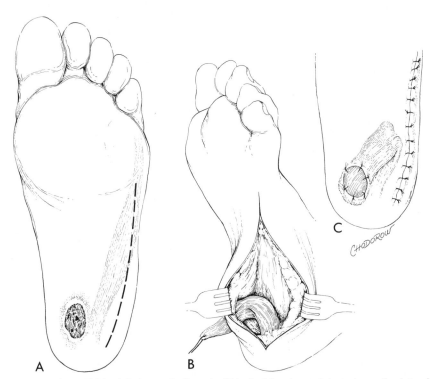

**FIGURE 86–39.** Abductor digiti minimi muscle flap. *A,* Skin incision located just above the lateral border of the plantar surface. *B,* Mobilized muscle passed posteromedially to fill the postexcisional defect. *C,* Muscle sutured in position prior to skin grafting.

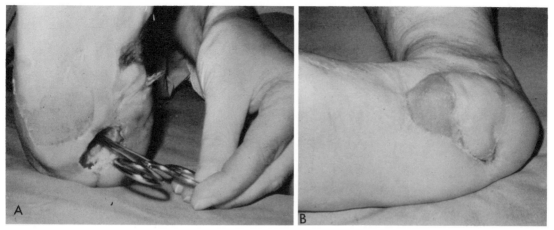

**FIGURE 86–40.**   Chronic ulcer of the heel. *A,* A large and deep ulcer overlying a defect following previous excision of the calcaneus. Note the previously unsuccessful local flaps. *B,* Appearance following filling of the defect with the mobilized abductor hallucis. The muscle was covered partly by a small rotation flap and a split-thickness skin graft.

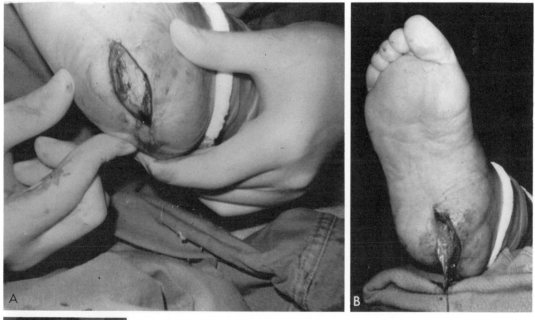

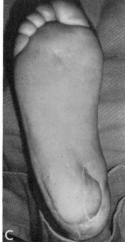

**FIGURE 86–41.**   Chronic calcaneal ulcer. *A,* Appearance following excision of ulcer. *B,* Mobilized abductor digiti minimi filling the defect. *C,* Postoperative appearance. Note that the incision is placed above the weight-bearing area of the plantar surface.

## Causes of Muscle Necrosis

1. A muscle lying between an indurated skin edge and a firmly applied dressing may undergo distal necrosis. Loose occlusive dressings are therefore routinely used.

2. Tension on a muscle will cause either necrosis of a portion of the muscle or dehiscence of the skin sutures, with a defect in either instance. It is preferable to accept a small uncovered area that will heal because of the increased blood supply provided by the flap.

3. Arterial disease can cause necrosis. In most instances, failure to palpate a peripheral pulse is due to the extensive subcutaneous fibrosis, but occasionally the underlying cause is peripheral arterial occlusive disease. In cases in which the arterial state is in doubt, plethysmography and/or arteriography may be indicated, in order to avoid performing surgery on ischemic tissues.

4. The crossing of muscle bellies may, at times, facilitate closure of a defect. This temptation should be resisted, for pressure across a muscle may cause distal necrosis.

5. A transposed abductor hallucis may be compressed by a firm upper medial shoe edge. When this muscle is transposed, either a soft shoe should be worn or the medial edge of a firm shoe should be removed (Ger, 1972).

6. The mobilization of tissues under tourniquet conditions and the inadvisability of preventing oozing by firm dressings render hematoma formation a distinct risk. To diminish this risk, it is advisable to obtain accurate hemostasis at surgery, provide drainage, preferably of the suction variety, and elevate the limb postoperatively. For similar reasons, it is also unwise to perform concomitant venous stripping operations. A large hematoma is capable of destroying a transposed muscle.

**Functional Disability Associated with Muscle Transposition.** It should be stated that in patients who are not completely independently mobile, muscle transpositions are functionally inconsequential.

With regard to muscle transpositions below the knee, it may generally be said that there does not appear to be any long-term difficulty in walking, but the rate of recovery varies with the muscles transposed. The most symptomatic transfer is that associated with the abductor hallucis muscle, where the loss of spring on ambulation is well appreciated by the patient and takes several months to return. Interference with running depends on the age of the patient. The younger patients, whose lesions were mostly post-traumatic, were able to run effectively.

**Fate of the Transposed Muscle.** Electromyographic and clinical studies (Ger, 1972) of transposed muscles show that the muscle retains its contractile power and that the bulk of the muscle persists as muscle. Even if this were not so and the muscle became fibrous tissue, the procedure would still have validity, e.g., coverage of an open tibial fracture, where primary healing can be obtained. However, it is preferable that the muscular tissue persist as such, so as to provide a soft padding for bone, a permanent hospitable host for the skin grafts, and a satisfactory blood supply.

## Closure of Defects of the Lower Extremity by Myocutaneous Flaps

JOHN B. McCRAW, M.D.

The concept that cutaneous blood supply is derived primarily from the underlying muscle is relatively new (Owens, 1955; Bakamjian, 1963). Orticochea (1972a, b) introduced the concept in lower extremity reconstruction using the gracilis muscle.

The viable myocutaneous vascular territories of the lower extremity have been defined by McCraw (1976a, b) and were discussed in Chapter 6. This work represents an extension of the contributions of Ger, which were outlined in the previous section. The gracilis, biceps femoris, rectus femoris, sartorius and gastrocnemius myocutaneous island flaps offer an additional method of lower extremity reconstruction.

**Definition of Terms.** A myocutaneous flap is a compound flap of muscle with its overlying fat and skin. An island myocutaneous flap is a flap supplied by only a muscular neurovascular pedicle without other muscular or cutaneous attachments. The dominant vascular pedicle is that set of vessels which is absolutely essential for the survival of any island myocutaneous flap. The flap rotation point is determined solely by the location of the dominant vascular pedicle.

The size of the myocutaneous flaps discussed includes the amount of muscle and skin that can be safely elevated as a viable island flap without a prior delay procedure. The cutaneous portion of the flaps can be expanded by a delay procedure, but the dimensions of such flaps are beyond the scope of this discussion.

**Rectus Femoris Myocutaneous Flap.** The rectus femoris is probably the most reliable

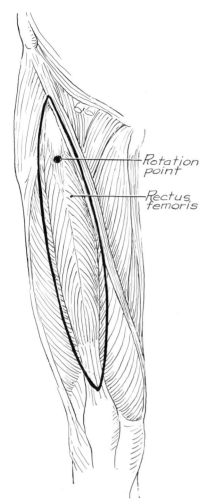

**FIGURE 86–42.** Rectus femoris myocutaneous flap. The flap rotation point lies 8 cm below the inguinal ligament.

quential. The dominant vascular pedicle is encountered approximately 8 cm below the inguinal ligament. Usually two prominent vascular pedicles are found in this area, and both must be preserved to maintain flap viability.

This is an extremely useful flap in the thigh and lower abdomen, but the functional deficit is more significant than with most muscle flaps. The use of this muscle results in moderate loss of knee extension, particularly in the last 20 degrees of extension. The functional significance of this is noted not in walking but in running or squatting. The flap has the advantage of carrying the intermediate cutaneous nerves of the thigh, which provides good sensation to the flap.

**Biceps Femoris Myocutaneous Flap.** The biceps femoris muscle supplies the largest cutaneous area in the posterior thigh and is expected to have normal sensation, since it carries the posterior cutaneous nerve of the thigh with

island myocutaneous flap in the lower extremity (Fig. 86–42). The entire muscle and its overlying skin can be elevated to the point of its insertion into the quadriceps mechanism. A flap with dimensions of 8 × 30 cm can be elevated reliably and the defect closed primarily. The proximal rotation point of the flap lies approximately 8 cm below the inguinal ligament and allows good upward mobility of the flap. The tip of the flap will reach above the umbilicus, the opposite pubic tubercle, the greater tuberosity, and intervening points in the thigh.

Flap elevation is begun distally where the rectus femoris tendon inserts into the quadriceps mechanism. The muscle is separated from the vastus lateralis and medialis, and the dissection is carried superiorly. The muscle is separated from the lateral border of the sartorius muscle, and the perforating vessels in the lower two-thirds of the muscle are inconse-

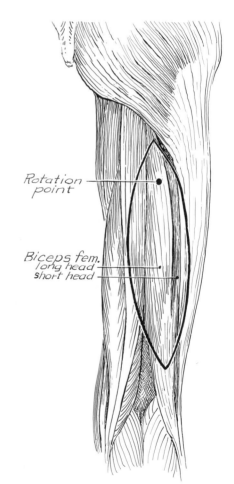

**FIGURE 86–43.** Biceps femoris myocutaneous flap. The flap rotation point lies 8 cm below the ischial tuberosity.

the flap. A 12 × 26 cm flap can be elevated on a proximal vascular pedicle with primary closure. The rotation point is usually 8 cm below the ischial tuberosity, and some variability causes a major problem with biceps femoris myocutaneous flaps (Fig. 86–43). Usually the dominant vascular pedicle is the first perforating vessel from the profunda femoris, but at times the second perforating vessel may be an important contributor to the distal muscle and cannot be divided. When the second perforating vessel proves to be a dominant vessel entering the midportion of the muscle, the superior rotation of the flap is considerably limited. Unfortunately, this is an all-or-none phenomenon in that division of this vessel usually results in some degree of distal muscle necrosis. Division of the second perforating vessel as a delay procedure is probably not feasible.

This flap provides coverage for the perineum, the mid-buttock region, and the greater tuberosity. Functional loss of the muscle is minimal, with mild weakening of knee flexion but no loss of knee stability; the short head of the bi-ceps femoris, the tensor, and the semitendinosus and the semimembranosus muscles compensate for loss of the biceps femoris muscle.

This is an excellent flap with normal sensation when the proximal vascular pedicle is the first perforating branch of the profunda femora artery; when it is not, the limitations of flap mobility make this an unusable flap.

**Gracilis Myocutaneous Flap.** The proximal two-thirds of the gracilis muscle can carry a flap that measures 6 × 20 cm with a rotation point that is 7 cm below the pubic tubercle. This flap provides small areas of coverage within a wide arc. The tip of the flap will reliably reach several inches above the pubic tubercle (Fig. 86–44), the anterior iliac spine, the lower sacrum, and intervening points. The details of flap elevation are discussed in Chapter 99.

The functional loss of this muscle is negligible, and the flap provides coverage for areas that are otherwise difficult to cover. The sensation in the flap is variable, and while it is usually fair to good, it is never excellent.

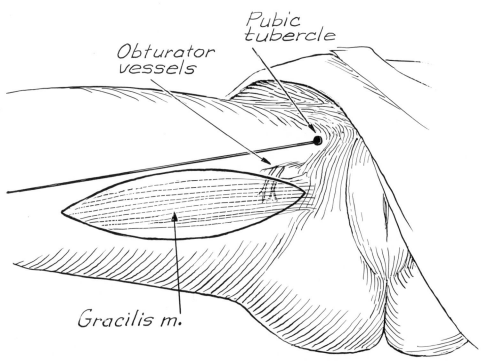

**FIGURE 86–44.** Gracilis myocutaneous flap.

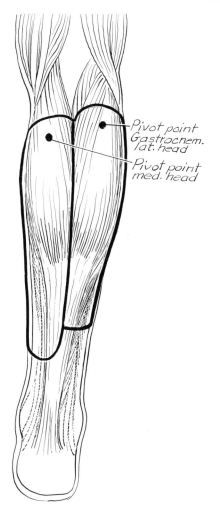

**FIGURE 86–45.** Medial and lateral gastrocnemius myocutaneous flaps. Flap rotation points are near the popliteal fossa.

**Medial Gastrocnemius Flap.** The medial head of the gastrocnemius can supply an area of skin that is usually 8 × 40 cm and extends from the anterior border of the muscle in a direct line inferiorly, with the lower margin of the flap lying approximately 5 cm above the medial malleolus and the posterior margin of the flap in the midline of the calf (Fig. 86–45).

Flap elevation is begun distally so that the saphenous nerve and the greater saphenous vein can be protected in their anterior location. The deep fascia of the calf is elevated with the flap up to the point where the gastrocnemius muscle is detached from its muscular insertion in the Achilles tendon superficial to the soleus muscle. It is separated from the lateral gastrocnemius muscle in the midline, and this should be done under direct vision so that the sural nerve is not injured. The proximal rotation point is quite high and lies at about the level of insertion of the semitendinosus tendon. This allows satisfactory upward mobility of the flap.

The flap provides excellent coverage of the pretibial area (Fig. 86–46) from a point about 8 cm above the medial malleolus extending the entire length of the anterior calf. In the superior direction the flap will cover the popliteal fossa, the anterior knee, and the lower 15 cm of the thigh for defects up to 8 cm in length.

The functional loss resulting from the use of this muscle is usually compensated for by the lateral gastrocnemius and soleus muscles for normal activities. There is a moderate decrease in the ability to push off, and a significant disability in running or in sustained ankle flexion. As with the lateral gastrocnemius and the rectus femoris, this is a muscle that should be used with caution in athletic individuals.

**Lateral Gastrocnemius Myocutaneous Flap.** The lateral gastrocnemius provides a flap that is substantially smaller than the medial gastrocnemius flap and measures 6 × 35 cm (see Fig. 86–45). The level of the rotation point is similar to the medial gastrocnemius flap.

Elevation of the flap is begun distally approximately 10 cm above the lateral malleolus, and the deep fascia is included with the flap. The flap extends 6 to 8 cm lateral to the midline of the calf. The sural nerve is protected during flap elevation and the muscle is separated from the Achilles tendon.

The flap provides similar coverage to the medial gastrocnemius flap on the lateral aspect of the calf and knee. For some reason it is not as well arterialized as the medial calf flap, but it does provide coverage for the lateral lower thigh, areas that are less amenable to traditional methods of flap coverage.

The functional loss is slightly less than the loss associated with the use of the medial gastrocnemius muscle. As expected, neither flap can carry sensory nerves when used as an island flap. Both of the flaps can be used as island flaps if a large area of attachment to the gastrocnemius muscle belly is maintained; consequently, the skin may be divided at the level of the knee joint but not in the area of the insertion of the gastrocnemius muscle, since this is a critical vascular cross-over point between a pure myocutaneous flap and a distal cutaneous flap carried by fascial interconnecting vessels. Like the medial gastrocnemius myocutaneous flap, the donor defect is so large that skin grafting is required.

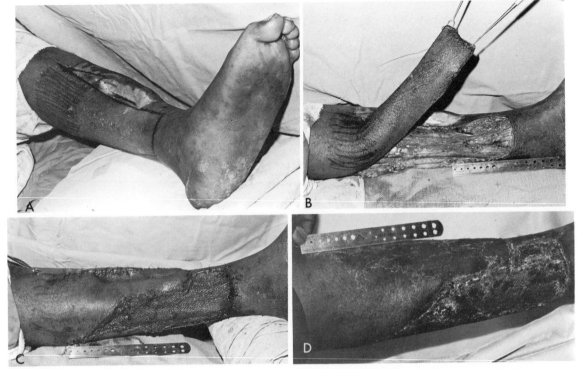

**FIGURE 86–46.** *A*, Medial gastrocnemius myocutaneous flap outlined adjacent to pretibial defect. *B*, Flap elevated without any delay. Portion of flap containing muscle is lined proximally. *C*, Immediate inset. Donor defect covered with unexpanded mesh graft. *D*, Healed flap and donor site graft at six weeks.

## SUMMARY OF FLAP RECONSTRUCTION OF THE LOWER EXTREMITY

In the preceding pages, the applications of local, distant, axial pattern, microvascular free, muscle, and myocutaneous flaps were discussed. While the simplest technique, usually a skin graft, remains the method of choice in resurfacing lower extremity defects, all of the flap techniques are part of the surgical armamentarium.

The flap possibilities listed according to anatomical sites, but *not necessarily according to preference,* are as follows:

*Thigh Region*
1. Local flaps, including abdominal rotation flaps
2. Distant flaps, e.g., tube and jump flaps
3. Microvascular free flaps
4. Sartorius, rectus femoris, vastus lateralis, and gracilis muscle flaps
5. Upper sartorius, rectus femoris, gracilis and biceps femoris myocutaneous flaps

*Knee Region*
1. Local flaps
2. Distant flaps, including cross-leg flaps
3. Microvascular free flaps
4. Sartorius and gastrocnemius (medial and lateral heads) muscle flaps
5. Lower sartorius, lower biceps femoris, and gastrocnemius myocutaneous flaps

*Pretibial Region*
1. Cross-leg flaps
2. Microvascular free flaps (anastomosed to anterior tibial vessels)
3. Soleus, gastrocnemius, and flexor digitorum longus muscle flaps
4. Island dorsalis pedis flap
5. Gastrocnemius myocutaneous flaps

*Lateral Aspect of Ankle and Heel*
1. Cross-leg and cross-foot flaps
2. Microvascular free flaps
3. Dorsalis pedis axial pattern flap
4. Peroneus tertius, peroneus brevis, soleus, and abductor digiti minimi muscle flaps

*Medial Aspect of Ankle and Heel*
1. Cross-leg and cross-foot flaps
2. Microvascular free flaps
3. Dorsalis pedis axial pattern flap
4. Abductor hallucis and flexor hallucis longus muscle flaps

*Sole of Foot*
1. Dermal overgrafting
2. Local flaps from non–weight-bearing surface

3. Cross-foot flap from opposite plantar arch
4. Cross-leg flaps with later cutaneous resurfacing [Millard (1969) crane principle] by full-thickness skin grafts from the dorsomedial aspect of the foot to avoid hair follicles on the plantar surface.
5. Abductor digiti minimi and abductor hallucis muscle flaps
6. Medial or lateral plantar artery island flaps
7. Dorsalis pedis axial pattern flap.

N.B.: If subcutaneous padding or sufficient granulation tissue is available in a plantar defect, skin grafting is preferable to transfer of a flap with hair-bearing skin.

## REFERENCES

Adams, W. M., Jr., Wisner, H. K., Larson, D. L., Lynch, J. B., and Lewis, S. R.: Steinmann pin fixation of extremities for cross-leg flap. Plast. Reconstr. Surg., 44:364, 1969.

Argamaso, R. V., Lewin, M. L., Baird, A. D., and Rothfleisch, S.: Cross-leg flaps in children. Plast. Reconstr. Surg., 51:662, 1973.

Bakamjian, V.: A technique for primary reconstruction of the palate after radical maxillectomy for cancer. Plast. Reconstr. Surg., 31:103, 1963.

Blackfield, H. M., and Hause, D. P.: Congenital constricting bands of the extremities. Plast. Reconstr. Surg., 8:101, 1951.

Cannon, B., Lischer, C. E., Davis, W. B., Chasko, S., Moore, A., Murray, J. E., and McDowell, A.: The use of open jump flaps in lower extremity repairs. Plast. Reconstr. Surg., 2:336, 1947.

Cockett, F. B.: Pathology and treatment of venous ulcers of the leg. Br. J. Surg., 43:260, 1955.

Connelly, J. R.: Reconstructive procedures of the lower extremity. In Grabb, W. C., and Smith, J. W. (Eds.): Plastic Surgery. A Concise Guide to Clinical Practice. Boston, Little, Brown and Company, 1973.

Constant, E., and Grabb, W.: Steinmann pin fixation of tibiae for cross-leg flap. Plast. Reconstr. Surg., 41:179, 1968.

Converse, J. M.: Orthopaedic aspects of plastic surgery. The early replacement of skin losses in war injuries of the extremities. Proc. R. Soc. Med., 34:791, 1941.

Converse, J. M.: Early skin grafting in war wounds of the extremities. Ann. Surg., 115:321, 1942.

Converse, J. M.: Plastic repair of the extremities by nontubulated pedicle skin flaps. J. Bone Joint Surg., 30A:163, 1948.

Converse, J. M.: Reconstructive Plastic Surgery, Philadelphia, W. B. Saunders Company, 1964, p. 1819.

Conway, H., Stark, R. B., Weeter, J. C., Garcia, F. A., and Kavanaugh, J. D.: Complications of decubitus ulcers in patients with paraplegia. Plast. Reconstr. Surg., 7:117, 1951.

Crawford, B. S.: The repair of defects of the lower limbs, using a local flap. Br. J. Plast. Surg., 10:32, 1957.

Crikelair, G. F., and Symonds, F. C.: The cross-leg pedicle in chronic osteomyelitis of the lower limb. Plast. Reconstr. Surg., 38:404, 1966.

Dehne, E., Metz, C. W., Deffer, P. A., and Hall, R. M.: Nonoperative treatment of the fractured tibia by immediate weight bearing. J. Trauma. 1:5, 1961a.

Dehne, E., Deffer, P. A., Hall, R. M., Brown, P. W., and Johnson, E. V.: The natural history of the fractured tibia. Surg. Clin. North Am., 41:1495, 1961b.

Dodd, H., and Cockett, F. B.: The Pathology and Surgery of the Veins of the Lower Limb. Baltimore, The Williams & Wilkins Company, 1956.

DuVries, H. L.: Surgery of the Foot. St. Louis, Mo., C. V. Mosby Company, 1959, pp. 207–218.

Fitzpatrick, T. B.: Dermatology in General Medicine. New York, McGraw-Hill, 1971.

Georgiade, N., Pickrell, K., and Maguire, C.: Total thigh flaps for extensive decubitus ulcers. Plast. Reconstr. Surg., 17:220, 1956.

Ger, R.: The surgical management of decubitus ulcers by muscle transposition. Surgery, 69:106, 1971.

Ger, R.: Surgical Management of Ulcerative Lesions of the Leg. Chicago, Year Book Medical Publishers, 1972.

Ger, R., and Adar, U.: The management of chronic cavities in the region of the hip joint. J. Bone Joint Surg., 55A:758, 1973.

Grabb, W. C. H., and Smith, J. W.: Plastic Surgery, 3rd Ed. Boston, Little, Brown and Company, 1968, p. 791.

Hamilton, F.: Old ulcers treated by anaplasty. N.Y. Med. J., 13:165, 1854.

Harashina, T.: Personal communication, 1974.

Harii, K.: Personal communication, 1974.

Hayes, H.: Cross-leg flaps after the age of fifty. Plast. Reconstr. Surg., 30:649, 1962.

Hayhurst, J. W., Mladick, R. A., and Adamson, J. E.: Experimental and clinical microvascular flaps. 1974 (in preparation).

Hueston, J. E., and Gunther, G. S.: Primary cross-leg flaps. Plast. Reconstr. Surg., 40:58, 1967.

Hynes, W.: "Shaving" in plastic surgery with special reference to the treatment of chronic radiodermatitis. Br. J. Plast. Surg., 12:43, 1959.

Kaplan, I.: Neurovascular island flap in the treatment of trophic ulceration of the heel. Br. J. Surg., 22:143, 1969.

Kiehn, C. L., Earle, A. S., and Des Prez, J. D.: Treatment of the chronic, painful metatarsal callus by a tendon transfer. Plast. Reconstr. Surg., 51:154, 1973.

Kisner, W. H., and Hendrix, J. H.: Keratosis palmaris et plantaris. Plast. Reconstr. Surg., 51:424, 1973.

Kitlowski, E. A.: Massive lymphangioma of leg. Plast. Reconstr. Surg., 19:246, 1957.

Kohler, H. G.: Congenital transverse defects of limbs and digits ("intrauterine amputation"). Arch. Dis. Child., 37:263, 1962.

Last, R. J.: Anatomy Regional and Applied. 5th Ed. Edinburgh, Churchill Livingstone, 1972.

Letterman, G. S., Schurter, M., and Prandoni, A. G.: Prophylactic anticoagulation in the cross-leg flap procedure. Plast. Reconstr. Surg., 27:520, 1961.

Linton, R. R.: Post-thrombotic ulceration of the lower extremity. Ann. Surg., 138:415, 1953.

Mathes, S., McCraw, J., and Vasconez, L.: Muscle transposition flaps for coverage of lower extremity defects: Anatomic considerations. Surg. Clin. North Am., 54:1337, 1974.

McCraw, J. B., and Furlow, L. T., Jr.: The dorsalis pedis arterialized flap. Plast. Reconstr. Surg., 55:177, 1975.

McCraw, J., Dibbell, D., Horton, C., Adamson, J., and Carraway, J.: Definition of new arterialized myocutaneous vascular territories. Presented before the American Association of Plastic Surgeons, Atlanta, Georgia, 1976a.

McCraw, J., Massey, F., Shanklin, K., and Horton, C.: Vaginal reconstruction with gracilis myocutaneous flaps. Plast. Reconstr. Surg., *58*:176, 1976b.

McGregor, I. A., and Jackson, I. T.: The groin flap. Br. J. Plast. Surg., *25*:3, 1972.

McGregor, I. A., and Morgan, G.: Axial and random pattern flaps. Br. J. Plast. Surg., *26*:202, 1973.

May, H.: Reconstructive and Reparative Surgery. 3rd Ed. Philadelphia, F. A. Davis Company, 1971, p. 719.

Millard, D. R.: The crane principle for the transport of subcutaneous tissue. Plast. Reconstr. Surg.,*43*:451, 1969.

Mir y Mir, L.: Functional graft of the heel. Plast. Reconstr. Surg., *14*:444, 1954.

Moberg, E.: Evaluation and management of nerve injuries in the hand. Surg. Clin. North Am., *44*:1019, 1964.

O'Brien, B. M., MacLeod, A. M., Hayhurst, J. W., and Morrison, W. A.: Successful transfer of a large island flap from the groin to the foot by microvascular anastomosis. Plast. Reconstr. Surg., *52*:271, 1973.

Orticochea, M.: A new method of total reconstruction of the penis. Br. J. Plast. Surg., *25*:347, 1972a.

Orticochea, M.: The musculocutaneous flap method: An immediate and heroic substitute for the method of delay. Br. J. Plast. Surg., *15*:106, 1972b.

Owens, N.: Compound neck pedicle designed for repair of massive facial defects. Plast. Reconstr. Surg., *15*:369, 1955.

Sarnat, B. G., and Kagan, B. M.: Prenatal constricting band and pseudoarthrosis of the lower leg. Plast. Reconstr. Surg., *47*:547, 1971.

Smith, P. J.: The vascular basis of axial pattern flaps. Br. J. Plast. Surg., *26*:150, 1973.

Snyder, G. B., and Edgerton, M. T.: The principle of the island neurovascular flap in the management of ulcerated anesthetic weight bearing areas of the lower extremity. Plast. Reconstr. Surg., *36*:518, 1965.

Stark, R. B.: The cross leg flap procedure. Plast. Reconstr. Surg., *9*:173, 1952.

Stark, R. B., and Kaplan, J. M.: Cross-leg flaps in patients over 50 years of age. Br. J. Plast. Surg., *25*:20, 1972.

Steiger, R. N., and Curtiss, P. H., Jr.: The use of a total thigh flap procedure for chronic infection of the hip. J. Bone Joint Surg., *50A*:1429, 1968.

Stern, O. S.: New fixation device for cross-leg flaps. Plast. Reconstr. Surg., *50*:194, 1972.

Taylor, G. I., Miller, G. D. H., and Ham, F. J.: The free vascularized bone graft. A clinical extension of microvascular techniques. Plast. Reconstr. Surg., *55*:533, 1975.

Thompson, N.: A clinical and histological investigation into the fate of epithelial elements buried following the grafting of "shaved" skin surfaces. Br. J. Plast. Surg., *13*:219, 1960.

Thompson, N., and Ell, P. J.: Dermal overgrafting in the treatment of venous stasis ulcers. Plast. Reconstr. Surg., *54*:290, 1974.

Vasconez, L.: Personal communication, 1974.

Webster, G. V., Petersen, R. A., and Stein, H. L.: Dermal overgrafting of the leg. J. Bone Joint Surg.,*40A*:796, 1958.

White, W. L., Dupertuis, S. M., Gaisford, J. C., and Musgrave, R. H.: Evaluation of 114 cross-leg flaps. Transactions of the International Society of Plastic Surgeons, 1st Congress. Baltimore, The Williams & Wilkins Company, 1957.

Witschi, T. H., and Omer, G. E.: The treatment of open tibial shaft fractures from Vietnam War. J. Trauma, *10*:105, 1970.

# CHAPTER 87

# LYMPHEDEMA

## STEPHEN R. LEWIS, M.D., AND DUANE L. LARSON, M.D.

Knowledge and understanding of the lymphatic system have evolved slowly because of the minute size and fragility of the lymphatic vessels. Asellius of Milan noted the intestinal lymphatics in the dog in 1627, but it was not until the early 1930's that the superficial intradermal lymphatic network in man was documented with the intracutaneous injection of dye by Carvalho, Rodriquez and Perenia (1931) and Hudack and McMaster (1932).

The use of radiographic lymphangiography as a practical clinical method became possible in 1954 when Kinmonth published his report describing cannulation of the dye-injected subcutaneous lymphatics and the injection of radiopaque fluid to identify these vessels by radiography. The latter development furnished a tool with which to study the lymphatic system for both the basic scientist and the clinician. A surge of interest in the lymphatic system also followed the studies in transplantation immunology showing the small lymphocyte as an important cell in host defense mechanisms.

## EMBRYOLOGY

Sabin (1913) demonstrated that the lymphatic system begins as a series of endothelial buds arising from various centers in the early weeks of embryonic life; by the end of the eighth week there is a fusion with a fairly extensive lymph sac. The sprouting of the protoplasm associated with nuclear division of the endothelium of the capillary wall is considered as a continuous growth pattern with invasion of the body by these lymphatic channels. Continued growth occurs with gradual uniting of the multiple areas of the lymphatics into a pattern similar to that of the blood vessels. Their invasion of the body is not as complete as that of the other components of the vascular system, for the central nervous system, bone marrow, eye, internal ear, and intralobular portion of the liver do not contain lymphatics. The lymphatics are similar to capillaries; however, the basement membrane, which is present in capillaries, is absent or poorly defined in lymphatics. The pattern of lymphatic growth includes the formation of a series of valves to maintain directional control of the lymph flow, finally emptying into the vascular compartment (Fig. 87–1). The distribution of lymphatics in the skin consists of a valveless two- or three-layered dermal plexus draining into a valved subdermal arcade which follows the course of the superficial veins.

Lymphedema, lymphangioma, and cystic hygroma probably represent congenital malformations of the lymphatic system at different levels.

## PHYSIOLOGY

The physiology of the lymphatics is still the subject of changing concepts because of the large number of new techniques which have been developed for studying the functional aspects of edema. It has been shown by Pappen-

3567

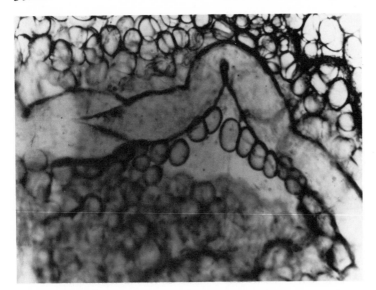

**FIGURE 87–1.**   A lymphatic valve in a lymphatic vessel of a rat.

heimer and Freund (1959) that the capillary wall is about 0.3 micron thick, and that the pores in the intercellular cement substance make up approximately 0.2 per cent of the surface area of the capillary wall. It is through these pores that small molecules of electrolytes and water easily filter. The passage of the solutes through the pores is by diffusion, which occurs readily because of the small distance involved in any direction. The protein molecules diffuse less readily, and, once in the interstitial space, they exert an increase in osmotic pressure which in turn draws additional water into the region. As the filtration flow of water shifts, the proteins of the plasma and tissue fluids come into a closer equilibrium. The protein that has left the vascular circulation must return via the lymphatics. Since the capillary leakage of proteins for 24 hours is half of the total circulating protein, this is an important vital function. It becomes apparent that the main physiologic role of the lymphatics is to carry from the tissue spaces substances of every molecular size, including all of the larger molecular particles.

Peripheral or edema fluid accumulates when the rate of capillary filtration exceeds the lymphatic return flow and the resorptive powers of the venous capillary bed. Factors controlling the equilibrium are capillary pressure, osmotic pressure of the blood, capillary permeability, and localized tissue pressure (Fig. 87–2). The difference between the osmotic pressure due to plasma colloids and electrolytes and that of the tissue colloids and electrolytes equals the effective osmotic pressure that allows water to be drawn back into the capillaries from the tissue fluids. This effective pressure falls progressive-

ly with the decrease of blood pressure from the arteriolar to the venous end of the capillary. When the hydrostatic pressure is greater than the effective osmotic pressure, there is an increase in the water leaving the capillary over that returning. The converse is also true; when

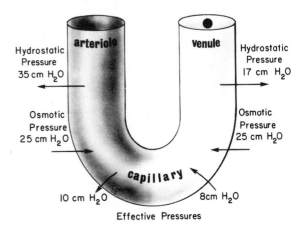

**Effective Pressures**

### Interstitial Compartment

LYMPHATICS ■

1.) Removal of excess water & solutes
2.) Return of plasma proteins to the vascular compartments

■ Diminution of lymphatic flow results in local accumulation of water, solutes, and especially proteins.

● Block or insufficiency at venous end results in increased venous pressure leading to a decrease or reversal of filtration flow, thereby producing accumulation of water and solutes in the interstitial compartment. (Peripheral Venous Disease)

**FIGURE 87–2.**   The physiology of diffusion of fluids in the capillary bed.

the effective hydrostatic pressure is less than the osmotic pressure, more water returns to the capillary. Any factor, either systemic or local, that causes an increase in the effective hydrostatic pressure, or a decrease of the osmotic pressure, disturbs the balance in favor of increasing the diffusion of water out of the capillary and increasing accumulation of water in the tissues until an equilibrium is reached. The variations in pressure caused by localized agents, such as heat or muscular activity, play a role in constantly shifting fluids in the extravascular compartments. The concentration of protein in the edema fluid may increase under certain circumstances and results in a rise in tissue osmotic pressure. Secondary to the rise in osmotic pressure, there is a further shift of water into the tissue spaces. The progressive accumulation of edema fluid generally shifts the protein concentration to levels of 4 g per 100 ml, thereby causing a change in the tissue environment. There is also the fact that obstruction of the venous return raises the venous capillary pressure and thus increases the interstitial fluid by limiting the absorption capacity of the capillary and increasing diffusion from the capillary. Obstruction in the lymphatic channels slows the removal of the high molecular weight filtrate, which normally moves from the foot to the neck in five minutes (Fig. 87–3). With the increase of molecular concentration, progressive lymphedema results.

Cannulation of the lymphatics of the lower extremity in normal subjects or in those without lymphedema demonstrated that the intralymphatic pressures are characteristically sub-

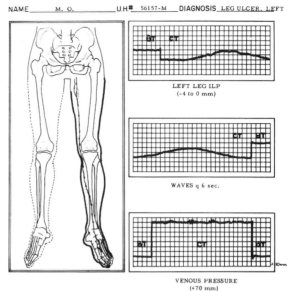

FIGURE 87–4. Normal intralymphatic pressures (negative range) associated with an early varicose ulcer.

atmospheric (Fig. 87–4). Studies of intralymphatic pressure readings in both clinical and experimental subjects following careful standardization showed a characteristic slow regular wave of minus 2 mm to minus 10 mm water, at approximately 6- to 8-second intervals, and this is not synchronous with respiration. Intralymphatic pressure becomes atmospheric or positive in the presence of either chronic or acute edema (Figs. 87–5 and 87–6). In his studies, Drinker (1942) showed that the pressure in the thoracic duct was slightly subatmospheric and that it could be influenced by the Valsalva maneuver.

The consistent recording of subatmospheric pressures in the lymphatics of the normal extremity explains the active flow phenomenon in the horizontal position during general anesthesia. The same finding has been demonstrated with radioisotopic techniques. Under normal conditions, the intralymphatic pressure in the lower extremities has been found to be subatmospheric, with a decreasing gradient as the thoracic duct is approached. Lower levels of negative pressure may be obtained with motion or massage of the leg. The subatmospheric pressure becomes more negative at the thoracic duct level on deep inspiration, but it becomes positive on expiration or during a Valsalva maneuver. Daily as well as hourly lymph flow may vary considerably because of the many factors influencing lymph flow (Figs. 87–7 and 87–8).

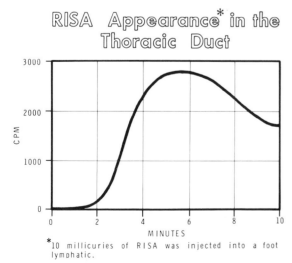

FIGURE 87–3. Normal appearance of RISA in the thoracic duct following injection into a foot lymphatic.

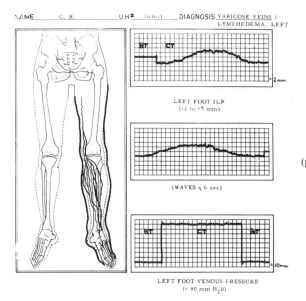

FIGURE 87-5. Increased intralymphatic pressures (positive range) associated with chronic venous stasis.

FIGURE 87-6. Increased intralymphatic pressures associated with congenital lymphedema.

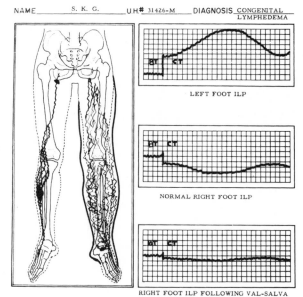

| PATIENT | AGE (YRS) | DISEASE | MINUTE OUTPUT | DAILY OUTPUT |
|---------|-----------|---------|---------------|--------------|
| MALE | 24 | RENAL | 5.6cc | 8 L |
| MALE | 23 | RENAL | 2.1cc | 3 L |
| FEMALE | 26 | RENAL | 3.5cc | 5 L |
| FEMALE | 34 | RENAL | 2.1cc | 3 L |
| MALE | 48 | LIVER | 2.4cc | 3.5 L |
| MALE | 11 | BURN (75% 1PBD) | 1.2cc | 1.8 L |
| FEMALE | 61 | BURN (55% 4PBD) | 0.6cc | 0.8 L |
| FEMALE | 75 | BURN | 1.7cc | 2.4 L |
| FEMALE | 60 | MELANOMA (TOE) | 1.0cc | 1.5 L |

FIGURE 87-7. Flow of thoracic duct lymph in disease states.

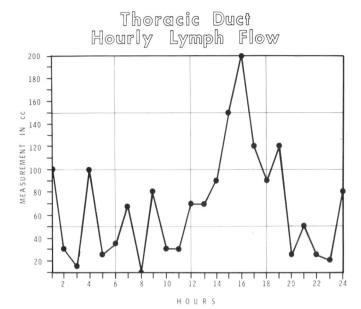

**Thoracic Duct
Hourly Lymph Flow**

**FIGURE 87–8.** Thoracic duct lymph flow varies hourly.

All of the patients in the author's series showed positive pressure readings when clinical edema was present. In patients in whom reversible edema was present, the intralymphatic pressure became negative as the edema subsided. In one patient with an inferior vena cava syndrome produced by a mediastinal tumor, there was generalized edema from the nipple down; the recorded intralymphatic pressure was 400 mm of water.

From these basic observations it is apparent that multiple factors influence the extent of lymphedema. These include capillary permeability, filtration, and osmotic pressure, all of which may be affected by local inflammatory or systemic factors, either of which may impair the venous or lymphatic flow.

## ANATOMY

**Technique of Lymphangiography.** The anatomical arrangement of the lymphatic channels can be determined by cannulating the dye-injected subcutaneous lymphatics and by injecting radiopaque media with a "C" clamp or electric pump (Fig. 87–9). The lymphatics in the sole of the foot and palm of the hand are more numerous than in any other part of the body with the exception of the intestinal tract. As the lymphatic channels within the dermis are situated so closely together, it is almost impossible to give an intradermal injection without injecting some of the material directly into the lymphatics. Following injection of 0.5 ml of 4

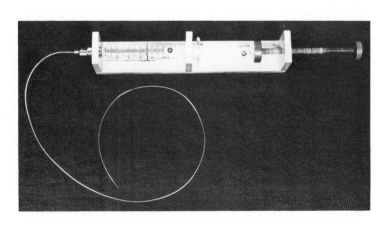

**FIGURE 87–9.** "C" clamp for injecting a radiopaque medium into the lymphatic.

per cent direct sky blue dye into the webbed spaces of the foot, lymphatic channels are identified by the bluish discoloration of the lymph in an incision made 2 or 3 inches proximal to the site of injection. The lymphatic vessel is cannulated with a 27- or 30-gauge needle from which the hub has been removed and a fine polyethylene catheter has been attached (Fig. 87–10). Ethiodol is then injected into the polyethylene catheter, which carries it directly into the lumen of the lymphatic. The electric microinfusion pump or a ''C'' clamp is used for injection purposes. Cinefluorography and radiographic studies are performed during and after the injection period to determine the anatomical lymphatic network by means of the radiopaque medium within the lumen of the lymphatic channel and lymph nodes.

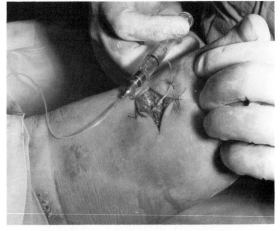

**FIGURE 87–10.**   Cannulation of a foot lymphatic.

### Lower Extremity

The lymphatic outflow tract of the lower extremity may be classified into the superficial lymphatic system (the greater saphenous lymphatics and the lesser saphenous lymphatics) and the deep lymphatic system.

**Superficial Lymphatics.** The superficial lymphatics in the leg appear as small channels of uniform diameter with characteristic beading 1 cm apart at valve sites (Fig. 87–11). The vessels bifurcate and communicate with one another by anastomosing branches but do not increase in size as they ascend the leg. There

are, apparently, two superficial lymphatic systems in the lower extremity. The greater saphenous lymphatic system is defined as comprising those lymph vessels which may be cannulated on the dorsum of the foot. These vessels accompany the greater saphenous vein as they ascend along the medial aspect of the leg eventually to drain into the superficial inguinal lymph nodes (Figs. 87–12, 87–13, and 87–14). The lesser saphenous lymphatic system differs from the greater saphenous venous system in that the former consists of two distinctly different sets of lymphatics. Those lymphatics cannulated on the posterior calf flow laterally around the knee and lower thigh to drain into the superficial

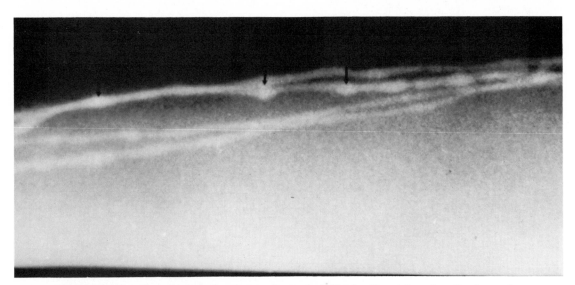

**FIGURE 87–11.**   Normal lymphatic valves as demonstrated by beading at the valve sites (arrows).

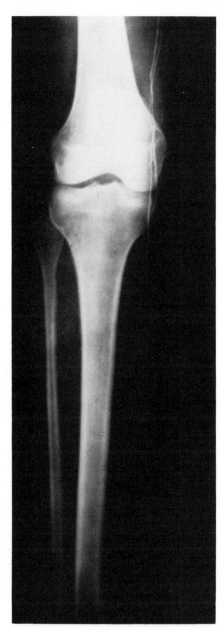

**FIGURE 87–12.** Normal lymphangiogram of the greater saphenous system (anteroposterior view).

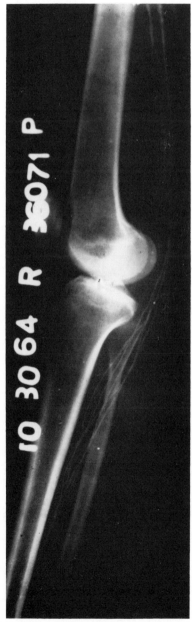

**FIGURE 87–13.** Normal lymphangiogram of the greater saphenous system (lateral view).

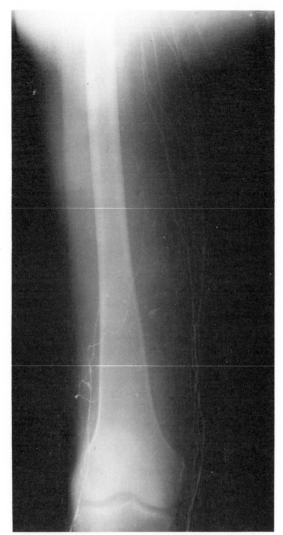

**FIGURE 87–14.** Normal lymphangiogram of the thigh lymphatics.

of the popliteal space, and traverse the lower one-third of the thigh beneath the medial posterior border of the femur (Figs. 87–16 and 87–17). The channels then pass medially and anteriorly to drain into the deep inguinal lymph nodes. The deep lymphatic system in the leg is in close proximity to the bones; consequently, one would anticipate a high incidence of injury to this system following fractures. Fortunately, however, the lymphatic system has excellent regenerative capacity.

Under normal conditions, the radiopaque medium in the deep lymphatic system does not flow into the superficial system; the only connections between the superficial and deep systems exist in the drainage of the posterolateral aspect of the foot and in association with pathologic conditions.

The inguinal lymphatics drain into the iliac lymphatics, thence into the periaortic nodes, and finally into the cisterna chyli (Figs. 87–18 and 87–19). The thoracic duct carries the lymph from the abdomen through the chest, to drain into the venous angle formed by the confluence of the internal jugular and subclavian veins in the neck (Figs. 87–20 and 87–21).

*Text continued on page 3578*

inguinal lymph nodes, while those from the posterolateral edge of the foot ascend the posterolateral side of the calf to drain into the popliteal nodes and then into the deep lymphatic system of the thigh.

**Deep Lymphatics.** The deep lymphatic channels accompany the posterior tibial artery, the two posterior tibial veins, and the tibial nerve and can be cannulated by making an incision just posterior to the medial malleolus (Fig. 87–15). The deep system is similar to that of the superficial system in that it contains numerous valves approximately 1 cm apart. The deep lymphatics ascend the leg just medial to the posterior border of the tibia, pass across the depth

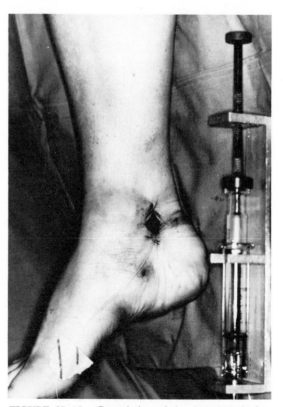

**FIGURE 87–15.** Cannulation of the deep lymphatics.

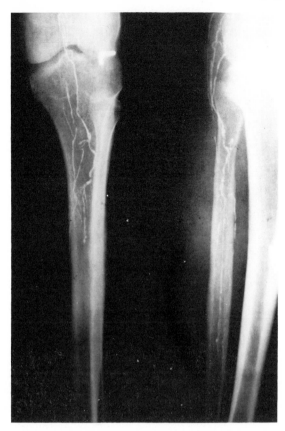

**FIGURE 87–16.** Normal lymphangiogram of the deep lymphatics (anteroposterior view).

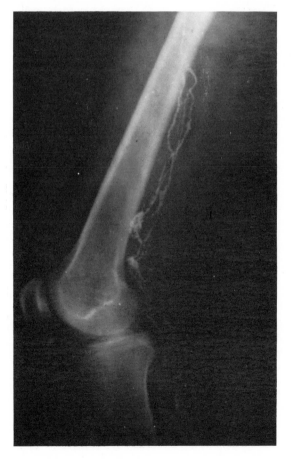

**FIGURE 87–17.** Normal lymphangiogram of the deep lymphatics and the popliteal lymph nodes (lateral view).

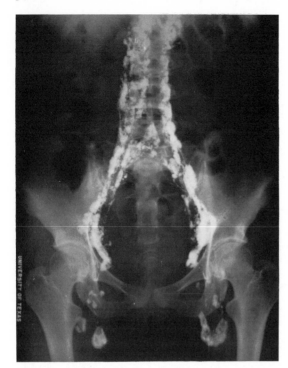

**FIGURE 87–18.**    The inguinal, iliac, and periaortic lymphatics (anteroposterior view).

**FIGURE 87–19.**    The inguinal, iliac, and periaortic lymphatics (lateral view).

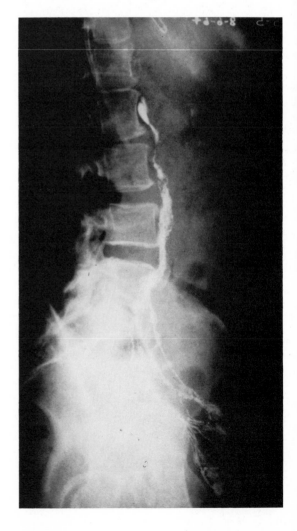

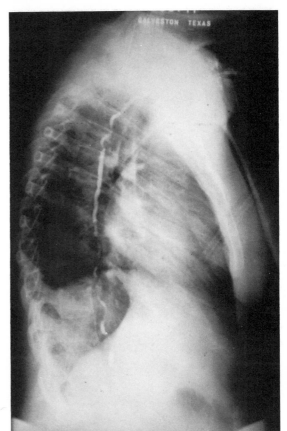

**FIGURE 87–20.** The thoracic duct (lateral view).

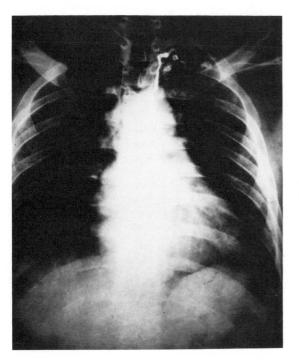

**FIGURE 87–21.** The thoracic duct (anteroposterior view). Note the retrograde flow into the supraclavicular nodes.

## Upper Extremity

In the upper limb, cannulation of the superficial lymphatics at the wrist reveals three groups of superficial lymphatic channels in the forearm: radial, median, and ulnar, and these accompany the veins (Fig. 87–22). The epitrochlear gland lies only in the pathway of the ulnar group, and its efferent vessels may be superficial or deep to the fascia during the ascent to the axillary nodes. The radial lymphatics cross anteriorly from the lateral to the medial side in the lower two-thirds of the upper arm to reach the axilla, but they may accompany the cephalic vein into a deltopectoral lymph node and thence to the supraclavicular nodes, thus bypassing the axilla. The median lymphatics drain directly to the axillary lymph nodes.

## PATHOPHYSIOLOGY OF EDEMA

Multiple factors may cause peripheral edema, and these may be on a local or a systemic basis. Peripheral edema results when the rate of capillary filtration exceeds the lymphatic return flow and the reabsorptive capacity of the venous capillary bed. The factors controlling the equilibrium are the capillary bed pressure, capillary permeability, local tissue pressure, and the oncotic pressure exerted by the plasma protein. Disturbances of the lymphatic and venous systems are among the most common causes of chronic peripheral edema.

### CLASSIFICATION OF REGIONAL EDEMA

Acute edema
    Traumatic (thermal, mechanical)
    Acute infectious (cellulitis)
    Acute thrombophlebitis
    Systemic disease (cardiac, renal, allergic)
Chronic edema
    Primary venous defect
        Venous stasis (varicose veins)
        Venous insufficiency (postphlebitic syndrome)
        Venous obstruction (surgical, neoplastic, thrombotic)
        Arterial-venous malformations
    Primary lymphatic defect
        Congenital lymphedema
            Aplastic lymphatics
            Hypoplastic lymphatics
            Varicose lymphatics
        Acquired lymphedema
            Neoplastic
            Parasitic (filariasis, yeast, fungi)
            Postsurgical
            Postradiation
            Chronic infections (streptococcal, staphylococcal, tuberculous, syphilitic)

### Acute Edema

Acute edema resulting from trauma, infection, thrombophlebitis, or systemic disease may be

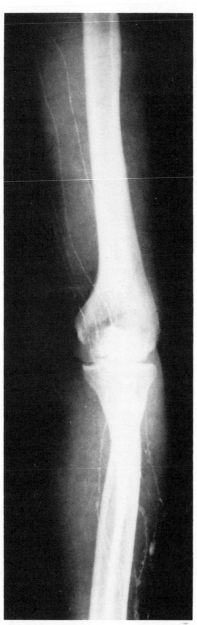

**FIGURE 87–22.** Normal lymphangiogram of the upper extremity.

secondary to an increase of protein concentration in the interstitial space, to an increased permeability of the capillary wall, to blockage of the lymphatics and veins, or to a decrease in plasma proteins. This type of edema usually subsides with treatment of the underlying cause.

### Chronic Edema

**Primary Venous Defect.** As was stated previously, if there is a venous blockage or insufficient flow of the venous system, edema will develop owing to the secondary increase in hydrostatic pressure in the venule. Venography of the leg is useful in the diagnosis of the defects of the venous system and also aids in the selection and evaluation of therapy. The examination is easily performed, and complications are few and minor. Experience, however, is necessary for reliable interpretation, since artifacts may lead to misinterpretation of the findings.

Occasionally, a patient may have both venous and lymphatic defects. Venograms and lymphangiograms can be done simultaneously. However, it is preferable to do the venograms first, and, when the dye has cleared the venous system, the lymphangiogram can be performed. By this means, one can avoid the loss of detail when the radiopaque dye-filled venous system is superimposed over the lymphatics. Superficial venography discloses varicose veins, incompetent valves of the superficial system, and frequently extreme tortuosity of the veins. Study of the deep venous system shows the patent vessels. If there is deep vein thrombosis, collateral venous channels will be seen.

Varicose veins associated with chronic edema may eventually produce irreversible changes in the skin and subcutaneous tissue, as well as abnormalities of the lymphatic vessels. The abnormalities of the lymphatics are the direct result of fibrosis in the skin and subcutaneous tissues, which is secondary to chronic edema. In the lower extremity with venous insufficiency or venous obstruction, increased edema formation occurs as a result of the change in the reabsorptive powers on the venule side of the capillary bed. Early in venous disease, the edema is reversible by elevation of the extremity; in such cases, lymphatic pressures revert to normal ranges as the edema subsides. However, if the venous disease progresses to a later stage, lymphedema and associated fibrosis of the subcutaneous tissue occurs, and the intralymphatic pressures in these patients is permanently elevated. Lymphangiographic studies demonstrate severe abnormalities beneath the ulceration and in the more distal portion of the lower extremity.

Arteriovenous malformations have also resulted in increased hydrostatic pressure in the venous system and may lead to the formation of chronic edema. Patients with this syndrome are difficult to manage, as local cellulitis leading to bacteremia and possibly septicemia is not uncommon.

**Primary Lymphatic Defect.** As was stated previously, the primary function of the lymphatic system is the removal of excess water and solutes and the return of plasma proteins to the vascular compartment; consequently, blockage of this system will result in regional edema. To determine accurately the lymphatic defect involved, a lymphangiogram of both the deep and superficial systems should be accomplished. To determine the progress of the disease, it is important that accurate methods be utilized to determine changes in the volume of the extremity or changes in the circumferential measurements.

Although the primary defect may exist in the lymphatics, the resulting chronic edema and secondary fibrosis of the subcutaneous tissue may, on occasion, lead to venous obstruction and venous stasis. Persistent or recurrent lymphedema leads to the invasion of the subcutaneous tissue and dermis by fibroblasts, followed by an overgrowth of connective tissue with associated thickening of the lymphatic capillaries. The subcutaneous adipose tissue may gradually be replaced by fibrosis to the extent that the previous nonpitting edema may eventually develop into a brawny edema associated with thickened, hairless, keratotic skin as seen in the late stages of lymphedema.

In the early stages of lymphedema, dye which is injected into the webbed spaces between the toes is seen to traverse slowly the channels in the subcutaneous tissues; the latter can easily be cannulated (Fig. 87–23). When there are elephantiasic changes, as in the late stages, or patients with congenital lymphedema (Fig. 87–24), the dye can no longer pass by way of the lymphatic trunks, and lymphatic cannulation is difficult or impossible.

CONGENITAL LYMPHEDEMA. In the author's series, there has been a family history of lymphedema in less than 5 per cent of the total number of cases. Some authors have subdivided lymphedema into the lymphedema praecox and tarda groups. It is the author's opinion that both groups represent congenital lymphedema and

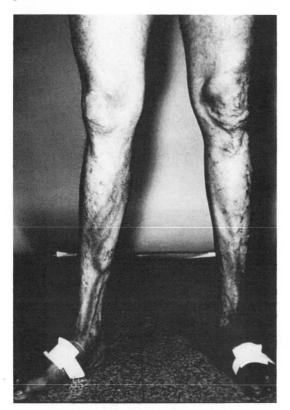

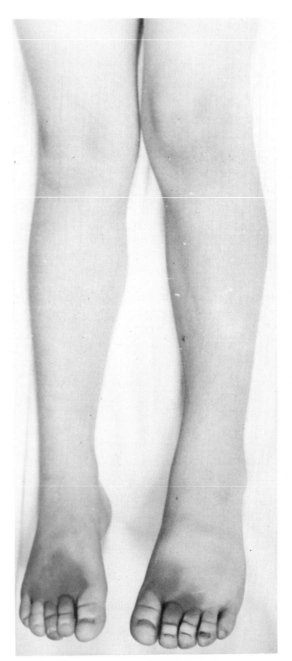

**FIGURE 87–23.** Sky blue dye fills the greater saphenous lymphatics following injection into the web spaces of the foot.

**FIGURE 87–24.** Congenital abnormalities of the lymphatics demonstrated 24 hours following injection of sky blue dye. Note the inability of the dye to ascend proximally.

that they differ only in the time of onset and in the severity of the lymphatic defect. Congenital lymphedema can be classified anatomically as aplastic, hypoplastic, or varicose lymphatics.

In *aplasia,* no main lymphatic trunks can be seen (Fig. 87–25). The dye spreads in the dermal plexus on the dorsum of the foot but fails to proceed any farther than the inferior portion of the ankle because of the absence of functioning lymphatic trunks. If an incision is made on the dorsum of the foot, no main lymphatic trunks are found. However, an occasional minute dermal lymphatic may be cannulated and a small amount of dye injected gently and slowly. On radiographic examination, only the lymphatics of the skin are seen. Only small subcutaneous lymphatic spaces are found on microscopic examination.

*Hypoplasia* is characterized by a deficiency in the number of lymphatic trunks (Fig. 87–26).

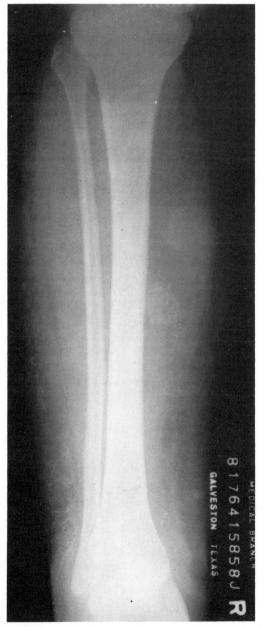

**FIGURE 87–25.** Congenital lymphedema of the aplastic type.

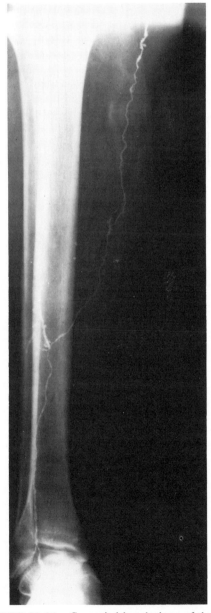

**FIGURE 87–26.** Congenital lymphedema of the hypoplastic type.

The blue dye spreads over the dorsum of the foot; however, it is gradually absorbed within two to four weeks, depending on the competence of the few available lymphatics. The lymphangiographic findings may show contrast material in only one or two lymphatic trunks. If a patient with this type of abnormality is followed, lymphedema often develops following some type of injury, or, as the child grows, the increased demand on the few lymphatic channels exceeds their capacity.

Some patients with lymphedema show lymphangiographic findings of an increased number of lymphatic channels which are extremely tortuous and dilated (*varicose* lymphatics) (Figs. 87–27 and 87–28). Dermal backflow, sec-

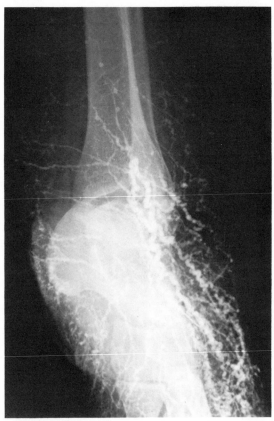

**FIGURE 87–28.** Varicose lymphatics (late changes).

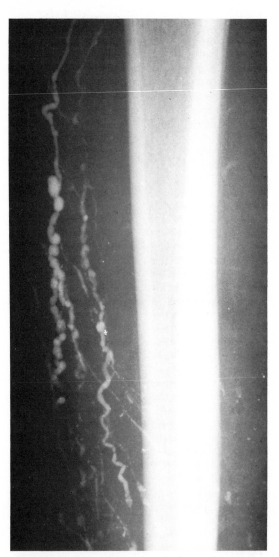

**FIGURE 87–27.** Varicose lymphatics (early changes).

ondary to valvular incompetency of the connecting lymphatics between the superficial lymphatic plexuses and the subcutaneous lymphatic trunks, is frequently associated with this condition. It is seen as a multitudinous number of small, stringy lines on lymphangiographic study. In normal subjects, there is no flow of lymph or contrast material into the dermal lymphatics, as valves direct the flow centrally.

Recurrent episodes of lymphangitis or cellulitis are common and represent one of the major complications of primary lymphedema. Trichophytosis occurs in approximately 10 per cent of patients, and medical therapy should include a recommendation to avoid additional insult to the extremity. Occasionally, ulceration secondary to trivial or major injury may cause a localized infection, and early therapy of ulcerations is imperative. In patients who have recurrent inflammatory episodes, one should consider the possibility of long-term antibiotic therapy, similar to that used in the treatment of rheumatic fever. It is our recommendation that those patients who are not allergic to penicillin should be treated with oral penicillin for a minimum of six months, if the lesions remain in a quiescent stage. Later, if an injury is incurred and any minimal inflammatory lesion appears, penicillin therapy or other appropriate antibiotic therapy should be resumed.

Occasionally, a familial history of lymphedema can be elicited (Fig. 87–29). Approximately 15 per cent of patients with primary lymphedema have an associated congenital abnormality. The most frequent associated anomaly in patients with primary lymphedema of the lower extremity involves the vascular system. There have been a few case reports of urinary tract abnormalities, and patients have been described with idiopathic retroperitoneal fibrosis. These anomalies support the concept that the disease is due to an inborn error in the development of the vascular system.

The newer methods of clinical lymphangiographic study have made possible a better understanding of the deficiency of the lymph channels. Volume displacement and circumferential measurement studies are indicated in all cases of primary lymphedema, in order to document the progress of the disease. Venograms and other studies of the local circulation may be of value, although in the majority of cases the venous and arterial circulation will be found to be normal.

On macroscopic examination, biopsy specimens show increased thickness of the skin (primarily the dermal elements) and the subcutaneous tissue. In the advanced cases, involvement of the subcutaneous tissue predominates; this tissue may be as much as 20 times thicker than the skin; the latter, in turn, will be three to five times thicker than normal. Watery fluid may be easily expressed from the involved tissues, and one may see pale, lobulated subcutaneous fat, surrounded by a thick fibrous septum. The skin surface is usually hairless and keratotic and may be slightly pigmented.

On microscopic examination, there is generally thinning of the epithelium overlying the thickened dermal papillae. Hyperkeratosis and acanthosis are frequently present. The dermal appendages are decreased in size and number, although the dermal and subcutaneous blood vessels are generally normal in appearance. Fibroblastic proliferation is seen throughout the microscopic specimen down to and including the deep fascia. There is an increase in collagen fibers in the dermal layer. The collagen may be poorly formed and may show evidence of edematous separation. There are frequently inflammatory cells in the superficial subcutaneous tissue, and there may be an infiltration of lymphocytes and plasma cells in the perilymphatic regions. Dilatation of the lymphatic trunks may be seen with associated perilymphatic lymphocytes and plasma cells. Subcutaneous fat is abundant. Collagenous hypertrophy of the dermis is present in the majority of cases. Superficial lymph vessels may be absent or considerably decreased in numbers. Fragmentation of the dermal and subcutaneous elastic fibers is present in all cases.

ACQUIRED LYMPHEDEMA. Acquired lymphedema is a type of peripheral edema which develops following trauma, infection, or disease. Sufficient blockage of the lymphatic channels by tumors to cause lymphedema is uncommon, except in the late phase of the dis-

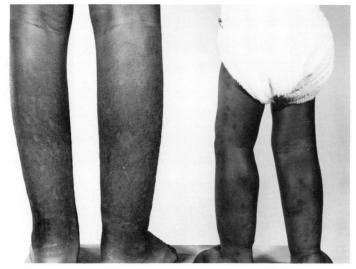

**FIGURE 87–29.** Familial bilateral edema of the lower extremities in a 27 year old mother and 2 year old daughter.

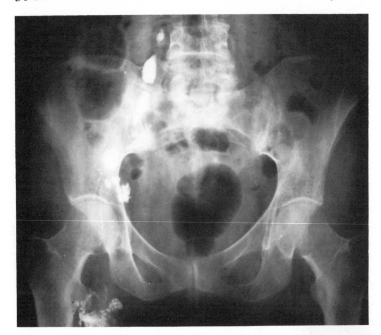

**FIGURE 87–30.** Lymphangiography showing inguinal metastasis with incomplete filling of the nodes on one side.

**FIGURE 87–31.** Verification of the diagnosis on examination of a node (see Fig. 87–30).

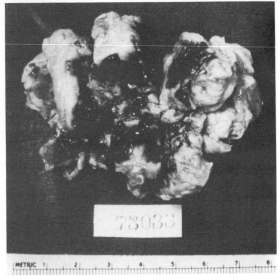

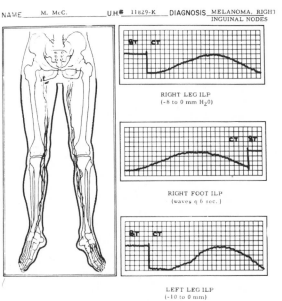

NAME ___ M. McC. ___ U.H# __11829-K__ DIAGNOSIS __MELANOMA, RIGHT__ INGUINAL NODES

RT   CT

RIGHT LEG ILP
(-8 to 0 mm H₂0)

CT   RT

RIGHT FOOT ILP
(waves q 6 sec.)

RT   CT

LEFT LEG ILP
(-10 to 0 mm)

**FIGURE 87–32.** Normal lymphangiogram and intralymphatic pressure recorded in a patient with melanoma involvement of the inguinal nodes.

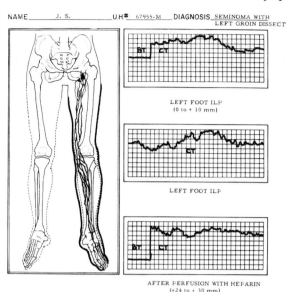

NAME_____J. S._____U.H.# 67955-M DIAGNOSIS SEMINOMA WITH LEFT GROIN DISSECT

LEFT FOOT ILP
(0 to + 10 mm)

LEFT FOOT ILP

AFTER PERFUSION WITH HEPARIN
(+24 to + 30 mm)

**FIGURE 87–33.** Increased intralymphatic pressure and development of lymphedema following mechanical obstruction of the lymph flow after surgical resection of the left inguinal nodes for a seminoma.

finding following recurrent lymphangitis and chronic lymphedema is that of varicose lymphatics. The majority of cases of varicose lymphatics in our series have been secondary to some type of chronic obstruction as a result of a congenital defect of the proximal lymphatic channels, longstanding recurrent chronic lymphangitis, severe fractures, or traumatic injuries of the lower extremity. Varicose lymphatics can be of congenital origin when valvular incompetence is present, such as is seen in the venous system. Congenital valvular incompetence is infrequent.

## LYMPHEDEMA OF THE UPPER EXTREMITY

Congenital primary lymphedema of the arm is extremely rare. Most cases of lymphedema of the upper extremity involve women and are secondary to cancer of the breast treated by radical mastectomy (Figs. 87–34 and 87–35). Following radical mastectomy, edema of vary-

ease when there is extensive spread of tumor (Figs. 87–30, 87–31, and 87–32). The lymphedema commonly associated with neoplastic disease is more often secondary to surgical extirpation of the lesion in association with the regional lymphatics (Fig. 87–33). Postoperative radiation therapy or the development of local infection results in additional fibrous tissue deposition with an increase in the incidence and severity of edema formation. The lymphedema seen in the lower extremity is frequently the result of an inguinal lymph node dissection or extensive radiation of the pelvis for malignant gynecologic tumors.

Filarial or tropical lymphangitis is caused by *Filaria bancrofti.* The microfilariae are carried in the blood and lymphatic channels, and they have a particular predilection for the lymph channels and nodes, which become obstructed by the adult worm. Fungal infections, such as actinomycosis, can also involve the lymph nodes, with resulting obstruction and secondary lymphedema.

An acute attack of lymphangitis may progress to chronic recurrent lymphangitis, if it is not adequately treated. With recurrent episodes of infection, progressive blockage of the lymphatics can occur. The most common organism encountered in recurrent lymphangitis is Streptococcus; Staphylococcus is only occasionally the offending organism. The lymphangiographic

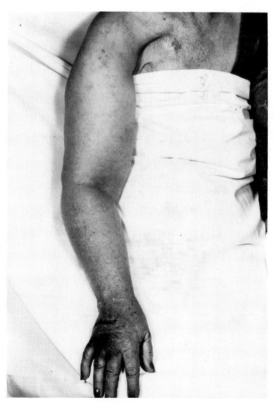

**FIGURE 87–34.** Lymphedema of the arm following radical axillary lymph node resection. Note the localization of the dye in the dorsum of the hand.

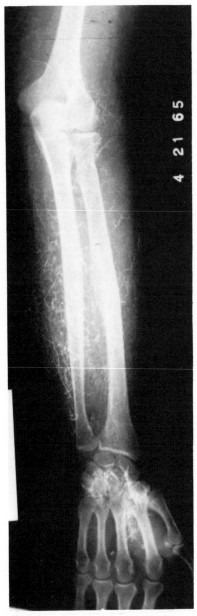

**FIGURE 87–35.** Abnormal lymphangiogram with tortuous lymphatics following axillary lymph node resection.

prognosis for this type of tumor is extremely poor. Treatment by amputation offers hope only in an occasional patient, and radiation therapy usually gives only temporary palliation. Edema following radical mastectomy may be noticed very early in the postoperative period, often secondary to infection, or it may herald recurrence of the tumor months or years after the surgery. Radiation therapy following surgery has been implicated as increasing the total number of patients with edema. It is apparent that delayed wound healing increases significantly the incidence of lymphedema (Britton, 1962). Localized early postoperative infection, skin necrosis, and prolonged drainage from the axilla have been considered contributing factors. Mechanical blockage due to scarring and complete removal of the lymph nodes in the lymph channels of the axilla probably account for the majority of cases of postmastectomy lymphedema. Secondary lymphedema may, if not treated, gradually undergo the same progressive changes in the skin and subcutaneous tissue observed in primary lymphedema.

## OBSTRUCTION OF THE THORACIC DUCT

**Cervical Level.** Ligation of the thoracic duct during a radical neck dissection is not an uncommon procedure. It has been the experience of many surgeons that this does not result in any deleterious effects. In two patients whose thoracic ducts were ligated at the time of radical neck dissection, lower extremity lymphangiograms three and five months later showed the usual lymphatic channels to the upper mediastinum, where the lymph flow was by way of the right lymphatic duct rather than the thoracic duct (Fig. 87–36). The development of collateral flow most likely accounts for the minimal sequelae following ligation of the thoracic duct.

**Cisterna Chyli Level.** The most common cause of obstruction at the level of the cisterna chyli is extrinsic pressure by tumor. Next in order of frequency are the idiopathic cases for which no real cause is ever found; however, with a thorough evaluation including lymphangiography, some of these may be shown to be secondary to congenital abnormalities. The least frequent cause is trauma. Chronic obstruction of the cisterna chyli can cause retrograde lymphatic flow and result in a rupture of the lymphatic system in the peritoneum with the development of chylous ascites (Fig. 87–37).

ing degrees occurs in approximately 50 per cent of patients. In approximately 10 per cent of the cases, edema is present in a relatively moderate degree, posing a cosmetic as well as a functional problem. Approximately 20,000 to 25,000 women per year are left with noticeably swollen arms following radical mastectomy. A fairly uncommon but noteworthy complication of prolonged lymphedema of the upper extremity is post-lymphedematous lymphangiosarcoma; the

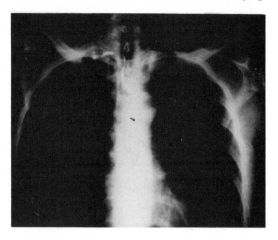

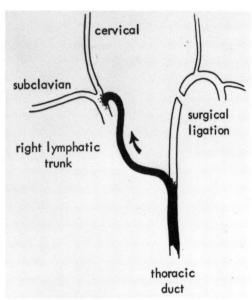

**FIGURE 87–36.** Lymph flow via the right lymphatic duct following thoracic duct obstruction.

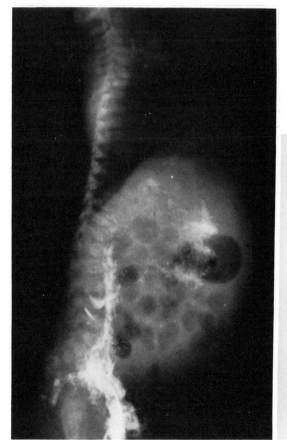

**FIGURE 87–37.** Chylous ascites with cisterna chyli obstruction.

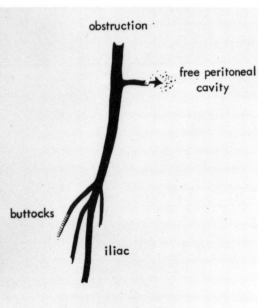

Collateral channels can also develop on the lower abdominal wall, carrying lymph flow to the inguinal lymph nodes on the contralateral side (Fig. 87–38). Collateral lymphatic vessels have also been noted to flow toward the buttocks. The ability to form numerous collateral lymphatic channels is probably the reason that conservative therapy for chylous ascites in children is so successful.

Radiopaque media may also flow retrograde through the mesenteric lymphatics into the lumen of the small bowel (Fig. 87–39) or flow retrograde into the pelvis of the kidney (Fig. 87–40).

**Iliac Level.** Obstruction of the iliac lymphatic vessels usually results in collateral lymphatic flow through the perineum to the contralateral side of the pelvis. Lymph flow may also be directed to the thigh, buttocks, or anterior abdominal wall. If the block is high in the pelvis, collateral flow may go to the posterolateral abdominal wall and return along the ribs to the posterior mediastinum.

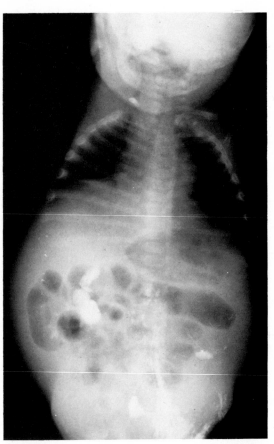

**FIGURE 87–39.** Retrograde lymphatic flow into the small bowel. Note the pooling of the dye in the intestinal lumina.

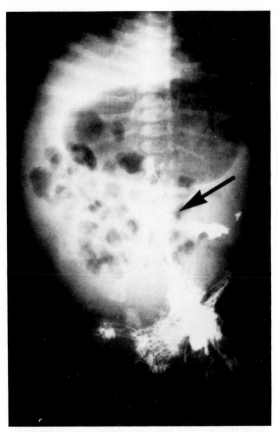

**FIGURE 87–38.** Collateral lymphatics associated with cisterna chyli obstruction.

Lymphatic obstruction gives rise to an increase in intralymphatic pressure, which may be sufficiently high to dilate the lymphatic vessels and cause eventual incompetence of the valves. The incompetent valves are associated with retrograde flow, which may result in seepage of vessel contents into the lumina or organs. If this occurs in the gastrointestinal tract, it is called protein-losing gastroenteropathy; if it occurs in the pelvis of the kidney, it is referred to as chyluria. When the intralymphatic pressure rises and is associated with a structural defect of the lymphatic vessel, a rupture of the vessel with free leakage of contents may result. Leakage into the peritoneal cavity would result in chylous ascites. Lymphatic block may also be associated with the establishment of collateral lymphatic channels and lymphaticovenous shunts (Fig. 87–41).

There have been numerous publications reporting lymphaticovenous shunts in the dog, rat, monkey, cat, sheep, and man. These have been

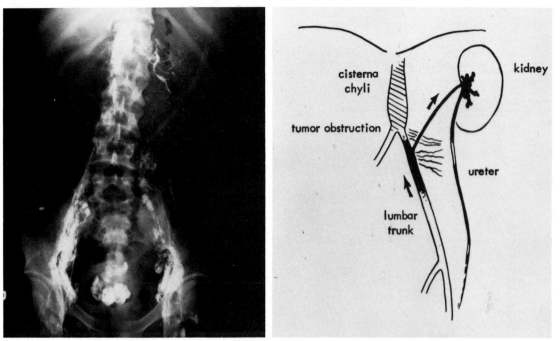

**FIGURE 87–40.** Retrograde lymphatic flow into the pelvis of the kidney.

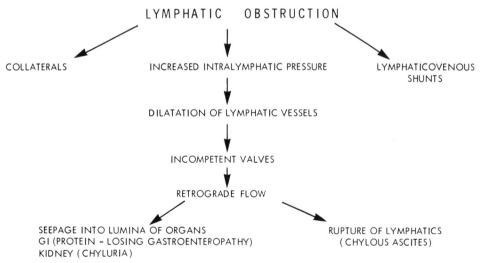

**FIGURE 87–41.** Consequences of lymphatic obstruction.

described as occurring with the hemiazygos vein, inferior vena cava, renal vein, azygos vein, intercostal vein, and portal vein. For lymph to drain into the venous system, the pressure in the vein at the level of communication must be lower than the pressure in the lymphatic. The author has demonstrated this by recording a lymphaticovenous shunt in the dog by lymphangiography and cinefluorography following experimental obstruction of the thoracic duct. As the rate of injection of the radiopaque media in the lymphatic was increased, the shunt opened and responded with an increased flow (Figs. 87–42 and 87–43). Clinical experience indicates that this occurs with chronic obstruction. Experimentally, the dye passes through a lymphatic into a lymph node and exits through a small vein.

Therapy for chyluria, chylous ascites, and protein-losing gastroenteropathy secondary to

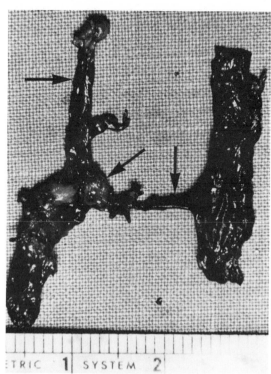

**FIGURE 87–43.** Lymphaticovenous shunt from the thoracic duct (left) through a lymph node (middle arrow) to the azygos vein (right).

obstruction of the thoracic duct depends primarily on the reduction of lymph flow through the thoracic duct. Lipids with fatty acids of carbon chain length greater than 12 are esterified in the intestinal mucosa and are transported almost exclusively by the thoracic duct. Fatty acids with a chain length less than 12 pass into the portal vein and are not found in the thoracic duct; therefore, feedings of medium-chain triglycerides to patients with intestinal lymphangiectasia and chylous ascites and with chyluria may be helpful.

## EXPERIMENTAL LYMPHEDEMA

Lymphedema is experimentally produced by injecting a mixture of Silastic fluid and a catalyst in the lymphatic to form an obstructing gel with minimal tissue reaction. This results in a lymphangiogram in the dog similar to that seen in the human with lymphatic obstruction (Figs. 87–44 through 87–47).

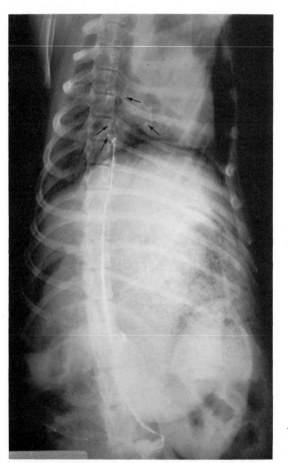

**FIGURE 87–42.** Lymphaticovenous shunt in the dog. Note the passage of dye from the thoracic duct (left) to the azygos vein (right).

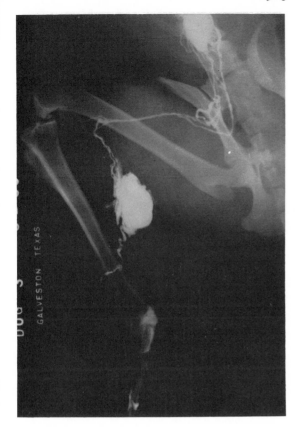

**FIGURE 87–44.** Normal lower extremity lymphangiogram in the dog (popliteal lymph node).

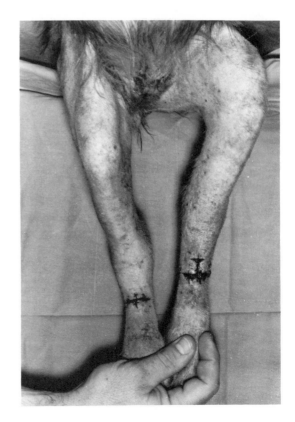

**FIGURE 87–45.** Experimental lymphedema in the dog.

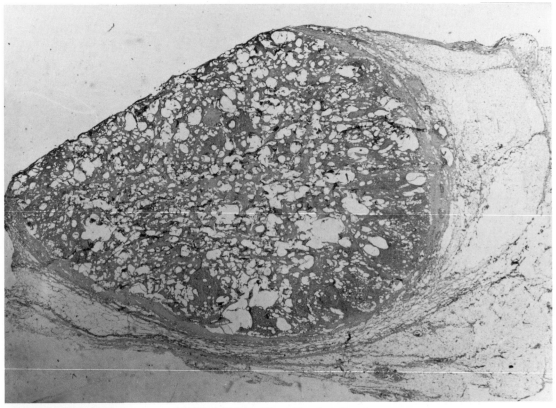

**FIGURE 87-46.**  Silastic in a lymph node.

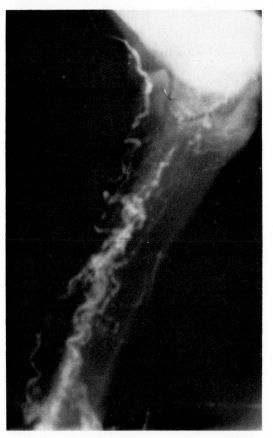

**FIGURE 87-47.**  Abnormal canine lymphangiogram showing tortuous, dilated lymphatics following experimental obstruction.

## TREATMENT OF LYMPHEDEMA

### Conservative Therapy

All patients with lymphedema should initially receive a trial of conservative therapy consisting of continuous pressure. Initial pressure therapy for lymphedema of the extremity consists of an Ace wrap rather than an elasticized bandage. The Ace wrap is preferred because of the change in size of the extremity following pressure, elevation, or bed rest. The pressure exerted by the Ace bandages varies from 25 to 40 mm of mercury. The patient is instructed to wrap the extremities with Ace bandages and to wear these continuously, even during sleep. Once the extremity has decreased in size, an elastic garment such as a sleeve or stocking can be worn. It is not infrequent that the patient finds an elastic garment too constrictive and must return to using the Ace wrap. A disadvantage of the Ace wrap is its tendency to roll about the knee, causing increased pressure in this area. The patient should be forewarned of this common problem, which may require a small strip of tape on the medial and lateral sides of the leg to prevent it from occurring. In many instances, constant pressure is all that is required to maintain a reasonably sized extremity. Intermittent pneumatic compression of an extremity by the use of mechanical devices, such as a Jobst pump, has also proved helpful to a number of patients. Diuretics are used periodically in promoting mobilization of the edematous fluid. A diuretic is usually added to the regimen when a pressure dressing has not achieved the desired result. Appropriate antibiotics, especially those used to control streptococcal and staphylococcal infections, are frequently indicated.

### Surgical Treatment of Lymphedema

**Lymphangioplasty.** Many attempts have been made by surgeons to establish new lymphatic pathways; however, all of these efforts have failed. Handley in 1908 buried silk threads in the subcutaneous tissue with a view to establishing an ascending flow of lymph by capillary action. Unfortunately, there was a high incidence of infection with extrusion of the buried foreign material. Rubber tubes, nylon thread, polyethylene tubes, and celloidin strips have also been used without success. These foreign materials generally resulted in increased formation of scar tissue. Long dermal strips from the lower abdomen were threaded subcutaneously down the leg to improve lymph drainage, and this technique also proved unsatisfactory (Fig. 87–48).

**Lymphatic Bridge Procedures with Pedicles.** Following the report by Gillies and Fraser (1935) of transferring a skin flap from a site containing normal lymphatics to an area of lymphatic obstruction, many surgeons have attempted to employ this principle to bypass lymphatic blocks in the leg and arm. Numerous skin flaps including tube flaps have been attempted, and all have left much to be desired. Several surgeons (Padgett, Wynn, Gillies, Mowlem, and Smith) have attempted bridging procedures with questionable results. The physiologic basis for the bridging surgical techniques exists only in the treatment of secondary or obstructive lymphedema. Furthermore, a flap that bypasses the obstruction and gains anastomosis between normally competent functioning lymphatics and competent blocked lymphatics must be designed. The failure rate increases if the flap blood supply is marginal and wound healing is retarded.

**Transposition of an Omental Flap.** Goldsmith and De Los Santos (1966, 1967) were the first to employ an omental flap. The surgical procedure consisted of developing an omental flap and transporting it below the inguinal ligament to the diseased extremity in a subcutaneous plane. The omentum has a rich lymphatic and vascular supply. Danese, Bower, and Howard (1962) were unable to demonstrate any lymphatic connections after the third month following surgery, and on exploration the omental flap was surrounded by thick fibrous fat. The author's experience has consisted of only one patient who was referred following this procedure complaining of intermittent severe abdominal discomfort. The omental flap had been introduced into the lower extremity several months previously, and the patient complained of intermittent abdominal distress and no improvement of the lymphedematous extremity. On exploration considerable fibrosis surrounded and infiltrated the omental flap. The procedure is fraught with problems, including abdominal wall hernias, bowel obstruction and wound dehiscence, and may be associated with high morbidity. Consequently, the technique should be used with caution.

**Lymphaticovenous Shunts.** Because the lymphatic circulation drains into the venous circulation, a number of surgeons have attempted

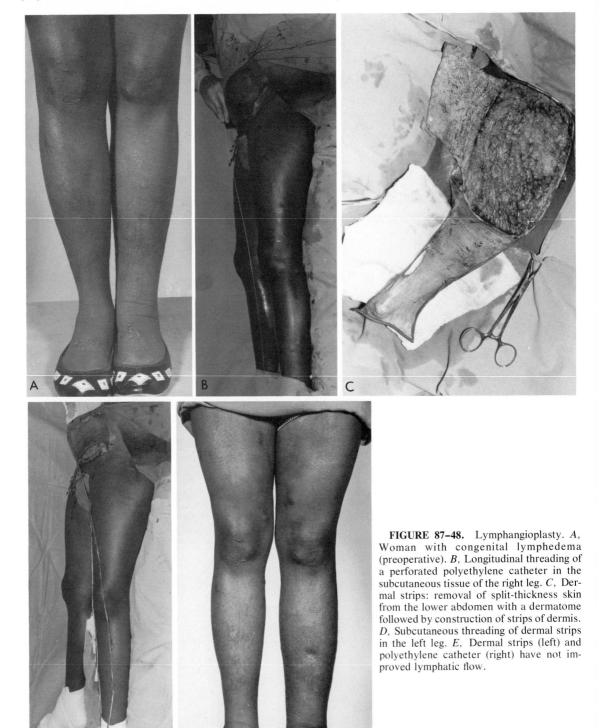

**FIGURE 87–48.** Lymphangioplasty. *A*, Woman with congenital lymphedema (preoperative). *B*, Longitudinal threading of a perforated polyethylene catheter in the subcutaneous tissue of the right leg. *C*, Dermal strips: removal of split-thickness skin from the lower abdomen with a dermatome followed by construction of strips of dermis. *D*, Subcutaneous threading of dermal strips in the left leg. *E*, Dermal strips (left) and polyethylene catheter (right) have not improved lymphatic flow.

to create a functional anastomosis between the lymph nodes and veins. Rivero, Calnan, Reis, and Taylor (1967) created a functional anastomosis between the popliteal lymph nodes and veins in dogs, but found obstruction after two to three months because of fibrosis. However, Nielubowicz, Olszewski, and Sokolowski (1968) were able to demonstrate patency in lymphaticovenous shunts in dogs one year after surgery. They also performed the procedure in four patients with secondary lymphedema and reported considerable improvement. Of the 17 patients with primary lymphedema who underwent the procedure, only half showed some improvement. This type of procedure should be considered only in patients with obstructive secondary lymphedema. Using microsurgical techniques, O'Brien (1975) has performed direct lymphaticovenous anastomoses for the relief of postmastectomy upper extremity lymphedema (see Chapter 14).

**Excision of Lymphedematous Tissue.** The most popular operations have been based on the excision of the elephantoid tissue. Charles in 1912 excised the skin, subcutaneous tissue, and deep fascia down to the muscle from below the knee to the ankle. He then applied a split-thickness skin graft. Kondoleon in 1912 excised strips of subcutaneous tissue down to and including the deep fascia and closed the wound primarily. Matas (1913) reported that the removal of the deep fascia allowed the lymphatics to form an anastomosing channel between the subcutaneous tissue and the deeper lymphatics. Sistrunk (1918) modified the Kondoleon operation by removing skin along with the subcutaneous tissue and fascia from the iliac crest to the external malleolus. Twelve days following the first procedure on the lateral aspect, a similar operation was done on the medial aspect.

It has been emphasized that the important aspect in obtaining successful results by this procedure was the use of elastic dressings after the operation. Seventy-two per cent of the patients who obtained a successful result had worn the elastic dressings, whereas only 40 per cent of those who failed to use postoperative elastic dressings showed any improvement. In 1936 Homans pointed out the value of elevation of the affected extremities for 3 to 4 days prior to operation in order to promote as much lymph drainage as possible. Homans recommended parallel incisions from below the knee to the malleolus with the removal of approximately 2.5 cm of skin. Undermining was then done, removing the subcutaneous tissue ante-

riorly and posteriorly to the periosteum and muscle. This produced an almost full-thickness type of skin graft covering one-half of the calf. Approximately three months later, a similar procedure was done involving the lateral aspect of the leg. Macey (1940) peeled back the skin and subcutaneous tissue including the deep fascia on one-half of the leg and applied thick split-thickness grafts over the denuded area. The overlying pad of tissue was sutured back in place to serve as a pressure dressing and was trimmed away after a period of approximately ten days. Poth, Barnes, and Ross (1947) described a similar procedure employing a one stage operation and excised all of the tissue except a narrow strip covering the anterior aspect of the tibia.

Miller (1975) has advocated staged subcutaneous excisions beneath skin flaps of the affected extremities. In a first stage, skin flaps, 1.5 cm in thickness, are elevated along the medial aspect of the limb, and all underlying subcutaneous tissue, including the investing fascia, is resected; any excess skin is also excised. The second stage is performed two months later along the lateral aspect of the extremity. Care is always taken to preserve the superficial nerves. Although the technique is not curative, it has reduced the size and improved the function of the affected limb.

The majority of operative procedures up to this time have included the utilization of skin from the diseased extremity. Pratt in 1953 recommended that the skin graft should be much thinner in order to avoid transplanting obstructed lymphatic structures in the grafted skin. He felt that the success of the operation required adequate preparation, radical excision including fascia, nontraumatic removal of the skin, and adequate postoperative support (Fig. 87–49). Kinmonth (1954) warned that one should never use the skin of a defective leg in the presence of dermal backflow, because obstructed dermal lymphatics are being replaced. The patients, therefore, are still subject to repeated attacks of infection. Numerous other reports have stressed the development of widespread hyperkeratinization, surface weeping of lymph, local breakdown and ulceration, cellulitis, keloid formation, and the recurrence of severe lymphedema in the skin-grafted surface. If surgical excision of all lymphedematous skin and subcutaneous tissue is to be performed, skin grafts should be removed from a nonaffected area of the body. It is also important to undermine and excise some of the subcutaneous tissue near the knee so as to avoid the pantaloon effect at the

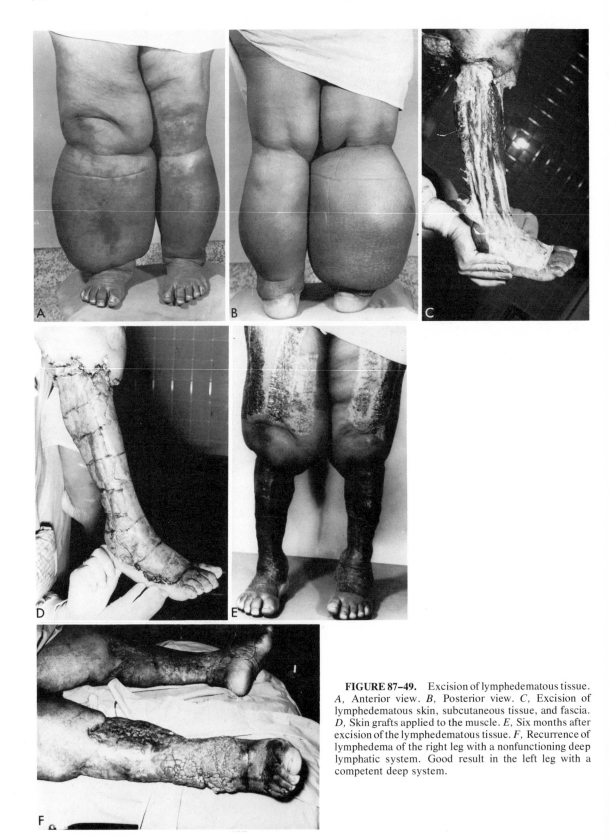

**FIGURE 87–49.** Excision of lymphedematous tissue. *A*, Anterior view. *B*, Posterior view. *C*, Excision of lymphedematous skin, subcutaneous tissue, and fascia. *D*, Skin grafts applied to the muscle. *E*, Six months after excision of the lymphedematous tissue. *F*, Recurrence of lymphedema of the right leg with a nonfunctioning deep lymphatic system. Good result in the left leg with a competent deep system.

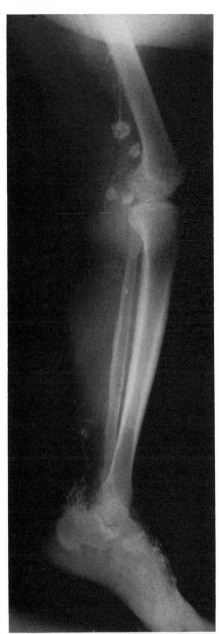

**FIGURE 87–50.** Superficial lymphatics of the foot drain into the deep system following radical excision.

junction of the remaining tissue in the skin-grafted area.

For the excision and graft to be completely successful, it is probably necessary that the deep lymphatic system be intact and functioning. Following excision, the superficial lymphatic system of the foot may drain into the deep lymphatic system (Fig. 87–50).

**Anastomosis of the Superficial to the Deep Lymphatic System.** Lanz (1911) first attempted

to anastomose the superficial and deep lymphatics by turning shaved flaps of deep fascia into the muscle. Kondoleon (1912) later excised strips of deep fascia in the hope of draining the superficial lymph into the deep lymphatic system. This operation was further modified by Sistrunk (1918) and Homans (1936). Late failure of these procedures was explained by Bertwistle and Gregg (1928) and by Peer (1954), who demonstrated that regeneration of the deep fascia reestablished the initial barrier.

To obviate the reestablishment of the deep fascia, Thompson (1962, 1967) maintained lymphatic connections by transposing a dermal flap through the fascia opening into the muscle. The Thompson buried dermal flap technique has a sound physiologic basis and appears to be a promising surgical procedure. The procedure consists of bed rest and compression bandaging of the limb for three days to reduce the edema. Antibiotic prophylaxis against Streptococcus and Staphylococcus organisms is also administered. Transfer of a medial flap is usually performed first, and if a further procedure is required, a lateral flap transfer is later carried out. The procedure on the medial aspect of the leg consists of excising thick split-thickness skin grafts, at the junction of the posterior one-third and the anterior two-thirds of the leg, until the deep dermal level is reached. Following this, an incision is made along the posterior edge of the dermal flap. Lymphedematous subcutaneous tissue is excised both anteriorly and posteriorly, care being taken to avoid compromising the circulation to the skin edges. A portion of the fascia overlying the muscle is excised, and the dermal flap is placed into the anterior muscle bed. Sutures are placed between the fascia and the dermal flap to hold it in position. The posterior skin edge is then sutured to the anterior edge of the dermal flap (Figs. 87–51 and 87–52). If one desires to perform a flap transfer later, this is done in a similar fashion, except that the dermal flap is situated between the anterior one-third and the posterior two-thirds of the leg; the dermal flap is based posteriorly. On the lateral aspect of the leg, a local pad of fat and fascia is left overlying the head of the fibula to protect the peroneal nerve.

In our first cases, the medial flap was based posteriorly, as described by Thompson. However, in subsequent cases the flap was based anteriorly in order to take advantage of the normal posterior lymph flow in the medial aspect of the leg. The dermal flow in lymphedema appears to be in all directions; therefore, the flap should

*Text continued on page 3601*

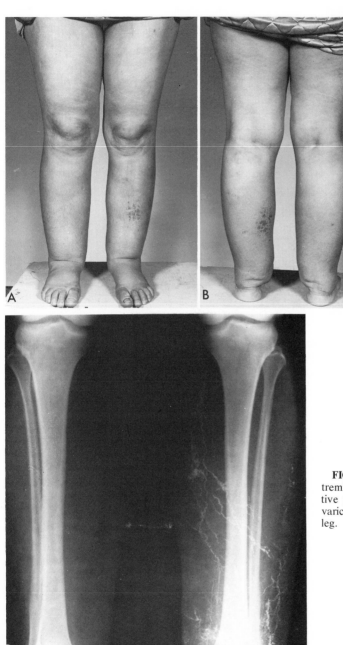

**FIGURE 87–51.** Lymphedema of the lower extremities. *A*, Preoperative frontal view. *B*, Preoperative posterior view. *C*, Lymphangiogram showing varicose lymphatics and dermal back-flow of the left leg.

*Legend continued on the opposite page*

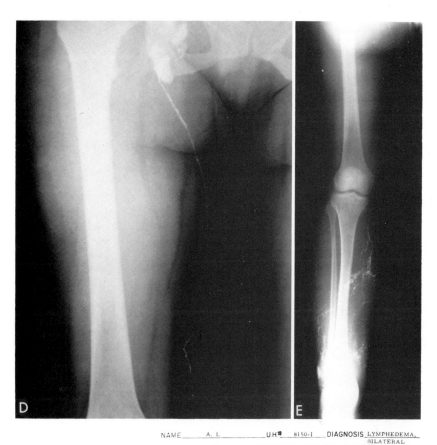

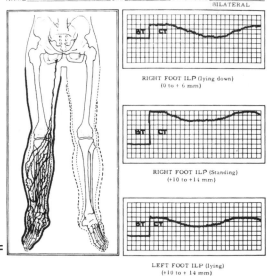

**FIGURE 87–51** *Continued.* *D,* Hypoplasia of the thigh lymphatics. *E,* Severe lymph stasis as one-half of the radiopaque media remains one month following injection. *F,* Abnormal positive lymphatic pressure readings.

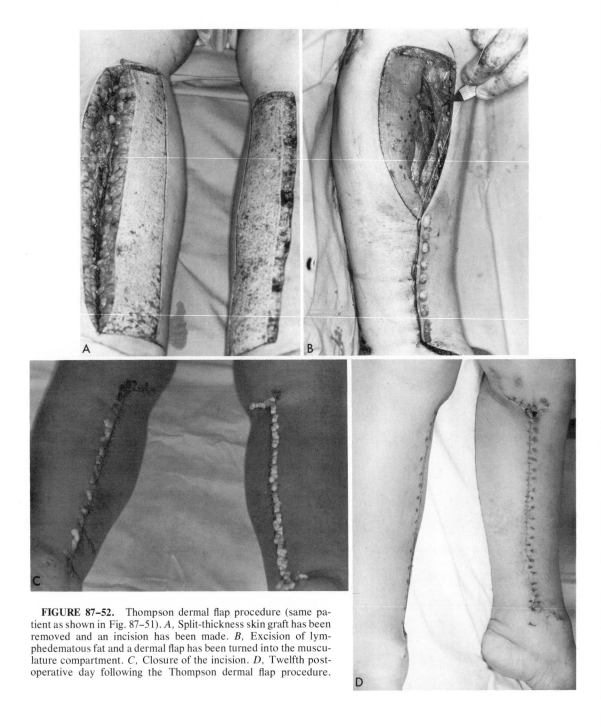

**FIGURE 87–52.** Thompson dermal flap procedure (same patient as shown in Fig. 87–51). *A*, Split-thickness skin graft has been removed and an incision has been made. *B*, Excision of lymphedematous fat and a dermal flap has been turned into the musculature compartment. *C*, Closure of the incision. *D*, Twelfth postoperative day following the Thompson dermal flap procedure.

drain regardless of the position of the base of the flap. Theoretically, the flow should be better if the flap is in the direction of normal lymph flow, i.e., based anteriorly in the medial aspect of the leg and posteriorly in the lateral aspect of the leg.

The turning of a dermal flap into the deeper tissues anastomoses the dermal lymphatics with the deeper lymphatic system (Fig. 87–53). This procedure is particularly useful when a valvular incompetence and dermal backflow are present. The advantages of this procedure include a shorter hospitalization and healing time. There is also a more pleasing immediate appearance, with an eventual acceptable contour of the extremity. If the procedure fails, one can then excise the lymphedematous skin and subcutaneous tissue and later apply split-thickness skin grafts.

A recent evaluation of the Thompson dermal flap technique (Sawhney, 1974) showed that the immediate postoperative reduction in size may be explained by the excision of edematous subcutaneous tissue and is proportional to the volume of excision. Thompson (1974) claims that, although the procedure may not be the final solution to the problem of lymphedema, recurrent episodes of lymphangitis and cellulitis are reduced in patients who have undergone the procedure.

## Summary of Treatment

The first stage in therapy should always consist of continuous elastic pressure by the use of Ace bandages and elastic garments. If a thorough trial of conservative therapy fails, the next procedure preferred by the author is the Thompson dermal flap technique. A medial flap is attempted first, and if further corrective surgery is indicated, a lateral flap is performed. At least three months should elapse between the two procedures. The lymphedematous

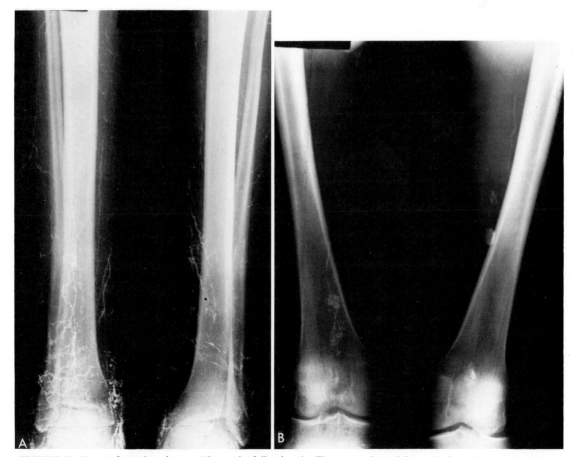

**FIGURE 87–53.** *A,* Lymphangiogram 18 months following the Thompson dermal flap technique. *B,* Lymphangiogram after injecting the dorsum of the foot lymphatic 18 months following a dermal flap technique. Note the flow via the deep lymphatics (popliteal lymph nodes).

process in some patients will continue to progress despite conservative therapy and the Thompson dermal flap procedure. Should this occur and the leg become so heavy that it restricts or limits mobility and ambulation, a final surgical procedure consisting in excising all lymphedematous tissue down to the muscle and applying moderately thick split-thickness skin grafts is indicated.

## REFERENCES

Bertwistle, A. P., and Gregg, A. L.: Elephantiasis. Br. J. Surg., *16*:267, 1928.

Britton, R. C.: Management of peripheral edema, including lymphedema of the arm after radical mastectomy. Cleveland Clin. Quart., 26:53, 1962.

Britton, R. C., and Nelson, P. A.: Causes and treatment of postmastectomy lymphedema of the arm. J.A.M.A., *180*:95, 1962.

Carvalho, R., Rodriquez, A., and Perenia, S.: La mise en évidence pour la radiographie du system lymphatique chez le vivant. Ann. Anat. Pathol., *8*:193, 1931.

Charles, R. H.: Elephantiasis scroti. *In* Latham, A., and English, T. C. (Eds.): A System of Treatment. Vol. 3. London, Churchill, 1912.

Danese, C., Bower, R., and Howard, J.: Experimental anastomoses of lymphatics. Arch. Surg., *84*:24, 1962.

Drinker, C. K.: The Lymphatic System. Lane Medical Lectures. Stanford, California, Stanford University Press, 1942.

Gillies, H., and Fraser, F. R.: The treatment of lymphoedema by plastic operation. Br. Med. J., *1*:96, 1935.

Goldsmith, H. S., and De Los Santos, R.: Omental transposition for the treatment of chronic lymphedema. Rev. Surg., 23:303, 1966.

Goldsmith, H. S., and De Los Santos, R.: Omental transposition in primary lymphedema. Surg. Gynec. Obstet., *125*:607, 1967.

Handley, W. S.: Lymphangioplasty; new method for relief of brawny arm of breast-cancer, and for similar conditions of lymphatic oedema. Lancet, *1*:783, 1908.

Homans, J.: The treatment of elephantiasis of the legs. A preliminary report. New Engl. J. Med., *215*:1099, 1936.

Hudack, S. S., and McMaster, P. D.: The lymphatic participation in human lymphatic vessels as seen in transparent chambers. Am. J. Anat., *51*:49, 1932.

Hudack, S. S., and McMaster, P. D.: Lymphatic participation in human cutaneous phenomena; study of minute lymphatics of living skin. J. Exp. Med., *57*:751, 1933.

Kinmonth, J. B.: Lymphangiography in clinical surgery and particularly in the treatment of lymphoedema. Ann. R. Coll. Surg., *15*:300, 1954.

Kondoleon, E.: Die operative Behandlung der elephantiastischer Odeme. Zentralbl. Chir., *39*:1022, 1912.

Lanz, O.: Eröffnung neuer Abfuhrwege bei Stauung im Bauch und untern Extremitäten. Zentralbl. Chir., *38*:153, 1911.

Macey, H. B.: A new surgical procedure for lymphedema of the extremities—Report of a case. Proc. Staff. Meet. Mayo Clin., *15*:49, 1940.

Matas, R.: The surgical treatment of elephantiasis and elephantoid states dependent upon chronic obstruction of lymphatic and venous channels. Am. J. Trop. Dis., *1*:60, 1913.

Miller, T. A.: Surgical management of lymphedema of the extremity. Plast. Reconstr. Surg., *56*:633, 1975.

Nielubowicz, J., and Olszewski, W.: Surgical lymphaticovenous shunts in patients with secondary lymphoedema. Br. J. Surg., *55*:440, 1968.

Nielubowicz, J., Olszewski, W., and Sokolowski, J.: Surgical lymphovenous shunts. J. Cardiovasc. Surg., *9*:262, 1968.

Nylander, G., and Tjernberg, B.: The lymphatics of the greater omentum; an experimental study in the dog. Lymphology, *2*:3, 1969.

O'Brien, B.: Personal communication, 1975.

Pappenheimer, A. M., and Freund, J.: Induction of delayed hypersensitivity to protein antigens. *In* Lawrence, H. S. (Ed.): Cellular and Humoral Aspects of the Hypersensitive States, New York, Hoeber-Harper, 1959.

Peer, L. A., Shahgholi, M., Walker, J. C., and Mancusi-Ungaro, A.: Modified operation for lymphedema of the leg and arm. Plast. Reconstr. Surg., *14*:347, 1954.

Poth, E. J., Barnes, S. R., and Ross, G. T.: A new operative treatment of elephantiasis. Surg. Gynecol. Obstet., *84*:642, 1947.

Pratt, G. H.: Surgical correction of lymphoedema: Application of new operative technique in lymph stasis and allied conditions. J.A.M.A., *151*:888, 1953.

Rivero, O. R., Calnan, J. S., Reis, N. D., and Taylor, L. M.: Experimental peripheral lympho-venous communications. Br. J. Plast. Surg., *20*:124, 1967.

Sabin, F. R.: The Origin and Development of the Lymphatic System. Baltimore, Johns Hopkins Press, 1913.

Sawhney, C. P.: Evaluation of Thompson's burned dermal flap operation for lymphoedema of the limbs: A clinical radioisotopic study. Br. J. Plast. Surg., *27*:278, 1974.

Sistrunk, W. E.: Elephantiasis treated by the Kondoleon operation. Surg. Gynecol. Obstet., *26*:388, 1918.

Thompson, N.: Surgical treatment of chronic lymphoedema of the lower limb. With preliminary report of new operation. Br. Med. J., *2*:1567, 1962.

Thompson, N.: The surgical treatment of chronic lymphoedema of the extremities. Surg. Clin. N. Am., *47*:445, 1967.

Thompson, N.: Personal communication, 1974.

## ADDITIONAL REFERENCES

Allen, E. V.: Lymphedema of the extremities: Classification, etiology, and differential diagnosis. A study of three hundred cases. Arch. Int. Med., *54*:606, 1934.

Allen, L.: On the penetrability of the lymphatics of the diaphragm. Anat. Rec., *124*:639, 1956.

Bard, P. (Ed.): Medical Physiology. 11th Ed. St. Louis, Mo., C. V. Mosby Company, 1956.

Barnes, J., and Trueta, J.: Absorption of bacteria, toxins and snake venoms from the tissues. Importance of the lymphatic circulation. Lancet, *1*:623, 1941.

Bauer, W., Short, C. L., and Bennett, G. A.: The manner of removal of proteins from normal joints. J. Exp. Med., *57*:419, 1933.

Bedell, W. C.: Treatment of edematous extremity with diuretics. J.A.M.A., *173*:109, 1960.

Beninson, J.: Stasis and dermatitis and stasis ulcer. *In* Conn, H. F. (Ed.): Current Therapy, 1958. Philadelphia, W. B. Saunders Company, 1958, p. 493.

Beninson, J.: Six years of pressure-gradient therapy. Angiology, *12*:36, 1961.

Beninson, J., and Ensign, D. C.: Leg ulcers in rheumatoid arthritis. J.A.M.A., *175*:437, 1961.

Best, C. H., and Taylor, N. B.: The Physiological Basis

of Medical Practice. 7th Ed. Baltimore, The Williams & Wilkins Company, 1961.

Biegeleisen, H. I.: New biopsy needle treatment of lymphedema. Am. J. Surg., *101*:786, 1961.

Blocker, T. G., Jr.: Surgical treatment of elephantiasis of the lower extremity. Plast. Reconstr. Surg., *4*:407, 1949.

Blocker, T. G., Jr., Smith, J. R., Dunton, E. F., Protas, J. M., Cooley, R. N., Lewis, S. R., and Kirby, E. J.: Studies of ulceration and edema of the lower extremities by lymphatic cannulation. Ann. Surg., *149*:884, 1959.

Blocker, T. G., Jr., Lewis, S. R., Smith, J. R., Dunton, E. F., Kirby, E. J., and Meyer, J. V.: Lymphodynamics. Plast. Reconstr. Surg., *25*:337, 1960.

Bowers, W. F., Schear, E. W., and LeGolvan, P. C.: Lymphangiosarcoma in the postmastectomy lymphedematous arm. Am. J. Surg., *90*:682, 1955.

Boyd, A. D., and Altemeier, W. A.: Lymphangiography in management of malignant neoplasms of the lower extremities. Arch. Surg., *86*:911, 1963.

Brush, B. E., Wylie, J. H., Jr., and Beninson, J.: Some devices for the management of lymphedema of the extremities. Surg. Clin. N. Am., *39*:1493, 1959.

Buonocore, E., and Young, J. R.: Lymphangiographic evaluation of lymphedema and lymphatic flow. Am. J. Roentgenol. Radium Ther. Nucl. Med., *95*:751, 1965.

Burch, G. E., and Sodeman, W. A.: The estimation of the subcutaneous pressure by a direct method. J. Clin. Invest., *16*:845, 1937.

Butcher, H. R., and Hoover, A. L.: Abnormalities of human superficial cutaneous lymphatics associated with stasis ulcers, lymphedema, scars and cutaneous autografts. Ann. Surg., *142*:633, 1955.

Cajori, F. A., Crounter, C. Y., and Pemberton, R.: The physiologic effect of massage; second contribution. Arch. Int. Med., *39*:281, 1927.

Calnan, J.: Lymphoedema; the case for doubt. Br. J. Plast. Surg., *21*:32, 1968.

Calnan, J., and Kountz, S. L.: Effect of venous obstruction on lymphatics. Br. J. Surg., *52*:800, 1965.

Clark, E. R., and Clark, E. L.: Observation on the growth of lymphatic vessels as seen in transparent chambers. Am. J. Anat., *51*:49, 1932.

Clark, E. R., and Clark, E. L.: Further observations on living vessels in the transparent chamber in the rabbit's ear; their relation to the tissue spaces. Am. J. Anat., *52*:273, 1933.

Clark, E. R., and Clark, E. L.: Observations on living mammalian lymphatic capillaries; their relation to the blood vessels. Am. J. Anat., *60*:253, 1937.

Clark, E. R., and Clark, E. L.: Observations on isolated lymphatic capillaries in the living mammal. Am. J. Anat., *62*:59, 1938.

Clark, E. R., and Clark, E. L.: Observations on the growth of lymphatic vessels from the tissues. Importance of the lymphatic circulation. Lancet, *1*:623, 1941.

Cohnheim, J.: Lectures on General Pathology. Translated from 2nd Edition by Alexander McKee. London, The New Sydenham Society, 1889, p. 502.

Courtice, F. C.: The effect of local temperature on fluid loss in thermal burns. J. Physiol., *104*:321, 1946.

Courtice, F. C., and Simmonds, W. J.: Absorption from the lungs. J. Physiol., *109*:103, 1949.

Crockett, D. J.: Protein levels of oedema fluids. Lancet, *2*:1179, 1956.

Crockett, D. J.: Lymphatic anatomy and lymphoedema. Br. J. Plast. Surg., *18*:12, 1965.

Cruse, R., Fisher, W. C., III, and Usher, F. C.: Lymphangiosarcoma in postmastectomy lymphedema. Surgery, *30*:565, 1951.

Danese, C. A., Georgalas-Bertakis, M., and Morales, L. E.: A model of chronic postsurgical lymphedema in dogs' limbs. Surgery, *64*:814, 1968a.

Danese, C. A., Papaioannou, A. N., Morales, L. E., and Mitsuda, S.: Surgical approaches to lymphatic blocks. Surgery, *64*:821, 1968b.

Devenish, E. A., and Jessop, W. H. G.: Nature and cause of swelling of upper limb after radical mastectomy. Br. J. Surg., *28*:222, 1940.

Diszauer, S., and Ross, R. C.: Lymphangiosarcoma in lymphoedema. Can. Med. Assoc. J., *76*:475, 1957.

Ditchek, T., Blahut, R. J., and Kittleson, A. C.: Lymphadenography in normal subjects. Radiology, *80*:175, 1963.

Doremus, W. P., and Salvia, G. A.: Lymphangiosarcoma in the postmastectomy lymphedematous arm. Am. J. Surg., *96*:576, 1958.

Drinker, C. K., and Yoffey, J. M.: Lymphatics, Lymph and Lymphoid Tissue. Their Physiologic and Clinical Significance. Cambridge, Harvard University Press, 1941.

Drinker, C. K., Field, M. E., and Homans, J.: The experimental production of edema and elephantiasis as a result of lymphatic obstruction. Am. J. Physiol., *108*:509, 1934.

Edwards, E. A.: Recurrent febrile episodes and lymphedema. J.A.M.A., *184*:102, 1963.

Eichner, E., and Bone, E. R.: In vivo studies on the lymphatic drainage of the human ovary. Surg. Gynecol. Obstet., *3*:287, 1954.

Elkins, E. C., Herrick, J. F., Grindlay, J. G., Mann, F. C., and DeForest, R. E.: Effect of various procedures on the flow of lymph. Arch. Phys. Med., *34*:31, 1953.

Eloesser, L.: Obstruction of lymph channels by scar. J.A.M.A., *81*:1867, 1923.

Emmett, A. J., Barron, J. N., and Veall, N.: The use of [131]I albumin tissue clearance measurements and other physiological tests for the clinical assessment of patients with lymphoedema. Br. J. Plast. Surg., *20*:1, 1967.

Field, M. E., and Drinker, C. K.: The rapidity of interchanges between the blood and the lymph in the dog. Am. J. Physiol., *98*:378, 1931.

Field, M. E., Drinker, C. K., and White, J. C.: Lymph pressure in sterile inflammation. J. Exp. Med., *56*:363, 1932.

Fischer, H.: A technic for radiography of lymph nodes and vessels. Lab. Invest., *6*:522, 1957.

Fischer, H., and Zimmerman, G. R.: Roentgenographic visualization of lymph nodes and lymph channels. Am. J. Roentgenol., *81*:3, 1959.

Fischer, H. W., Lawrence, M. S., and Zimmerman, G. R.: Contrast radiographic demonstration of a lymph node metastasis. J.A.M.A., *175*:139, 1961.

Fitts, W. T., Jr., Keuhnelian, J. G., Raydin, I. S., and Schor, S.: Swelling of the arm after radical mastectomy: A clinical study of its causes. Surgery, *35*:460, 1954.

Foldi, M.: Lymphedema. *In* Kugelmass, I. N. (Ed.): Diseases of Lymphatics and Lymph Circulation. Springfield, Ill., Charles C Thomas, Publisher, 1969.

Forbes, G.: Lymphatics of the skin with a note on lymphatic watershed areas. J. Anat., *72*:399, 1937-1938.

Foster, J. H., and Kirtley, J. A.: Unilateral lower extremity hypertrophy. Surg. Gynecol. Obstet., *108*:35, 1959.

Francis, K. C., and Lindquist, H. D.: Lymphangiosarcoma of the lower extremity involved with chronic lymphedema. Am. J. Surg., *100*:617, 1960.

Freeman, L. M.: Lymphatic pathways from the intestine in the dog. Anat. Rec., *82*:543, 1942.

Gager, L. T.: Lymphatic obstruction; nonparasitic elephantiasis. Am. J. Med. Sci., *166*:200, 1923.

Gergely, R.: The roentgen examination of the lymphatics in man. Radiology, *71*:59, 1958.

Ghormley, R. K., and Overton, L. M.: The surgical treatment of severe forms of lymphedema (elephantiasis) of the extremities: A study of end results. Surg. Gynecol. Obstet., *61*:83, 1935.

Glenn, W. W. L., Gilbert, H. H., and Drinker, C. K.: The treatment of burns by the closed plaster method, with certain physiological considerations implicit in the success of this technique. J. Clin. Invest., *22*:609, 1943.

Glucksmann, A.: Local factors in the histogenesis of hypertrophic scars. Br. J. Plast. Surg., *4*:88, 1951.

Goffrini, P., Bobbie, G., Peracchia, G., and Pellegrino, F.: Anatomical lymphographic comparative method for studying lymph node pathology. Arch. Ital. Chir., *87*:613, 1961.

Gough, M. H.: Primary lymphoedema; clinical and lymphangiographic studies. Br. J. Surg., *53*:917, 1966.

Guthrie, D., and Gagnon, G.: Prevention and treatment of postoperative lymphedema of the arm. Ann. Surg., *123*:925, 1946.

Hall-Smith, S. P., and Haber, H.: Lymphangiosarcoma in postmastectomy lymphedema (Stewart-Treves syndrome). Proc. R. Soc. Med., *47*:174, 1954.

Halsted, W. S.: The swelling of the arm after operations for cancer of the breast. Elephantiasis chirurgica; its cause and prevention. Bull. Johns Hopkins Hosp., *32*:309, 1921.

Harkins, G. A., and Sabiston, D. C., Jr.: Lymphangioma in infancy and childhood. Surgery, *47*:811, 1960.

Herrmann, J. B., and Gruhn, J. G.: Lymphangiosarcoma secondary to chronic lymphedema. Surg. Gynecol. Obstet., *105*:665, 1957.

Hilfinger, M. F., Jr., and Eberle, R. D.: Lymphangiosarcoma in postmastectomy lymphedema. Cancer, *6*:1192, 1953.

Hogeman, K.: Personal communication, 1963.

Hugo, N. E.: Recent advances in the treatment of lymphedema. Surg. Clin. N. Am., *51*:111, 1971.

Jacobsson, S., and Feldman, A.: Estimation of lymph flow in the extremities. Arch. Surg., *82*:117, 127, 1961.

Katzenstein, R., Mylon, E., and Winternitz, M. C.: The toxicity of the thoracic duct fluid after release of tourniquets applied to the hind legs of dogs for the production of shock. Am. J. Physiol., *139*:307, 1943.

Keeley, J. L., Schairer, A. E., and Pesek, I. G.: Edema of the lower extremities. Mod. Med., *30*:97, 1962.

Kettle, J. H.: Lymphangiosarcoma following postmastectomy lymphoedema. Br. Med. J., *1*:193, 1957.

Kinmonth, J. B.: Vascular surgery. Chronic edema of the leg. *In* Carling, E. R., and Ross, J. P. (Eds.): British Surgical Practice: Surgical Progress. London, Butterworth, 1952.

Kinmonth, J. B., Harper, R. A. K., and Taylor, G. W.: Lymphangiography by radiological methods. J. Fac. Radiol. (Lond.) *6*:217, 1955a.

Kinmonth, J. B., Taylor, G. W., and Harper, R. K.: Lymphangiography: A technique for its clinical use in the lower limb. Br. Med. J., *1*:940, 1955b.

Kinmonth, J. B., Taylor, G. W., Tracy, G. D., and Marsh, J. D.: Primary lymphedema: Clinical and lymphangiographic studies of 107 patients in which the lower limbs were affected. Br. J. Surg., *45*:1, 1957.

Kruse, R. D., Kruse, A., and Britton, R. C.: Physical therapy for the patient with peripheral edema: Procedures for management. Phys. Ther. Rev., *40*:29, 1960.

Ladd, M. P., Kottke, F. J., and Blanchard, R. S.: Studies of the effect of massage on the flow of lymph from the foreleg of the dog. Arch. Phys. Med., *33*:604, 1952.

Linton, R. R.: Peripheral vascular diseases. New Engl. J. Med., *260*:370, 1959.

Macey, H. B.: Surgical procedures for lymphedema of the extremities. J. Bone Joint Surg., *30A*:339, 1948.

McLachlin, A. D., McLachlin, J. A., Jory, T. A., and Rawling, E. G.: Venous stasis in the lower extremities. Ann. Surg., *152*:678, 1960.

McMaster, P. D.: Changes in the cutaneous lymphatics of human beings and in the lymph flow under normal and pathological conditions. J. Exp. Med., *65*:347, 1937.

McMaster, P. D.: Lymphatic participation in cutaneous phenomena (Harvey Lecture). Bull. N. Y. Acad. Med., *18*:731, 1942.

McMaster, P. D.: Conditions in the skin influencing interstitial fluid movement, lymph formation and lymph flow. Ann. N. Y. Acad. Sci., *46*:743, 1946.

McMaster, P. D., and Hudack, S. S.: The participation of skin lymphatics in repair of the lesions due to incisions and burns. J. Exp. Med., *60*:479, 1934.

McSwain, B., and Stephenson, S.: Lymphangiosarcoma of the edematous extremity. Ann. Surg., *151*:649, 1960.

Malek, P., Kolc, J., and Belan, A.: Problems of lymphography of the deep lymphatic system of the pelvis and lower limbs. Cesk. Roentgenol., *13*:54, 1959.

Martorell, F.: Tumorigenic lymphedema. Angiology, *2*:386, 1951.

Mason, P. B., and Allen, E. V.: Congenital lymphangiectasis (lymphedema). Am. J. Dis. Child., *50*:945, 1935.

Milroy, W. F.: Chronic hereditary edema: Milroy's disease. J.A.M.A., *91*:1172, 1928.

Mowlem, R.: Hypertrophic scars. Br. J. Plast. Surg., *4*:113, 1951.

Moyer, C. A., and Butcher, H. R., Jr.: Stasis ulcers; an evaluation of the effectiveness of three methods of therapy and the implication of obliterative cutaneous lymphangitis as a creditable etiologic factor. Ann. Surg., *141*:577, 1955.

Ochsner, A., Longacre, A. B., and Murray, S. D.: Progressive lymphedema associated with recurrent erysipeloid infections. Surgery, *8*:383, 1940.

Olszewski, W., Machowski, Z., Sokolowski, J., and Nielubowicz, J.: Experimental lymphedema in dogs. J. Cardiovasc. Surg., *9*:178, 1968.

Pappenheimer, A. M., and Freund, J.: Induction of delayed hypersensitivity to protein antigens. *In* Lawrence, H. S. (Ed.): Cellular and Humoral Aspects of the Hypersensitive States. New York, Hoeber-Harper, 1959.

Politowski, M., Bartkowski, S., and Dynowski, J.: Treatment of lymphedema of the limbs by lymphatic-venous fistula. Surgery, *66*:639, 1969.

Pullinger, B. D., and Florey, H. W.: Proliferation of lymphatics in inflammation. J. Pathol. Bacteriol., *45*:157, 1937.

Reichert, F. L.: The regeneration of lymphatics. Arch. Surg., *13*:871, 1926.

Reynolds, H.: Stasis dermatitis and stasis (varicose) ulcer. *In* Conn, H. F. (Ed.): Current Therapy, 1962. Philadelphia, W. B. Saunders Company, 1962, p. 433.

Rienhoff, W. F., Jr.: Use of muscle pedicle flap for prevention of swelling of the arm following radical operation for carcinoma of the breast. Preliminary report. Bull. Johns Hopkins Hosp., *60*:609, 1937.

Rouvière, H.: Anatomie des Lymphatiques de l'Homme. Paris, Masson & Cie, 1932.

Sage, H. H., and Gozun, B. V.: Lymphatic scintigrams: A method for studying the functional pattern of lymphatics and lymph nodes. Cancer, *11*:200, 1958.

St. Francis Hospital: Instructions for Pressure Therapy. Evanston, Ill., April, 1963.

Sappey, M. P. C.: Anatomie, Physiologie, Pathologie des Vaisseaux Lymphatiques Considerès chez l'Homme et les Vertebres. Paris, A. Delahaye & E. Lacrosnier, 1874.

Schatz, I. J., Podolsky, S., and Frame, B.: Idiopathic orthostatic hypotension. J.A.M.A., *186*:537, 1963.

Schirger, A., Harrison, E. G., and James, J. M.: Management of idiopathic lymphedema. Mod. Med.,*31*:115, 1963.

Singleton, A. O., and Singleton, E. B.: Disease of the lymphatics. *In* Lewis' Practice of Surgery. Vol. III. Hagerstown, Md., W. F. Prior Co., 1957.

Smedal, M. I., and Evans, J. A.: The cause and treatment of edema of the arm following radical mastectomy. Surg. Gynecol. Obstet., *111*:29, 1960.

Smith, C. A.: Studies on lymphedema of the extremities. Ann. Surg., *156*:1010, 1962.

Smith, J. R.: Motion Picture: Lymphatic Cannulation. USAF Hospital, Lackland AFB, Texas.

Smith, J. R., Dunton, E. F., Protas, J. M., Blocker, T. G., Jr., Cooley, R. N., and Lewis, S. R.: Cannulation of the lymphatics of the lower extremity. Surg. Forum, *9*:881, 1959.

Smith, J. W., and Conway, H.: Selection of appropriate surgical procedures in lymphedema: Introduction of the hinged pedicle. Plast. Reconstr. Surg., *30*:10, 1962.

Smith, R. D., Spittell, J. A., and Schirger, A.: Secondary lymphedema of the leg. Mod. Med., *31*:90, 1963.

Sonneland, J.: Postmastectomy edema of the arm. West. J. Surg., *70*:230, 1962.

Starling, E. G.: The influence of mechanical factors on lymph production. J. Physiol., *16*:224, 1894.

Starling, E. G.: Tissue fluid formation and absorption. J. Physiol., *19*:312, 1895.

Stewart, F. W., and Treves, N.: Lymphangiosarcoma in postmastectomy lymphedema: Report of 6 cases in elephantiasis chirurgica. Cancer, *1*:64, 1948.

Stillwell, G. K., Redford, J. W. B., and Krusen, F. H.: Further studies on the treatment of lymphedema. Arch. Phys. Med., *28*:435, 1957.

Taylor, G. W.: Lymphoedema. Postgrad. Med. J. (London), *35*:2, 1959.

Taylor, G. W., Kinmonth, J. B., and Dangerfield, W. G.: Protein content of edema fluid in lymphedema. Br. Med. J., *1*:1159, 1958.

Thomas, C. G.: Lymphatic dissemination of radio-gold in the presence of lymph node metastases. Surg. Gynecol. Obstet., *103*:151, 1956.

Threefoot, S. A.: The collection of lymph from intact peripheral cutaneous lymphatics of man. J. Lab. Clin. Med., *50*:720, 1957.

Turner-Warwick, R. T.: Lymphatics after mastectomy. Ann. R. Coll. Surg., *24*:101, 1957.

Wakim, K. G., Martin, G. M., and Krusen, F. H.: Influence of centripetal rhythmic compression on localized edema of an extremity. Arch. Phys. Med., *35*:98, 1955.

Watson, J.: Chronic lymphedema of the extremities and its management. Br. J. Surg., *31*:31, 1953.

Webb, R., Jr., and Starzl, T. E.: The effect of blood vessel pulsation on lymph pressure in large lymphatics. Bull. Johns Hopkins Hosp., *93*:401, 1953.

Wells, H. S., Youmans. J. B., and Miller, D. G., Jr.: Tissue pressure (intracutaneous, subcutaneous and intramuscular) as related to venous pressure, capillary filtration and other factors. J. Clin. Invest., *17*:489, 1938.

West, J. P., and Ellison, J.: A study of the causes and prevention of edema of the arm following radical mastectomy. Surg. Gynecol. Obstet., *109*:359, 1959.

White, J. C., Field, M. E., and Drinker, C. K.: On the protein content and normal flow of lymph from the foot of the dog. Am. J. Physiol., *103*:34, 1933.

Wiliams, R. W.: Filariasis research at Rangoon. WHO Chron., *22*:219, 1968.

Yoffey, J. M.: Regeneration of lymphatics. Proceedings of the 15th International Surgical Congress, Lisbon, 1954.

Yoffey, J. M., and Courtice, F. C.: Lymphatics, Lymph and Lymphoid Tissue. 2nd Ed. Cambridge, Harvard University Press, 1956.

*Part Five*

# THE TRUNK

# CHAPTER 88

# CHEST WALL RECONSTRUCTION

SHERRELL J. ASTON, M.D., AND
KENNETH L. PICKRELL, M.D.

The reconstruction of thoracic wall defects must provide pleural and structural continuity to support the mechanisms of respiration, a covering for the vulnerable intrathoracic contents, and, when possible, an acceptable external appearance.

The anatomical structure of the thorax is designed to facilitate ventilation of the lungs by the coordinated motion of the bony framework and associated soft tissues and at the same time to provide optimal conditions for the function of the cardiocirculatory system. Normal ventilation of the lungs requires relatively effortless chest wall and diaphragmatic excursions. Therefore, any defect or loss of thoracic cage integrity may reduce cardiorespiratory function.

A description of pathophysiology of the tracheal-bronchial tree and gaseous exchange at the alveolar level is beyond the scope of the present chapter. Loss of chest wall rigidity normally provided by the osteocartilaginous struts of the ribs and sternum results in a flail portion of the thoracic cage with paradoxical motion of the chest wall. With a closed chest defect, the degree of ventilatory embarrassment parallels the size of the chest wall lacking structural stability. In general, injury to the thinner, more mobile anterior chest wall produces more severe physiologic deficit than injury of similar magnitude to the posterior chest wall. Fracture or loss of ribs, both anteriorly and

posteriorly, results in a flail chest with severe respiratory impairment.

The normal subatmospheric pressure within the thoracic cavity (inspiration $-4$ to $-10$ cm of water; expiration $-2$ to $-4$ cm of water) is indicative of the need for pleural integrity and stability. Loss of the intrathoracic negative pressure secondary to a chest wall defect produces a partial or total pneumothorax, depending upon the volume of air within the pleural space. The transmission of pressure changes across the mediastinum may result in ventilatory compromise of both lungs and potential respiratory failure.

## INJURIES OF THE THORAX

All trauma affecting the thoracic cage, whether a simple contusion or a violent compression with penetration and laceration, whether due to blunt force or to penetration and perforation by sharp objects or projectiles, is likely to result in serious damage to the intrathoracic organs. Cutaneous emphysema and pneumo- and hemothorax are of frequent occurrence; rupture of the bronchi, the lung, the mediastinum, or the diaphragm is not rare. Fractures may occur in any component part of the thorax. In cases of severe chest injury, the services of a thoracic surgeon should be obtained, for proper initial treatment determines the subsequent clinical course and, in most instances, the final result.

Most perforating wounds of the thorax injure the pleura; they may also extend into or involve intrathoracic organs. From a mechanical standpoint, it does not matter much whether the injury is due to a broken rib or to perforation by a sharp projectile or instrument. The usual result is pneumothorax of varying degree and, perhaps somewhat less frequently, hemothorax of parietal or pulmonary origin. Collapse of the lung, mediastinal displacement, and embarrassment of the circulation and respiration are often associated features. These may terminate in irreversible shock and death. Depending on the mechanism of injury, there may be other problems of varying nature and degree, such as secondary hemorrhage, infection, pneumonia, or pulmonary gangrene.

*Hemoptysis* is always indicative of pulmonary trauma. If it occurs primarily, it points to serious lung trauma; if it occurs secondarily, it may be a sign of pulmonary disintegration.

*Pneumothorax* is usually associated with hemothorax as hemopneumothorax. If it occurs from a small thoracic wound and without evidence of gross contamination, early closure of the wound with expansion of the lung and gradual absorption may be anticipated. The external open pneumothorax may be immediately fatal, especially in the case of a very large opening. If death does not result, the air and blood are sucked back and forth with each respiration or attempt at coughing, thus preparing the way for infection. When there has been extensive loss of tissue, the services of a plastic surgeon may be of value in transferring a flap to close the defect. A sucking wound should be closed at once, if by no other means than an airtight dressing, until definitive treatment is undertaken.

In the case of *combined injuries of the thorax and abdomen,* the picture may be clouded by the preponderance of symptoms distracting attention from the major injury (Fig. 88–1). For example, a tense or rigid abdomen may be present without serious abdominal injury; on the other hand, there may be instances of severe subdiaphragmatic injury in which the thoracic symptoms are unduly in evidence. Usually, however, the character of the injury presents sufficient evidence for proper evaluation and formulation of a treatment plan. Roentgenographic examination is of great assistance.

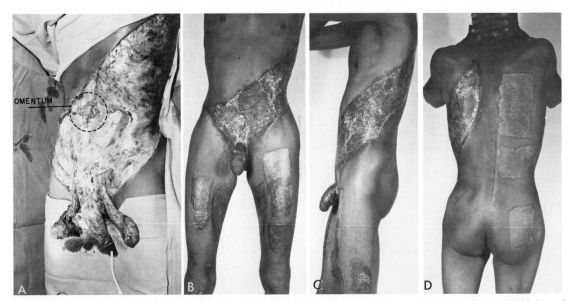

**FIGURE 88–1.** *A,* Photograph taken in the operating room, showing a 26 year old man with an extensive avulsing injury of the thorax, abdominal wall, and genitalia. The injury was received when the patient was caught by a hook in a conveyor belt, which fed him into large rollers. The rollers produced many fractured ribs, while the hooks caused the avulsion and a rupture of the abdominal wall with protrusion of the omentum and intestine.

The omentum was resected; the intestine was replaced; the traumatic dehiscence was repaired; the testes were implanted into subcutaneous pockets in the thighs; and five sheets of split-thickness skin grafts were applied to the denuded abdomen and genitalia. Five days later, six additional split-thickness skin grafts were applied to the upper abdomen, flank, and thorax. Postoperative photographs *B, C,* and *D* were taken six weeks after injury. The scrotum was reconstructed after the method of Baxter (1949) at a later date.

# RECONSTRUCTION OF CHEST WALL DEFECTS

The majority of thoracic wall defects are caused by surgical extirpation of primary or metastatic chest wall tumors, pulmonary or breast malignancies invading the chest wall, and radiation-induced ulcers. In most instances fear of not being able to reconstruct the chest wall should not prevent the surgeon from performing an adequate radical tumor excision. Likewise, when large dose radiation therapy is indicated, the radiotherapist should not be inhibited by the fear of causing postradiation changes which may require chest wall reconstruction. Fortunately, current regimens of radiation therapy have greatly reduced the incidence of radionecrosis so prevalent in earlier years from unscreened radium and low voltage radiation therapy.

**Preoperative Planning.** As in all reconstructive surgery, preoperative planning between the extirpative and reconstructive surgeons should establish the limits of resection necessary for adequate tumor ablation and optimal chest wall reconstruction. Resection of the chest wall beyond the limits of feasible reconstruction would obviously leave the patient doomed to a respiratory death. In planning chest wall reconstruction, the surgeons must consider the etiology of the defect. Small benign or low grade malignancies and minimal to moderate radiation tissue damage may result in a relatively minor defect where sufficient integumentary and bony structures remain, so that reconstruction can be effected by either wound coaptation, a local flap, or occasionally a skin graft. Invasive tumors and large or deep areas of radiation necrosis may produce a more extensive defect with only integumentary loss, only skeletal loss, a combination of integumentary and skeletal loss, and possibly associated diaphragmatic loss (Martini, Starzynski and Beattie, 1969). Closure of such a chest wall defect will therefore require a more involved operative procedure.

The two major goals of reconstructing chest wall defects are (1) to provide a permanent pleural seal when there is a full thickness chest wall defect, and (2) to provide chest wall stability to prevent significant paradoxical respiratory motion.

**Extent of Radiation Damage.** The extent of radiation damage is of major concern in determining the amount of chest wall to be resected or in planning the reconstruction of an area of chronic radionecrosis. Wide excision of all heavily irradiated tissue is mandatory to prevent poor healing between an adequately vascularized flap and the inadequately vascularized margins of the recipient bed (Routledge, 1954; Rintala, 1967) (Fig. 88–2). The host bed of irradiated areas is poorly vascularized and provides little nutrition to a flap designed and placed on its surface. Rees and Converse (1965) emphasized that it is not always possible to determine with accuracy the area of radiation damage preoperatively. It is only at the time of surgery, when active bleeding is observed, that one can be sure that the resection has been extended into an adequately vascularized area. Deep radiation changes with scarring and fibrosis of the pleura, lung, pericardium, or myocardium may occasionally be helpful in sealing the pleural space.

**Local Flaps.** Closure of the skin is the most important layer of closure. When there is an adequate amount of viable tissue available, a local flap is preferred for the closure of thoracic wall defects. A local rotation or advancement flap applied over the pleura, lung, or pericardium provides excellent coverage for small defects without mediastinal instability or significant paradoxical chest wall motion. Even following en bloc resection of two or three ribs and intercostal muscles with preservation of the pectoral muscles, subcutaneous tissue, and skin, there will be no significant paradoxical motion once stiffening and healing of the soft tissue flap has occurred (Groff and Adkins, 1967; Korlof, Nylén, Olsson, Skoog and Strombeck, 1973).

When possible, it is preferable to outline a local flap utilizing the best regional blood supply available and delay the flap for three weeks. A bipedicle flap will help ensure flap survival when such design is possible; however, a bipedicle flap is limited in its mobility. When the flap is transposed or rotated to postradiation avascular areas, it must survive on its own blood supply (Brown, Fryer and McDowell, 1951). The flap should also be sufficiently large to overlap into the adjacent vascularized areas after excision of the area of radiation damage.

Numerous local rotation flaps based on the lateral thoracic, internal mammary, acromiothoracic, or intercostal arteries can be designed, depending upon the defect to be corrected and the ingenuity of the surgeon (Figs. 88–3 and 88–4). Occasionally, radical reconstructive surgery is necessary. Starzynski, Snyderman, and Beattie (1969) described a technique of arm amputation and used a filleted arm flap in treat-

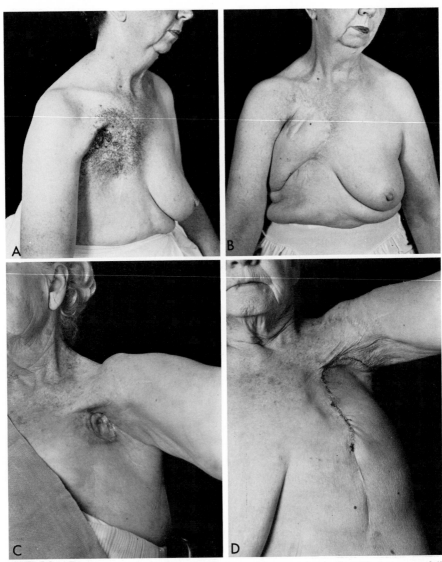

**FIGURE 88–2.** *A,* Extensive cutaneous postirradiation dermatitis occurring in the skin ten years following radical mastectomy and irradiation therapy. A large dorsal flap was elevated, and a sheet of Silastic was interposed beneath the flap to act as a separator or barrier. *B,* The entire area of involvement of the chest wall and axilla was excised, and the back flap was transferred to resurface the denuded area. Postoperative photograph taken three years later. *C,* A 75 year old woman with postirradiation ulceration and necrosis of the axilla. Portions of the second, third, fourth, and fifth ribs were resected, together with the underlying pleura. *D,* The area was resurfaced using a flap transferred from the back.

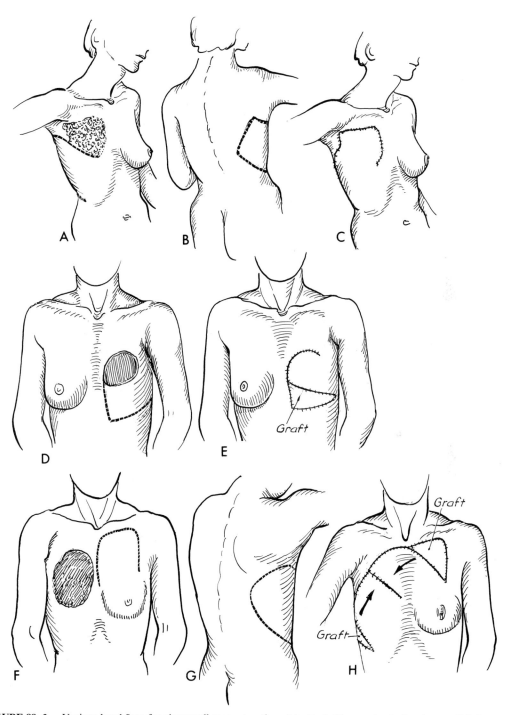

**FIGURE 88–3.** Various local flaps for chest wall reconstruction. *A to C,* Axillary and anterior chest wall defect covered by a dorsal flap. *D, E,* Anterior chest wall defect covered by a transposition flap. *F, G, H,* Large anterior chest wall defect covered by a dorsal and anterior chest wall transposition flap. Note that split-thickness skin grafts were used to cover the defect remaining after flap transposition.

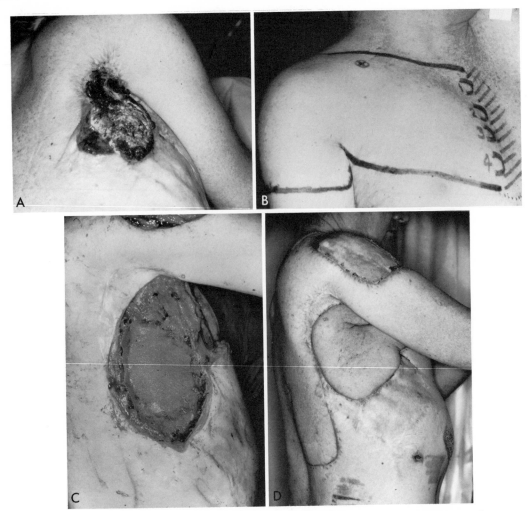

**FIGURE 88–4.** *A,* Recurrent squamous cell carcinoma in the posterolateral aspect of the thorax. Note the surrounding area of healed skin grafts, which necessitates the use of a distant flap. *B,* Outline of a deltopectoral flap with a paddle extension over the deltoid region. The latter was delayed as a preliminary procedure. *C,* Intraoperative view following full-thickness resection of the chest wall and insertion of a Marlex mesh. *D,* Appearance of the flap two weeks following surgery. A superiorly based dorsal flap which had been delayed was not used in the chest wall reconstruction. (Courtesy of Dr. Joseph G. McCarthy, Institute of Reconstructive Plastic Surgery).

ing two patients with chest wall radiation burns. The upper extremity of one of the patients was flail from previous surgical and irradiation treatment of breast carcinoma; the second patient's upper extremity was functional prior to being used to cover a major chest wall defect.

Applying the concept of preserving the axial vessels as in the deltopectoral flap (Bakamjian, Culf and Bales, 1967) and groin flap (McGregor and Jackson, 1972), Tai and Hasegawa (1974) described a medially based transverse abdominal flap incorporating the superior epigastric artery and vein. The length to width ratio of the flap may be 1 to 2.5 or less. The safe limit of the flap

laterally is the posterior axillary line unless the flap has been delayed. The long axis can be transverse or oblique according to the location of the defect. Undermining of the flap is usually done between the superficial and deep fascia unless there is a parietal pleural defect. For the latter problem, the deep fascia is removed with the flap to replace the resected pleura.

### Distant Flaps

GREATER OMENTUM. Dupont and Menard (1972) described extra-abdominal transposition of the greater omentum pedicled on the right or left gastroepiploic vessels (depending upon the site of the chest wall defect) to reconstruct areas of postradiation necrosis (Fig. 88–5). The omentum was sutured into the defect and covered with a split-thickness skin graft in a single operative procedure. In one of their patients, a defect of the third, fourth, and fifth right ribs was reconstructed with Marlex mesh, which in turn was covered by the greater omentum surfaced with a skin graft. Although the authors reported excellent results with this technique, more conventional flap coverage is preferred whenever possible.

THE BREAST FLAP. In females with one normal breast of adequate size, a flap can be constructed to close a chest wall defect, providing closure of the skin and intermediate layers as well (Fig. 88–6). Pickrell, Kelley, and Marzoni (1948), Rees and Converse (1965), Latham

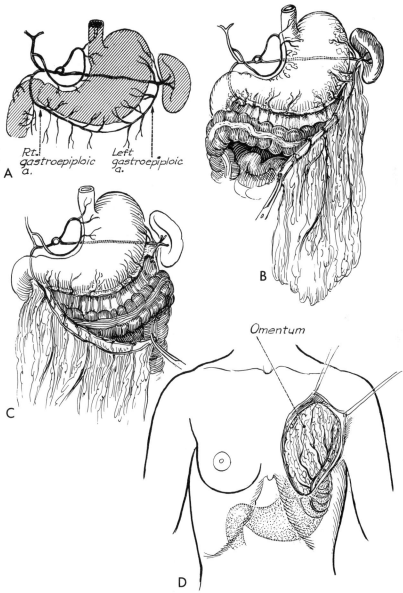

**FIGURE 88–5.** Closure of a chest wall defect with greater omentum. *A,* The main arterial supply of the greater omentum. *B, C,* Greater omentum can be pedicled on the right or left gastroepiploic artery, depending on the site of the defect to be closed. The omental flap is freed from the stomach at the muscularis layer in order to maintain the integrity of the vascular gastroepiploic arch. *D,* The greater omentum transferred to the thoracic defect through the superior portion of the abdominal wall incision or through a separate stab wound. A subcutaneous tunnel may be utilized to pass the omentum to the defect. (After Dupont, C., and Menard, Y.: Transposition of the greater omentum for reconstruction of the chest wall. Plast. Reconstr. Surg., *49:*263, 1972.)

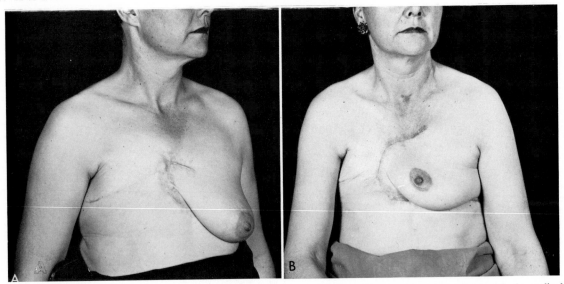

**FIGURE 88–6.** *A,* A recurrent carcinoma of the sternum and ribs in a 47 year old woman who had had a radical mastectomy one year previously. The patient had received a full course of irradiation postoperatively. An en bloc excision of the sternum and third, fourth, fifth, sixth, and seventh ribs was performed. The operative defect was covered and closed by transposing the left breast on a superior pedicle. *B,* Four years after operation.

(1966), and others have employed the entire breast rotated as a flap to cover large adjacent defects. Beardsley (1950) utilized a complete breast to cover a tantalum plate inserted to provide stability following resection of the sternum for sarcoma. Schepelman (1924), who is credited with first using the contralateral breast as a rotation flap, split the breast to gain additional flap width. Maier (1947), Urban (1951), Whalen (1953), and Rees and Converse (1965) have likewise reported success with this method.

When the breast is to be rotated to cover a defect, a flap can be filleted from the breast tissue, or the gland can be rotated as a compound flap to supply additional bulk. An incision is made transversely across the anterior chest along the inframammary crease and extended into the axilla (Fig. 88–7). The breast is elevated at the level of the prepectoral fascia and undermined widely, care being taken to preserve a superior lateral pedicle containing the acromiothoracic and lateral thoracic arterial branches. A split-thickness skin graft repairs the secondary defect resulting from medial rotation of the flap and avoids tension on the suture line with the attendant risk of vascular compromise of the flap.

The extra flap width provided by dividing the breast is frequently advantageous (Figs. 88–8 and 88–9, *A, B*). The technique employs the transverse inframammary fold incision, with a vertical incision dividing the breast either ob-

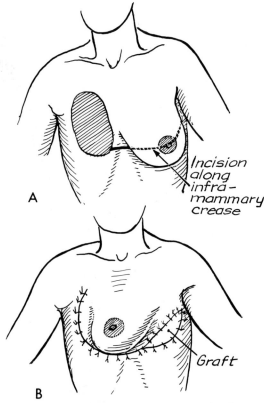

**FIGURE 88–7.** Reconstruction of an anterior chest wall defect by rotation of the contralateral breast. A generous superior pedicle containing the lateral thoracic arterial branches is preserved. A split-thickness skin graft is used to repair the lateral defect produced by rotation of the breast.

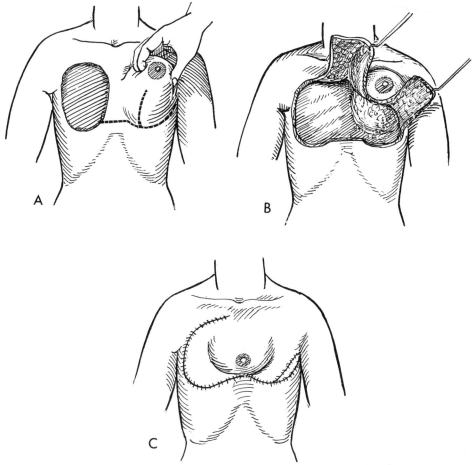

**FIGURE 88–8.** Technique of partially splitting the contralateral breast in order to provide extra flap surface area. Additional flap width is gained at the expense of length. A skin graft is used lateral to the flap to prevent tension on the suture line. (After Rees, T., and Converse, J.: Surgical reconstruction of defects of the thoracic wall. Surg. Gynecol. Obstet., *121*:1066, 1965.)

liquely or vertically in the midline, depending upon the defect to be closed. The vertical incision extends up to the areola, circumferentially around the areola, and then in a superior direction. The areola and nipple can be removed or retained if additional tissue is needed (Whalen, 1953). A branch of the internal mammary artery supplies the medial section of the breast, and the lateral portion is supplied by the lateral thoracic artery (Maliniac, 1943). A local transposition flap can be used in addition to the breast flap for coverage of large defects (Fig. 88–9, *C, D*).

OTHER FLAPS. When the contralateral breast is inadequate or the tissue is unsuitable for a local flap, a more innovative technique is required. A tubed thoracoabdominal flap can be "walked up" to the area of the defect or planned defect (Fig. 88–10). This, of course, will require several operative procedures to tube the flap and migrate it to the recipient area (Rees, 1961).

Converse, Campbell, and Watson (1951) described a large jump flap carried from the abdomen on the forearm to cover a large postradiation defect with exposure of the underlying pericardium (Fig. 88–11).

The technique of microvascular free flaps will also find application in chest wall reconstruction (see Chapter 14).

**Closure of the Pleural Space.** Permanent closure of the pleural space is mandatory. Use of flaps of parietal pleura, muscle, and pericardium in combination with split-thickness skin grafts has been described, but these methods produce an unstable chest wall with inadequate coverage

*Text continued on page 3621*

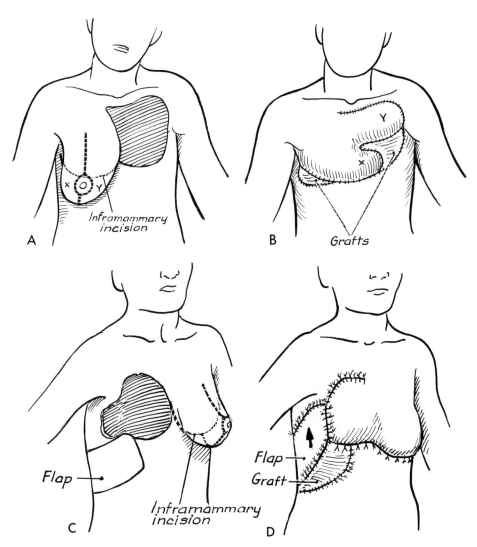

**FIGURE 88–9.**  *A, B,* Complete split breast flap technique with cleavage of the breast extending from the infra-mammary crease to the superior limit of breast tissue. The nipple in this case has been discarded, but it can be retained if additional tissue is needed. This technique provides the largest amount of readily available tissue for defect closure. *C, D,* The complete split breast technique used in conjunction with a local transposition flap to close a defect of the anterior thoracic wall with extension into the axilla. (After Whalen, W. P.: Coverage of thoracic wall defects by a split breast flap. Plast. Reconstr. Surg., *12*:64, 1953.)

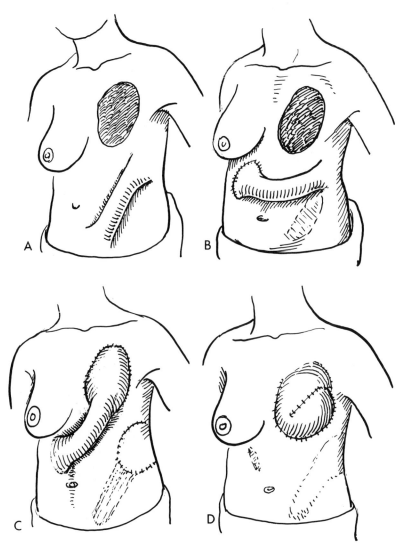

**FIGURE 88–10.** A full thickness defect of the anterior chest wall with exposed pericardium. *A,* Construction of a thoracoabdominal tube. *B,* Inferior end of tube migrated to the epigastrium. *C,* Lateral tube attachment migrated to the defect. *D,* Inferior inset of tube transposed to the area of the defect. (After Rees, T. D.: Radiation necrosis of the chest wall, full-thickness reconstruction with pedicle flap and diced homologous cartilage over the pericardium complicated by cardiac arrest. Plast. Reconstr. Surg., *28*:67, 1961.)

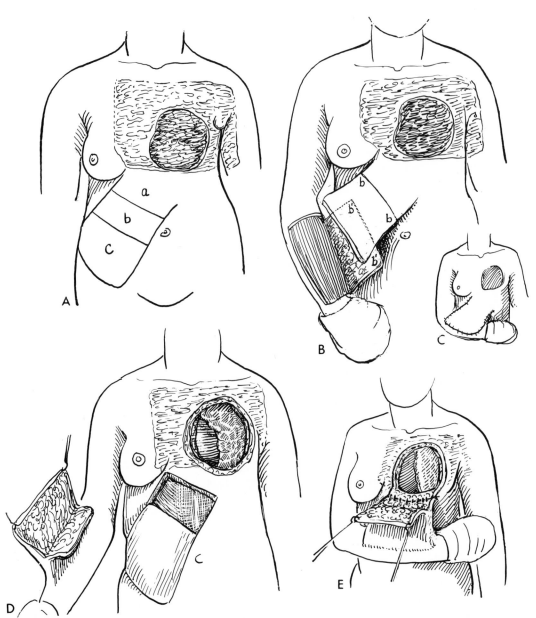

**FIGURE 88–11.**    The closed carried flap for closure of a thoracic defect. *A,* Chest wall defect, pericardium exposed. The shaded area represents the scarred, previously irradiated skin. Flap outlined. Portion *a* will remain attached to the abdomen; portion *b* is the intermediary part of the flap; portion *c* will be attached to the forearm. *B,* The abdominal and hinge forearm flaps are raised and are in position for suturing. *C,* The closed carried flap established. A split-thickness skin graft is used to cover the secondary abdominal wall defect after elevation of the flap. *D,* Devitalized tissue excised, exposing the pericardium and the lung. The proximal end of the flap is detached from the abdomen. *E,* The distal end of the forearm flap sutured to the inferior end of the thoracic wall defect.

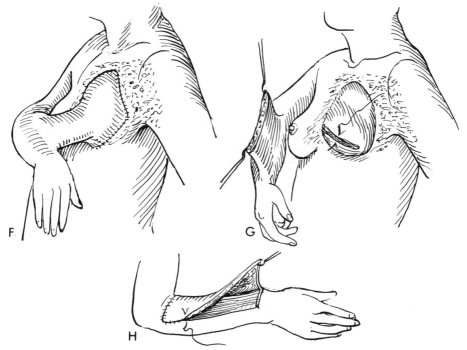

**FIGURE 88–11** *Continued.* *F,* Suture of the flap to the thoracic defect completed. *G,* The flap cut from its attachment to the chest. *H,* The forearm flap returned to its original position. (From Converse, J., Campbell, R., and Watson, W.: Repair of ulcers situated over the heart and brain. Ann. Surg., *133*:95, 1951.)

of the underlying viscera (Heuer, 1932; Pickrell, Baker and Collins, 1947; Campbell, 1950) (Fig. 88–12). In earlier years, integrity of the pleural space was maintained by staged chest wall resection, so as to produce adhesions of the lung to the edges of the planned surgical defect prior to extirpative surgery (Heblom, 1933; Nathan, Kingsley and Paulson, 1971). Closure of the pleural space by suturing the fibrous pericardium to the adjacent chest wall defect, or obliteration of the pleural space by suturing the visceral pleura to the wound margins is not recommended.

Decompression of the pleural space by underwater seal drainage with associated positive pressure mechanical ventilatory assistance, when necessary, is the current method of choice for sealing the pleural space. However, when a flap is used to reconstruct the defect, the application of suction to such a pleural drain is not advised, since it may perpetuate a pleural leak around the margins of the flap (Lister and Gibson, 1973).

Closure of the pleural cavity and stabilization of the chest wall using fascia lata sutured to the edge of the parietal pleural defect have received a great deal of support (Winkel, 1935; Southwick, Economou and Otten, 1956) and have been frequently used for closure of defects following resection of the internal mammary lymph nodes in association with a radical mastectomy (Urban and Baker, 1952). Watson and James (1947) noted the advantages of fascia lata: (1) it eliminates the need for a foreign body if the surgeon feels closure of the chest wall at the pleural level is indicated; (2) it is readily available; (3) it makes the wound airtight; (4) it adds support; and (5) it is firm enough to prevent a postoperative pulmonary herniation.

Dunavant (1955) reported successful closure of a chest wall defect with a full-thickness skin graft. Pickrell, Baker, and Collins (1947) and Vianna (1952) utilized sliding skin flaps to close defects created by mammary carcinoma extirpation.

Tamoney and Stent (1964) advocated autogenous dermal grafts to close the pleural cavity because (1) a dermal graft is relatively easy to obtain in large quantities; (2) it does not compromise the primary surgical procedure; (3) it is easy to handle; (4) it lacks antigenicity or

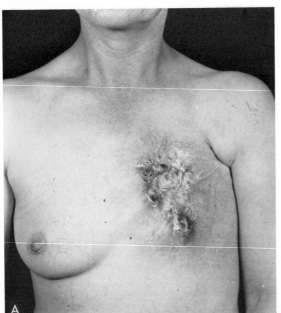

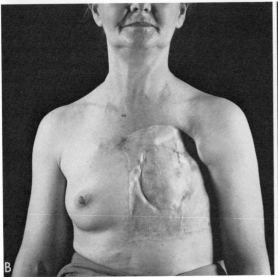

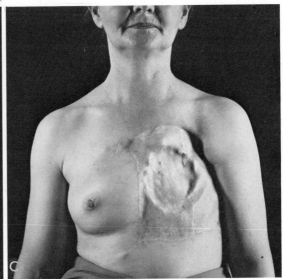

**FIGURE 88–12.** *A*, A large, recurrent carcinoma of the chest wall following radical mastectomy and irradiation therapy. The patient could not tolerate additional irradiation. The lesion was widely excised, together with the underlying ribs and sternum. Split-thickness skin grafts were applied directly to the pericardium and chest wall. *B*, Position of the graft-covered pericardium in forced expiration. *C*, The grafted pericardium is drawn inward at the beginning of inspiration. Photographs *B* and *C* were taken more than three years after operation.

carcinogenicity; and (5) it will withstand infection or loss of overlying tissue.

When the deep layer has been closed by fascia lata, dermis, or suturing of the pleura to the wound edges, an overlying stabilizing or filler layer may be necessary with large defects. Campbell (1950) and Southwick and his associates (1956) used a latissimus dorsi muscle flap with its primary blood and nerve supply preserved to cover such a thoracic wall defect (Fig. 88–13). When a bronchial fistula accompanies a chest wall defect, closure may be extremely difficult. The fistula must be closed first (Figs. 88–14 and 88–15).

**The Rib as a Stabilizing Factor.** Flaps of ribs (Janes, 1939), periosteum (Blades and Paul, 1950), or both have been advocated to provide chest wall stabilization. Economou, Southwick, and Slaughter (1961) described and utilized a method of autogenous sliding rib grafts to provide chest wall stability. Pers and Medgyesi (1973) have described transposition of a part of the serratus anterior muscle with three split ribs attached to cover a full thickness chest wall defect (Fig. 88–16). The pleura was not replaced, and the muscle rib transplant was covered by a large local skin flap.

Brodkin and Peer (1958) advocated diced autogenous or homologous cartilage supported on tantalum mesh to stabilize the chest wall. Rees (1961) utilized diced homologous cartilage grafts just beneath the skin flap in order to provide a fibrocartilaginous shield over the underlying pericardium.

Maier (1947) advocated grafts of periosteum with or without attached segments of rib or cartilage. Mauer and Blades (1946) reported that they obtained the best results with rib, periosteum, and muscle. They described closure of defects by cutting ribs tangentially at the edge of the chest wall defect, with the ribs then

*Text continued on page 3627*

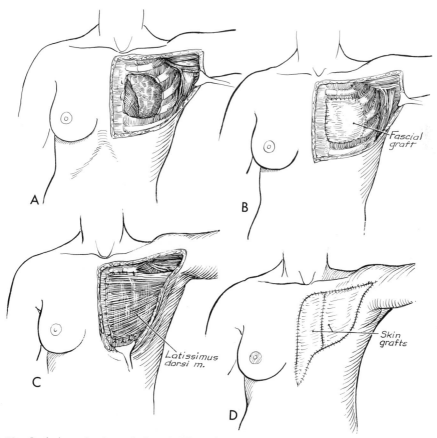

**FIGURE 88–13.** Latissimus dorsi muscle flap. *A,* Thoracic defect after resection of a three-rib segment of the anterior chest wall. *B,* Fascia lata sutured to the edges of the defect. *C,* Latissimus dorsi transplanted with its primary nerve and blood supply preserved. *D,* Split-thickness skin grafts placed on the muscle to complete the procedure. (After Campbell, D.: Reconstruction of the anterior thoracic wall. J. Thorac. Surg., *19:*456, 1950.)

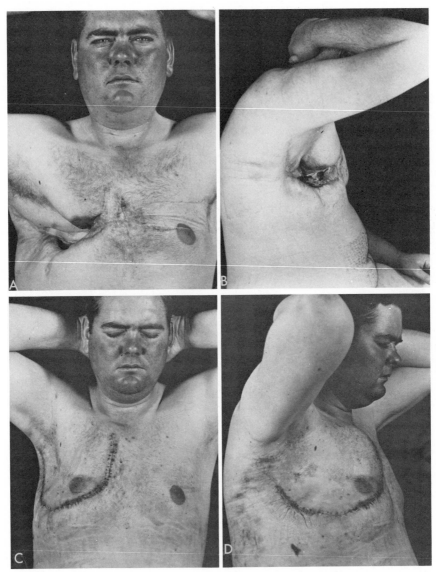

**FIGURE 88–14.** *A, B,* A 26 year old man with a severe deformity of the chest and a bronchial fistula following a penetrating wound of the right chest five years previously. It was impossible for the patient to go swimming and even dangerous to take a tub bath. Four attempts to close the defect had been unsuccessful. The bronchial fistula was closed, and a pectoral muscle flap was transposed to fill the defect. *C, D,* Primary healing occurred, and the patient was discharged on the eleventh postoperative day.

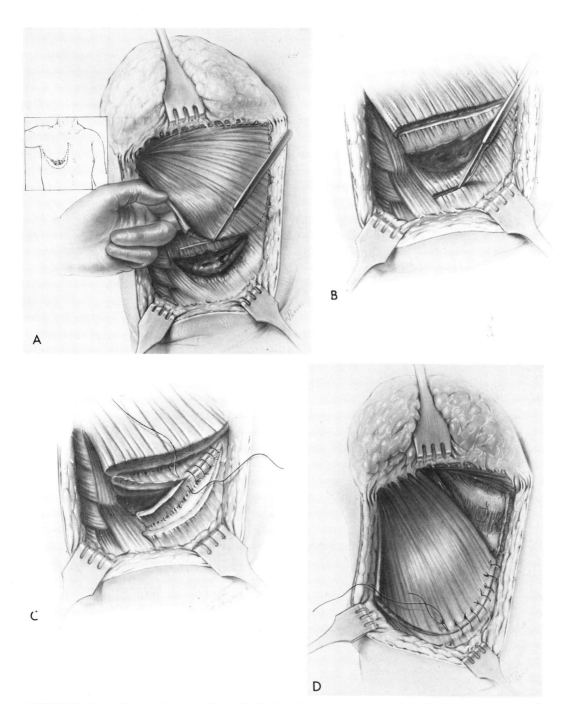

**FIGURE 88–15.** *A,* Same patient as in Figure 88–14. Inset shows the horseshoe-shaped incisions used to excise the scars resulting from the previous operations. A large skin and subcutaneous tissue flap was mobilized superiorly to the clavicle. The pectoralis major was incised beginning about 3 cm above the superior border of the pulmonary cavity and continued upward, as shown by the dotted line, along the right lateral border of the sternum; the clavicular attachment was freed superiorly. *B,* The pectoralis was incised about 3 cm above and below the margins of the pulmonary cavity. The bronchial fistula was closed using interrupted sutures of chromic catgut. The short muscle flaps were mobilized toward each other to obliterate the cavity. *C,* The muscle flaps were approximated using interrupted silk sutures. *D,* The pectoral muscle flap was transposed laterally and inferiorly in order to obtain the necessary length to cover completely and reinforce the first line of sutures. The flap was anchored in its new position to the originally incised inferior muscle margin. The skin and subcutaneous tissue flap was sutured to the inferior incised margin with interrupted silk sutures in layers.

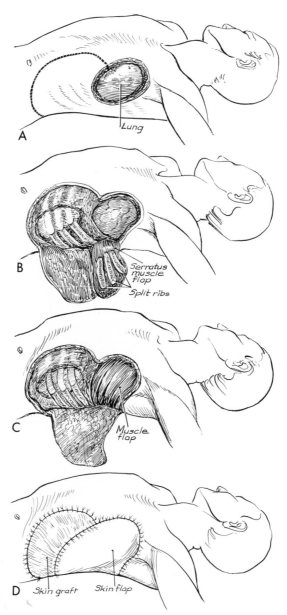

**FIGURE 88–16.**   Muscle-rib flap closure of a lateral thoracic defect. *A,* Defect with exposed lung. *B,* Serratus muscle–split rib flap developed. *C,* Muscle-rib flap closing the thoracic defect. *D,* Large local skin flap used to cover the muscle-rib flap. (After Pers, M., and Medgyesi, S.: Pedicle muscle flaps and their applications in the surgery of repair. Br. J. Plast. Surg., *26*:313, 1973.)

displaced up or down and fixed to an adjacent rib (Fig. 88–17). Prioleau (1945) described closure of a 10 × 10 cm anterior, precordial, full thickness chest wall defect by paravertebral thoracoplasty and a sliding full thickness flap of chest wall.

**Prosthetic Implants.** Numerous inorganic materials, including tantalum plates (Beardsley, 1950), tantalum mesh (Morrow, 1950), stainless steel mesh (Stephenson and Mosley, 1956),

Teflon (Hardin and Harrison, 1957), Lucite (Hardin, Kittle and Schafer, 1952), fiberglass cloth (Hardin and Kittle, 1956), Ivalon (Fitch and Fries, 1958), polymethylmethacrylate (LeRoux, 1964), and Marlex polyethylene (Usher, 1961), have been used to provide chest wall closure, stabilization, and reconstruction. All of these prostheses must, of course, be covered by a soft tissue flap. The main complications associated with these implants have been infection, migration, fragmentation, and extru-

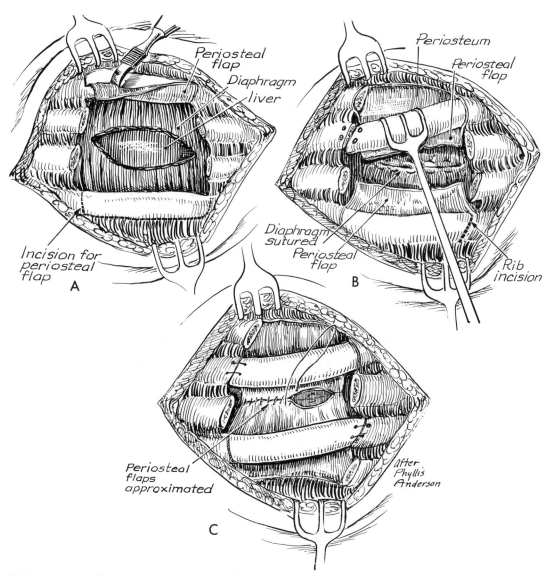

**FIGURE 88–17.** Rib and periosteal flap closure of thoracic defects. *A,* Full thickness chest wall defect. Periosteum being elevated from the ribs for periosteal flaps. *B,* Rib cut tangentially and displaced to the cut end of the adjacent rib. Drill holes placed through the cut ends of the ribs for suture stabilization. *C,* Periosteal flaps approximated under tension over the chest wall defect. The displaced ribs are secured to the tangentially cut ends by chromic catgut sutures. (After Mauer, E., and Blades, B.: Hernia of the lung. J. Thorac. Surg., *15*:77, 1946.)

sion. Marlex mesh (Graham, Usher, Perry and Barkley, 1960) has given the most favorable long-term results, as it has high tensile strength, elicits little foreign body reaction, and is readily incorporated into the chest wall by infiltration of fibrous tissue through its interstices. Leininger, Barker, and Langston (1972) described the building of a horizontal and vertical latticework of synthetic sutures placed in such a fashion as to bridge the skeletal defect of the chest wall. Extracostal muscle flaps were then used to cover the latticework chest wall.

The authors limit the use of inorganic implants to patients with massive defects or to critically ill patients in whom only temporary thoracic wall stability is indicated. Autogenous living tissue is preferred to close chest wall defects whenever possible.

## RECONSTRUCTION OF STERNAL DEFECTS

Most defects of the anterior midline of the chest wall are secondary to primary or metastatic tumors, post-thoracotomy wound infections, which occasionally result in sternal dehiscence, and trauma. Rarely do patients sustaining trauma of such magnitude survive to require the services of the reconstructive surgeon.

Tumors of the sternum are relatively uncommon; when present, they are usually malignant (Groff and Adkins, 1967; Martini, Starzynski and Beattie, 1974). Metastatic carcinomas from the breast and kidney are the most frequent sternal tumors (Heuer, 1932; Kinsella, White and Koucky, 1947; Griswold, 1947). Primary sternal tumors are almost always malignant. The vast majority are chondrosarcomas and osteogenic sarcomas. The other primary sternal tumors are mainly tumors of reticuloendothelial origin—Ewing's sarcoma, myelomas, and lymphomas. Benign primary sternal tumors are rare but do occur—chondromas, osteochondromas, eosinophilic granulomas, aneurysmal bone cysts. The majority of sternal tumors, particularly primary tumors, require radical resection including the adjacent chest wall. Such resections may produce significant chest wall instability and pulmonary complications. The magnitude of the reconstructive procedure obviously will depend upon the extent of the resection.

The anterior sagittal sternum is analogous to the tie beam in a common gable roof (Starzynski, Snyderman and Beattie, 1969). The entire sternal body and all four sternebrae (including the second through seventh costal cartilages) may be resected, including the lower half of the manubrium if the first costal arches and clavicles remain joined to the manubrium (Fig. 88–18). The defect can be reconstructed, but tracheostomy and assisted ventilation frequently will be necessary immediately following such extensive resection. Although the respiratory deficit is moderately severe, adequate respiration can be expected with the help of the accessory respiratory muscles above and the intercostal, the pectoralis major and minor, and the serratus anterior muscles inferiorly and laterally. A defect involving loss of the upper portion of the sternum and the first to the fifth costal cartilages, the ribs, clavicles, and manubrium produces a significant

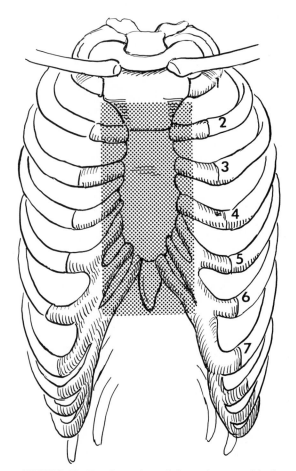

**FIGURE 88–18.** Resection of the entire sternal body, lower half of the manubrium, and the second through the seventh costal cartilages. The articulation of the first rib with the manubrium, which is the most stable of the costal arches, is retained. The sternocleidomastoid and scalene muscles, in addition to the pectoralis, intercostal, and serratus anterior muscles, remain functionally intact.

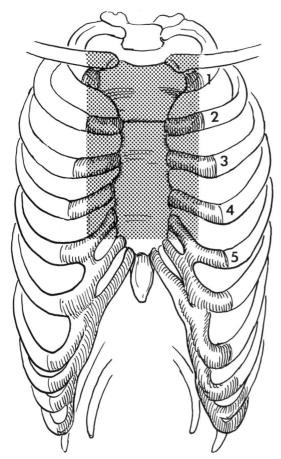

**FIGURE 88–19.** Resection of the upper sternum, clavicle, manubrium, and first through fifth costal cartilages leaves only the sixth and seventh costal cartilages attached to the median tie-beam. The function of the upper anterior accessory muscles of respiration is completely lost. Although the remaining respiratory muscles are surprisingly efficient, the morbidity from respiratory insufficiency with this type of resection is high. A stable reconstruction is difficult.

anatomical and respiratory deficit (Fig. 88–19). The only continuity in such a defect is maintained by the sixth and seventh costal arches joined to the fourth sternebrae. Reconstruction is feasible; however, the respiratory deficit is severe and requires long periods of artificial ventilation with associated high morbidity and mortality rates.

Holden in 1878 described resection of a portion of the sternum for sarcoma. Richardson (1913) reported resection of the manubrium and medial ends of the clavicles for an enchondroma. The bony defect was covered by approximation of the pectoralis fascia. Heuer (1932) resected the lower two-thirds of the sternum, approximated the pectorialis muscle fascia in the midline, and fashioned an external cardboard breastplate to help reduce the paradoxical motion of the anterior chest wall. Small local resections, curettage, cauterization, and radiation therapy were the principal modes of treatment of sternal tumors until modern methods of anesthesia and positive pressure ventilatory support were developed.

Kinsella, White and Koucky (1947) resected the entire gladiolus and the inferior portion of the manubrium and clavicles *en bloc* to treat a sternal giant cell tumor. The sternal defect was reconstructed by using tibial bone graft struts arranged in a ladder configuration, with the spaces between the struts filled with bone chips lying on a sheet of fascia lata sutured to the edge of the thoracic wall defect (Fig. 88–20).

Griswold (1947) divided the sternum at the junction of the body and the manubrium, resected the third, fourth, fifth, sixth, and seventh costal cartilages bilaterally, and obtained satisfactory postoperative chest wall stabilization

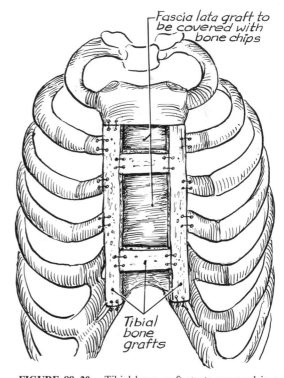

**FIGURE 88–20.** Tibial bone graft struts arranged in a ladder configuration to stabilize the anterior chest wall. Soft tissue flaps including pectoral muscles were approximated in the midline to close the wound. (After Kinsella, T., White, S., and Koucky, R.: Two unusual tumors of the sternum. J. Thorac. Surg., *16*:640, 1947.)

with a tantalum plate. Bone grafts for sternal reconstruction are subjected to constant to-and-fro motion and are often absorbed when placed in the older debilitated patient. A tantalum plate for midline chest wall reconstruction has also been advocated.

Bisgard and Swenson (1948) resected the gladiolus and the costal cartilages of ribs three, four, and five bilaterally for a round cell sarcoma. A portion of the right seventh rib was removed and sectioned to construct three rib grafts, which were mortized into the transected ends of ribs three, four, and five (Fig. 88–21).

Myre and Kirkland (1956) suggested that bone grafts and prosthetic materials were not necessary to stabilize the chest wall following subtotal resection of the sternum and a portion of the attached costal cartilages. These authors strongly advocated that the defects be covered by pectoralis fascia, subcutaneous tissue, and skin which would be stiffened by the ingrowth of fibrous tissue with limitation of paradoxical motion.

**Total Resection of the Sternum.** Brodkin and Linden (1959) resected a chondrosarcoma and reported the first known case of total resection of the entire sternum in one stage for malignant disease. Stabilization of the chest wall was obtained by a plate of iliac bone wired to the clavicles and first ribs. The lower remaining ribs were stabilized by skin strips placed vertically between contiguous ribs and horizontally between adjacent ribs. Tension on the skin strips diminished during the postoperative period, resulting in unsatisfactory stability of the lower chest wall.

Baue (1963) reported the first case of total resection of the sternum in the United States. The patient, a 62 year old female, had metastatic follicular adenocarcinoma of the thyroid with a large mass overlying the manubrium and body of the sternum accompanied by invasion of the sternum. The primary tumor had been treated by total thyroidectomy two years earlier. A sheet of Marlex mesh was cut to fit the surgical defect, sutured to the ribs and intercostal muscles, and covered by dissecting and approximating the pectoralis major muscles in the midline (Fig. 88–22). The author reported that even in the immediate postoperative period there was no paradoxical motion. Arnold, Meese, D'Amato and Maughon (1966) performed a total sternectomy for localized Hodgkin's disease which originated in the right internal mammary lymph node chain and appeared as a primary sternal tumor. The chest wall opening was covered with Marlex mesh in the manner described by Baue (1963).

Larson, Lick, and Maxeiner (1969) resected a sternal chondrosarcoma *en bloc,* including the manubrium, medial clavicles, and sternum down to the level of the fifth intercostal space. A large sheet of fascia lata was sutured in place under tension to cover the defect; a rib strut was placed obliquely across the defect superficial to the fascia lata and wired above to the left second rib and below to the right fifth rib. Bone chips were placed on the surface of the fascia lata, and the pectoralis muscle fascia was approximated in the midline (Fig. 88–23). Alonso-Lej and deLinera (1971) resected the entire sternum, the medial third of both clavicles, the costal cartilages, and the anterior end of the first five ribs bilaterally to remove a chondromyxoid

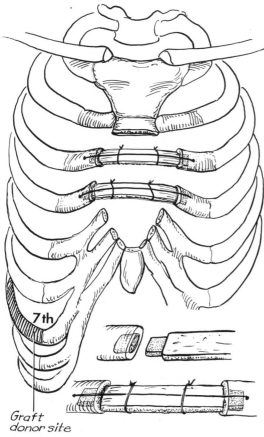

7th

Graft
donor site

**FIGURE 88–21.** Bony continuity of the thoracic cage reestablished by seventh rib bone grafts mortised into the medial ends of the transected ribs. More than one rib can be used as a graft donor site if necessary. (After Bisgard, J., and Swenson, S.: Tumors of the sternum: Report of a case with special operative technique. Arch. Surg., *56*:570, 1948.)

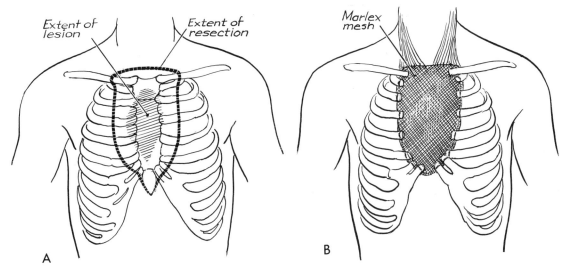

**FIGURE 88-22.** Reconstruction following total resection of the sternum. *A,* The extent of the total sternal resection. *B,* Reconstruction was accomplished with Marlex mesh sutured to the margins of the defect and covered with the pectoralis muscles approximated in the midline. (After Baue, A.: Total resection of the sternum. J. Thorac. Cardiovasc. Surg., *45*:559, 1963.)

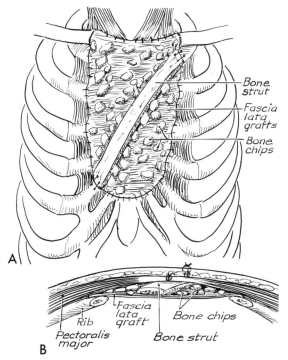

**FIGURE 88-23.** Technique of reconstruction following resection of the entire manubrium, clavicles, gladiolus, and costal cartilages down to the fifth intercostal space. *A,* Fascia lata seals the mediastinum, the rib bone strut gives stability, and the bone chips potentially allow regrowth of an anterior bony shield. *B,* Cross section shows the midline approximation of the pectoralis fascia. (After Larson, R., Lick, L., and Maxeiner, S.: Technique for chest wall reconstruction following sternal chondrosarcoma. Arch. Surg., *98*:668, 1969.)

fibroma. Reconstruction of the surgical defect was performed with Marlex mesh, acrylic resin, and flaps of pectoralis muscles.

Frøysaker and Hall (1970) reported excellent results in three patients after subtotal sternal resection using a modification of the techniques of Kinsella, White, and Koucky (1947) and Larson, Lick, and Maxeiner (1969). Fascia lata or Dacron mesh was sutured to the edge of the defect; transverse rib grafts were placed between adjacent ribs; bone chips were placed on the fascia lata or Dacron mesh, and a superficial layer of fascia lata or Dacron mesh was placed over the rib grafts and bone chips (Fig. 88-24). Longacre, Maurer, and Keirle (1974) reported reconstruction of a large anterior midline chest wall defect by suturing a synthetic mesh, Mylar, to the edges of the pleural opening and then fashioning a "new sternum" with split rib grafts wired to horizontally placed split rib grafts for stability.

Martini and associates (1974) reported wide surgical excision of primary malignant tumors of the sternum in eight patients. These authors suggested that, unless the entire sternum is involved by tumor, a part of the sternum with its attachments to the remaining rib cage should be preserved to reduce postoperative paradoxical motion. Ox fascia and Marlex mesh were the preferred materials for obliteration of bony defects produced by resection. The decision to leave a portion of a sternum involved with a malignant tumor must be carefully evaluated.

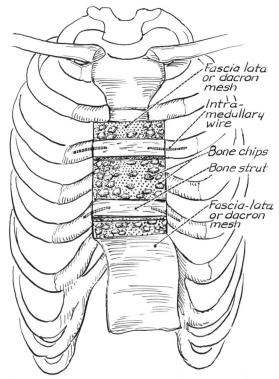

Fascia lata
or dacron
mesh

Intra-
medullary
wire

Bone chips

Bone strut

Fascia-lata
or dacron
mesh

**FIGURE 88–24.** Technique of sternal reconstruction utilizing anterior and posterior layers of fascia lata or Dacron mesh with the rib strut supported by intramedullary wires. (After Frøysaker, T., and Hall, K.: Reconstruction of the chest wall. Scand. J. Thorac. Cardiovasc. Surg., 4:183, 1970.)

## STERNAL DEHISCENCE

Milton described the median sternotomy in 1897; however, it was not until Gibbons (1954) developed successful total cardiopulmonary bypass, allowing open cardiac surgery to "become of age," that this rather simple and excellent exposure of the heart and great vessels became popular. Complications following this incision can be disastrous.

Infection of a median sternotomy wound requires emergency treatment. Cardiac surgery patients are particularly in danger because of the potential secondary infection of suture lines of the great vessels, prosthetic grafts of the great vessels, or intracardiac prostheses. Superficial wound infection may be treated by drainage, debridement, and parenteral administration of antibiotics. Infection extending into the anterior mediastinum may occasionally be treated with tube drainage, parenteral administration of anti-

biotics, and irrigation of the wound with antibiotic solution. Ineffective control of the infection by this conservative method will necessitate reopening the sternum for adequate drainage and debridement (Jiminez-Martinez, Arguero-Sanchez, Perez-Alvarez, and Mina-Castanada, 1970; Bryant, Spencer and Trinkle, 1969). Sternal osteomyelitis, requiring resection of the involved portion of the sternum, may occur following such a wound infection.

Brown and associates (1969) reviewed 748 patients, and Sanfelippo and Danielson (1972a) reviewed 272 patients on whom median sternotomies had been performed. In both series major wound dehiscence (separation of all layers of the wound requiring surgical closure) was related to reopening of the incision for hemorrhage, external cardiac massage for cardiac arrest, postoperative positive pressure ventilation, and tracheostomy. A properly performed median sternotomy should split the sternum precisely in the midline without fracture of either side. There should be minimal insertion of foreign bodies (bone, wax, hemostatic agents, and nonabsorbable sutures). Hemostasis should be complete, and the wound should be closed with firm sternal approximation. Failure to adhere to these technical considerations is frequently associated with early wound dehiscence. Disruption of the sternum following closure by stainless steel wires with the latter cutting through the bone is well known. Lambert, Mitchel, Adam and Skiekh (1971) and Taber and Madaras (1969) have described methods of closure of the sternum designed to prevent this complication with wire sutures.

Peristernal nylon bands applied and tightened with a special tie gun have been advocated for sternal closure (LeVeen and Piccone, 1968). Sanfelippo and Danielson (1972b) reviewed a series of 55 patients closed by this method and found the complication rate prohibitive. These authors advocate stainless steel wire as the suture of choice for closure of median sternotomies.

Sternal dehiscence requires immediate surgical closure, preferably utilizing interrupted peristernal surgical wires in adults and nonabsorbable synthetic sutures in small children to provide chest wall stabilization. Occasionally an infected wound may be allowed to granulate or heal by secondary intention by applying a chest binder to provide chest wall stability if the pleural spaces remain sealed. When a significant portion of the sternum is lost, one of the methods of reconstruction described earlier will be necessary.

## CHEST WALL DEHISCENCE

Disruption of chest wall closures following thoracotomy allows free communication of the pleural cavity with a potential large space between the overlying musculature and the subcutaneous space when soft tissue continuity remains intact. When there is concomitant soft tissue dehiscence, there is obviously free contact of the pleural space with the external environment. The physiologic deficit associated with paradoxical motion of the chest wall, pneumothorax, and occasionally extension of the lung out of the pleural space are obvious (Gorlin, Knowles and Storey, 1957; Gibbons, 1962).

The high morbidity associated with this complication is in part related to delay in diagnosis and treatment. Boyd, Gonzalez, and Altemeier (1966) noted that frequently the factors causing a delayed diagnosis are failure of the physician to think of the diagnosis and camouflage of the underlying defect by continuity of the overlying soft tissues or a large bulky dressing, preventing recognition of the paradoxical chest wall motion. Primary wound infection as a cause of disruption of lateral thoracotomies is unusual. However, an empyema resulting from exposure of the pleural cavity to the contaminated environment is a real possibility.

Prevention is the obvious best treatment. Boyd, Gonzalez, and Altemeier (1966) showed that closure of an intercostal thoracotomy in young patients by closely spaced, pericostal, heavy chromic catgut sutures is feasible. In older patients who undergo resection of a rib, because of a more rigid and brittle chest wall, heavy nonabsorbable sutures in addition to heavy chromic catgut pericostal sutures should be used to approximate the periosteum of the resected rib bed.

When a dehiscence is diagnosed, early secondary wound closure is mandatory. Ribs should be approximated with a nonreactive, nonabsorbable suture, preferably stainless steel, and the muscle and fascia layers closed with catgut. There is no place for wound packing in a thoracotomy dehiscence following a primary thoracotomy closure.

## PECTUS EXCAVATUM

Pectus excavatum (funnel chest) is a depression of the anterior chest wall involving the sternum and costal cartilages beginning at, or inferior to, the manubriogladiolar junction and extending to the xiphoid process. Most often posterior angulation of the sternum begins at its junction with the manubrium, and the narrowest vertebrosternal distance is at the level of the xiphisternal junction (Figs. 88–25 through 88–28). Occasionally, the deformity is so severe that the sternum reaches the vertebral bodies, or the sternum may actually pass to one side of the vertebral bodies into the paravertebral gutter (Ravitch, 1951).

Pectus excavatum is usually noted soon after birth. The rate and degree of progression is inconstant. In some patients the deformity is not noticed at birth and becomes obvious only some months later. Occasionally, an older patient may report that the deformity became obvious only in early adolescence. When the deformity progresses beyond the adolescent years, it is characteristically associated with lumbodorsal scoliosis, slumped shoulders, and a protruding abdomen.

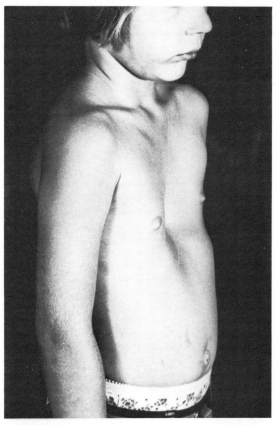

**FIGURE 88–25.** Pectus excavatum deformity beginning at the level of the manubriosternal junction. The narrowest vertebrosternal distance is at the level of the xiphisternal junction. (Courtesy of Dr. Mark M. Ravitch, Pittsburgh, Pennsylvania.)

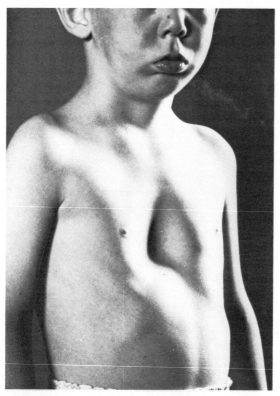

**FIGURE 88–26.** Pectus excavatum deformity beginning at the level of the second costochondral junction. (Courtesy of Dr. Mark M. Ravitch, Pittsburgh, Pennsylvania.)

Numerous suggestions as to the etiology of pectus excavatum have been made: arrested development of the sternum, nutritional disturbances and developmental retardation, failure of ossification of the lower sternum, aplasia of the sternum, congenitally short rectus muscles, mediastinal tumors, mediastinitis, pressure on the anterior chest wall in utero, birth injuries, hereditary syphilis, fibrous bands at the lower end of the sternum, muscular pull of the diaphragm, and shortened central tendon of the diaphragm (Ebstein, 1882; Féré and Schmid, 1893; Troisier and Monnerot-Dumaine, 1930; Nageotte-Wilbouchewitch, 1935; Ochsner and DeBakey, 1939; Lindskog and Felton, 1955; Fish and coworkers, 1954). The present concepts most readily accepted are related to overgrowth of the costal cartilages forcing the sternum posteriorly (Hausmann, 1955). Overgrowth of the costal cartilages with protrusion of the sternum would explain the occurrence of pectus excavatum and pectus carinatum in different members of the same family (Sweet, 1944; Becker and Schneider, 1962). Whatever the etiology, it is currently accepted that the involved cartilages must be excised in order to correct the deformity (Haller, Peters, Mazur and White, 1970).

**Etiology.** The etiology of the deformity is unknown, and little is understood about its pathogenesis. A familial tendency does exist, with four generations of the anomaly reported in one family and six involved members of another family documented (Troisier and Monnerot-Dumaine, 1930). Males have pectus excavatum three times more often than females.

The anterior chest wall of the newborn is very flexible and always shows some paradoxical motion of the lower portion of the sternum during increased negative intrathoracic pressure with gasping and crying. Congenital pulmonary deformities and poor pulmonary compliance accentuate the retraction. Some infants may have a normal respiratory system but have abnormally soft or underdeveloped costochondral cartilages and therefore excess anterior chest wall retraction with inspiration. Such newborn sternal retractions are not pectus excavatum, although some of these infants will, no doubt, develop the deformity (Fish, Baxter and Moran, 1954; Jensen, Schmidt, Caramella and Lynch, 1970).

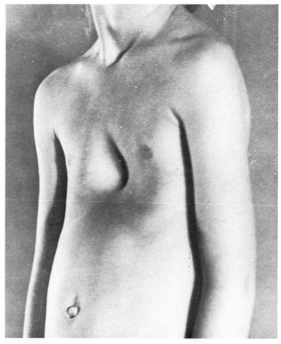

**FIGURE 88–27.** Severe cavitary pectus excavatum beginning at the third costochondral junction. (Courtesy of Dr. Mark M. Ravitch, Pittsburgh, Pennsylvania.)

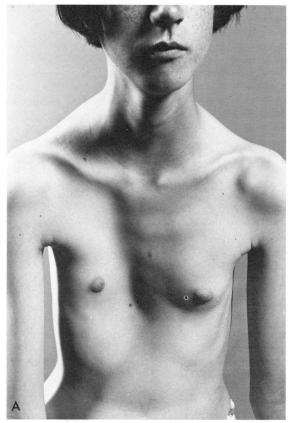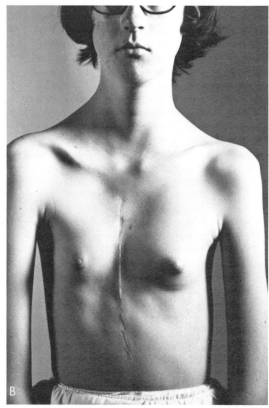

**FIGURE 88–28.** *A,* Adolescent female with pectus excavatum demonstrating chest wall asymmetry, rotation of the axis of the sternum, and hypoplasia of the right breast. *B,* Following structural correction of the bony thorax. (Courtesy of Dr. Mark M. Ravitch, Pittsburgh, Pennsylvania.)

**Symptoms.** The majority of patients with pectus excavatum are essentially asymptomatic, although adolescents and young adults may have slight dyspnea, palpitations, or mild limitation of activity. Patients with the most severe pectus excavatum deformities complain more often of limitation in their ability to perform strenuous exercises and may actually suffer respiratory and cardiac insufficiency.

**Cardiopulmonary Function.** Most studies of cardiopulmonary function in patients with pectus excavatum report normal heart rate, venous pressure, blood pressure, circulation time, oxygen saturation, arterial-venous difference, vital capacity, and maximal breathing capacity in the majority of patients (Becker and Schneider, 1952; Brewer, 1958). Likewise, evaluation of patients with cardiac catheterization has yielded normal or nearly normal intracardiac pressures and cardiac output in most patients (Fabricius and coworkers, 1957; Reusch, 1961). Although some abnormal cardiac catheterizations have

been reported (Ravitch, 1951; Lindskog and Felton, 1955; Lyons, Zuhdi and Kelly, 1955), Brown and Cook (1951), in extensive studies of the respiratory status, found maximum breathing capacity reduced 50 per cent in 9 of 11 patients with pectus excavatum. The electrocardiogram is normal in most patients, but a few show mild axis changes or right bundle branch block thought to be secondary to cardiac displacement rather than intrinsic cardiac disease (Wachtel, Ravitch and Grishman, 1956; Brewer, 1958; Haller, Peters, Mazur and White, 1970).

Many patients with mild symptoms, primarily limitation of strenuous activity, receive significant symptomatic benefit from surgical correction, but the physiologic basis for improvement has been questioned because of reported normal, or near normal, cardiac catheterization studies.

It is clear that pectus excavatum, by displacement and compression of the heart, may cause cardiac symptoms to appear in adolescent or young adult life with lesser degrees of exercise tolerance. Occasionally severe cardiac stress occurs, with arrhythmias and cardiac failure (Ravitch, 1951). Ravitch (1951, 1956) reviewed the recorded experience with pectus excavatum and cardiac disorders up until the time of his reports. The suggested mechanisms responsible for cardiac disability are (1) a decreased return of blood to the right heart; (2) cardiac arrhythmias secondary to atrial compression; (3) restriction of diastolic filling; and (4) a decrease of respiratory reserve. These findings are limited to patients with severe pectus excavatum.

Beiser and associates (1972) obtained normal data on cardiac catheterization of the right side of the heart and found normal hemodynamic responses to supine exercise in patients with pectus excavatum deformity. However, the cardiac output and stroke volume response to mild upright exercise differed from the normal. The cardiac output and stroke volume during intense upright exercise was reduced in five of six patients. After operative repair in three patients, cardiac output during intense upright exercise increased an average of 38 per cent, and hemodynamic response to mild upright exercise also changed toward normal. The investigators hypothesized that the sternal deformity is most severe at its caudal end, and upright position of the torso interferes with pumping capacity as the heart descends into the portion of the thorax most compromised by the depression of the lower sternum. This finding is significant since most exercise studies performed on patients with pectus excavatum during cardiac catheterization have been performed in the supine position. Bevegard (1962) had previously found anomalies with patients studied in the upright position. The stroke volume was considerably smaller during exercise in the sitting position as compared to exercise in the supine position. The author suggested an alteration in the abdominothoracic pumping mechanism secondary to the anterior chest wall deformity. Thus the discrepancy between the symptomatic status of the patients and catheterization data may be due to the position in which the patients were studied.

**Roentgenographic Studies.** The most common finding on anterior-posterior projection is an increase in the extension of the cardiac silhouette into the left chest, although patients with wide pectus excavatum deformities may show a "flattened" heart on the lateral film and extension to the right and left on the anteroposterior film.

The deformity seen on radiography will obviously vary with the degree of the bony abnormality. The normal distance from the anterior surface of the vertebral column to the posterior surface of the sternum averages approximately 9 cm in adult women and 10.5 cm in men (Roesler, 1934; DeLeon, Perloff and Twigg, 1965).

Fabricius, Davidsen, and Hansen (1957) defined pectus excavatum deformity as being "slight" when the distance was over 7 cm, "marked" when the distance was 5 to 7 cm, and "severe" when the distance was less than 5 cm. Ben-Menachem, O'Hara, and Kane (1973) reported radiographic paradoxical cardiac enlargement during inspiration in children with pectus excavatum and stressed the necessity of inspiratory and expiratory films to evaluate heart size adequately.

**Indications for Surgical Correction.** Surgical correction is required for cosmetic reasons and in more advanced cases because of cardiorespiratory dysfunction. While most patients are relatively asymptomatic, the psychologic implications resulting from an anterior thoracic wall deformity may be significant to the patient or his parents. This is adequate indication for surgical correction (Becker and Schneider, 1962; Haller and coworkers, 1970; Jensen and coworkers, 1970; Johnson, 1972; Vidne and Levy, 1973).

Although in the past it was felt by some that affected individuals were suffering primarily from the psychologic standpoint, the now well-established cardiopulmonary restriction which may develop along with drooped shoulders, protuberant abdomen, kyphosis, and scoliosis are clear indications for surgical correction. Likewise, the deformity is unpredictably progressive, and surgical correction is indicated in (1) infants with severe deformity, (2) infants with an observed progression of the deformity, (3) children and young adults with deformity, and (4) adults who are symptomatic. It is generally believed that surgery should be performed in the younger group between 2 and 6 years of age before disturbance of the child's developing personality and before the development of orthopedic problems (Vidne and Levy, 1973).

**Operative Procedure.** Surgical correction of pectus excavatum began with Meyer's (1911) and Sauerbruch's (1928) attempts to alleviate cardiorespiratory symptoms. Lexer (as reported by Hoffmeister, 1927) performed the first bilateral resection of costal cartilages and transverse sternal osteotomy and reversed the anterior-posterior surfaces of the sternum. Ochsner and DeBakey (1939) reviewed the techniques of surgical correction of pectus excavatum up until the time of their report. Brown (1939) established the basis for most present day techniques with bilateral resection of the costal cartilages, excision of the xiphoid, division of the attachments of the diaphragm and rectus muscles, transverse cuneiform osteotomy at the manubriosternal junction, stabilization by wiring the fifth costal cartilage to the sternum, and traction on the sternum by wires placed in the gladiolus.

Although current methods vary, it is generally agreed that limited operations designed to free the diaphragm from the anterior chest wall are not adequate and should be abandoned. The sternum must be returned to its normal anatomical position and stabilized.

Most methods involve a midline vertical skin incision or, frequently, a transverse submammary curvilinear incision severing muscle attachments from the sternum and costal cartilages; resection of deformed cartilages; transverse sternal osteotomy; and elevation of the sternum. The authors favor the procedure described by Ravitch (1949) with the revisions made in 1965 and 1970 (Ravitch, 1965, 1970; Haller and coworkers, 1970).

OPERATIVE TECHNIQUE. The chest is arched forward by placing a folded towel between the scapulae. A vertical skin incision in the midline of the sternum provides maximum exposure. A transverse curvilinear submammary skin incision is frequently used and is particularly indicated in young females. Flaps of skin, subcutaneous tissue, and pectoralis major muscles are elevated bilaterally and cephalad to expose the entire area of the deformity (Fig. 88–29, *A, B*). Injury to the perichondrium must be avoided in elevating the flaps.

Longitudinal incisions are made through the perichondrium of the involved cartilages, and transverse incisions are made at both ends of the longitudinal incisions so that rectangular flaps of perichondrium can be reflected (Fig. 88–29, *C*). An upper flap of perichondrium is first released by grasping the upper edge of the incised perichondrium and by dissecting with a Joseph nasal periosteal elevator or with a blunt staphylorrhaphy elevator. The lower edge of the perichondrium is elevated in a similar fashion. The perichondrium is quite thin over the upper and lower borders of the rib, and careful dissection in these areas is required to avoid disruption. It may be possible to pass a blunt instrument behind the cartilage, leaving the perichondrium intact, and to divide the cartilage at the two ends (Fig. 88–29, *D*). In other instances it is difficult to strip the perichondrium behind the cartilage. A Kocher clamp is used to hold the cartilage while it is incised in its midportion until one half of the cartilage is lifted from the underlying perichondrium. The perichondrium is dissected from both halves of the cartilage, and the two ends of the cartilage are divided medially and laterally to remove the specimen. The deformed cartilages are resected for the full length of their deformity. The costochondral junction is preserved when possible. In infants and small children, the resection will include 3 to 5 cm of the lower cartilages and only 1 to 2 cm of the upper cartilages. In older children and young adults, the deformity usually extends laterally into the bony rib. As few as three cartilages may be removed, but usually four and frequently five on each side must be resected.

An unsatisfactory postoperative result can occur if the cartilages are not resected far enough laterally or if a sufficient number of cartilages is not excised. When all deformed cartilages have been removed, the next higher cartilages, usually the second or third, are transected from in front and medially to behind and laterally to allow overlap of the medial fragment upon the lateral when the sternum is lifted to its corrected position. Suture fixation of the overlapped cartilages is established later in the procedure.

With the sternum elevated by a bone hook, the xiphoid process is divided from the sternum and allowed to retract (Fig. 88–29, *E, F*). A finger is inserted into the mediastinum through the opening made by division of the sternum and xiphoid, and the reflected pleura is displaced laterally on both sides. When the sternum is raised by upward traction on the bone hook, it is possible to cut the intercostal bundles away from the sternum on both sides, preferably medial to the internal mammary vessels, so as to isolate the sternum as a peninsula attached only above (Fig. 88–29, *F*).

A posterior transverse osteotomy of the sternum is performed at the next higher interspace above the transected normal cartilage. A wire is passed around the sternum at the desired level of the osteotomy, the sternum is elevated, and a sharp osteotome scores the posterior surface of the sternum until the sternum is fractured forward (Fig. 88–29, *G, H*). A block of rib bone may then be placed in the defect resulting from the posterior osteotomy (Fig. 88–29, *K*). If a bone block is used, it should be sutured in place with a suture through it or around the sternum to prevent it from being dislodged into the mediastinum postoperatively. The posterior sternal osteotomy came into practice because it was

*Text continued on page 3641*

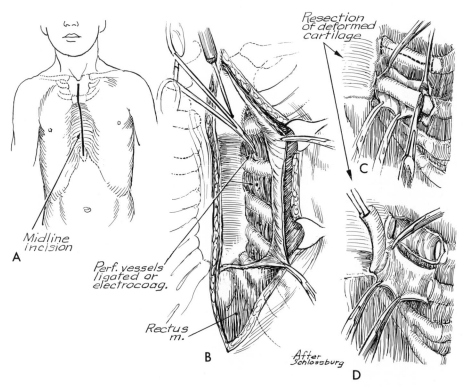

**FIGURE 88–29.** Correction of pectus excavatum (Ravitch technique). *A,* A midline incision gives better exposure with less dissection and smaller flaps. A transverse submammary incision does not provide adequate exposure in older patients or in those whose defect begins at the manubriosternal junction. *B,* Flaps of skin, subcutaneous fat, and pectoralis major muscle are dissected, exposing the deformed ribs and cartilages. *C,* Rectangular perichondrial flaps are developed to provide access to the deformed cartilage. *D,* The deformed cartilages are resected for the full extent of their deformity.

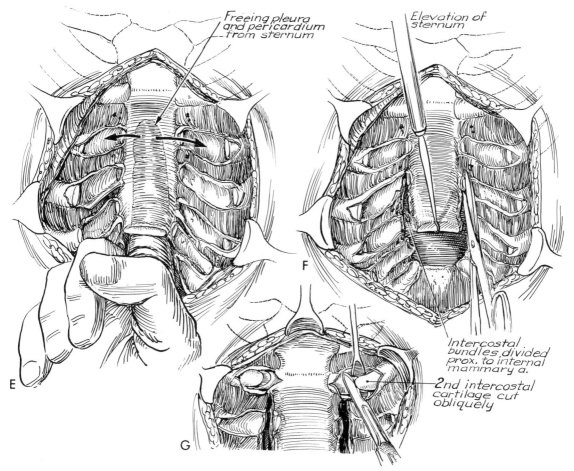

**FIGURE 88–29** *Continued.* *E,* The xiphoid is divided from the sternum, and blunt finger dissection separates the posterior surface of the sternum from the pleura and pericardium. *F,* The sternum is retracted upward, and the intercostal bundles are divided medial to the internal mammary vessels. *G,* The next higher cartilage above the level of the deformity is divided obliquely for later three-point fixation.

*Legend continued on the following page*

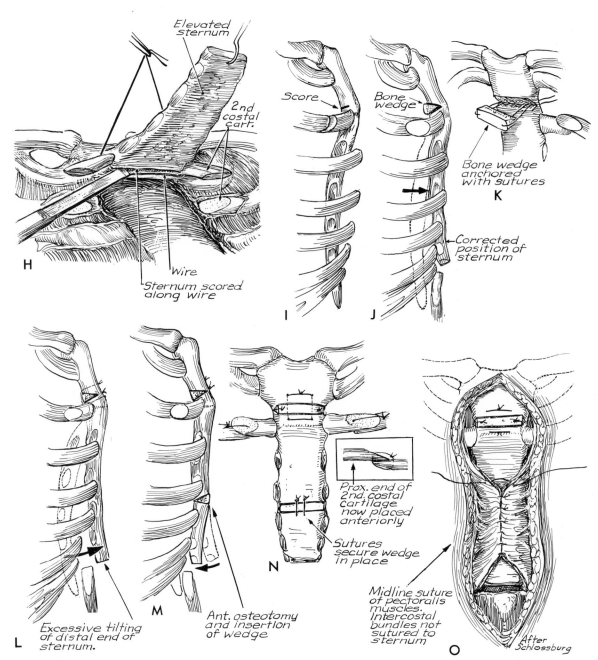

**FIGURE 88–29** *Continued.*   *H, I,* A posterior transverse osteotomy is performed at the next higher interspace above the transected normal cartilage. The wire passed around the sternum gives a guideline to the exact site of the desired osteotomy. *J, K,* A bone block is placed in the osteotomy defect produced by anterior movement of the sternum. The bone block can be held in place with sutures placed either through it or around the sternum. *L, M,* When the distal sternum points excessively anteriorly following the superior transverse osteotomy, a distal anterior transverse osteotomy is performed and stabilized with a bone block. *N,* The superior osteotomy is secured by using silk sutures placed through-and-through the sternum across the osteotomy site. The beveled, transected, normal cartilages are secured as shown to provide "tripod fixation" of the sternum in its new position (two cartilages and anterior periosteum). *O,* The pectoral muscles are sutured together and to the sternum in the midline. The intercostal bundles are not sutured back to the sternum because of a tendency to recreate the deformity. (After Ravitch, M. M.: General Thoracic Surgery. Philadelphia, Lea and Febiger, 1972.)

noted that in some patients undergoing an anterior cuneiform osteotomy and fracture of the posterior cortical lamella, the posterior periosteum stripped back, allowing the distal sternal fragment subsequently to assume a stepped-back or recessed position. After posterior osteotomy, any tendency to progression of the original deformity will produce a desired anterior tilting of the distal segment of the sternum (Fig. 88–29, *L*). In some patients, especially older children, the sternum may be rather sharply rotated toward the right, i.e., counterclockwise. This can usually be corrected by dividing the right half of the osteotomy completely and twisting the sternum back into position.

The sternum is held in a somewhat overcorrected position by two or three mattress sutures of heavy braided silk placed through the bone anteriorly *across* the level of the posterior osteotomy (Fig. 88–29, *N*). A saddler's awl or a heavy gauge Reverdin needle can be helpful in passing sutures through the sternum. The transected, overlapped, unaffected cartilages are sutured into their new position. This establishes a natural internal fixation referred to as "tripod fixation" because the sternum is supported by its anterior periosteum as well as the two cartilages. The pectoral muscles are sutured, and the sternal periosteum is sutured in the midline (Fig. 88–29, *O*). The intercostal bundles are not sutured back to the sternum because of a tendency to reproduce the deformity. Likewise, the xiphoid process is not sutured back to the sternum. A large suction catheter is placed retrosternally in the mediastinal space, and 20 to 30 cm of water suction is applied. The subcutaneous tissue and skin are closed in layers.

Occasionally, the sternum of a patient is so scaphoid that, when the osteotomy has been performed and maintained by sutures, the distal end of the sternum projects forward, requiring a transverse osteotomy in the distal portion of the sternum to allow it to fall downward in order to correct the exaggerated anterior curvature.

A chest X-ray film is taken immediately after completion of the operation, and if a pneumothorax is present, it is aspirated. Some paradoxical motion of the anterior chest wall may be present in the first few postoperative days, but this is of little physiologic significance. Postoperative activity is not limited in the usual patient. Meticulous pulmonary toilet is necessary. Wound problems such as hematoma and infection are infrequent but may occur.

Wada and Ikeda (1972) reported favorable results in 225 patients in whom the "sternoturnover procedure" was performed and in 56 patients in whom "funnel costoplasty" was performed. The sternoturnover procedure is performed through a longitudinal or transverse inframammary incision (Fig. 88–30). Skin, subcutaneous tissue, and pectoral muscle flaps are elevated. Blunt dissection separates the sternum from the mediastinal tissues. Likewise, the mediastinal tissues and pleura are dissected from the cartilages and ribs using blunt manual dissection. The ribs or cartilages and intercostal muscles are transected bilaterally at the costal arches and cephalad along the margin of the deformity.

The sternum is elevated, and both internal mammary arteries are ligated and divided. The sternum is transected just above the level of the beginning of the deformity, removed en bloc, and turned over; its convex side is flattened by wedge resection and turned to fit the defect in the thoracic wall. The sternum is sutured in position with stainless steel wire, and each costal cartilage or rib is sutured with heavy silk. When there is mild asymmetry, the reversed sternum can be shifted to one side parallel to the sternal axis or obliquely positioned after trimming. It is important that the reversed sternum fits snugly into a suitable position. As noted by Ravitch (1965), the indications for the sternoturnover procedure are probably limited to patients with unusually wide defects in whom the required resections would not be tolerated. Infection in this large graft could be disastrous.

Wada and Ikeda (1972) developed the funnel costoplasty for patients with deep asymmetrical funnel chest, usually involving the right side in adults (Fig. 88–31). In this procedure the deformed cartilages and ribs are mobilized by transecting their sternal attachments. Cartilages and ribs are straightened by multiple partial incisions or wedge resections and sutured to the sternum anteriorly to form a new and elevated costal contour.

INTERNAL AND EXTERNAL FIXATION. Various internal fixation devices have been used in an attempt to stabilize the sternum postoperatively and to prevent recurrence of pectus excavatum. These devices include stainless steel struts (Rehbein and Wernicke, 1957; Adkins and Gwathmey, 1958; Ravitch, 1965; Jensen and coworkers, 1970; Vidne and Levy, 1973), stainless steel wire mesh (May, 1961), Kirschner wires or Steinmann pins (Mayo and Long, 1962; Peters and Johnson, 1964), and rib bone struts (Sweet, 1944; Brodkin, 1948; Adkins and Gwathmey, 1958).

Jensen, Schmidt, Caramella, and Lynch (1970) used a preformed stainless steel strut

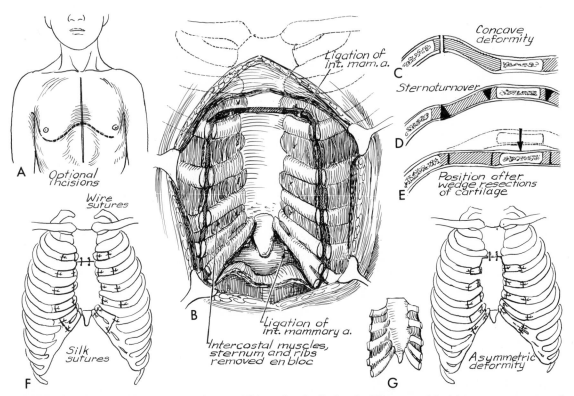

**FIGURE 88–30.**   Sternoturnover procedure. *A,* Either a longitudinal and midline sternal incision or a transverse and inframammary incision may be used. *B,* The ribs or cartilages and intercostal muscle bundles are transected bilaterally at the costal arches cephalad along the margin of the deformity. The internal mammary arteries are ligated and transected bilaterally. The sternum is ready for elevation and removal en bloc. *C, D, E,* The convex side of the sternum is flattened by wedge resections and trimmed to fit the defect in the thoracic wall. *F,* The sternum is sutured in place with stainless steel wire, and each costal cartilage or rib is sutured with heavy silk. *G,* In mild asymmetry, the reversed sternum is either shifted to one side parallel to the sternal axis or obliquely positioned after trimming. (After Wada, J., and Ikeda, K.: Clinical experience with 306 funnel chest operations. Internat. Surg., 57:707, 1972.)

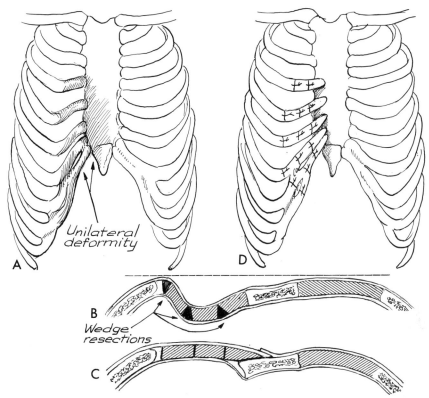

**FIGURE 88–31.** Funnel costoplasty. *A,* Deep, unilateral, asymmetrical funnel chest. *B, C,* The deformed ribs and cartilages are straightened by multiple wedge resections and detachment of the cartilages from the sternum. *D,* The recontoured ribs are sutured to the sternum anteriorly. (After Wada, J., and Ikeda, K.: Clinical experience with 306 funnel chest operations. Internat. Surg., *57:*707, 1972.)

(Strib)* manufactured especially for anterior chest wall stabilization (Fig. 88–32). A transverse incision exposes the underlying deformed chest wall. Short incisions are made through the overlying pectoral muscles to expose each costochondral junction. Periosteal flaps are developed, and a wedge of cartilage is removed from each deformed cartilage and from the web at the costal arch. The xiphoid process is freed from its rectus muscle attachments, and the sternum is freed of all posterior attachments up to the deformity. Wedge osteotomy of the anterior sternum is performed with an osteotome. The sternum is retracted forward, and wedges of cartilage are removed from the posterior surfaces of the medial end of each cartilage where they join the sternum. If necessary, a second osteotomy of the sternum is performed. A stainless steel strut is placed from one midaxillary line to the other between the endothoracic fascia and the pleura posterior to the sternum, and, when adjusted in contour, it supports the

___

*Medic-Made, Inc., Minneapolis, Minnesota.

sternum. The strut is removed after 12 to 18 months.

Vidne and Levy (1973) resected the deformed cartilages, performed an anterior cuneiform osteotomy of the sternum, and placed a stainless steel strut retrosternally in a fashion similar to that of Jensen and his coworkers (1970). These authors removed the strut after approximately six months.

Barnard and DeWet Lubbe (1973) resected the deformed cartilages, mobilized the sternum, and performed an osteotomy through the posterior cortex of the sternum. A medium-sized Kirschner wire was slightly bent with an anterior convexity and inserted between the anterior and posterior tables of the sternum at the level of the fifth costal cartilage. The laterally protruding ends of wire partially overlapped the bony anterior thoracic wall to which they were fixed with silk sutures. The authors indicated that they do not remove the wire unless some need arises to do so.

External devices to maintain or overcorrect the position of the sternum during the early

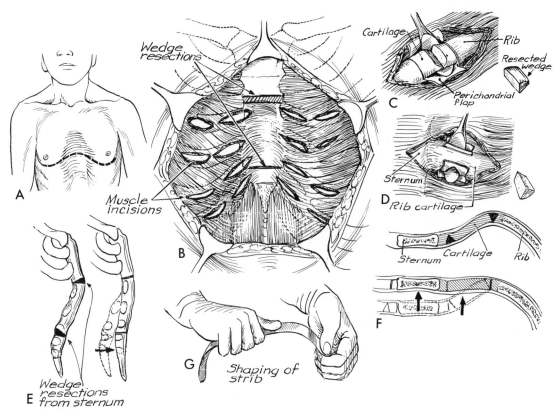

**FIGURE 88–32.** Stabilization of corrected pectus excavatum deformity using Strib internal fixation. *A,* Submammary incision extending from the anterior axillary line to the anterior axillary line, with the back of the incision turned up toward the axilla and the center curved cephalad to aid in exposure of the upper sternum. *B,* Skin, subcutaneous fat, and fascia flaps are elevated superiorly and inferiorly, exposing the pectoral muscles. Short incisions through the muscles expose each costochondral junction. *C, D,* Subperichondrial dissection exposes the cartilages, and wedges of cartilage are removed from each deformed cartilage as well as the web at the costal arch. The costochondral junction is not disturbed in children, as this is the growth line of the rib. *E,* The posterior aspect of the sternum is freed of all attachments up to the level of the deformity. Wedge osteotomies of the sternum are performed, preserving the posterior periosteum to serve as a hinge. *F,* Reversed wedges are excised from the medial ends of the cartilages as they join the sternum, permitting straightening of the ribs. Cartilage wedges and lengths may be revised at this time to permit the desired positioning of the sternum. *G,* A Strib of the required length is selected by measuring the distance from one midaxillary line across the anterior chest to the opposite midaxillary line, and is hand bent.

*Legend continued on the opposite page*

postoperative course have been advocated. In general, this consists of a wire placed through or around the sternum, brought through the skin, and tied over a fixation device of some sort (Lester, 1946; Fish and coworkers, 1954; Lindskog and Felton, 1955). The discomfort of these prostheses and supports, the increased risk of infection with prostheses penetrating the skin, and the short period of time usually advocated for use of these prostheses have led to their unpopularity. They are currently seldom used.

Rib graft buttresses (Dormer, Keil and Schissel, 1950; Adkins and Gwathmey, 1958) have been abandoned because of bone softening and resorption, as well as the lack of a sufficient variety in sizes and curvature of ribs.

Experience with silicone implants for breast augmentation stimulated the choice of this material for correction of purely cosmetic deformities in adults (Masson, Payne and Gonzalez, 1970; Stanford and coworkers, 1972) (Fig. 88–33). Whereas these implants were initially fabricated by the surgeon after a plaster model of the deformity was made, such implants can now be custom-ordered to fill the defect precisely. Synthetic implants should be used only in adult patients and only if there are no cardiopulmonary symptoms, as the anatomical deformity is not changed by this method. As with the use of all prosthetic materials, complications of bleeding, infection, and extrusion of the implant must be anticipated.

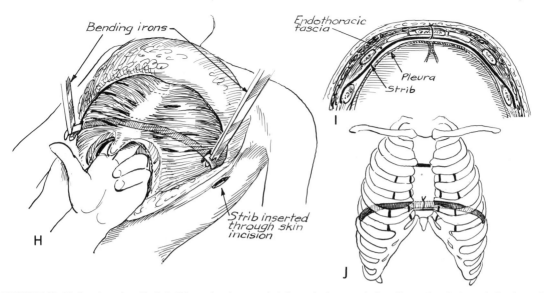

**FIGURE 88–32** *Continued.* *H, I, J,* Dissection is extended through the muscle bundles and endothoracic fascia to the pleura, and the Strib is guided across the mediastinum between the pleura and endothoracic fascia. Specially designed bending irons are used to form the ends of the strut around the adjacent ribs. Final contour adjustment is made by bringing the sternum and Strib into continuity and securing it in position with a heavy catgut suture. (After Jensen, K., Schmidt, R., Caramella, J., and Lynch, M.: Pectus excavatum: The how, when and why of surgical correction. J. Pediatr. Surg., 5:4, 1970.)

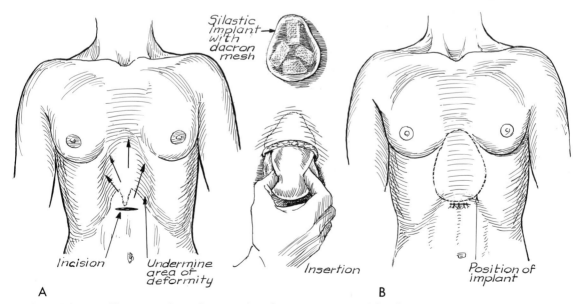

**FIGURE 88–33.** Silcone prostheses for correction of pectus excavatum deformity. *A,* Incision is made just below the xiphoid; sharp dissection elevates the fascia over the sternum and pectoralis muscle, creating a pocket somewhat larger than the silicone implant. *B,* The incision is closed with a double layer of sutures.

## PECTUS CARINATUM

Pectus carinatum (pigeon breast) is a protrusion deformity of the anterior chest wall and is regarded as the opposite of pectus excavatum deformity. Pectus excavatum occurs approximately ten times more frequently than pectus carinatum. Hippocrates (1849) described the deformity and noted that patients in whom "the chest becomes sharp pointed and not broad become affected with difficulty of breathing and hoarseness; for the cavities which inspire and expire do not attain proper capacity." In some patients a rigid chest develops; there is an increased anteroposterior diameter fixed in almost full inspiration, with insufficient respiratory efforts made only by the diaphragm and the muscles of respiration. There is alveolar hypoventilation and increased pulmonary circulatory resistance (Fishman, Turino and Bergofsky, 1958; Bergofsky, Turino and Fishman, 1959). The lungs lose compliance, and there is progressive emphysema and a tendency to pulmonary infection (Welch and Vos, 1973).

**Etiology.** The etiology of the deformity is unknown. Suggested theories include abnormal fusion of sternal segments (Currarino and Silverman, 1958), defective ossification (DeOliviera, Sambhi and Zimmerman, 1958), rickets (Brodkin, 1958), and various influences of the diaphragm on chest wall development (Brodkin, 1948, 1958; Chin, 1957; Lester, 1961). Sweet's (1944) explanation of the overgrowth of the costal cartilages with forward protrusion of the manubrium, gladiolus, and xiphoid is reasonable and would explain to some extent how pectus carinatum is caused by an anterior growth of the cartilages and pectus excavatum by a posterior growth.

**Types.** Brodkin (1949) recognized and described two types of protruding chest deformities: chondrogladiolar and chondromanubrial. *Chondrogladiolar* prominence is characterized by forward projection of the lower anterior thorax and body of the sternum so that the level of the junction of the sternum and xiphoid is the most prominent point of the anterior chest wall (Fig. 88–34). Associated with the protrusion is the lateral depression of the anterior chest wall, which may be deep enough to decrease the thoracic cavity and produce cardiorespiratory symptoms (Ravitch, 1960). This type of deformity is said to appear more often (Brodkin, 1949; Welch and Vos, 1973), although some reports do not agree (Lam and Taber, 1971). *Chondromanubrial* prominence is characterized by projection of the manubrium and the adjacent first and second cartilages, with a vertical or posteriorly directed gladiolus (Fig. 88–34). Although he did not call the deformity "pectus carinatum," Ravitch (1952) reported correction of this type of defect in a patient with cardiac symptoms.

Robicsek, Sanger, Taylor, and Thomas (1963) noted a third type of pectus carinatum, *lateral* pectus carinatum, either unilateral or bilateral. This deformity is rare.

**Symptoms and Signs.** Symptoms in most patients are vague and vary from retarded growth, exertional dyspnea, or chronic dyspnea to asthmatic attacks and palpitation (Robicsek and coworkers, 1963). Many patients are only minimally aware of their limitations and become more aware after surgery has produced an improved status (Lester, 1953).

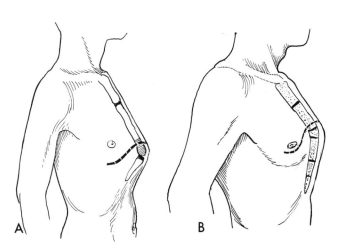

**FIGURE 88–34.** *A,* Chondrogladiolar type of pectus carinatum with forward projection of the lower anterior thorax and body of the sternum. The level of the junction of the sternum and xiphoid is the most prominent point of the anterior chest wall. The broken line indicates the level of the incision for surgical correction.

*B,* Chondromanubrial type of pectus carinatum with forward projection of the manubrium and adjacent first and second ribs. The gladiolas may be directed vertically or posteriorly. The broken line indicates the level of the incision for surgical correction.

### Surgical Techniques

CORRECTION OF CHONDROGLADIOLAR DEFORMITY. Several operative methods of correction have been described, indicating that no single method is totally satisfactory. Lester (1953) resected approximately 2 cm of the sternal end of each cartilage below the second cartilage; the xiphoid was freed from the sternum, and subperiosteal resection of the sternum was extended out from the level of the second rib. When necessary, the rib ends were also resected.

Chin (1957) detached the xiphoid from the sternum, leaving the rectus abdominis muscle attached to the xiphoid, sternal ends of the sixth and seventh ribs in children (ribs three through seven in adults were resected superichondrially); a slot osteotomy was performed on the anterior sternum at the level of the fourth costal cartilage, and the detached xiphoid process was sutured into the slot osteotomy with the idea that the posterior pull of the xiphoid would correct the deformity.

Ravitch (1960) described a two-stage resection of the costal cartilages in one patient and a one-stage bilateral resection of cartilages, combined with a distal osteotomy, in another patient to correct the manubriogladiolar type of deformity. In the patient undergoing the two-stage resection (Fig. 88–35), the right pectoral muscles and rectus muscles were reflected from the opera-

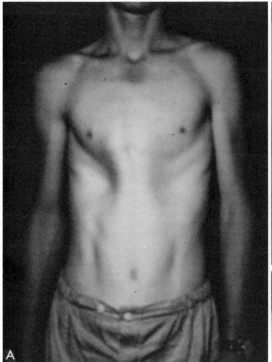

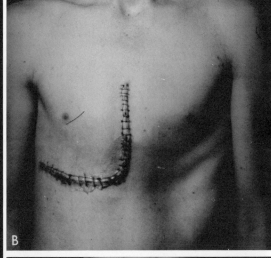

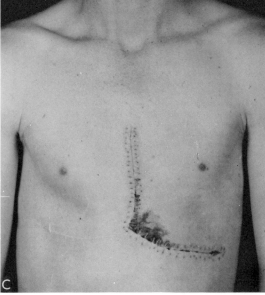

**FIGURE 88–35.** Pectus carinatum deformity. *A,* Chondrogladiolar type deformity with projection of the lower anterior thorax and body of the sternum. There is associated lateral depression of the anterior chest wall. The pectus carinatum correction in this patient was one of the first performed by Ravitch; the operation involved two stages. *B,* Patient in early postoperative course after correction of deformity of the right side of thorax. *C,* Eight months later following correction of the deformity of the left side. (Courtesy of Dr. Mark M. Ravitch, Pittsburgh, Pennsylvania.)

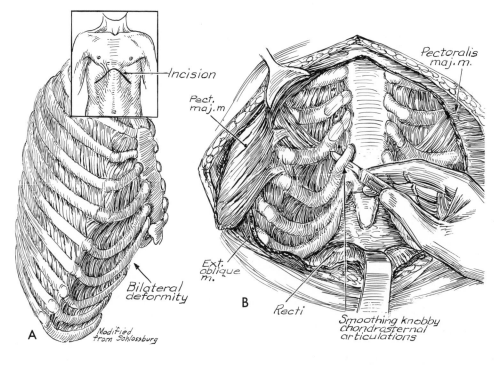

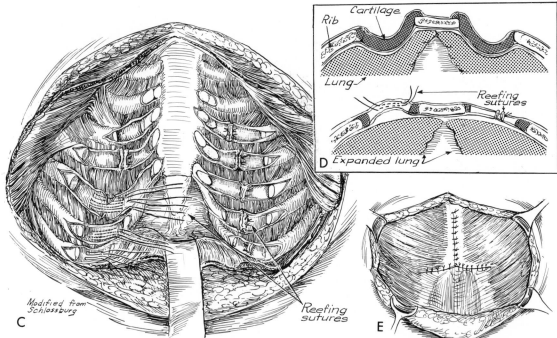

**FIGURE 88–36.**   Ravitch technique for correction of chondrogladiolar type of pectus carinatum. *A, B,* A transverse curvilinear incision is used to elevate flaps down to and including the pectoral muscles. The rectus muscle attachments are divided. Cartilaginous irregularities and knobby projections of the chondrosternal articulations are sharply smoothed out. *C, D,* The posteriorly curved, deformed cartilages are resected subperichondrially. The redundant perichondrium is tightened by mattress silk reefing sutures so that the new cartilage will grow in a straight line from the ribs to the sternum. *E,* The pectoral muscles and recti are reattached to the sternum. (After Ravitch, M. M.: General Thoracic Surgery. Philadelphia, Lea and Febiger, 1972.)

tive field; knobby lesions of costal cartilages four, five, and six, which were exaggerating the prominence of the sternum, were excised; and subperiosteal resection of cartilages five, six, seven, eight, and nine was performed. The redundant perichondrium was tightened with reefing sutures, and the pectoral and rectus abdominis muscles were sutured in place. The left side was similarly repaired eight months later. The patient tolerated the one-sided operation so well that the next patient operated on by Ravitch was resected bilaterally at one stage. In discussing the paper of Welch and Vos (1973), Ravitch noted that he performs all pectus carinatum deformities in one stage without sternal osteotomy (Fig. 88–36).

Robicsek, Sanger, Taylor, and Thomas (1963) described correction of manubriogladiolar prominence by subperiosteal resection beginning at the third costal cartilage, transverse osteotomy of the sternum at the beginning of the abnormal forward curvature (usually just below the angle of Louis), resection of the lower protruding end of the sternum, and suture of the

previously detached xiphoid process with stainless steel wire to the new end of the sternum (Fig. 88–37). The rectus muscles pulled the sternum downward, correcting the deformity.

Lam and Taber (1971) described correction of chondrogladiolar prominence by resection of cartilages three through seven and osteotomy of the anterior table of the upper portion of the sternum to permit the protruding sternum to be fractured backward. These procedures were combined with an osteotomy of the anterior table of the lower sternum at the level of the sixth cartilage, with removal of a wedge of bone, permitting the tip of the sternum to be elevated. The wedge of bone from the lower osteotomy was placed into the gaping upper osteotomy line to maintain the new angulation.

CORRECTION OF CHONDROMANUBRIAL DEFORMITY. Ravitch (1952) reported correction of an unusual chondromanubrial type of deformity without calling it pectus carinatum (Fig. 88–38). Bilateral subperichondrial resection of five cartilages was done; the xiphisternal junction was divided; and two osteotomies were per-

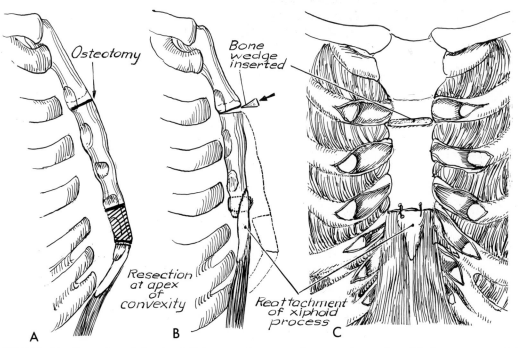

**FIGURE 88–37.** Correction of chondrogladiolar type of pectus carinatum with resection of the lower sternum. *A,* The costal cartilages have been resected subperichondrially; a transverse sternal osteotomy has been performed at the level of the second rib, leaving the posterior periosteum intact, and the protruding lower end of the corpus sterni has been resected. *B, C,* The lower end of the transected corpus sterni has been smoothed out and joined to the xiphoid with stainless steel wires. A bone wedge taken from the excised portion of the lower sternum is placed in the gap produced at the osteotomy by posteriorly directing the sternum. (After Robicsek, F., Sanger, P., Taylor, F., and Thomas M.: The surgical treatment of chondrosternal prominence (pectus carinatum). J. Thorac. Cardiovasc. Surg., 45:691, 1963.)

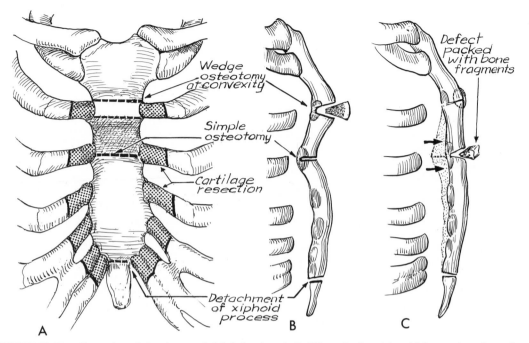

**FIGURE 88–38.** Correction of chondromanubrial deformity. *A, B,* Bilateral subperichondrial resection of costal cartilages, division of xiphisternal junction, and two osteotomies. The superior wedge osteotomy at the level of greatest convexity allows the posteriorly directed sternal segment to be lifted anteriorly, thereby fracturing the posterior cortical lamella, restoring a more normal alignment. *C,* Anterior tilting of the lower portion of the corpus sterni thus produced is corrected by a simple osteotomy, with bone fragments used to splint the osteotomy site. The manubrium and gladiolus are stabilized by stainless steel sutures. (After Ravitch, M. M.: Unusual sternal deformity with cardiac symptoms. J. Thorac. Surg., *23*:138, 1952.)

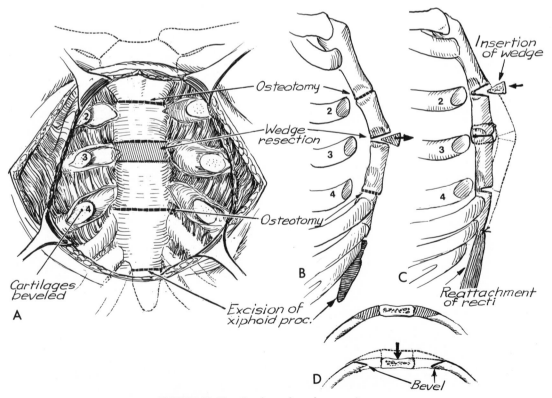

**FIGURE 88–39.** *See legend on the opposite page.*

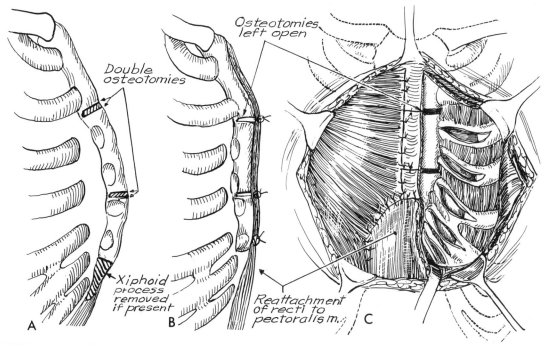

**FIGURE 88–40.** Correction of chondrogladiolar type of pectus carinatum with stabilization by rectus fascia apex flaps. *A,* Following symmetrical bilateral cartilage resection preserving the perichondrial sheaths, double anterior table osteotomies are made at the level of the first and third sternal segments, and the xiphoid process is resected. *B, C,* The pectoral muscles are reattached to the sternum in the midline and the rectus muscle apex flaps are advanced into the pectoral defect anterior to the sternum. (After Welch, K., and Vos, A.: J. Pediatr. Surg., 8:659, 1973.)

formed. The superior osteotomy at the level of the greatest prominence of the convex deformity permitted the sternum to be lifted anteriorly, thereby fracturing the posterior cortical lamella and restoring normal alignment. This resulted in an anterior tilting of the lower portion of the body of the sternum, which was corrected by an osteotomy at the appropriate level to allow the sternum to be fractured posteriorly. The lower osteotomy was packed by fragments from the wedge osteotomy, and the corrected position was maintained without sutures. The manubrium and gladiolus were sutured together across the superior osteotomy. No traction or splinting was employed postoperatively.

Lam and Taber (1971) (Fig. 88–39) reported resection of the second, third, and fourth cartilages subperichondrially and excision of a cuneiform segment 2 cm wide from the prominence of the convexity of the sternum. Transverse osteotomies above and below the resection permitted the sternum to be fractured into a flat position, which was maintained by sutures at the resection site.

Welch and Vos (1973) (Fig. 88–40) reported symmetrical bilateral subperichondrial cartilage resection and double anterior table osteotomies at the first and third sternal segments. The pectoral muscles were approximated to the sternum in the midline, and a triangular flap of the apex of the rectus fascia was placed into the corresponding pectoral defect anterior to the sternum.

Other techniques described for the correction

**FIGURE 88–39.** Correction of chondromanubrial deformity with resection of the center of convexity. *A, B,* Protruding costal cartilages of ribs two, three, and four resected. Transverse osteotomies above and below the level of the deformity, a wedge resection at the level of the sternal prominence, and detachment of the xiphoid process permit the sternum to be straightened. *C,* Sternum stabilized by stainless steel wire at the site of sternal resection, bone wedge in upper osteotomy, and reattachment of xiphoid process. (After Lam, C., and Taber, R.: Surgical treatment of pectus carinatum. Arch. Surg., *103*:191, 1971.)

of the chondromanubrial type of chest protrusion represent essentially slight modifications of the Ravitch technique and will not be detailed.

## TUMORS OF THE CHEST WALL

### Benign Tumors

Except for surface lesions to be described later in the text, such as lipomas and other benign conditions of the breast, the largest category of benign tumors is the neurogenic type. These tumors are generally asymptomatic and are usually discovered on routine X-ray films of the chest, which disclose a smooth, discrete density whose convex surface is central, while the tumor is based upon the chest wall peripherally. Neurofibromas and ganglioneuromas are generally located posteriorly and are related to the intercostal nerves or sympathetic chain.

Although chondromas of the rib cage may appear histologically benign, as noted by Mallory (1938), they frequently manifest a predisposition to local implantation, with the ultimate development of malignancy and widespread metastases. Therefore, a chondroma must be treated, like any malignant lesion, by radical resection at the outset, because of its propensity to implantation and local recurrence. Chondromas frequently appear during adolescence and early adulthood. Other benign chest wall tumors include fibrous dysplasia of the ribs and lipomas arising beneath the fascia propria of the chest wall musculature.

### Malignant Tumors

The more common malignant chest wall tumors include osteogenic sarcoma, Ewing's sarcoma of the ribs, malignant mesenchymoma, neurogenic sarcoma (Fig. 88–41), hemangioendothelial sarcoma (Fig. 88–42), plasma cell myeloma, and chondrosarcoma, the commonest and most insidious of all. Chondrosarcomas may initially be histologically benign, allowing recurrence before the true malignant nature of the tumor is recognized.

The incidence of metastatic tumors from distant primary lesions is greater by far than that of primary malignant tumors of the chest wall.

**Surgical Considerations.** All primary chest wall tumors should be excised early and adequately. This will involve a thoracotomy approach, the pleural space being entered two or more interspaces above or below the tumor to evaluate the nature of the tumor and the extent of the pleural involvement. If one is reasonably secure in the belief that the tumor is benign, a thorough local excision is performed and the specimen is sent for study by frozen section. A radical reexcision may be performed, if warranted, after receipt of the laboratory report and personal conference with the pathologist. If the tumor clinically appears to be malignant, a primary radical excision should be performed, resecting at least one uninvolved rib and intercostal bundle above and below the tumor, together with a wide portion of the surrounding skin, including the chest wall or upper abdominal skin and musculature.

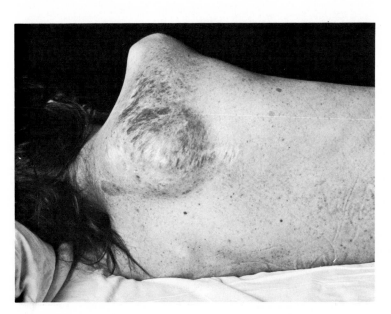

**FIGURE 88–41.** An 18 year old girl with a neurogenic fibrosarcoma of the upper back which had extended into the thoracic cage and vertebrae. Note the café au lait spots and peripheral subcutaneous nodules. The patient's admission was prompted by weakness of the legs which progressed to complete paralysis within a week. At operation the tumor was found to extend into the chest and to involve the second, third, fourth, and fifth dorsal laminae. Because of diffuse pleural seeding, complete removal was not possible. Pathologic studies disclosed that fibrosarcomatous degeneration had probably occurred in a neurofibroma.

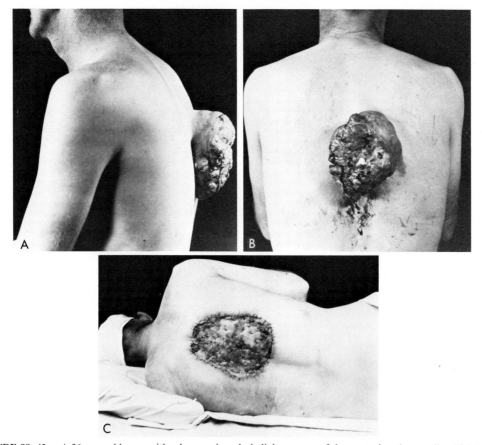

**FIGURE 88–42.** A 36 year old man with a hemangioendothelial sarcoma of the posterior chest wall, which had grown from a walnut-sized mass to its present dimensions in two years. Repeated hemorrhages from the tumor finally prompted admission. Roentgenograms disclosed no involvement or destruction of the spine or ribs. The tumor was widely excised, and the defect was covered with thick split-thickness skin grafts. Postoperative photographs were taken prior to removal of sutures. The patient was alive and well five years later.

## Carcinoma of the Breast and Chest Wall

During recent years there has been a considerable accumulation of literature on the surgical treatment of breast cancer. Extended radical mastectomy, modified radical mastectomy, simple mastectomy, partial mastectomy, and "lumpectomy" all have their strong proponents and, as well, their opponents. The status of radiation therapy, chemotherapy, and immunotherapy as adjuncts to surgical treatment is no less uncertain. Likewise, the role of the regional nodes in terms of host defense mechanisms is at present uncertain.

The National Surgical Adjuvant Breast Project has been collecting data for the past 15 years in a coordinated effort to determine the important factors relative to cure or extended survival following treatment of breast cancer. All factors being equal, the five- and ten-year survival rates are more dependent on the extent of the cancer when the patient is first treated than on which surgical procedure is performed.

There is a linear increase in the incidence of metastatic disease in the regional lymph nodes with increase in tumor size. Thirty per cent of patients who are clinically negative for nodal metastases show microscopic involvement when the lymph nodes are studied following dissection. When more than three axillary lymph nodes are positive, the survival rate dramatically decreases. When the axillary nodes are positive, one-quarter of the patients have positive internal mammary nodes and one-third have positive interpectoral nodes. Postoperative radiation is helpful in treating local or distant recurrent disease but has no influence on the distant recurrence rate or overall survival rates. Simple mastectomy, radical mastectomy, modified radical mastectomy, and extended radical mastectomy all have five-year survival rates of 75 to 85 per cent if the patient has histologically negative nodes when first treated.

Recurrent local disease occurs in 30 per cent of patients following radical mastectomy and may appear as single or several nodules of tumor in the skin, subcutaneous tissue, or ribs. Occasionally, the recurrent disease presents as multiple nodules *en cuirasse* or as the carcinomatous dermatitis referred to as inflammatory or erysipeloid cancer. Treatment of recurrent local tumor may be by radiation, surgery, or a combination of radiation and surgery.

At present, the classic Halsted radical mastectomy remains the standard for comparison of all other procedures. It is based on sound surgical and pathologic principles and is applicable in the majority of patients in whom clinical evidence fails to disclose that the disease has already progressed beyond the scope of curability or operability.

### Benign Tumors of the Skin of the Thorax

**Fibroma.** A fibroma is a benign, solid, fibrous tumor which develops particularly in the subcutaneous tissues. It is encapsulated, freely movable, and varies considerably in consistency. Some fibromas are firm and elastic, whereas others have a soft, loose structure and are more vascular. In many parts of the body, fibromas are combined with other growths: fibroadenomas of the breast, fibromyomas of the uterus, fibro-osteoma (ossifying fibroma; fibrous dysplasia of the facial bones particularly, but occurring peripherally also). In many of these hyphenated tumors, the fibrous element has been suspected of being, in part at least, a secondary responsive reaction.

**Keloid.** A keloid is a dense fibrous tissue tumor of the skin which occurs at the site of injury (see Chapter 16). That the fibrous tissue represents an overgrowth is evidenced by the fact that a keloid extends not only above the surface of the skin but also laterally to involve areas which were not involved in the original trauma (Fig. 88–43). This characteristic is of special significance in the clinical differentiation of keloids from hypertrophied scars. The color of the keloid may vary from red to pink to white, and the lesion may have multiple telangiectatic vessels coursing on its surface.

Keloids occur most frequently in Negroes and brunette Caucasians. There is individual susceptibility, for they may occur in one or two

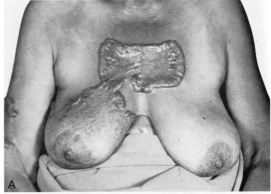

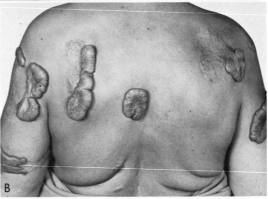

**FIGURE 88–43.** *A,* Extensive butterfly keloid of the sternum, which grew to its present size in two months following an abrasion. The frequency of such keloids in this location in females may be associated with the increased cutaneous tension due to the weight of the breasts. *B,* Scattered keloids of the back which followed minimal trauma.

members of a family while the others are spared. In addition, there is a well recognized regional susceptibility; the deltoid region, the sternal area, and the face and neck are particularly susceptible.

**Neurofibroma.** This tumor is one of nerve sheaths and not of axis cylinders. It is usually multiple and in its typical form is recognized as von Recklinghausen's disease. Many soft, pedunculated, skin-covered tumors are scattered over the surface of the body (Figs. 88–44 and 88–45). Acoustic neuromas, tumors within the chest or within the spinal canal, and fibromas growing along nerve sheaths (e.g., the sciatic, the obturator, or the vagus nerves) (Altany and Pickrell, 1956) may be associated with the cutaneous tumors of von Recklinghausen's disease.

**Pachydermatocele.** Pachydermatocele (elephant skin) is a type of pendant fibroma of the skin and subcutaneous tissue which occurs in conjunction with von Recklinghausen's disease.

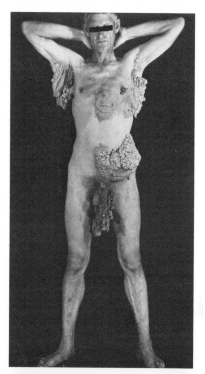

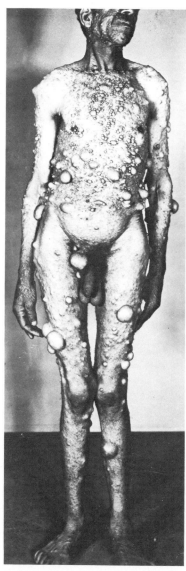

**FIGURE 88–44.** Diffuse nodular neurofibromatosis in a 50 year old man. Only the larger masses were excised.

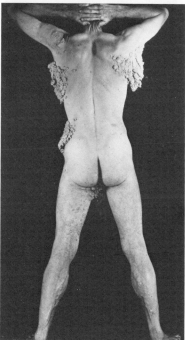

**FIGURE 88–45.** Neurofibromatosis of von Reckling-hausen. The cutaneous tumors in this 45 year old man ranged from small nodules to tremendous hanging masses which were treated by excision and skin grafting in stages. Because of the multiplicity of the cutaneous nodules, only the larger ones were removed.

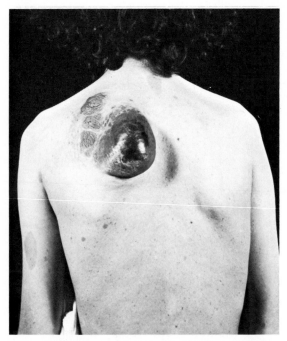

**FIGURE 88–46.** A 14 year old girl with a pachydermatocele of the back which had been present since birth. Her emergency admission was prompted because of a sudden hemorrhage (dark area) into previously pendant, flabby tumor. The tumor was excised and grafted. Note the many café au lait spots and nodules.

These large, pendant tumors (Fig. 88–46) vary in color from light to dark brown; the skin shows a soft corrugation, with creases separating patches of thickened skin which is devoid of lymphatic circulation. The tumors are soft but not compressible. Though they are usually very vascular, no bruit can be detected. The growths may take a curious form in which they hang from the side of the forehead, face, or neck (see Fig. 88–45). The disease, which often has a familial tendency, represents both a malformation and a new growth.

**Lipoma.** A lipoma is a tumor of adipose tissue occurring most frequently upon the surface of the body; it may also occur on or in the thoracic cage or the back (Fig. 88–47), or it may form an immense retroperitoneal mass. Typically, a lipoma is a sessile tumor of a consistency soft enough to give a sensation much like fluctuation. This results from the thinness of the capsule and the softness of the adipose tissue itself; usually the skin over the tumor is unchanged, although the mass may be adherent to it. Its outline is occasionally well circumscribed, while in other cases its borders are so vague that it is distinguished with difficulty from the normal surrounding fat. Its size may vary from that of a

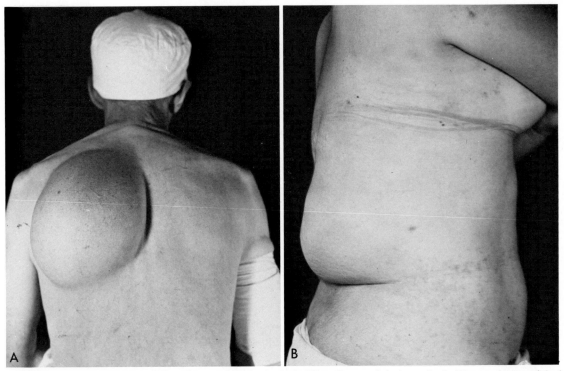

**FIGURE 88–47.** *A,* A football-sized lipoma of the back. *B,* A diffuse lipoma of the lower back. The specimen weighed more than five pounds.

walnut to that of a loaf of bread. The tumor is most often found on the shoulders, the axilla, the back, or the buttocks. Very rarely, an increase of subcutaneous fat on the entire body is related to the sensory nerves, so that pressure becomes painful—adiposis dolorosa (Dercum's disease).

**Lymphangioma.** Lymphangiomas are tumors of lymph vessels. Many are present at birth and are congenital collections of proliferating lymph vessels, quite like cavernous hemangiomas. They are seen commonly in the tongue (macroglossia), the lips (macrochelia), and the cheeks and neck (cystic hygroma). They may appear, however, in other parts of the body, notably the thorax (Fig. 88–48) and the hands and feet. In the latter locations, they may resemble lipomas, neurofibromas (von Recklinghausen's disease), or cavernous angiomas, being soft tumors of indefinite outline. Lymphangiomas are classified as simple, cavernous, and cystic.

*Lymphangioma simplex* presents cystic areas which project above the surface of the skin and are surrounded by irregular nodules. The cysts may be quite translucent and straw-colored or blue. The blue color is attributed to the rupture of dilated blood vessels into the cysts. The lesion is common in the upper half of the body, on the scalp, face, neck, shoulders, upper extremities, and chest. The term *lymphangioma complex* would better describe the lesion. Histologically, lymphangioma simplex shows multiple vesicles lined with endothelial cells. *Cavernous lymphangiomas* are usually multiple and may be reddish in color and have a spongy compressibility. They may have hemangiomatous elements in their structure—hence, the pathologic classification hemangiolymphangioma. The *cystic lymphangioma* differs from the cavernous lymphangioma in that it is not compressible, and it occurs as a single lesion of the neck or extremities.

The treatment of all such conditions, which in themselves are benign, is dependent upon whether or not the tumor is disabling or unsightly. Their vagueness of outline and their involvement of adjacent structures often make a clean excision difficult; however, they should be removed, either en bloc or by serial excisions.

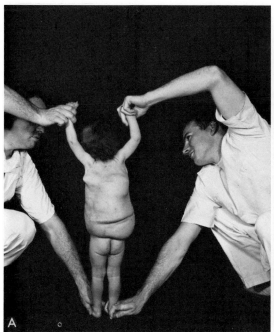 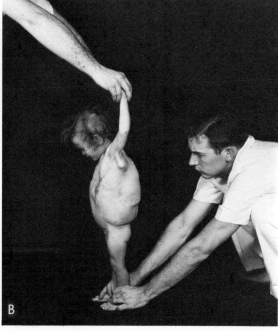

**FIGURE 88–48.** A 3 year old child with an enormous lymphangioma involving the entire torso. At birth a soft, cystic, compressible tumor occupied only the left side; however, within three months the right side became involved, and despite three operations the tumor continued to increase in size. Six drums of split-thickness skin were removed from the surface and refrigerated. The lymphangioma, which was about 15 cm thick, was then removed from the posterior and lateral sides of the torso. The stored skin was applied one week later.

# REFERENCES

Adkins, P. C., and Gwathmey, C.: Pectus excavatum; surgical treatment. J. Thorac. Surg., *36*:697, 1958.

Alonso-Lej, F., and deLinera, F. A.: Resection of the entire sternum and replacement with acrylic resin. J. Thorac. Cardiovasc. Surg., *62*:271, 1971.

Altany, F., and Pickrell, K.: Neurilemomas of the vagus nerve. A.M.S. Arch. Surg., *73*:793, 1956.

Arnold, H. S., Meese, E. H., D'Amato, N. A., and Maughon, J. S.: Localized Hodgkin's disease presenting as a sternal tumor and treated by total sternectomy. Ann. Thorac. Surg., *2*:87, 1966.

Bakamjian, V. Y., Culf, N. K., and Bales, H. W.: Versatility of the deltopectoral flap in reconstructions following head and neck cancer surgery. *In* Transactions of the International Congress of Plastic Surgeons, 4th Congress. Amsterdam, Excerpta Medica, 1967, p. 808.

Barnard, P. M., and DeWet Lubbe, J. J.: Pectus excavatum. A modified technique of internal fixation. S. Afr. Med. J., *47*:649, 1973.

Baue, A. E.: Total resection of the sternum. J. Thorac. Cardiovasc. Surg., *45*:559, 1963.

Beardsley, J. M.: The use of tantalum plate when resecting large areas of the chest wall. J. Thorac. Surg., *19*:444, 1950.

Becker, J., and Schneider, K.: Indications for surgical treatment of pectus excavatum. J. A. M. A., *180*:22, 1962.

Beiser, D., Epstein, S., Stampfer, M., Goldstein, R., Noland, S., and Levitsky, S.: Impairment of cardiac function in patients with pectus excavatum, with improvement after operative correction. New Engl. J. Med., *287*:267, 1972.

Ben-Menachem, Y., O'Hara, E., and Kane, H.: Paradoxical cardiac enlargement during inspiration in children with pectus excavatum: A new observation. Br. J. Radiol., *46*:38, 1973.

Bergofsky, E., Turino, G., and Fishman, A.: Cardiorespiratory failure in kyphoscoliosis. Medicine, *38*:263, 1959.

Bevegard, S.: Postural circulatory changes after and during exercise in patients with a funnel chest with special reference to factors affecting stroke volume. Acta Med. Scand., *171*:695, 1962.

Bisgard, J. D., and Swenson, S. A., Jr.: Tumors of the sternum: Report of a case with special operative technique. Arch. Surg., *56*:570, 1948.

Blades, B. B., and Paul, J. S.: Chest wall tumors. Ann. Surg., *131*:976, 1950.

Boyd, A. D., Gonzalez, L. L., and Altemeier, W. A.: Disruption of chest wall closure following thoracotomy. J. Thorac. Cardiovasc. Surg., *52*:47, 1966.

Brewer, L. A.: Discussion of article by K. J. Welch: Satisfactory surgical correction of pectus excavatum deformity in childhood. J. Thorac. Surg., *36*:697, 1958.

Brodkin, H. A.: Congenital chondrosternal depression (funnel chest) relieved by chondrosternoplasty. Am. J. Surg., *75*:716, 1948.

Brodkin, H. A.: Congenital chondrosternal prominence (pigeon breast): A new interpretation. Pediatrics, *3*:286, 1949.

Brodkin, H. A.: Pigeon chest: Congenital chondrosternal prominence. A.M.A. Arch. Surg., *77*:261, 1958.

Brodkin, H. A., and Linden, K.: Resection of the whole of the sternum and the cartilaginous parts of costae I-Iv. A case report. Acta Chir. Scand., *118*:1315, 1959.

Brodkin, H. A., and Peer, L. A.: Diced cartilage for chest wall defects. J. Thorac. Surg., *28*:97, 1958.

Brown, A. H., Braimbridge, M. V., Panagopoulos, P., and

Sabar, E. F.: The complications of median sternotomy. J. Thorac Cardiovasc. Surg., *58*:189, 1969.

Brown, A. L.: Pectus excavatum (funnel chest). J. Thorac. Surg., *9*:164, 1939.

Brown, A. L., and Cook, O.: Cardiorespiratory studies in pre- and postoperative funnel chest (pectus excavatum). Dis. Chest, *20*:378, 1951.

Brown, J. B., Fryer, M. P., and McDowell, F.: Permanent pedicle-blood carrying flaps for repairing defects in avascular areas. Ann. Surg., *134*:486, 1951.

Bryant, L. R., Spencer, F. C., and Trinkle, J. K.: Treatment of median sternotomy infection by mediastinal irrigation with an antibiotic solution. Ann. Surg., *169*:914, 1969.

Campbell, D. A.: Reconstruction of the anterior thoracic wall. J. Thorac. Surg., *19*:456, 1950.

Chin, E. F.: Surgery of funnel chest and congenital sternal prominence. Br. J. Surg., *44*:360, 1957.

Converse, J. M., Campbell, R. M., and Watson, W. L.: Repair of large radiation ulcers situated over heart and brain. Ann. Surg., *133*:95, 1951.

Currarino, G., and Silverman, F.: Premature obliteration of sternal sutures and pigeon breast deformity. Radiology, *70*:532, 1958.

DeLeon, A., Jr., Perloff, J., and Twigg, H.: The straight back syndrome: Clinical cardiovascular manifestation. Circulation, *32*:193, 1965.

DeOliviera, M., Sambhi, M., and Zimmerman, H.: The electrocardiogram in pectus excavatum. Br. Heart J., *20*:495, 1958.

Dormer, R., Keil, P., and Schissel, D.: Pectus excavatum. J. Thorac. Surg., *20*:444, 1950.

Dunavant, W. D.: Full thickness skin graft in the closure of a defect of the thoracic wall. J.A.M.A., *159*:1202, 1955.

Dupont, C., and Menard, Y.: Transposition of the greater omentum for reconstruction of the chest wall. Plast. Reconstr. Surg., *49*:263, 1972.

Ebstein, W.: Ueber die Trichterbenst. Dtsch. Arch., *30*:411, 1882.

Economou, S. G., Southwick, H. W., and Slaughter, D. P.: Chest repair following mammary lymphadenectomy. Arch. Surg., *83*:231, 1961.

Fabricius, J., Davidsen, H., and Hansen, A.: Cardiac function in funnel chest: Twenty-six patients investigated by cardiac catheterization. Dan. Med. Bull., *4*:251, 1957.

Féré, C., and Schmid, E.: De quelques déformations du thorax et en particulier du thorax en entonnoir et du thorax en gouttière. J. Anat. Physiol. (Paris), *29*:564, 1893.

Fish, H. G., Baxter, R. H., and Moran, R. E.: A conservative treatment of pectus excavatum in the young. Plast. Reconstr. Surg., *14*:324, 1954.

Fisher, B., Slack, N., Cavanaugh, P. T., Gardner, B., and Ravdin, R.: Postoperative radiotherapy in the treatment of breast cancer. Ann. Surg., *172*:711, 1970.

Fishman, A., Turino, G., and Bergofsky, E.: Disorders of the respiration and circulation in subjects with deformities of the thorax. Mod. Concepts Cardiovasc. Dis., *27*:449, 1958.

Fitch, E. A., and Fries, J. G.: Ivalon as a chest wall prosthesis—An 18 months follow-up. J. Thorac. Surg., *36*:262, 1958.

Frøysaker, T., and Hall, K. U.: Reconstruction of the chest wall. Scand. J. Thorac. Cardiovasc. Surg., *4*:183, 1970.

Gibbons, J. H.: Application of a mechanical heart and lung apparatus to cardiac surgery. Minn. Med., *37*:171, 1954.

Gibbons, J. H.: Surgery of the Chest. Philadelphia, W. B. Saunders Company, 1962.

Gorlin, R., Knowles, J. H., and Storey, C. F.: Effects of thoracotomy on pulmonary function. J. Thorac. Surg., *34*:242, 1957.

Graham, J., Usher, F. C., Perry, J. L., and Barkley, H. T.:

Marlex mesh as a prosthesis in the repair of thoracic wall defects. Ann. Surg., *151*:469, 1960.

Griswold, R. A.: Osteochondrosarcoma of the sternum: Use of tantalum plate as a prosthesis. Arch. Surg.,*55*:681, 1947.

Groff, D. B., and Adkins, P. C.: Collective Review: Chest wall tumors, Ann. Thorac. Surg., *4*:260, 1967.

Haller, A., Peters, G., Mazur, D., and White, J.: Pectus excavatum: A 20 year surgical experience. J. Thorac. Cardiovasc. Surg., *60*:375, 1970.

Hardin, C. A., and Harrison, J. H.: Teflon weave for replacing tissue defects. Surg. Gynecol. Obstet., *104*:584, 1957.

Hardin, C. A., and Kittle, F. C.: Repair of surgical defects of the chest wall with fiberglass. Am. Surg.,*22*:139, 1956.

Hardin, C. A., Kittle, F. C., and Schafer, P. W.: Reconstruction methods for surgical defects of chest wall. Including the use of preformed lucite plates. Am. Surg., *18*:201, 1952.

Hausmann, P. F.: The surgical management of funnel chest. J. Thorac. Surg., *29*:636, 1955.

Heblom, C. A.: Tumors of the bony chest wall. Ann. Surg., *98*:528, 1933.

Heuer, G. J.: The tumors of the sternum: Report of removal of a large mediastinal sternal chondromyxoma. Ann. Surg., *96*:830, 1932.

Hippocrates: Genuine Works. Sydenham Society, 1849.

Hoffmeister, W.: Operation der angeborenen Trichterbrust. Beitr. Klin. Chir., *141*:214, 1927.

Holden, J. S.: Sarcoma of the sternum. Br. Med. J., *11*:358, 1878.

Janes, R. M.: Primary tumors of the ribs. J. Thorac. Surg., *9*:145, 1939.

Jensen, K., Schmidt, R., Caramella, J., and Lynch, M.: Pectus excavatum: The how, when and why of surgical correction. J. Pediatr. Surg., *5*:4, 1970.

Jiminez-Martinez, M., Arguero-Sanchez, R., Perez-Alvarez, J. J., and Mina-Castaneda, P.: Anterior mediastinitis as a complication of median sternotomy incisions: Diagnostic and surgical considerations. Surgery, *67*:929, 1970.

Johnson, L. P.: Criteria for the management of moderate funnel chest deformities in children. Am. Surg., *38*:498, 1972.

Kinsella, T. J., White, S. M., and Koucky, R. W.: Two unusual tumors of the sternum. J. Thorac. Surg., *16*:640, 1947.

Korlof, B., Nylén, B., Olsson, P., Skoog, T., and Strombeck, J.: Resection of the thoracic wall and local flap repair for recurrences of mammary carcinoma. Br. J. Plast. Surg., *26*:322, 1973.

Lam, C., and Taber, R.: Surgical treatment of pectus carinatum. Arch. Surg., *103*:191, 1971.

Lambert, C. J., Mitchel, B. F., Adam, M., and Skiekh, S.: A modified technique for severe median sternotomy closure. Surgery, *69*:393, 1971.

Larson, R. E., Lick, L. C., and Maxeiner, S. R.: Technique of chest wall reconstruction following resection of chondrosarcoma. Arch. Surg., *98*:668, 1969.

Latham, W. D.: Operative treatment for postradiation defects of the chest wall. Am. Surg., *32*:700, 1966.

Leininger, B. J., Baker, W. L., and Langston, H. T.: A simplified method of chest wall reconstruction. Ann. Thorac. Surg., *13*:258, 1972.

LeRoux, B. T.: Maintenance of chest wall stability. Thorax, *19*:397, 1964.

Lester, C.: The surgical treatment of funnel chest. Ann. Surg., *123*:1003, 1946.

Lester, C.: Pigeon breast (pectus carinatum) and other protrusion deformities of developmental origin. Ann. Surg., *137*:482, 1953.

Lester, C.: Surgical treatment of protrusion deformities of the sternum and costal cartilages (pectus carinatum, pigeon breast). Ann. Surg., *153*:441, 1961.

LeVeen, H., and Piccone, V.: Nylon band chest closure. Arch. Surg., *96*:36, 1968.

Lindskog, G., and Felton, W.: Pectus excavatum. Surg. Gynecol. Obstet., *95*:615, 1952.

Lindskog, G., and Felton, W.: Considerations in the surgical treatment of pectus excavatum. Ann. Surg., *142*:654, 1955.

Lister, G. D., and Gibson, T.: Destruction of the chest wall and damage to the heart by x-irradiation from an industrial source. Br. J. Plast. Surg., *26*:328, 1973.

Longacre, J. J., Maurer, E. P., and Keirle, A. M.: Immediate skeletal reconstruction of an extensive bilateral defect of the anterior chest wall. Plast. Reconstr. Surg., *53*:593, 1974.

Lyons, H., Zuhdi, M., and Kelly, J., Jr.: Pectus excavatum (funnel chest), a cause of impaired ventricular distensibility as exhibited by right ventricular pressure pattern. Am. Heart J., *50*:921, 1955.

Maier, H. C.: Surgical management of large defects of the thoracic wall. Surgery, *22*:169, 1947

Maliniac, J. W.: Arterial supply of the breast. Arch. Surg., *47*:329, 1943.

Mallory, T. B.: Chondroma of rib. New Engl. J. Med., *218*:886, 1938.

Martini, N., Starzynski, T. E., and Beattie, E. J.: Problems in chest wall resection. Surg. Clin. North Am., *49*:313, 1969.

Martini, N., Huvos, A. G., Smith, J., and Beattie, E. J.: Primary malignant tumors of the sternum. Surg. Gynecol., Obstet., *138*:391, 1974.

Masson, J. K., Payne, W. S., and Gonzalez, J. B.: Pectus excavatum: Use of preformed prosthesis for correction in the adult. Case report. Plast. Reconstr. Surg., *46*:399, 1970.

Mauer, E., and Blades, B.: Hernia of lung. J. Thorac. Surg., *15*:77, 1946.

May, A. M.: Operation for pectus excavatum using stainless steel wire mesh. J. Thorac. Cardiovasc. Surg., *42*:122, 1961.

Mayo, P., and Long, G.: Surgical repair of pectus excavatum by pin immobilization. J. Thorac. Cardiovasc. Surg., *44*:53, 1962.

McGregor, I. A., and Jackson, I. T.: The groin flap. Br. J. Plast. Surg., *25*:3, 1972.

Medgyesi, S.: Investigation into the carrying ability of pedicled bone grafts during transplantation. Acta Orthop. Scand., *39*:1, 1968.

Meyer, L.: Zur chirurgischen Behandlung der angeboren en Trichterbrust. Verh. d. Berl. Med. Ges., *42*:364, 1911.

Milton, H.: Mediastinal surgery. Lancet, *1*:872, 1897.

Morrow, A. G.: The use of tantalum gauze in the closure of full-thickness defects of the chest wall. Surgery, *28*:1016, 1950.

Myre, T. T., and Kirklin, J. W.: Resection of tumors of the sternum. Ann. Surg., *144*:1023, 1956.

Nageotte-Wilbouchewitch, M.: Inadequacy of growth tables: Importance of thoracic perimeter with respiratory amplitude; diameter of funnel-shaped chest. Bull. Soc. Pediatr. Paris, *33*:627, 1935.

Nathan, M. J., Kingsley, W. B., and Paulson, D. L.: Staged radical pulmonary and chest wall resection for metastatic osteosarcoma. Ann. Thorac. Surg., *12*:305, 1971.

Ochsner, A., and DeBakey, M.: Chone-chondrosternon. J. Thorac. Surg., *8*:469, 1939.

Pers, M., and Medgyesi, S.: Pedicle muscle flaps and their applications in the surgery of repair. Br. J. Plast. Surg., 26:313, 1973.

Peters, R., and Johnson, G., Jr.: Stabilization of pectus deformity with wire strut. J. Thorac. Cardiovasc. Surg., 47:814, 1964.

Pickrell, K. L., Baker, H. M., and Collins, J. P.: Reconstructive surgery of the chest wall. Surg. Gynecol. Obstet., 84:465, 1947.

Pickrell, K. L., Kelley, J. W., and Marzoni, F. A.: The surgical treatment of recurrent carcinoma of the breast and chest wall. Plast. Reconstr. Surg., 3:156, 1948.

Prioleau, W. H.: Full-thickness closure of large thoracotomy due to chemical destruction of chest wall. J. Thorac. Surg., 14:433, 1945.

Ravitch, M. M.: The operative treatment of pectus excavatum. Ann. Surg., 129:429, 1949.

Ravitch, M. M.: Pectus excavatum and heart failure. Surgery, 30:178, 1951.

Ravitch, M. M.: Unusual sternal deformity with cardiac symptoms. J. Thorac. Surg., 23:138, 1952.

Ravitch, M. M.: The operative treatment of pectus excavatum. J. Pediatr., 48:465, 1956.

Ravitch, M. M.: The operative correction of pectus carinatum (pigeon breast). Ann. Surg., 151:705, 1960.

Ravitch, M. M.: Technical problems in the operative correction of pectus excavatum. Ann. Surg., 162:29, 1965.

Ravitch, M. M.: Discussion of article by Haller and coworkers. J. Thorac. Cardiovasc. Surg., 60:381, 1970.

Rees, T. D.: Radiation necrosis of the chest wall, full-thickness reconstruction with pedicle flap and diced homologous cartilage over the pericardium complicated by cardiac arrest. Plast. Reconstr. Surg., 28:67, 1961.

Rees, T. D., and Converse, J. M.: Surgical reconstruction of defects of the thoracic wall. Surg. Gynecol. Obstet., 121:1066, 1965.

Rehbein, F., and Wernicke, H.H.: The operative treatment of the funnel chest. Arch. Dis. Child. (Lond.), 32:5, 1957.

Reusch, C. S.: Hemodynamic studies in pectus excavatum. Circulation, 24:1143, 1961.

Richardson, W. G.: Enchondroma of the manubrium sterni successfully removed by operation. Br. Med. J., 1:985, 1913.

Rintala, A.: Local radiation burns. Acta Chir. Scand. Suppl. 376, 1967.

Robicsek, F., Sanger, P., Taylor, F., and Thomas, M.: The surgical treatment of chondrosternal prominence (pectus carinatum). J. Thorac. Cardiovasc. Surg., 45:691, 1963.

Roesler, H.: The relation of the shape of the heart to the shape of the chest: With special reference to the anteroposterior dimension and the morphology of various normal heart types. Am. J. Roentgenol. Radium Ther. Nucl. Med., 32:464, 1934.

Routledge, R. T.: The surgical problem of local post-irradiation effects. Br. J. Plast. Surg., 7:134, 1954.

Sanfelippo, P. M., and Danielson, G. K.: Complications associated with median sternotomy. J. Thorac. Cardiovasc. Surg., 63:419, 1972a.

Sanfelippo, P. M., and Danielson, G. K.: Nylon bands for closure of median sternotomy incisions: An unacceptable method. Ann. Thorac. Surg., 13:404, 1972b.

Sauerbruch, E. F.: Die Chirurgie der Brustorgane. 3rd ed. Berlin, G. Springer, 1928.

Schepelman, E.: Zur plastiche nach mammoamputation. Zentralbl. Gynaekol., 48:1902, 1924.

Smith, P. J., Foley, B., McGregor, I. A., and Jackson, I. T.: The anatomical basis of the groin flap. Plast. Reconstr. Surg., 49:41, 1972.

Southwick, H. W., Economou, S. G., and Otten, J. W.: Prosthetic replacement of chest wall defects. Arch. Surg., 72:901, 1956.

Stanford, W., Bowers, D., Lindberg, E., Armstrong, R., Finger, E., and Dibbell, D.: Silastic implants for correction of pectus excavatum. Ann. Thorac. Surg., 13:529, 1972.

Starzynski, T. E., Snyderman, R. K., and Beattie, E. J.: Problems of major chest wall reconstruction. Plast. Reconstr. Surg., 44:525, 1969.

Stephenson, K. L., and Mosley, J. M.: Reconstructive problems of chest and breast. Am. J. Surg., 92:26, 1956.

Sweet, R.: Pectus excavatum: Report of two cases successfully operated upon. Ann. Surg., 119:922, 1944.

Taber, R. E., and Madaras, J.: Prevention of sternotomy wound disruptions by the use of figure-of-eight pericostal sutures. Ann. Thorac. Surg., 8:367, 1969.

Tai, Y., and Hasegawa, H.: A transverse abdominal flap for reconstruction after radical operations for recurrent breast cancer. Plast. Reconstr. Surg., 53:52, 1974.

Tamoney, H. J., and Stent, P. A.: Dermal graft for chest wall repair. Surg. Gynecol. Obstet., 118:289, 1964.

Troisier, J., and Monnerot, D.: Thorax en entonnoir et doight Renté. Deux tableaux généalogique. Bull. Mém. Soc. Med. Hop. Paris, 54:311, 1930.

Urban, J.A.:Radical excision of the chest wall for mammary cancer. Lancet, 4:1263, 1951.

Urban, J. A., and Baker, H. W.: Radical mastectomy in continuity with en bloc resection of the internal mammary lymph node chain. Cancer, 5:992, 1952.

Usher, F. C.: Knitted Marlex mesh. An improved Marlex prosthesis for repairing hernias and other tissue defects. Arch. Surg., 82:771, 1961.

Vianna, J. B.: Partial resection of the anterior thoracic wall with skin flap reconstruction. J. Int. Coll. Surg., 18:193, 1952.

Vidne, B., and Levy, M. J.: Surgical treatment for pectus excavatum. Israel J. Med. Sci., 9:1565, 1973.

Wachtel, F., Ravitch, M. M., and Grishman, A.: The relationship of pectus excavatum to heart disease. Am. Heart J., 52:121, 1956.

Wada, J., and Ikeda, K.: Clinical experience with 306 funnel chest operations. Internatl. Surg., 57:707, 1972.

Watson, W. L., and James, A. G.: Fascia lata grafts for chest wall defects. J. Thorac. Surg., 16:399, 1947.

Welch, K., and Vos, A.: Surgical correction of pectus carinatum (pigeon breast). J. Pediatr. Surg., 8:659, 1973.

Whalen, W. P.: Coverage of thoracic wall defects by a split breast flap. Plast. Reconstr. Surg., 12:64, 1953.

Winkel, A. H.: Hernia of lung. J. Thorac. Surg., 4:627, 1935.

# CHAPTER 89

# PLASTIC SURGERY OF THE BREAST

## THOMAS D. REES, M.D.

Reconstruction of the Female Breast
After Radical Mastectomy
*H. Höhler, M.D.*

In addition to being an important functional organ, the female breast must be considered in the perspective of present-day social consciousness as a structure of considerable psychologic significance. Since the era of classic Greek art, the female breast has been a symbol of femininity. Deformities of the size and shape of this structure assume importance above and beyond those of a functioning secondary sexual organ. To have physically acceptable breasts is a normal desire, and the psychologic implications of this desire must not be underestimated.

Plastic surgery of the breast is now generally accepted by the medical profession and demanded by the lay public. Deforming operations or amputations of the breast are justifiable only in the therapy of breast cancer. Modern reconstructive techniques have made possible the restitution of adequate contour following surgery for benign lesions, reduction and augmentation mammaplasty, and in some instances following cancer ablation.

### HISTORY

Surgical consciousness of preserving or reconstructing cosmetically acceptable breasts has been evident since 1669 when Durstan reported the first attempt at a breast reconstruction, in which he performed essentially a mastectomy to correct ptotic breasts. Following his report almost 200 years elapsed until Velpeau (1854) published his study of mastoptosis.

Czerny (1895) was the first to "deal in the plastic manner with defects of breasts." He removed a fibroadenoma from the breast and substituted a lipoma from the same patient "with good results." Michel and Pousson (1897) described removing a pie-shaped section from the upper half of the breast in a young woman with bilateral hypertrophy. They employed two crescentic incisions in the upper anterior portion of the breast, removing a full-thickness wedge of tissue down to the aponeurosis of the pectoralis major muscle, but did not attempt gland reduction per se. The breast was anchored to the aponeurosis of the pectoralis major muscle. They reported a satisfactory result in this case.

In 1898 Verchère described excision of a triangular portion from the lateral part of the upper half of the breast. Guinard (1903) is credited with operating on a patient with marked macromastia by partial removal of breast tissue through semicircular incisions in the submammary fold. Morestin (1903) described the removal of a small benign tumor from the breast through a buttonhole incision in the hairy part of the axilla. At this presentation in 1903 by Morestin, Guinard also reported his famous case. In 1907, Morestin described a large discoid resection via a submammary (Thomas) incision in a patient with macromastia. Accordingly it was suggested by Joseph that the technique of discoid breast resection should be credited to these two surgeons and known as the Morestin-Guinard method.

Dehner's mastopexy technique (1908) consisted of the removal of a semilunar section from the superior aspect of both breasts. The fascia of the pectoralis muscles was split and the breasts attached to the periosteum of the third rib.

The so-called Thomas submammary incision had been described in 1882 by Dr. Gaillard Thomas, a New York surgeon. This incision was originally used for tumor excision. It was revived by Girard in 1910 for use in mastopexy, in which he made a submammary incision, separated the gland from the pectoral fascia, and suspended the posterior surface of the breast from the pectoralis fascia and the second rib.

Several years later, Passot (1925) reported his now well known incision, utilizing the Thomas principle. The priority for nipple transposition through a buttonhole incision in the skin flap is somewhat clouded but is generally credited to Villandre, who performed this step in 1911. Auber (1923), of Marseilles, was actually first to report the technique. Transposition of the nipple was performed by Dufourmentel in 1916, but a report was not published by him until 1927. Passot (1925) preferred nipple transposition in conjunction with his adaptation of the Thomas incision.

Shortly after Auber's paper there appeared the report by Kraske (1923), in which he described a technique of nipple transposition which was apparently used by Lexer in 1912. This consisted of nipple transposition and excision of the lower midline quadrant of breast tissue.

In 1916 Kausch reported a case in which he excised hypertrophic breast tissue through crescentic incisions around the areola; though of ingenious design, the result was marred by scarring. Complete separation of the skin covering the breast on its anterior surface, permitting easy maneuverability of the underlying breast tissue is first credited to Axhausen (1926). He also favored nipple transposition.

Other important contributions to breast reconstructive techniques were made by Thorek (1922), Lotsch (1923), Dartigues (1924, 1928), Joseph (1925), Mornard (1926), and Noël (1928).

The Biesenberger operation was reported in 1928. He described excision of the lateral portion of the gland with rotation of the remaining glandular pedicle attached to the nipple and formation of a skin brassiere. The Biesenberger

technique was probably most widely practiced throughout the world as the operation of choice for the nipple transposition technique, until Strömbeck introduced his technique in 1960.

Joseph (1925) deserves credit for suggesting a two-stage pedicle technique to preserve maximum blood supply to the breast.

Credit for documenting the technique of free nipple grafting belongs to Thorek (1922). There is evidence that free nipple transplantation was practiced before Thorek by Lexer and Dartigues (Maliniac, 1959). However, Dartigues did not publish his work until 1928. Maliniac (1959) credits Lexer with having done this operation as early as 1912. The operation reported by Thorek was essentially a partial mammary amputation, utilizing a Passot type of incision and transplanting the nipples as free composite grafts of areola, muscle, and ductile tissue. Later, Thorek (1946) reported 25 years' experience with free nipple transplantation. The technique has been widely adopted in America and was championed by Adams (1944, 1947), Conway (1952, 1958), Marino (1952), Longacre (1953), and May (1956). However, the Strömbeck principle has generally obviated the need for free nipple grafts except in cases of enormous hypertrophy or marked ptosis (Felix and associates, 1970).

Many authors have contributed to the literature on this subject by describing their personal experience and variations in technique. Gillies and McIndoe (1939) provided a detailed description of the Biesenberger technique as further modified by them. Bames (1948, 1950, 1953), Aufricht (1949), Maliniac (1950), Tamerin (1951), Conway (1952, 1958), Marino (1952, 1957), Penn (1955, 1960), May (1956), Wise (1956, 1963), McIndoe and Rees (1958), Pitanguy (1960, 1967), Strömbeck (1960, 1968), Skoog (1963), Dufourmentel and Mouly (1961, 1965), McKissock (1972), Wiener and coworkers (1973), and others have made contributions. A monumental analysis of 500 personal cases of breast reduction mammaplasty was reported by Ragnell (1957).

The chronology thus far has referred to breast reduction mammaplasty or mastopexy. Another area of breast reconstruction is augmentation mammaplasty. Longacre (1953, 1954, 1956, 1959) described his techniques for reconstruction of the hypoplastic gland, either congenital or acquired, by local de-epitelized pedicle flaps. Another form of augmentation mammaplasty, the transplantation of free dermis-fat or fat-fascia grafts to supply the necessary bulk for contour, has been reported by Berson (1945), Bames (1950, 1953), and Conway and Smith

(1958). A comprehensive review of this technique was published by Watson (1959).

The third type of breast augmentation is the insertion of a permanent prosthesis. The most suitable substances currently in use for this purpose are the various types of silicone prostheses. Experience with sponge implantations has been reported by Pangman and Wallace (1954), Edgerton and McClary (1958), Edgerton, Meyer, and Jacobson (1961), Conway and Dietz (1962), and Pickrell (1962). Cronin and Gerow (1964) first described a subcutaneous prosthesis containing a gel form of dimethylpolysiloxane (silicone) contained in a Silastic envelope. The latter prosthesis, or variations of it, has gained ubiquitous approval by plastic surgeons the world over as the most satisfactory material thus far developed. Recent development of the round, "soft" prostheses with thin Silastic envelopes has further improved the results.

The Ashley prosthesis was described in 1970 and 1972. It also consists of a silicone envelope filled with silicone gel, but it has an outer layer of fine-celled sponge which is useful in tissue adherence. Arion (1965), Tabari (1969), Jenny (1969), and Rees, Guy, and Coburn (1973), have developed inflatable balloon devices, which are essentially silicone bladders. The balloons are inserted through small periareolar or submammary incisions and inflated with dextran, PVP, or saline to the desired volume. They are of particular advantage in patients with breast asymmetry.

## SURGICAL ANATOMY OF THE BREAST

The adult female breast is a glandular structure which varies considerably in size and shape. The breast normally occupies an area extending from the second through the sixth ribs, and from the sternum to the anterior axillary line. The axillary tail (of Spence) can be palpated along the lateral border of the pectoralis muscle toward the axilla.

Except at the nipple and areola, the gland is located subcutaneously, and a rather well defined layer of areolar and adipose tissue lies between the gland proper and the overlying skin. This plane lends itself well to blunt or sharp dissection for elevating flaps in mammaplasty; it is moderately vascular.

The parenchyma of the gland is enveloped by a capsule or fascial layer that is continuous with the pectoral fascia. This same fascia subdivides the gland into lobules, and a few strands extend to the overlying skin; these are divided in raising skin flaps. The slips of fascia are more numerous in the upper hemisphere of the gland, where they are known as the suspensory ligaments of Cooper.

The posterior surface of the gland lies on the pectoralis major muscle. Between the intimately attached fascia of the gland and the outer fascia of the muscle is a layer of adipose tissue. This plane is relatively avascular except for a few perforating vessels and is of importance as the plane in which foreign implants are inserted in mammary augmentation operations. Implants are actually positioned outside the gland, lying between the gland and the pectoralis major muscle.

The areola with its central eminence, the nipple, varies in size and color, from pink to dark brown. It is rich in vascular supply from a dermal plexus of veins and arteries. Care must be taken to preserve these vessels in nipple transposition operations.

The nipple eminence is formed by the emergence of 15 to 25 mammary ducts which dilate to form ampullae just before opening to the surface. The nipple and areola are covered by a modified mucous membrane lubricated by the glands of Montgomery (sebaceous glands) located beneath the areola.

The mammary ducts extend radially from the nipple and divide into a variable number of secondary tubules which terminate by forming the lobules or acinar structures of the breast. The tubules and acini vary numerically in different individuals and at different periods, depending on such factors as menstrual phases or pregnancy. These epithelial structures constitute the parenchyma of the gland. The stroma of the gland is composed of a mixture of fatty tissue separated by the fascial septa described above.

**Blood Supply.** The arterial supply of the breast is abundant and arises from three main sources: (1) the posterior intercostal arteries that branch off the descending aorta; (2) the large lateral thoracic artery and the variable external mammary artery branching from the axillary artery; (3) the internal mammary artery arising from the subclavian. It is important in breast surgery to realize that there is a rich anastomosis between the smaller branches of these three major arterial sources. Many parts of the mammary gland are supplied by two and sometimes three of the main sources. The rich vascular plexus supplying the areola and nipples is an example of a vital surgical area that receives contributions or ramifications from all three systems. It is the overlapping of vascular supply that provides a margin of safety in breast reconstruction. It is also important to realize that there are variations in blood supply, although these are not usually of clinical importance.

The medial portion of the gland often derives its major supply from the penetrating or intercostal branches of the internal mammary artery. The anterior lateral cutaneous branches of the intercostal arteries are widely distributed to the entire gland, whereas the branches of the lateral thoracic artery mainly supply the lateral portion of the gland. It is emphasized that the three primary sources form two rich anastomotic systems, a superficial plexus about the areola and a deep plexus in the gland proper. The venous drainage of the breast generally follows the course of the arteries.

The lymphatic drainage of the breast is abundant and of major significance in neoplastic surgery, but of minor significance in plastic surgery. Postoperative lymphedema in reconstructed breasts is rarely a problem.

The mammary gland contains a superficial (subareolar) plexus and a deep (fascial) plexus of lymphatics similar to those of the blood supply. The superficial plexus drains mainly to the axillary and pectoral muscle nodes. From the axilla, the drainage is to the subclavian nodes.

The deep plexus drains via perforating channels, through the pectoralis muscles to the deep pectoral nodes and then to the subclavian nodes. The remainder of the deep plexus drains medially along the internal mammary artery to the mediastinal nodes.

Other lymphatic drainage pathways are of lesser significance and include pathways to the abdominal lymphatics and sometimes a superficial cross drainage to the opposite breast.

**Nerve Supply.** The cutaneous sensory nerves to the breast are derived from the supraclavicular branch of the cervical plexus and also from the anterior and lateral perforating branches of the second, third, fourth, and fifth intercostal branches. The deep nerve supply to the gland proper is derived almost entirely from the fourth, fifth, and sixth intercostal branches.

Often in the course of a mammaplasty, the cutaneous sensory distribution to the nipple and areolar areas, as well as the sympathetic innervation, is divided. However, after varying periods of time, usually six months to one year, sensation and erectile function of the nipple return. Usually there is little or no loss of either sensation or erectile function of the nipple in nipple transposition operations, whereas after free nipple transplantation a complete loss of

these functions occurs initially, with gradual but variable return of function.

## CLASSIFICATION OF BREAST DEFORMITIES

A classification of breast deformities requiring plastic surgery includes breasts that are too large, too small, absent, asymmetric, or of faulty position. Deformities resulting from surgery for benign or malignant lesions must also be included. Such a classification is, of course, an

TABLE 89–1.  *Classification*

I. Candidates for Reduction Mammaplasty or Mastopexy
  Type 1—Long, flabby breasts with or without glandular hypertrophy (adolescent type)
  Type 2—Broad, heavy, obese breasts
  Type 3—Pendulous, saclike breasts following pregnancy and/or weight reduction
  Type 4—Virginal hypertrophy (true gynecomastia)
  Type 5—Asymmetry (unilateral macromastia)

II. Candidates for Augmentation Mammaplasty
  1. Aplasia
  2. Hypoplasia
  3. Idiopathic involution (usually following pregnancy)
  4. Asymmetry

III. Candidates for Glandular Ablation and Reconstruction of the Mammary Eminence (Benign and/or Premalignant Disease)
  1. Multiple fibroadenomas of menopause
  2. Advanced or intractable mammary dysplasia
    a. Severe mastodynia
    b. Cystic mastitis (advanced)
    c. Adenosis (Schimmelbush's disease)
  3. Residual lactation mastitis
  4. Lobular carcinoma in situ
  5. Questionable mammograms (repeated)
  6. Intraductile carcinoma in a young woman requiring radical mastectomy on one side
  7. To be considered in a young woman with a strong family history

IV. Candidates for Mammary Reconstruction Following Ablation of Cancer by Excision and/or Irradiation
  1. Radiation necrosis (nonhealing wounds)
  2. Severe psychiatric disturbances, after suitable time Postcancer reconstruction is undertaken only after careful evaluation of the individual case or in the presence of nonhealing radiation ulcers. Reconstruction can be considered sooner than five years when the original tumor was apparently localized and without positive regional nodes or other evidence of metastases.

V. Candidates for Excisional Biopsy and/or Plastic Repair
  1. Developmental anomalies
    a. Polymastia
    b. Polythelia
  2. Persistent gynecomastia in men

oversimplification. A more detailed breakdown is provided in Table 89–1.

The most common type of breast deformity requiring plastic surgery is the broad, heavy, obese type (type 2 in Table 89–1). In a series of 347 cases (McIndoe and Rees, 1958), 201 were of this type. The second most common group requiring breast reduction mammaplasty is type 3, the pendulous, saclike breast, frequently following pregnancy or weight reduction.

The incidence of underdeveloped breasts in the general public is difficult, if not impossible, to ascertain. There is little doubt that this physical impediment is very common and may possibly be present in as much as 30 per cent of the adult female population.

## BREAST REDUCTION MAMMAPLASTY AND MASTOPEXY

**Indications for Operation.** Discomfort due to excessive weight of one or both breasts is the chief indication for a mammary reduction operation in the majority of patients. Heavy, pendulous breasts are a severe handicap, mentally and physically. As the deformity progresses, the social adjustment of the afflicted patient may be seriously affected. Conway (1952) has shown that kyphosis and arthritis of the cervical spine may develop secondary to postural attitudes to compensate for excessively large breasts. Uncomfortable grooving of the shoulders can occur at the site of brassiere supports. Increased moisture in the submammary crease often results in intertrigo which is difficult to treat. Mammary hypertrophy may be associated with painful, chronic mastitis. This can often be relieved in proportion to the amount of breast tissue excised.

In severe forms of mammary dysplasia, especially when "cancer phobia" is present following multiple biopsy procedures and a strong family history of malignant breast disease, total glandular ablation with reconstruction of the mammary eminence should be seriously considered, as proposed by Maliniac (1950) and Longacre (1959) and recently championed by Freeman (1962, 1969), Lewis (1965), Bader, Pellettiere, and Curtin (1970); Goulian and McDivitt (1972), and Wiener and associates (1973).

Asymmetry of breasts with unilateral hypomastia is another deformity requiring mammaplasty (Rees and Dupuis, 1968). Marked discrepancy in the size of the breasts can result in scoliosis. One must also be cognizant of the possibility of serious emotional problems resulting from such a deformity.

Financial hardships inflicted on these patients by the added expense of custom-made brassieres, blouses, and dresses should not be ignored.

As previously emphasized, except in mammary cancer, mammectomy or amputation is almost never a justifiable procedure.

**Preoperative Planning and Selection of Operation.** The general physical condition of the patient is carefully evaluated before surgery. Mammaplasty, though not a life-threatening operation, can nevertheless be one of considerable magnitude and may involve prolonged anesthesia.

A detailed and careful examination of the breasts and axillary regions is important to rule out unrecognized breast disease. Mammograms and thermograms should also be considered as diagnostic adjuncts. Preoperative assessment of the individual problem is always indicated, particularly in breast reduction surgery. No one operative procedure is the panacea, and the operative technique is selected to fit the case at hand.

Controversy has arisen between advocates of transposition of the nipple on a pedicle and those who transplant the nipple as a free composite graft. Surgeons who feel strongly in favor of nipple transposition believe that to destroy lactation, particularly in the young woman, is physiologically and psychologically unsound. Nipple transposition is criticized on the bases that: (1) Blood supply may be impaired with danger of nipple slough. This complication is particularly a danger in the reduction of massive breasts with a resulting long nipple pedicle. (2) Most patients seeking reduction mammaplasty are little, if at all, concerned about maintaining functional lactation. (3) A free nipple transplant is almost always successful if properly executed. In regard to the danger of sloughing of the nipple, it should be noted that of the 347 cases reviewed by McIndoe and Rees (1958), partial nipple loss occurred in only four patients and total nipple loss in one. All nipple losses were secondary to hematoma.

Maliniac (1950, 1959) has strongly criticized the free nipple transplant operation as constituting a potential carcinogenic hazard by interfering with ductile egress. He cited opinions by Warren, Geschickter, Huggins, and Treves as his basis of argument. This view is not accepted by most surgeons. The supporting evidence lies mostly in the realm of individual opinion rather than scientific fact based on clinical studies and statistics. Instances in which malignancy has been reported following breast plastic surgery appear to be coincidental when examined by statistical analysis.

It is only reasonable that both the technique of free nipple transplantation and that of nipple transposition have a proper place in the surgeon's armamentarium. In cases of gigantomastia with marked ptosis or enormous breasts, an operation of the nipple transposition type is unduly hazardous to nipple survival. In these extreme cases, the procedure of choice is free nipple transplantation. The maintenance of the lactating function is of no importance in such patients.

Nipple transposition by the pedicle technique has stood the test of time and is the procedure of choice in moderate to severe degrees of hypertrophy. The nipple transposition operation usually results in a more desirable conical-shaped breast than free nipple grafting, with the Passot incision usually used. The nipple transposition operation reported in large series of cases by Gillies and McIndoe (1939), Ragnell (1946, 1957), McIndoe and Rees (1958), Strömbeck (1960, 1968), Pitanguy (1967), Beare (1967), Dufourmentel and Mouly (1965), Rees and Rhoads (1970), and McKissock (1972) has not proved unduly hazardous, particularly if every precaution to prevent postoperative hematoma is observed.

A second consideration of importance in planning breast reduction mammaplasty is electing a one- or two-stage operating technique. The one-stage operation is generally favored and is the ideal in any reconstructive procedure. A two-stage operation is indicated only when the surgeon feels that a single-stage operation will unduly compromise blood supply (Bames, 1948; Maliniac, 1950; Ragnell, 1957). A certain number of patients will require a secondary "trim up" or scar revision. If one utilizes free nipple transplantation in the excessively oversized breasts and a nipple transposition technique in less large breasts, there is rarely an indication for two-stage planning.

Three basic operations are presented in this chapter for dealing with oversized breasts unassociated with premalignant changes. These operations, or slight variations of them, are most commonly in use throughout the world today. They have stood the test of time and usage. The operations to be described are: (1) operation for reduction of minimal to moderately enlarged breasts; (2) operation for reduction of moderate to very large breasts (nipple transposition); (3) operation for excessively large breasts—gigantomastia (free nipple transplantation). Operations for correction of simple mastoptosis are also included.

### Techniques

POSITION ON OPERATING TABLE. The patient is placed on the operating table with the table "break" so located that the patient may be elevated to a semi-sitting position from time to time to facilitate marking and planning, and for final visual confirmation of the nipple sites and gland dependency.

Hands are tucked beneath the flanks with fingers extended to prevent pressure points over the joints. A foot plate is necessary.

It is important that the shoulders be "squared" and symmetrical. An ether screen or other device is necessary to isolate the anesthetist from the sterile field.

LOCATING THE NIPPLE SITES. Several techniques are available for preoperative determination of nipple location. Ideally, the nipples are located somewhat lateral to the midclavicular line (in the line of axis of the breast cone) and point upward and outward. Penn (1955) came to the conclusion that the nipples and the supraclavicular notch form a triangle in which each limb measures approximately 21 cm in the normal sized female. Pennisi, Klabunde, and Pletsch (1969) also provided a helpful guide for nipple location. No one set of measurements, however, can be applied to every individual. Location of the nipples depends not only on the length of the torso but also on the body habitus of the individual and the dimensions of the thoracic cage. Nipple measurements should vary after considering these factors. It is preferable to make the temporary preoperative nipple measurements with the patient in a standing or sitting position with the breasts dependent. The large breast caliper and draftsman's compass are helpful tools. New nipple sites are located at 19 cm to 24 cm from the sternal notch (McIndoe and Rees, 1958). This line is bisected by a line from the xiphoid, measuring 12.5 to 17 cm, depending on the size of the thorax.

Measurements can be done on the day before operation, the area being lightly scratched with a pin or marked with indelible ink. At the time of operation, with the patient on the operating table, the measurements are rechecked. Final placing of the nipples after mammaplasty is best measured visually by the surgeon with the aid of temporary dye marks. It is wise to locate the nipple sites slightly lower than these ideal and theoretical points, inasmuch as they tend to migrate upward in the ensuing months following surgery.

OPERATION FOR MILD TO MODERATE MACROMASTIA. Mild to moderate degrees of macromastia and mastoptosis can be satisfactorily corrected by several standard operative procedures. Preference remains with the individual surgeon. Free nipple transplantation is definitely not the procedure of choice in this less severe deformity. The simplified operation of Aries, as described by Pitanguy (1960), has the advantage of minimal tissue disturbance and avoids a scar in the inframammary crease where occasionally troublesome scar hypertrophy may occur. Penn (1960) pointed out that radial breast scars usually heal better than peripheral scars paralleling the breast crease.

Most surgeons have found the Strömbeck technique or its variations to be easily adaptable for the correction of minor degrees of ptosis and hypertrophy. This adaptation of the technique was pointed out by Kahn, Hoffman, and Simon (1968). Ptosis can also be corrected by a combination of mastopexy and the insertion of a silicone implant (Regnault, 1966).

Goulian and Conway (1969), however, pointed out the inadvisability of attempting to correct ptosis with implants alone. In such a case, implants may increase the ptosis or compound the deformity in a most bizarre way. Mastopexy should always be the principal operative procedure to correct ptosis, with or without prosthetic implants.

Ptosis is often the primary problem in the moderately hypertrophic breast. Mammary tissue is resected according to the need. Pitanguy pointed out that the vertical pull of a pendulous breast causes thickening of the connective tissue, and thus a vertical incision is less conspicuous than a transverse incision. In larger breasts, the excess of skin to be removed makes the transverse limb of the inverted T incision necessary. Penn (1960) obviated this by a tonguelike flap with two radially placed incisions, eliminating the submammary crease scar.

The technique of Dufourmentel and Mouly (1965, 1968), is also particularly well suited to correct the small, ptotic breast. They placed the incision in a radial line extending laterally towards the axilla, so that it lies within the clothing line of even the extreme modern dress styles.

After suitable preparation and positioning, the new nipple location is established according to the technique of preference. In the Aries-Pitanguy technique, a vertical ellipse of skin and gland is marked below the nipple (Fig. 89–1, *A*). The areola is then dissected, leaving a dermal ring attached circumferentially around the nipple (Fig. 89–1, *B*). The gland is undermined in a subcutaneous plane only to the width necessary to permit an upward shifting of the gland to the desired level (Fig. 89–1, *C*). Extensive undermining is avoided. Limited undermining also permits a downward shift of the excess skin and a plumping out or filling of the superior portion of the breast by forcing the tissue cephalad. The wedge defect formed by the glandular excision is sutured with 2–0 chromic catgut (Fig. 89–1, *C, D, E*). Finally, the excess skin is removed below the nipple to form a skin brassiere, and the vertical incision is tailored and sutured about the nipple (Fig. 89–1, *F*).

The vertical scar may extend for a short distance below the submammary crease, depending on the extent of the operation (Fig. 89–2). Should more extensive dissection and skin excision be necessary than originally contemplated, the horizontal limb of the inverted T incision may be utilized in the final adjustments of the skin brassiere.

Pitanguy (1961) has ingeniously adapted his technique further in the patient with small ptotic breasts in whom not only contour but bulk is required. In this instance he designed a lozenge-shaped incision, but instead of excising the excess of skin, it is de-epithelized and buried beneath the lateral skin flaps, which are sutured vertically (Fig. 89–3).

The Strömbeck technique which will subsequently be described can also be followed step by step to reshape the small ptotic breast, as can the technique of Dufourmentel and Mouly (1965, 1968). The vertical dermal pedicle technique described by McKissock (1972) and modified as a single superiorly based pedicle by Wiener and associates (1973) can also be employed.

OPERATION FOR MODERATE TO SEVERE MACROMASTIA. The majority of patients requesting breast reduction surgery fall into this category. In addition to marked hypertrophy of breast tissue, there usually is associated ptosis. Most operations devised for mammary reduction have dealt with correction of the large, ptotic breast. The incision that has proved most useful is the inverted T incision of the classic Biesenberger operation. Useful variations of this incision have been reported by Penn (1960) and Strömbeck (1960). Pedicle transposition of the nipple with an intact sensory and ductal structure is the procedure of choice, particularly

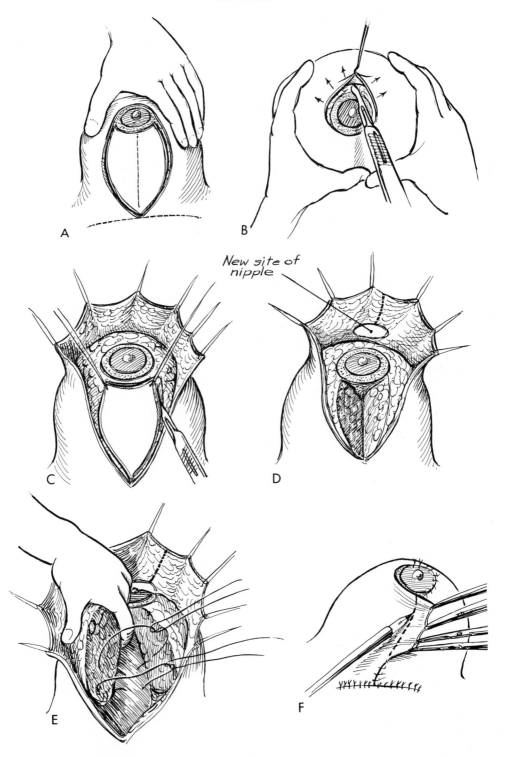

New site of
nipple

**FIGURE 89–1.**    The Aries-Pitanguy technique. *A*, A redundant inferior wedge of skin and fat is removed from below the nipple to the inframammary crease. *B*, The periareolar skin is undermined far enough to permit elevation of the areola to its new position. Extensive undermining is avoided. *C*, Excision of the wedge. In those patients with ptosis, the wedge includes only epithelium, and glandular tissue is not resected. *D*, Wedge excision completed. *E*, Approximation of the edges of the excised area with buried sutures. *F*, Excision of excess skin.

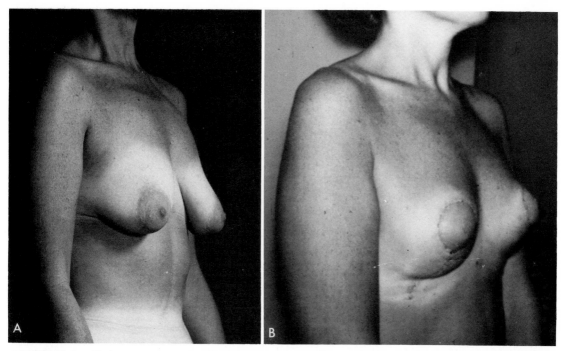

**FIGURE 89–2.** Moderate macromastia and mastoptosis corrected by Aries-Pitanguy technique. Limited undermining of the skin flaps was done. Note the slight extension of the vertical incision below the submammary crease which is necessary to avoid the horizontal limbs of the incisions.

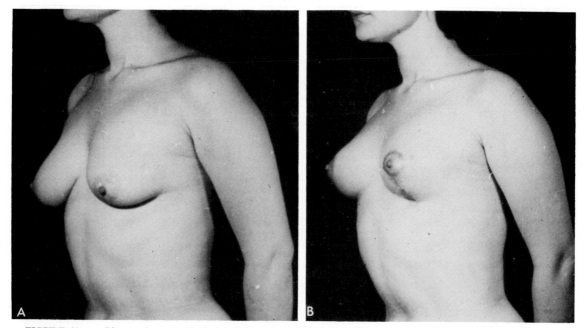

**FIGURE 89–3.** Pitanguy's method of elevating and shaping the small ptotic breast. This method is similar to the technique shown in Figure 89–1, except that an inferior wedge of tissue is de-epithelized and imbricated to provide augmentation to the small breast, rather than resecting the excess skin and fat. (Courtesy of Dr. I. Pitanguy.)

in the younger woman, and is readily adapted to all cases except those of gigantomastia.

The design of mammary tissue excision to reduce bulk varies according to the preferences of the surgeon. In general, the choice between excision of superior and inferior or lateral and medial wedges of tissue, or the S-shaped, lateral excision of Biesenberger, is unimportant provided the remaining portion of the gland has an intact blood supply. The arterial supply of the mammary gland is from the long thoracic artery, the penetrating branches of the internal mammary, and the branches from the intercostals. There is considerable discussion in the literature as to which of these branches is of primary importance in maintaining the blood supply to the gland and nipple region; thus different authors recommend different designs of glandular excision. It seems reasonable to assume that all sources of arterial supply are important but that the main requisite is that sufficient blood supply from a major source be left intact to provide nutrition for the remaining glandular substance.

*The Biesenberger operation (as further modified by McIndoe).* This operation is appropriate for moderate to marked degrees of hypertrophy and ptosis. However, because of the worldwide acceptance of the Strömbeck principle and the variations reported by Skoog (1963), Pitanguy (1967), Beare (1967), McKissock (1972), and Wiener and associates (1973), the Biesenberger technique is rapidly being relegated to surgical history. The operation is described here because of its influence on the course and development of reduction mammaplasty and because it is still used to good advantage by many surgeons. An interesting comparison of the results of some of the various procedures was made by Gupta (1965). Figure 89–4 demonstrates the steps in this operation.

With the patient in the classic position on the operating table with arms akimbo and the torso elevated so as to place the breasts in a dependent position, the new nipple sites are located, measured, and marked as previously described. An upside down T incision is outlined with the vertical component of this incision extending from the point of the new nipple location, around the areola (a 5-cm circumference), and extended down the inferior surface of the gland to the submammary crease. These incisions are not directly in the midclavicular line but deviate in a slightly lateral direction. The submammary or horizontal component of this incision is temporarily marked to conform to the submammary crease. It is important that the shoulders be kept squared so that nipple positions are accurately determined.

Depending on the shoulder width, the size of the thoracic cage, and the age of the patient, the nipples are situated 19 to 24 cm from the sternal notch and 11 to 13 cm from the xiphoid. The intersection of the two circles described by the

calipers roughly settles the point, but it is clear that the operator's judgment will have much to do with final positioning. The internipple distance is usually 25 to 27.5 cm, so that the nipples eventually are situated at the apex of the breast cone, pointing forward and outward. After skin markings have been made, the nipples are tightly stretched peripherally by the assistant, and the areola is circumscribed with a compass or a ring. The diameter of the areola varies from 3.5 to 5 cm, depending on the size of the breast to be constructed.

With the nipple in a stretched position, the incision is started around the nipple, with the knife beveled in an outward direction, just above the dermis level, to preserve the periareolar plexus of nerve and vessels and the areolar smooth muscle fibers. This is an important step upon which depend the viability and sensitivity of the nipple. The beveled undermining extends for a distance of about 2 cm all the way around the nipple and then deeper into the underlying fat. The vertical skin incision is made down to the submammary groove and upward to the predetermined position of the new nipple. Medial and lateral skin flaps are completely dissected away from the underlying substance of the breast by large dissecting scissors and blunt dissection. The uncovering of the breast is extensive, particularly upward where it should reach to the region of the second rib. The entire breast substance having thus been denuded, the requisite amount of breast tissue is resected in an S-shaped fashion laterally according to the Biesenberger technique. Great care must be taken to preserve the medial attachment of the breast pedicle, which McIndoe described as a "mesentery." The mesentery contains important arterial and venous branches to the breast. The freed portion of the breast pedicle is rotated superiorly and sutured into position with loose, approximating sutures of 2–0 chromic catgut to fashion a cone of breast tissue and fat.

The superior angle of the vertical incision (the site of the new nipple location) is grasped with a skin hook on which forward traction is placed. The underlying breast cone is lightly molded, and a smooth, curved intestinal clamp (Doyen) is applied over the redundant skin. Tension is adjusted by pulling this skin through the clamp. This step is highly important, since it results in the formation of a skin brassiere. The tension on which the skin is put must be accurately determined by the operator, taking care that it is not so tight as to provide circulatory embarrassment and not so loose as to allow postoperative slumping. The excess of skin is marked along the clamp with marking dye and sharply excised. The vertical edges are carefully approximated with fine silk or nylon sutures. An excess of submammary skin now lying transversely in the submammary groove is excised as economically as possible. These horizontal skin edges are anchored to the costal fascia by four heavy mattress sutures of silk which secure the submammary, transverse incision to the chest wall and complete the formation of the skin brassiere. This step also helps to prevent postoperative "dishing" or sagging of the breast. The remainder of the longitudinal limb of the incision is closed with fine nylon or silk sutures.

A careful rechecking of the measurements of the new nipple location is done with the calipers from the sternal notch and the xiphoid to ensure symmetry. The operator also rechecks the new nipple position visually, from the foot of the table, with the patient in a semi-sitting position. If satisfactory, a circle of skin of the same size as the circumscribed areola is marked at the uppermost apex of the vertical incision. This circle of skin is excised. The nipples are brought through the buttonhole wound and sutured into position with fine silk or nylon sutures. The circumareolar sutures must be carefully placed to include the full thickness of the areola and surrounding skin flaps for accurate

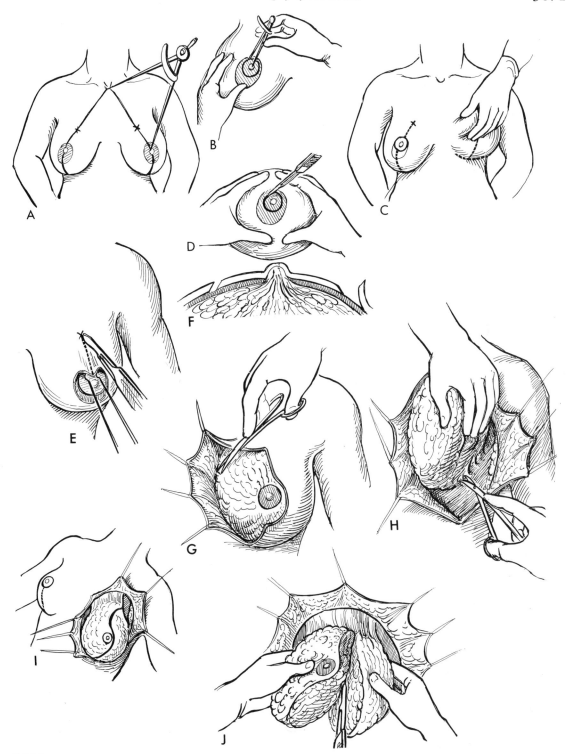

**FIGURE 89–4.** The Biesenberger-McIndoe technique. *A, B, C,* The new nipple sites are located with large calipers. The distance from the sternal notch is 17 to 18 cm, depending on the size of the thoracic cage. An inverted incision is marked. *D, E, F,* The dissection around the areola (5 cm in diameter). Care is taken to preserve the subdermal vascular supply. *G, H,* The breast is extensively denuded. *I, J,* A lateral S-shaped segment of breast representing the redundant gland is resected.

*Legend continued on the following page*

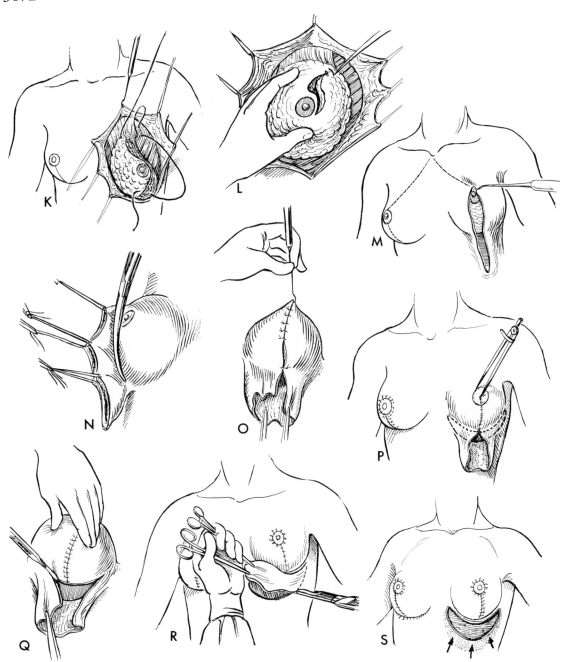

**FIGURE 89–4** *Continued.* *K, L,* The breast is rotated laterally and sutured to form a conical breast parenchyma. *M* to *S,* The remainder of the operation consists of the careful formation of a skin brassiere. Excess skin is resected, and the inverted T-incisions are closed with interrupted sutures.

approximation. Soft rubber tissue drains or Hemovac catheters may or may not be utilized, depending on the surgeon's preference. A compression dressing is applied.

Postoperatively, drains are removed within 48 hours and the sutures removed in stages from the seventh to the twelfth postoperative day (Fig. 89–5).

*The Strömbeck operation.* Another operation that is particularly suitable for reduction of the moderately enlarged breast was devised by Strömbeck (1960). Few operations introduced in the field of plastic surgery in the past 20 years have been as widely accepted and embraced by surgeons as the Strömbeck mammaplasty. This is largely because this technique has simplified reduction mammaplasty for the young surgeon, and, by eliminating the need for extensive undermining of skin flaps, it has significantly reduced the complication rate of hematoma and skin slough. Other techniques which also obviate undermining and are very similar, in principle, at least, to the Strömbeck method have been reported by Skoog (1963), Pitanguy (1967), Beare (1967), McKissock (1972), and Wiener and associates (1973). These may technically be considered modifications of the Strömbeck principle but were independently developed. They all have the virtues of reducing dead space and maintaining adequate blood supply to the gland, areola, and nipple, as well as the skin.

Strömbeck adapted the preoperative pattern planning introduced by Wise (1956), in which a brassiere pattern is utilized in the preoperative planning with skin markings. The circumference of the attachment or base of the female breast is approximately the same in normal, hypertrophic, and ptotic breasts and can therefore be standardized in pattern form.

The Strömbeck procedure is essentially a nipple transposition operation but with the distinct advantage that skin flaps are not undermined. It is a two-pedicle procedure with a medial and lateral pedicle containing the blood supply from the internal mammary and lateral thoracic arteries and with the nipple located in the midportion of the pedicle. The nipple attachment and blood supply are not disturbed.

The operation is done in one stage. A further

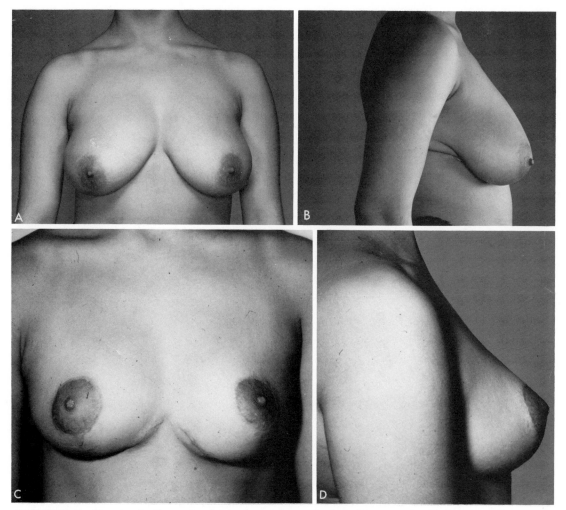

**FIGURE 89–5.** Breast reduction and reshaping in a patient with virginal hypertrophy (McIndoe modification of the Biesenberger technique). This operation is particularly adaptable to young patients with moderate degrees of hypertrophy. *A, B,* Preoperative appearance. *C, D,* Postoperative appearance.

advantage is that the skin overlying the gland is de-epithelized, thus maintaining a dermal covering over the entire breast pedicle. The lateral skin margins are approximated, inverting the dermis along with breast tissue. The gland is molded into shape by suturing the skin brassiere. Strömbeck originally reported a series of 37 patients (69 breasts) in whom he had performed this one-stage operation without necrosis of the skin, nipple, or gland in a single case. In 1968 he reported a personal experience involving more than 500 patients in whom there was a minimal complication rate.

As seen in Figure 89–6, *A, B, C,* preoperative skin markings are made using a standard pattern. The nipple is circumcised, and the skin sur-

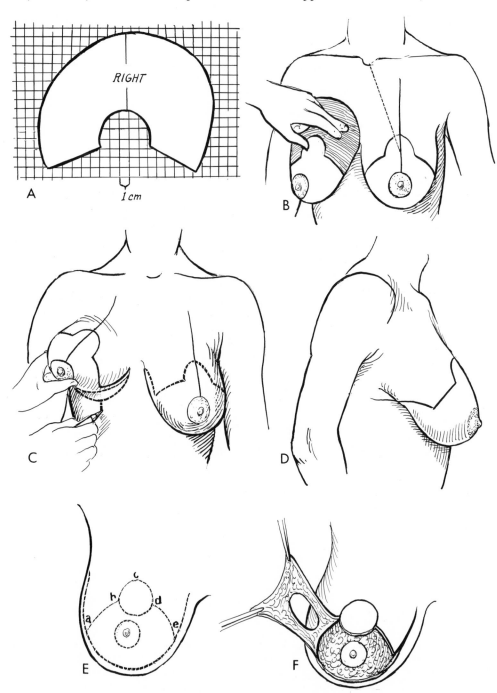

**FIGURE 89–6.** *See legend on the opposite page.*

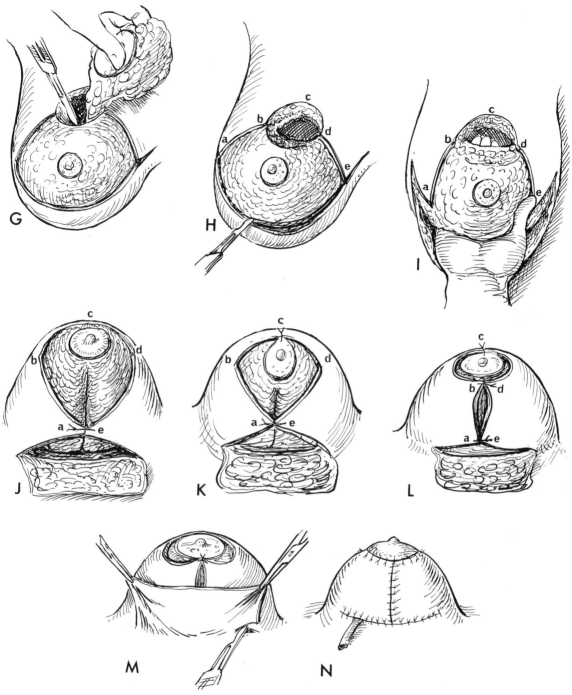

**FIGURE 89–6.** The Strömbeck technique. *A, B,* A standard preformed pattern is used to mark the skin incisions. These incisions can be slightly varied to conform to the configuration of the individual. *C,* The vertical marking below the inframammary line is important for orientation in the final suturing. *D, E, F,* The skin surrounding the areola and including the excess areolar width is dissected as a thick split-thickness skin graft to preserve the nerve and vascular supply to the nipple. *G, H, I,* A core of breast tissue is removed down to the pectoralis fascia, and an inferior curvilinear incision is also made to the level of the pectoralis fascia. The central segment is undermined to establish a bipedicle flap of breast tissue. *J, K, L,* The vertical limb is sutured as shown. This step elevates the areola to its new position. *M, N,* The remaining redundant skin and breast are resected, and the horizontal limb is sutured to establish the inframammary groove. The absence of extensive undermining of skin flaps is a significant safety factor in this technique. The closure usually seems to be excessively tight; however, this is to be expected and is not a matter of concern.

rounding the nipple and lying between the skin markings is removed as a split thickness layer, leaving the deep dermis attached to the breast tissue (Fig. 89–6, *E, F*). A full thickness button of tissue at the upper portion of the wound, representing the new nipple site, is excised down to the pectoralis muscle (Fig. 89–6, *G*). The lower horizontal incision is made (Fig. 89–6, *H*). It may be necessary to undermine the gland from the underlying muscle, thus creating a bipedicle glandular flap containing the nipple and areola (Fig. 89–6, *I*). Sutures are placed through the skin edges at the predetermined markings at points a and e, representing the lower pole of the vertical incision (Fig. 89–6, *J*). The areola is fixed by a suture at the midpoint of the new nipple location, and the skin margins are approximated around the areola and along the vertical suture line (Fig. 89–6, *K, L*). Excess gland and skin is excised from the submammary crease, and the wound is sutured. A small rubber drain or suction catheter is used (Fig. 89–6, *M, N*). If the dermis pedicle is tight in very large reductions, it can be divided close to the dermal edge on one or both sides.

One of the main virtues of this operation is that plicating or shaping sutures in the gland parenchyma are not necessary. Inasmuch as little or no undermining of skin flaps is done, "dead space" serving as a potential area for the formation of hematoma and serum collection is avoided. Since the gland is not sutured, the risk of glandular or fat necrosis caused by constricting buried sutures is also avoided.

Figure 89–7 represents pre- and postoperative photographs of a patient with moderate mammary hypertrophy and ptosis in whom the Strömbeck technique was done. The obvious advantages of this operation, particularly its

safety, are the reasons for its popularity. Variations of the technique to suit different sizes and shapes of the female breast were described by Strömbeck in 1968.

Four other operations for reduction mammaplasty and the correction of ptosis are gaining wide acceptance in recent years: those of Pitanguy (1967), Dufourmentel and Mouly (1965), McKissock (1972), and Wiener and associates (1973). The Pitanguy procedure (Fig. 89–8) differs somewhat from the operation of Strömbeck in design and execution; however, the basic concept is the same. Undermining is minimal, and the nipple and areola are attached to a dermis pedicle (Fig. 89–9).

The operation of Dufourmentel and Mouly also maintains a rich vascular bridge via the dermis to the nipple and areola. Excess parenchyma is excised laterally, and only one scar of the skin results, which extends radially towards the axilla and is camouflaged by the covering brassiere.

The operation of McKissock (Fig. 89–10) utilizes a nipple dermal pedicle designed in a vertical direction with a broad inferior component. Excess breast tissue is excised as medial and lateral wedges. Increased blood supply is assured by the inferior and superior attachments of the vertical dermal pedicle. This operation is simple and has gained wide acceptance at this time.

Wiener (Fig. 89–11) further modified the operations of Skoog and McKissock. He basically utilizes a vertical pedicle but severs the inferior attachment to provide upward mobility of the nipple.

OPERATION FOR SEVERE MACROMASTIA (GIGANTOMASTIA). In extreme hypertrophy of the breast (gigantomastia), unquestionably

*Text continued on page 3684*

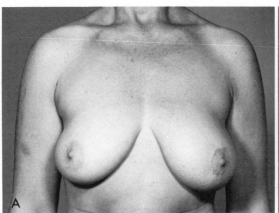 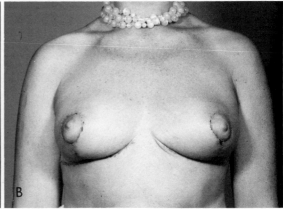

**FIGURE 89–7.**   Moderate hypertrophy and ptosis of the breasts reconstructed by the Strömbeck technique. Note the excellent conical result achieved.

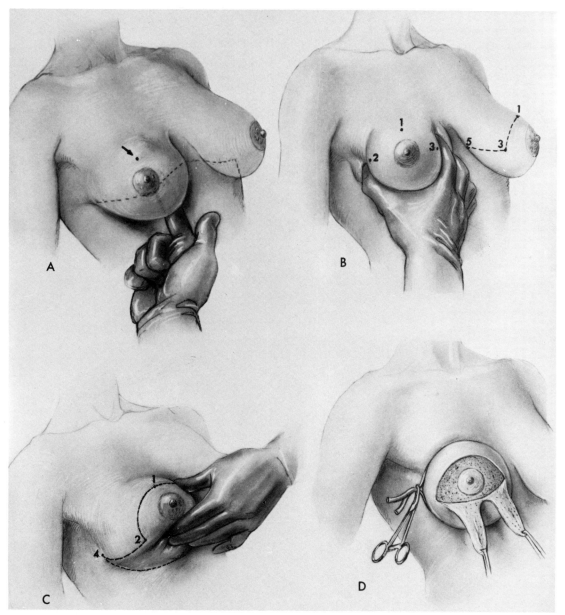

**FIGURE 89–8.** The Pitanguy technique of breast reduction is similar in principle to that of Strömbeck. Point 1 is located in the mid-mammary line and is indicated by the protruding finger placed in the inframammary sulcus (*A*). Points 2 and 3 are rough measurements calculated by holding the breast and estimating the amount of tissue to be resected according to the breast size or degree of ptosis (*B, C*).

Distance of the lines 1–2 and 1–3 is usually 6 to 7 cm. Line 2–4 is drawn with traction exerted on point 1. This line represents the axillary extension of the dissection. Line 3–5 represents the medial resection of the lower quadrant of the breast.

*Legend continued on the following pages*

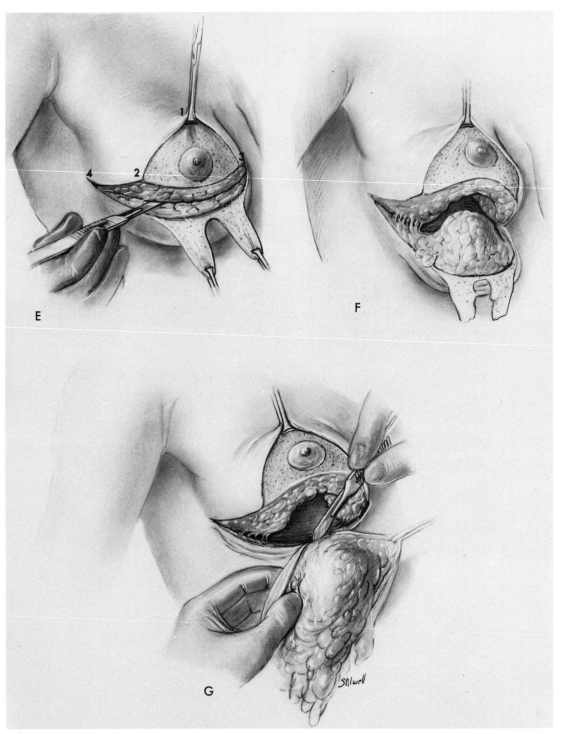

**FIGURE 89–8** *Continued.* The initial dissection is similar to that of Strömbeck. The skin around the areola is de-epithelized. The lower portion of the breast is dissected as indicated in *F*. The glandular resection is in the shape of a boat keel and is extended almost to the subcutaneous fat in the superior pole of the breast.

*Legend continued on the opposite page*

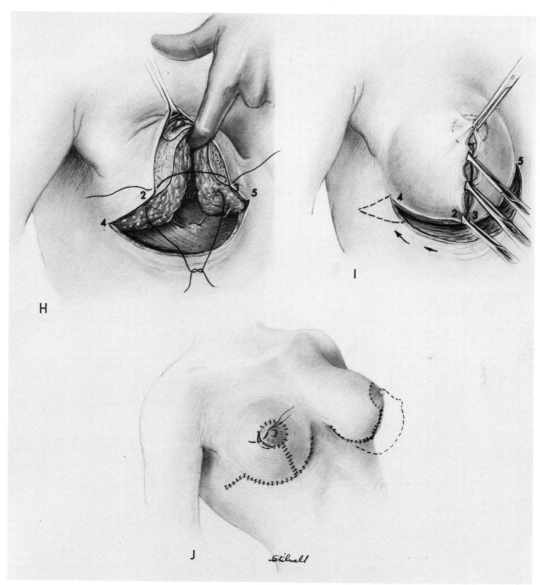

**FIGURE 89–8** *Continued.* Points 2 and 3 (*H*) are sutured together. Various minor readjustments can be made at this point in the procedure, following which the breast wounds are sutured. (After Pitanguy, Surgical treatment of breast hypertrophy. Br. J. Plast. Surg., *30*:78, 1967.)

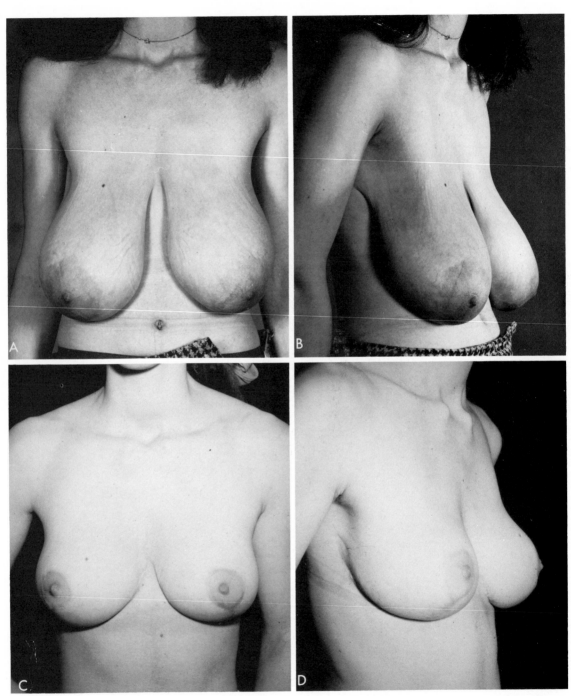

**FIGURE 89–9.** Pitanguy technique. Preoperative photographs of a patient with marked ptosis and hypertrophy (*A, B*) corrected with the Pitanguy technique. *C, D,* Postoperative views.

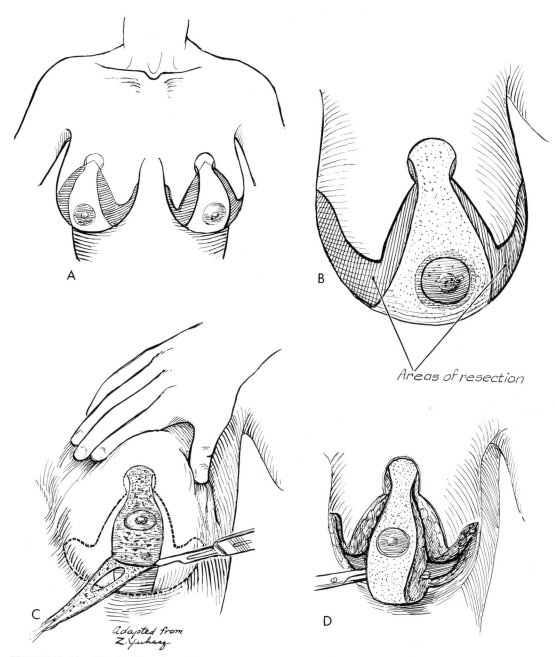

Adapted from
Z. Yuhasz

**FIGURE 89–10.** The McKissock (vertical dermal flap) operation. *A, B,* The preliminary steps are similar to those in a Strömbeck operation except that the areola is maintained on a vertical dermal pedicle and the breast resection is done medially and laterally to the pedicle. *C,* The vertical pedicle is de-epithelized. *D,* The vertical pedicle is developed as a flap but remains attached superiorly and inferiorly.

*Legend continued on the following pages*

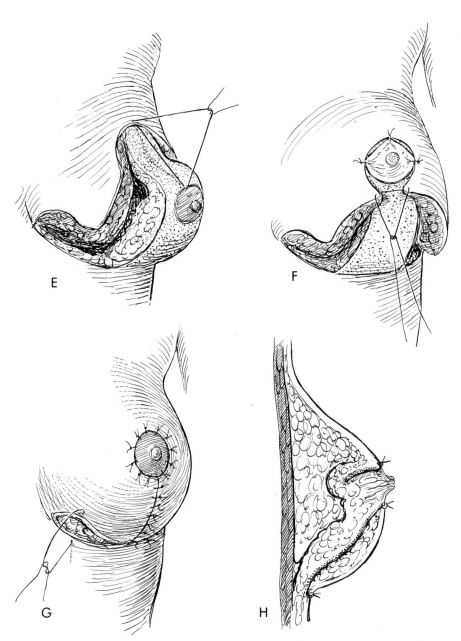

**FIGURE 89–10** *Continued.* *E,* The areola is readily elevated to its new position while the dermal pedicle folds under. Note the broader inferior pole of the pedicle. *F, G, H,* The breast skin flaps are sutured over the dermal areolar pedicle, which becomes buried.

*Legend continued on the opposite page*

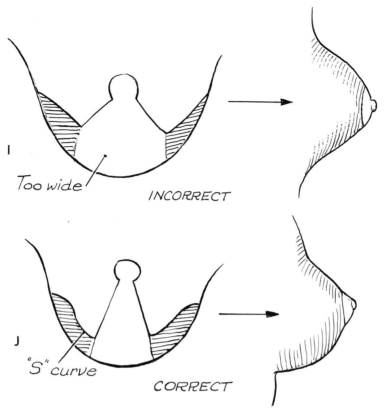

FIGURE 89–10 *Continued.* Important steps in planning the final breast shape include the width of the pedicle (*I*) and the formation of a gentle S-curve of the lateral incision (McKissock).

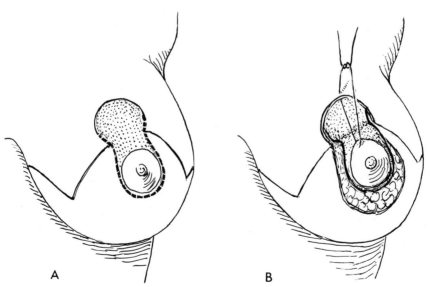

FIGURE 89–11. Wiener technique. The areola and nipple are attached to a superiorly based dermal flap which permits upward mobility.

the safest procedure is that of a partial breast amputation and free transplantation of the nipples (Thorek, 1922; Conway, 1952). Preserving nipple function in these cases is an absurdity, since the deformity per se is so disabling that the prime concern is to relieve the patient of excess poundage. In some instances of extreme hypertrophy of the breast, there is an associated factor of benign or premalignant breast disease. When this complication exists, the aim is to remove all breast tissue and fashion the remaining subcutaneous tissue and de-epithelized skin flaps into filler substance to establish a new mammary eminence.

The operation, partial mammectomy with free nipple transplantation, has been described in detail by Thorek (1922, 1946), Adams (1944, 1947), Conway (1952), and Felix and associates (1970).

Free grafts of nipple and areola consist of epidermis, dermis, muscular layers, and some ductal elements. When this technique is properly executed and the grafts are transferred to a recipient bed of dermis, the survival rate is excellent. Surgical technique must be meticulous to avoid trauma. Nipple erectile function and sensation return in varying periods of time. These grafts are vascularized as composite grafts by penetration of new vessels from the underlying dermal bed and surrounding skin edge.

Figure 89–12, *A* depicts the variation in measurements in the dependency as well as in the width of the breasts at their bases. Utilizing the nipple as the midpoint, vertical lines are marked parallel to the midsternal line along the longitudinal axis of the breast. As seen in Figure 89–12, *C, D, E,* and *F,* the Passot type of horizontal incision is located by holding one hand in the submammary fold and marking a curvilinear, horizontal incision on the anterior surface of the breast. This incision is approximately at the level of the submammary fold. The marking of the incision on the undersurface of the breast is made just slightly above the inframammary crease, and a rounded "dart" is included centrally. According to Conway, the staggering of the inferior incision permits formation of a conical bulge in the reconstructed breast in its midportion. Darts are planned at the extreme medial and lateral angles of the incision to compensate for inequalities in the length of the anterior and posterior incisions.

The nipple is measured (Fig. 89–12, *H*) and removed by the usual technique of stretching the nipple peripherally, drawing a ring of suitable diameter, usually 3 to 5 cm, and incising the areola through all of its layers and removing it as a composite graft of smooth muscle, ductile tissue, areolar skin, and nipple (Fig. 89–12, *I, J*). The posterior incision is made, followed by the anterior incision and amputation of the desired amount of breast tissue (Fig. 89–12, *K, L, M, N*). The amount removed is recorded by weighing or volumetric displacement. The width of the mammary gland is further reduced by removing a wedge-shaped portion in the center (Fig. 89–12, *O*). The lateral and medial elements are approximated with sutures of catgut (Fig. 89–12, *P*). The skin incision is approximated by fine sutures of nylon or silk after discrepancies in length of the two incisions are corrected by excising medial and lateral darts. After the incision is sutured, the new nipple site is again checked. Preoperative markings are utilized, and the center of the graft is usually placed approximately 11 cm medial to the vertical line shown in Figure 89–12, *B*. The recipient bed for the graft is prepared by excising a circular split-thickness graft of skin of the same diameter as the nipple graft. The composite areolar graft is then sutured in place and secured with a tie-over dressing.

Figure 89–13, *A* to *F*, demonstrates a variation on the free nipple transplant technique advocated by Conway for the repair of the small ptotic breast.

Figure 89–12, *X* and *Y*, shows the technique of invaginating mammary tissue into a submammary pocket in the long, flat, ptotic breast.

The success of composite nipple grafts approaches perfection, provided that they are properly applied to a recipient bed of dermis as described in the operative procedure; dermis is probably the most vascular tissue in the body when one considers its rich anastomotic system of blood vessels (Fig. 89–14).

Free nipple grafting can also be easily adapted to the general plan of glandular reduction of Strömbeck, Skoog, or Pitanguy (Felix and associates, 1970). The nipples and areola are transplanted as free grafts rather than as transposition pedicles delivered through buttonhole incisions in the skin flaps as the final step in the operation. Hoopes and Jabaley (1969) suggested another acceptable alternative in the correction of gigantomastia. They advocated resection of virtually all breast parenchyma and reconstruction of the skin envelope over a mammary prosthesis. This technique bears careful consideration in very large breasts, despite the obvious hazards in wound healing that are well recognized in subcutaneous mastectomy with immediate prosthetic implantation.

*Text continued on page 3688*

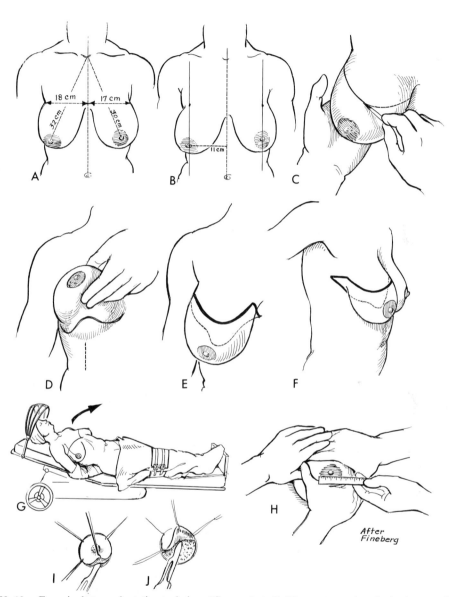

**FIGURE 89–12.** Free nipple transplantation technique (Conway). *A, B,* The postoperative nipple sites are planned with the patient in the sitting position. *C, D, E, F,* A Passot type of horizontal breast incision line is also marked preoperatively. *G,* The patient is placed on the operating table, and the table is elevated to a sitting position for reexamination of the nipple locations during the procedure. *H, I, J,* A 5-cm areolar graft is removed as a full-thickness composite graft.

*Legend continued on the following page*

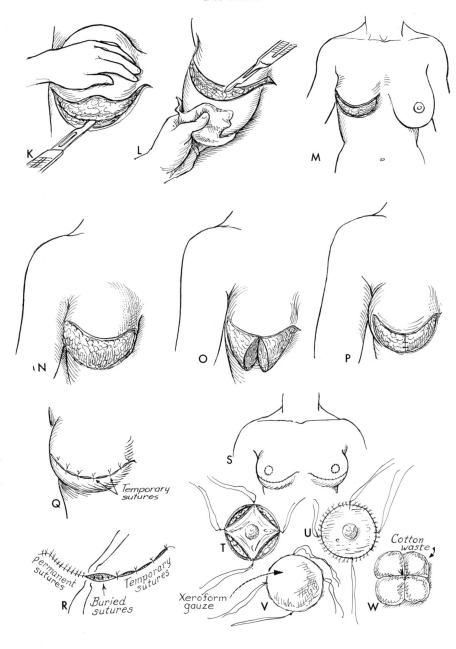

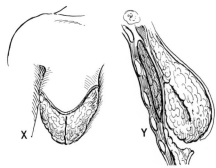

**FIGURE 89–12** *Continued.*   *K* to *Q,* The redundant skin and breast are resected, as well as a central wedge of parenchyma to narrow the breast, if necessary. The horizontal incision is sutured. *R* to *W,* A definitive wound suturing is done, and, after the nipple sites are checked, the nipple and areola graft is sutured to a dermal bed. A tie-over dressing is used for fixation and pressure. *X, Y,* A variation of this technique in the flattened breast in which an excess of breast parenchyma is preserved and ''tucked under'' the superior breast segment to provide bulk.

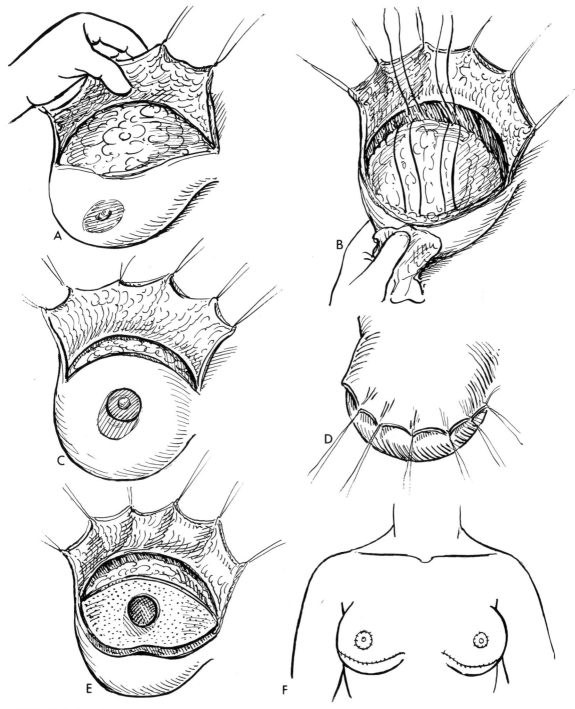

**FIGURE 89–13.** Conway technique for small ptotic breasts. *A,* A skin flap is elevated over the superior portion of the breast through a horizontal incision. *B,* Mattress sutures plicate the breast parenchyma and elevate it. *C, D, E,* The skin flap determines the position of the final suture line, and the inferior horizontal incision is marked. The central elliptical segment is de-epithelized and buried beneath the skin flap. *F,* The nipples can be brought out through buttonhole incisions or transplanted as grafts.

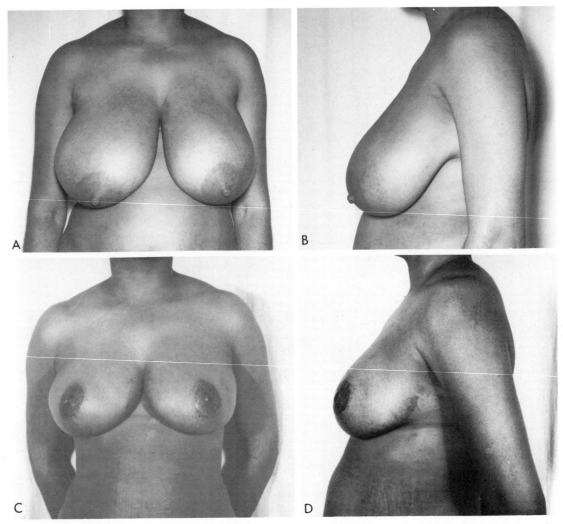

**FIGURE 89–14.** A case of gigantomastia in which reduction and reshaping were done by the free nipple transplant technique and the Passot type of incision. Note that a true conical shape is difficult to achieve by the horizontal incisions of Passot. *A, B,* Preoperative appearance; *C, D,* postoperative appearance.

**Complications of Reduction Mammaplasty and Mastopexy.** The complications of breast reduction mammaplasty and mastopexy have been discussed by Rees and Flagg (1972). These include immediate and late complications and another group of problems that can be termed "untoward results." Certain predisposing factors are known to contribute to untoward results or complications. These include generalized arteriosclerosis, occlusive vascular disease, diabetes, and, perhaps most important of all, obesity. The obese patient is very prone to complications of all types, including wound breakdown, fat necrosis, and infection. Pregnancy is, without further emphasis, a definite contraindication

to surgery. Strömbeck (1964) drew a direct correlation between the complication rate and the amount of tissue resected in the reduction. When massive amounts of tissue were resected, the complication rate rose steeply. In his series of 436 cases, 24 per cent of 25 breasts from which 1000 grams or more of tissue were resected developed complications, as compared with 2.5 per cent of 40 breasts in which only 200 grams were resected. These figures are in keeping with the author's experience.

The Biesenberger technique, in which the skin flaps were widely undermined, yielded a significantly higher rate of complications, such as skin slough and nipple necrosis, than do the newer techniques based on the Strömbeck principle, in which little or no undermining of the skin is done.

Minor postoperative complications include cyanosis of the nipple and areola, localized infection, local wound separation or slough, and the formation of inclusion cysts. These problems are usually self-limiting and are easily managed by conservative measures and careful attention to detail in wound management. Cysts resulting from buried dermis in the Strömbeck technique usually undergo spontaneous resolution, although incision and/or excision may occasionally be necessary.

Retraction of the nipple can occur after use of the Strömbeck or Pitanguy techniques when the reduction has been considerable. Such retraction usually corrects itself with time; however, on occasion surgical release may be required. The newer vertical dermal pedicle operation of McKissock (1972) may well prove to avoid the problem of the retracted nipple.

Major complications include significant slough of the wound margins or of the nipple and areola. When the slough is not extensive, conservative management is indicated. This involves allowing the slough to separate and secondary healing to occur. Significant wound sloughs should be debrided, and secondary wound closure with tension sutures may be accomplished. Nipple slough is corrected by free grafts of labia minora at a subsequent operation, and this technique affords a quite reasonable color match (Adams, 1949).

Hematoma is the most common complication and often is the primary cause of further wound complications (McIndoe and Rees, 1958). Hematomas should be promptly evacuated when recognized and secondary wound closure with drainage carried out.

Massive wound infection is rare following the advent of antibiotic therapy. When such infections occur, they are best treated with appropriate antibiotic coverage and incision and drainage.

Fat necrosis is a most aggravating and troublesome complication because of protracted wound healing and persistent drainage that occur. Fat necrosis is most often associated with localized hematoma, abscess formation, or occlusion of the segmental blood supply. If fat necrosis is extensive, it is usually associated with skin slough. In this case, aggressive debridement and secondary wound closure are indicated; however, if the necrotic area is small and associated with localized drainage through a small sinus tract, it is usually wiser to adopt a more conservative attitude. Irrigations of the sinus tract and gentle expression of the liquid fat can be done at frequent intervals until healing occurs, which may require several weeks.

Another serious but fortunately rare complication is gangrene of mammary tissue as a result of circulatory interference, secondary to excessive dissection and mobilization of breast parenchyma or torsion of the breast pedicle. This distressing complication is best managed by excision of the slough, drainage of the wound, and secondary wound closure.

Long-term untoward results following mammaplasty include breast asymmetry, unsightly scars, keloids, and upward migration of the nipples. These problems may require secondary corrective surgery with careful repair. Keloids are apt to occur in those with a keloid diathesis and are most common if the inframammary incisions cross the midline. They are best treated in this location with intralesional steroid injections, X-ray, and sometimes excision and repair (see Chapter 16).

## AUGMENTATION MAMMAPLASTY

**Indications.** The indications for augmentation mammaplasty lie almost completely within the realm of psychologic need. Modern advertising techniques, increased social consciousness of physical acceptability, and current social attitudes of frankness toward sexual relationships have taken an emotional toll in the woman who believes herself to be inadequately equipped physically to meet the subtle social standards identifying her sex. Attitudes of self-righteousness toward this overt propaganda are not realistic and, further, do nothing to solve the problems. "Flat-chested" women can become so emotionally handicapped that it is almost impossible for them to assume a normal role in courtship or marriage. Their natural reaction to men is subverted to one of timidity and defense. When women thus handicapped do marry, there is a significant incidence of sexual frigidity which may be traced to feelings of personal inadequacy. This complex of reactions may jeopardize the marriage. The surgeon dealing with these problems must have a sympathetic and understanding attitude rather than one of misguided intolerance.

The female desire for normal sized and contoured breasts is intense. A psychosocial evaluation of a group of 65 patients seeking augmentation mammaplasty was described by Edgerton and McClary (1958) and Edgerton, Meyer, and

Jacobson (1961). The initial study (1958) included 37 patients. In the overall evaluation of 65 patients (1961), several characteristics were evident. The majority of patients they studied were married Protestant women around 30 years of age. Most patients were involved in major domestic problems with stressful marriages (separation or impending separation or divorce). A frequent history of divorce, separation, and second marriages was noted (see also Chapter 21).

These investigators were impressed that patients seeking augmentation mammaplasty are "active, competitive, 'on-the-go' people who are physically graceful, often pretty and socially at ease." A history of major unhappiness in childhood was elicited in the majority.

It is the experience of most surgeons interested in augmentation mammaplasty that most patients so helped are very satisfied with the postoperative results. It is quite apparent that surgery does not solve the basic emotional problems of these patients. Continued psychiatric investigation is necessary, but the fact remains that the majority of patients are pleased, and surgery must therefore be considered of benefit.

Small breasts are due to (1) primary aplasia or hypoplasia, (2) surgery for benign or malignant disease, (3) sudden weight reduction in a patient with breasts smaller than normal to begin with, and (4) idiopathic involution, usually following pregnancy.

Since the development in recent years of the newer "natural feel" and shaped silicone prosthesis of Cronin and Gerow (1964), Arion (1965), Jenny (1969), and Ashley (1970), the results of augmentation mammaplasty have improved markedly. Recent improvements in the quality control of inflatable prostheses and the development of the soft, round, Silastic gel prostheses have considerably improved the naturalness of the results of augmentation mammaplasty. Because of this, the acceptance of this technique and the public demand for it have grown at a tremendous rate. Many thousands of these operations are done each year. A growing volume of meaningful data is accumulating about the long-term results following the implantation of such prostheses.

**Methods of Augmentation Mammaplasty.** There are essentially four methods of augmenting the female breast: (1) percutaneous injection of foreign substances, such as paraffin and, more recently, silicone preparations; (2) implantation of local flaps of dermis and fat; (3) implantation of free dermis-fat-fascia grafts; (4) implantation of a prosthetic material, such as the inflatable or silicone gel–filled prostheses.

INJECTION TECHNIQUE. Responsible surgeons are aware of the hazard of the paraffin injection technique introduced by Gersuny (1889). For many years this technique has been condemned, but it is still practiced in the Far East. Paraffin injected into the subcutaneous tissue not only is subject to change in shape and contour but also may produce troublesome granuloma. Silicone preparations have been used for this purpose in the Far East and Europe. Conway and Goulian (1963) reported their experience with Silastic, a form of silicone rubber. However, they later abandoned the technique because of the high incidence of complications.

Silicone (dimethyl polysiloxane) fluid in its pure manufactured form and in mixture with various adulterants, such as vegetable oils, has been used as an injectable material for mammary augmentation. This technique enjoyed considerable vogue for several years. However, few plastic surgeons supported the method. Long-term results have proved that the injection of such compounds into the breast is fraught with difficulties and untoward results. The formation of multiple nodules and/or cysts has frequently occurred, making breast examination very difficult and possibly masking the appearance of a neoplasm. Chronic edema of the breast, as well as the skin, has been seen in some patients. Furthermore, there is a tendency for breasts injected in this way to become heavy and ptotic. There is no significant evidence at this time that mammary augmentation by silicone injection is related to the formation of malignancy.

Another valid objection to the injection technique is that it is virtually impossible to remove the injected material should this be necessary. Implants can be removed in the event of problems.

Mammary augmentation by the injection of foreign body fluids is condemned at this time, until at least the problems discussed above can be solved and a suitable material developed. Complications of silicone breast injections were reported by Nosanchuk (1968), Boo-Chai (1969), and Chaplin (1969).

FLAPS OF DERMIS-FAT. Reconstruction of the mammary eminence with local flaps of de-epithelized tissue is an acceptable technique and the procedure of choice in some instances. These techniques have been developed by Maliniac (1950), Marino (1952), Longacre (1953, 1954, 1956, 1959), O'Conor (1964), and Goulian and McDivitt (1972).

Dermis-fat pedicle reconstruction is of particular value following subcutaneous removal of all mammary tissue for benign or premalignant conditions. Usually there is ample skin remaining from which the de-epithelized flaps can be fashioned. This technique has the added advantage of an intact blood supply, ensuring minimal absorption of bulk that is often seen in grafts of dermis-fat. Maliniac (1950) has adapted this technique for constructing an acceptably contoured breast in the very long, pendulous, or "pancake" type of breast in which very little breast tissue is present. Longacre has pointed out a second advantage: the resiliency of the dermis establishes a firm breast and one that approaches the normal in contour and consistency.

Some authorities consider chronic cystic mastitis to be a condition favorable for the development of carcinoma (Cheatle and Cutler, 1931; Warren, 1940; Ewing, 1940; Geschickter, 1943; Copeland and Geschickter, 1950). The presence of cystic mastitis can mask carcinoma in its early stages. In severe cases, total ablation of mammary tissue may therefore be indicated. Since this procedure may be advised in the age group between 30 and 45, where removal of the breast may produce severe psychic disturbance, the problem of reconstruction following resection becomes important. Longacre (1953) gave three indications for ablation of mammary tissue and reconstruction with dermis-fat flaps: (1) chronic cystic mastitis, (2) mastodynia, and (3) virginal hypertrophy. O'Conor (1964) also considered the procedure to be occasionally indicated as prophylaxis for bilateral cancer and for the prevention of cancer in the opposite breast, as well as in certain cases of gigantomastia. Figure 89–15 demonstrates the technique of reconstructing the breast. Skin flaps from the lower portion of the breast are designed. These are subsequently de-epithelized and implanted subcutaneously to replace the resected mammary tissue. The nipple is transplanted as a composite graft. A similar technique is utilized in reconstructing breasts that are deformed by scar tissue, as, for example, following burns. When the donor site of the dermis-fat pedicle is short of skin, a split-thickness skin graft can be utilized to resurface this region.

In the small breast of the so-called "nipple type" with a well-developed nipple and areola but insufficient mammary tissue beneath, Longacre has utilized dermis-fat flaps from the inferior hemisphere of the breast which are attached by a central pedicle (Fig. 89–15, *A, B*). The medial and lateral "wing" flaps are then brought together, placed in a subcutaneous pocket, and

the donor site is converted to a linear closure in the submammary fold (Fig. 89–15, *C*). Longacre (1956) also adapted this technique in reconstructing the so-called flat, discoid type of breast by fashioning the dermis-fat flaps from the inferior aspect of the breast in the shape of two wings with a central attachment. These flaps also are de-epithelized as seen in Figure 89–15. In this deformity there is no need for transfer of the nipple. The dermis-fat flaps are simply buried beneath the breast tissue and anchored to the fascia of the chest wall. The lower margin of the wound is undermined and advanced in order to establish a suture line and residual scar in the submammary fold (Fig. 89–16).

In 1959, Longacre summarized his ten years' experience with the various designs of his technique for mammary reconstruction with dermis-fat flaps. He has abandoned the procedure of subtotal resection of the mammary gland for hypertrophy in favor of a prophylactic resection of all the mammary tissue and reconstruction of the mammary elements by flaps. In most instances the nipple is transferred as a composite graft. He reported no signs of absorption or breakdown of the transplanted tissue in 32 patients.

In suitable patients there is no doubt that the surgical indications and technique are sound (Fig. 89–17). The main disadvantage of the dermis-fat flap technique is in individuals who have virtually no mammary tissue and minimal skin available to fashion flaps for implantation.

DERMIS-FAT GRAFTS. The use of grafts of dermis-fat or dermis-fat-fascia to fill the mammary eminence was first reported by Berson (1945) and subsequently reported by Bames (1950). A comprehensive paper, arousing renewed interest in this procedure, was published by Watson (1959). Dermis-fat grafts for reconstruction of the mammary eminence, either in the congenital hypoplastic breast or following glandular excision of the mammary tissue, remain more normal in consistency than foreign implants. Blood supply is rapidly established within the dermis portion of the graft via the rich vascular network of the dermis.

The disadvantages of fat grafts are (1) unsightly donor scars, usually in the buttocks; (2) absorption of the grafts (up to 50 per cent of the total bulk of the graft); and (3) the possibility of fat necrosis with chronic drainage. Most surgeons have abandoned this procedure because of these disadvantages in favor of the Silastic implants now available. The operation has its place in the armamentarium of the surgeon

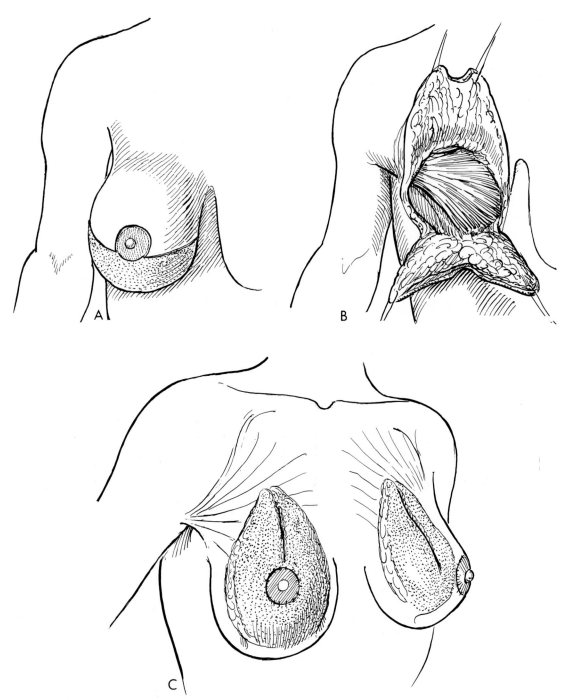

**FIGURE 89–15.** The dermis-fat flap technique (after Longacre). *A,* The inferior portion of the breast is de-epithelized. *B,* The superior segment containing the nipple is elevated as a flap at the level of the pectoral fascia, and a bipronged flap is fashioned of the de-epithelized lower segment. *C,* The flaps of dermis-fat are inserted beneath the gland to provide bulk. In this technique the nipple is often transplanted as a graft.

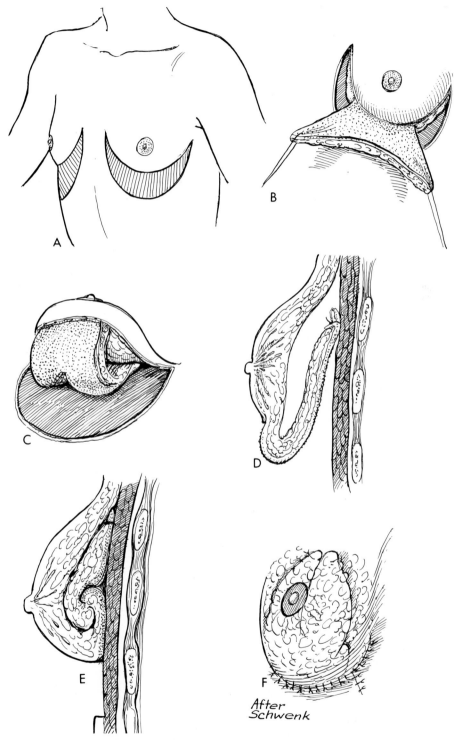

**FIGURE 89–16.** A variation of the dermis-fat flap technique for augmentation of the flat discoid breast (after Longacre). *A, B,* A crescentic design beneath the areola is de-epithelized, and a bipronged flap of dermis-fat is fashioned with a central pedicle. *C, D, E, F,* The flap is rolled into a pocket, which is dissected above the pectoral fascia of the breast, and the infra-mammary incision is sutured. The lower wound edge is undermined and advanced if necessary.

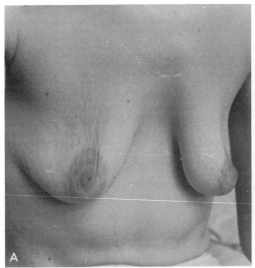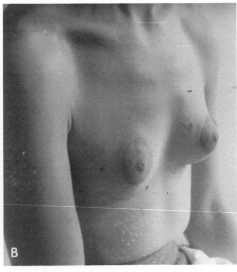

**FIGURE 89–17.**   Preoperative and postoperative photographs of a patient reconstructed by the dermis flap technique (Longacre). Reconstruction of small ptotic ("pancake") breasts by the de-epithelized flap technique. Local flaps are denuded of epithelium and buried to provide bulk.

interested in breast augmentation. The procedure shown in Figure 89–18 is essentially that of Bames as described by Watson.

The patient is placed in a prone position on the operating table, and two crescentic pieces of tissue are removed from the buttocks, their size being determined by the surgeon's estimate of the amount of tissue required (Fig. 89–18, *A, B*). These crescentic pieces of tissue include skin, subcutaneous tissue, and fascia, depending on the surgeon's preference. Some surgeons prefer to place the long axis of the ellipse in the inferior crease of the buttocks (Fig. 89–18, *B*).

Epithelium is then removed as a split-thickness graft (Fig. 89–18, *C*). This may be done prior to the actual excision of the grafts by using a pattern dermatome technique. After removal of the grafts, the donor wounds are closed. It is advisable to use tension sutures of a nonreactive material such as wire which may be left in place for ten days to two weeks. The patient is then turned on the operating table. After suitable preparation and draping, incisions are made inferolaterally in the submammary crease. The breast and subcutaneous tissues are undermined, and the dermis-fat grafts are inserted, establishing the desired contour. There is a difference of opinion as to whether the dermis portion of the graft should lie in juxtaposition to the skin flaps or to the pectoral fascia. Watson felt that the dermis is best placed in juxtaposition to the skin flaps (Fig. 89–18, *E*). The wounds are then sutured (Fig. 89–19).

The most important part of the operation is delicate and atraumatic handling of the grafts. Undue trauma will result in delayed healing and partial necrosis of the transplants. Liquefaction of the fat portion of the graft with persistent drainage is a troublesome complication. This condition may be aggravated by infection or hematoma and may result in ultimate loss of the graft. Some authors (Conway and Smith, 1958) report a 50 per cent complication rate in dermis-fat grafts.

Watson (1970) reported 52 cases of dermis-fat transplants for mammary augmentation, of which 5 were unilateral, representing a total of 99 grafts. Of those followed for more than one year, the maximum shrinkage rate was less than 15 to 20 per cent. A minority showed no shrinkage at all. Watson no longer advocates this method for augmentation, however. He found that over the course of 10 to 15 years, the grafts became increasingly fibrotic, tended to show areas of soap formation and calcification, and not infrequently required removal (Watson, 1975). He has therefore abandoned this method of treatment in favor of augmentation with the improved prosthetic products which are now in current use.

PROSTHETIC IMPLANTS FOR AUGMENTATION MAMMAPLASTY.   Ivory and other inert materials have been unsuccessfully utilized as implants in past years. More recently plastic resins have been used for implantation by orthopedic, vascular, and chest surgeons with a high degree of success. About 1951 plastic surgeons became interested in the use of polyvinyl sponge as a

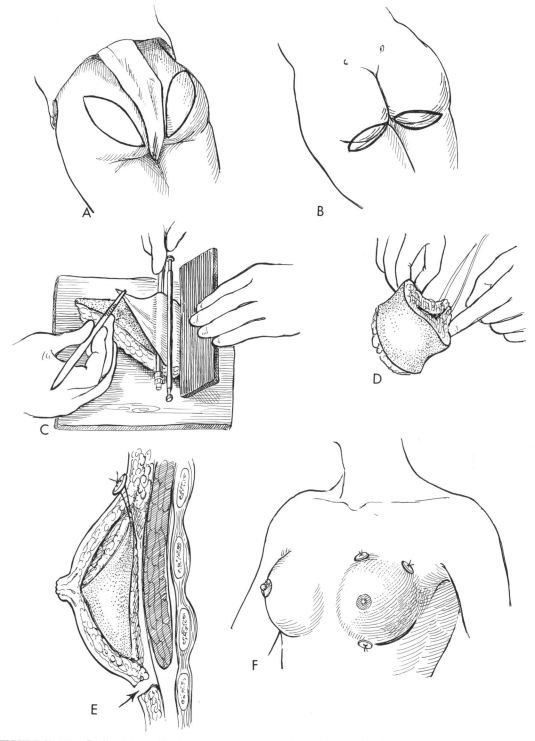

**FIGURE 89–18.** Grafts of dermis-fat for mammary augmentation as described by Watson. *A, B,* Crescentic wedges of skin and fat are excised from the buttocks; the design varies according to the configuration of the individual. *C,* A split-thickness skin graft is removed from the graft. *D, E, F,* The dermis-fat graft is folded on itself and inserted into a submammary pocket with the dermis side up. Several stabilizing sutures are brought through the skin and tied over buttons.

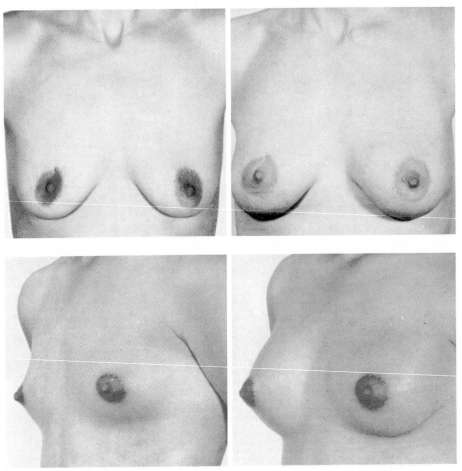

**FIGURE 89–19.** Preoperative (left) and postoperative (right) photographs of free dermis-fat grafts. (From Watson, J.: Some observations on free fat grafts: with reference to their use in mammaplasty. Br. J. Plast. Surg., *12*:263, 1959.)

breast implant material. This interest was stimulated by reports of the work of Grindlay and Clagett (1949) and Grindlay and Waugh (1951) on polyvinyl sponge implants in dogs. Their studies demonstrated the formation of a thin, penetrating fibrous capsule about the sponge implants. Surrounding the fibrous capsule zone an area of avascular, areolar tissue forms. Their work on Ivalon (polyvinyl) sponges, as well as the studies of Moore and Brown (1952), showed the sponge to be relatively inert and nontoxic and producing a minimum of inflammatory reaction. Polyvinyl sponge, however, does tend to undergo change after implantation for long periods.

Oppenheimer, Oppenheimer, and Stout (1952) were able to produce sarcomatous tumors in rats by implantation of many different types of plastic materials. Dukes and Mitchley (1962) produced similar tumors in rats by implanting polyvinyl (Ivalon) sponge. However, Edgerton and McClary (1958) and others doubt whether these atypical "sarcomas" are comparable to human cancers, and none has been reported to date in humans.

Ivalon sponge (Clay-Adams) was first used by Pangman in 1951 for mammary augmentation.

Etheron, or polyether, was the most widely used sponge for implantation. This substance is a solid polymer formed by the reaction of organic duocyanate with polyols (resins) in the presence of water and catalysts. The sponge is formed by the liberation of $CO_2$ which expands the solid polymer into a foam. Etheron had the distinct advantages of (1) producing a minimal foreign body reaction, (2) remaining softer and thus more natural than Ivalon, (3) contracting (shrinking) 30 to 50 per cent of its inserted bulk (Conway and Dietz, 1962), and (4) producing fewer postoperative complications.

An inner sponge of Silastic surrounded by a capsule of Teflon was advocated by Edwards (1963). The Teflon shell apparently prevented fibrous ingrowth and thus limited postoperative shrinking.

Sponge implants for breast augmentation have been almost universally abandoned in favor of the newer type of silicone bag implants. The reasons for this will be discussed subsequently.

The implants currently favored are similar in many respects. They consist of the basic capsular structure of Silastic (silicone) which is filled with silicone gel or some other material (saline, PVP, or dextran). Some of these implants (Cronin and Gerow, 1964) have patches of Dacron as part of the outer shell to induce attachment to the chest wall, while another type has an outer cellular coating of urethan (Ashley, 1970) to aid in fixation.

The most popular implant now in use is the silicone gel–filled Silastic envelope, which has undergone several modifications since it was first described by Cronin and Gerow (1964). The silicone prostheses have proved to have many advantages: (1) they do not shrink; (2) they remain relatively soft; (3) tissue reaction is minimal; (4) symmetry is more assured; and (5) the infection and drainage rate is minimal.

The Simaplast implant described by Arion (1965) consists of an inflatable silicone bag which can be inserted through a very small incision and then inflated with PVP, dextran, or saline to the desired size. This prosthesis is used by many surgeons. These bags have also been known to "deflate" on occasion. Tabari (1969) discussed his experiences with the use of Simaplast prostheses.

The Ashley prosthesis (1970) is also a silicone shell filled with dimethyl polysiloxane gel, as is the Cronin prosthesis; however, it has the advantage of being compartmentalized into three separate sections divided by septa.

Both the Cronin and the Ashley prostheses are available in several different sizes to suit the occasion.

Jenny (1969) has advocated a balloon type of prosthesis similar to the Simaplast one. This is a silicone bladder with a valve similar to that of an old-fashioned football. It is inserted through a small semicircular areolar incision and inflated to the desired size with saline solution. This prosthesis, after a short-term follow-up, seems to result in a soft and remarkably natural-feeling breast. The scar is almost totally camouflaged within the darkly pigmented areola. Significant long-term follow-up data are not yet available. Among the questions still to be answered with

this prosthesis are the incidence of rupture or deflation and whether or not the silicone capsule can act as a dialyzing membrane. Transection of the breast parenchyma has also been criticized by some as a possible source of problems.

The Akiyama prosthesis (Mutou, 1970) is a silicone bag which is filled with dimethyl polysiloxane fluid after insertion.

Research and development aimed at producing better and more natural prostheses continue; however, it is unlikely that the "perfect" trouble-free prosthesis will ever be manufactured, because of the basic tolerance problems common to all implants. The entire problem was comprehensively reviewed by Williams (1972) and Grossman (1973), and the status of the inflatable implants by Rees, Guy, and Coburn (1973). Suffice it to say that the choice of prosthesis for each patient should be individualized, depending upon the physical habitus of the patient, the goal of the operative procedure, and whether the operation is a primary or secondary procedure. Gel-filled prostheses seem preferable in subcutaneous mastectomy and as a secondary replacement for other types, while the inflatables are indicated in correction of asymmetry and in minimal to small augmentation. Inflatable implants unquestionably provide a more normal flow to the breast than other types, but this advantage is thought by some to be offset by a deflation rate of approximately 2 per cent and occasional wrinkling of the prosthetic capsule, a complication which can occur when the natural fibrous capsule surrounding the implant contracts.

The preoperative preparation of implants is extremely important in the prevention of wound complications. The manufacturer's instructions in this regard should be scrupulously followed. One of the most important precautions is a thorough washing of the implants.

Other materials have been used for implantation with varying degrees of success. These include Polystan (polyethylene) (Gonzalez-Ulloa, 1960) and polyester (polyurethane).

The operative procedure for prosthesis implantation is relatively simple (Fig. 89–20). There are, however, one or two important technical considerations. Meticulous aseptic technique is essential. Skin preparation should begin five days preoperatively with pHisoHex washes daily. Final surgical preparation is with aqueous Zephiran or Betadine.

The exact location of the incision varies. However, the inframammary site is commonly used (Fig. 89–21), and the inflatable prostheses can be introduced through a circumareolar incision

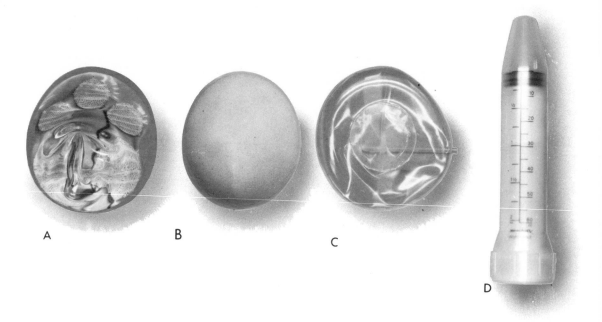

**FIGURE 89–20.**    The three most widely used prostheses for mammary augmentation. *A,* The silicone gel prosthesis of Cronin. This prosthesis is available with or without Dacron backing. *B,* The Ashley prosthesis, which is covered by a thin layer of sponge and divided into three compartments. The Ashley prosthesis is particularly suited for augmentation following subcutaneous mastectomy. *C, D,* The inflatable silicone balloon prosthesis with a 50-ml syringe for filling. This prosthesis, first described by Jenny, seems to give the most natural results to date. However, long-term evaluation is lacking.

(Fig. 89–22). Edgerton and McClary's (1958) "trick" of developing a superiorly based fat flap by beveling the incision downward to obtain a staggered closure has merit. The size of the pocket is measured preoperatively by ruler or caliper to mark its periphery. It is helpful to mark this area circumferentially with blue dye. When the pocket is formed, complete hemostasis is obtained. The procedure is facilitated by hypotensive anesthesia during the dissection. The pressure is allowed to rise after the pocket is formed. Meticulous atraumatic wound closure is important. Nonreactive, deep, dermal sutures are indicated. The skin is closed with a subcuticular suture of 3–0 nylon and augmented with interrupted sutures of 5–0 nylon. The interrupted sutures are removed on the seventh postoperative day and the subcuticular sutures on the tenth to twelfth postoperative day (Figs. 89–23 and 89–24).

Therapeutic doses of a suitable, wide-spectrum antibiotic are given postoperatively for ten days. The shoulders can be immobilized for three or four days by a type of Velpeau bandage.

Many surgeons utilize suction drainage (Hemovac) for 24 to 48 hours. The tubes should be brought out in the axilla, so that the residual small scars will be hidden by the brassiere line.

If suction drains are used, a light but supportive chest dressing may be used. If suction drains are not used, a more bulky pressure dressing is required.

All dressings for augmentation can be replaced on the third or fourth postoperative day by a soft but supportive elastic sleeping brassiere that fastens in the front.

Activities requiring active arm motion, such as lifting or driving, are sharply limited for the first week postoperatively and restrained for another two weeks. After three weeks, there are no limitations on physical activities.

**Complications of Augmentation Mammaplasty.** Complications associated with the dermis-fat flap reconstruction are generally those discussed under reduction mammaplasty and are managed as previously described. Dermis-fat grafts may be threatened by wound infection, the most serious complication. Vigorous antibiotic therapy should be immediately instituted and open drainage avoided unless abscess formation occurs. Intractable infection with prolonged drainage from sinus tracts may necessitate removal of the dermis-fat implants.

Another particularly troublesome complication of these grafts is sterile fat necrosis with

*Text continued on page 3703*

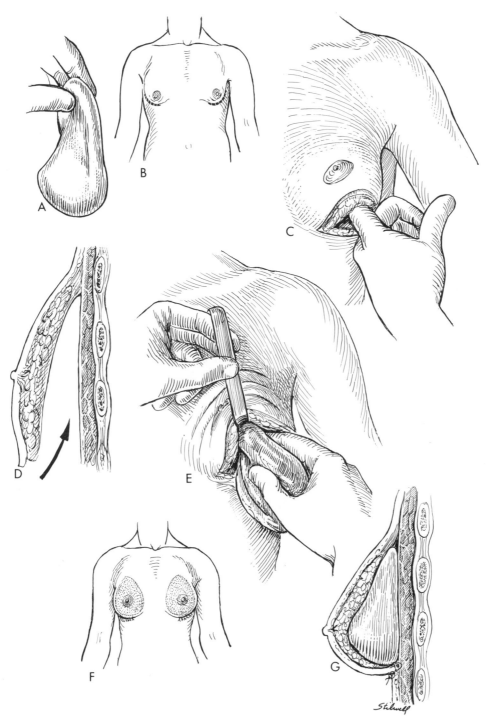

**FIGURE 89–21.**  Method of insertion of the silicone gel (Cronin) prosthesis. *A,* The prosthesis is a silicone rubber bag containing gel. It is pliable and natural-feeling. The prosthesis is available with or without Dacron patches to fix it to the chest wall. *B,* The incisions are located in the submammary crease laterally towards the axilla. *C,* A pocket is dissected between the gland and the pectoralis fascia. *D,* The pocket should be sized exactly to fit the prosthesis. It must not be too small, as a certain amount of contraction occurs. *E,* With the aid of a retractor, the prosthesis is inserted. It should be carefully unfolded and positioned. *F, G,* The prosthesis is in place, and the wound is sutured with a two-layered closure.

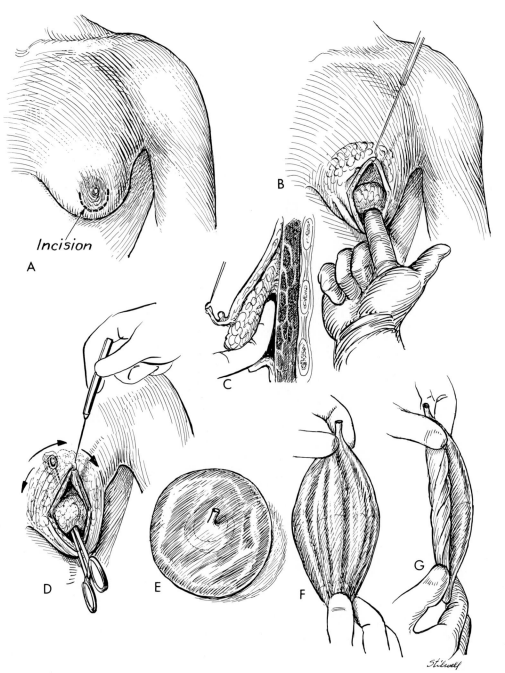

**FIGURE 89–22.** Method of mammary augmentation with the inflatable silicone balloon prosthesis. *A,* A semi-circular incision is made around the areolar border. *B, C,* The dissection is carried inferiorly around the inferior pole of the breast in small glands and down to the pectoralis fascia. *D,* Using blunt dissection, a suitable-sized pocket is created to accommodate the prosthesis. *E, F, G,* The empty balloon prosthesis of silicone rubber is rolled into a tubular shape. *H,* Dissection and hemostasis are facilitated by use of a fiberoptic retractor. *I, J, K,* The rolled-up prosthesis is inserted into the retromammary pocket and unfolded. It must not be handled by sharp instruments. *L, M,* The balloon is inflated to the desired size with normal saline solution. Manufacturers supply recommended volume scales to achieve the desired size. *N, O, P, Q,* A stylet is used to insert a plug into the neck of the prosthesis after any remaining air is aspirated, and the neck is inverted, presenting a smooth surface. *R, S,* The wound is sutured in layers. The skin is closed with a subcuticular suture. *T,* An alternate approach is shown whereby the gland is incised. This technique becomes necessary in larger breasts. The inflatable prosthesis can also be inserted via the usual retro-mammary incision.

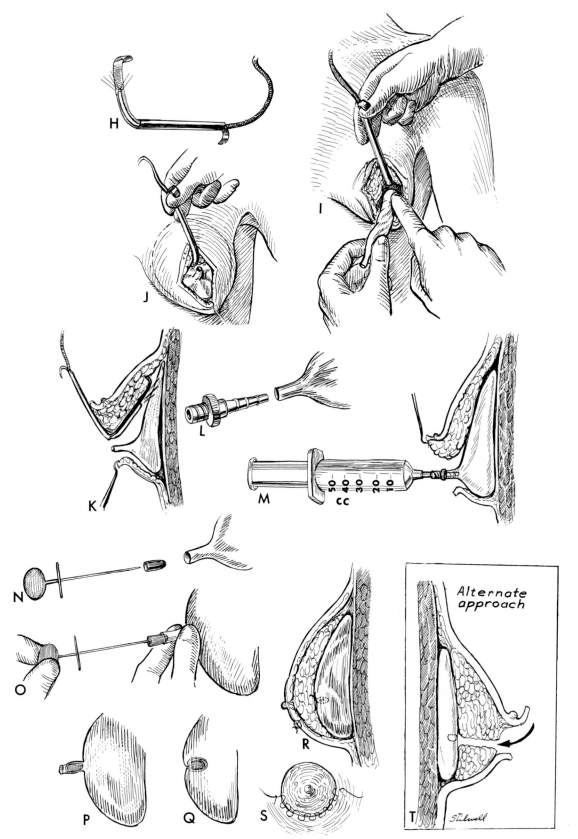

**FIGURE 89–22.** *See legend on the opposite page.*

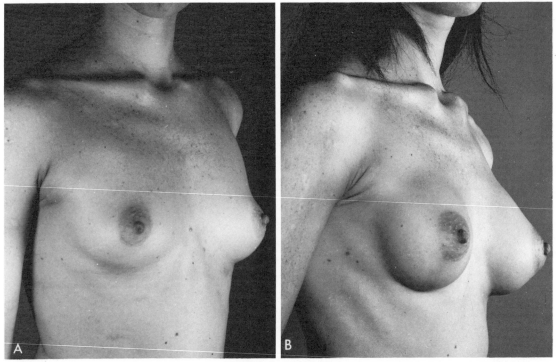

**FIGURE 89–23.**    Mammary augmentation by the implantation of the Cronin silicone gel prosthesis. Preoperative (*A*) and postoperative (*B*) views. The "new" Cronin prostheses were used in this patient. Note the natural curve of the breast along the inferior pole and the more normal contour of the superior pole.

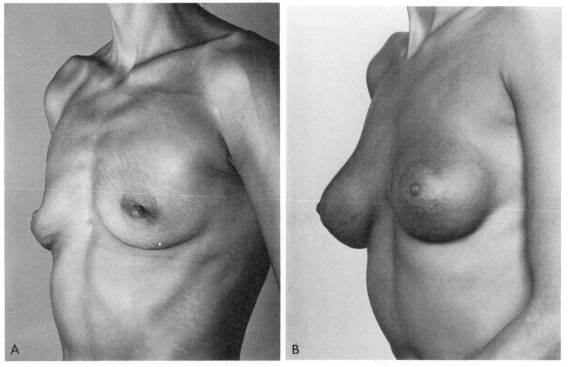

**FIGURE 89–24.**    *A*, Preoperative photograph of a patient with small, slightly ptotic breasts following pregnancy. Note the striae. *B*, Six months after mammary augmentation with inflatable silicone balloon prostheses. Note barely noticeable circumareolar incision. To inflate the balloon, 175 ml of saline was used.

continuous drainage that may result in eventual total loss of the bulk of the graft. Loss of the bulk, up to 50 per cent of dermis-fat grafts, can usually be anticipated within one to two years' time, even in the absence of open drainage or fat necrosis.

The complications of breast augmentation mammaplasty have been reviewed by several authors, including Kelly, Jacobson, Fox, and Jenny (1966); Broadbent and Woolf (1967); Gurdin and Carlin (1967); Dempsey and Latham (1968); Goulian and Conway (1969); DeCholnoky (1970); Silver (1972); and Grossman (1973). These complications are what one might expect following the implantation of foreign materials in the subcutaneous tissue or from the augmentation by dermis flaps or free grafts of dermis-fat. Complications following the implantation of polymers often depend on the physical and chemical nature of the implant, and their incidence is directly related to the nature of the implant. Thus, the various sponge implants which were formerly in use gave rise to a much higher incidence of drainage, infection, shrinkage, and capsule formation than the encapsulated gel implants now generally in use. The newer implants, which are mostly composed of outer capsules of silicone rubber (Silastic) containing a filler substance of silicone gel or saline, are much less prone to infection, shrinkage, asymmetry, or undue hardness than were the porous sponges, which were subject to difficulties in cleaning from impurities and which by their very nature were prone to fibrous tissue invasion associated with contraction and hardness. Such contraction was often of unequal degrees, so that asymmetry could result.

It should be pointed out that the complication rate following the now increasingly popular operation of subcutaneous mastectomy and prosthetic replacement is considerably higher than that following the usual implantation to correct mammary hypoplasia. This is particularly true if the prosthetic replacement is done at the same time as the glandular resection, for such a technique is stretching the limit of the blood supply to the skin flaps to the utmost and thus introducing another hazard to the operative procedure. This easily leads to circulatory complications, such as tissue necrosis, a complication rarely encountered following simple mammary augmentation. This complication was well documented by Kelly and associates (1966) and Freeman (1967).

The comprehensive review based on an analysis of 10,941 operations reported by DeCholnoky (1970) is worth reading by all interested in augmentation mammaplasty. He reported an overall infection rate of 2.5 per cent in all methods of augmentation mammaplasty, of which 1.7 per cent occurred in the immediate postoperative period and 0.8 per cent occurred late. As expected, the infection rate following subcutaneous mastectomy with implants was higher (5 per cent). The next highest incidence of infection was with the "open pore" type of implants (sponges), in which the infection rate was 3 per cent. *Staphylococcus aureus* and *albus* were usually the causative organisms.

Postoperative fluid accumulation is hardly a complication, as it occurs frequently to some degree following all types of implants but usually disappears spontaneously. Aspiration is rarely indicated; however, prolonged fluid accumulation may on occasion require aspiration and antibiotic administration.

DeCholnoky reported a leakage of 3 per cent in the balloon type prosthesis, and this was attributed to perforation of the prosthesis or to loss of the occluding plug. Another explanation may be dialysis of the inclusion material through the balloon membrane, although this is probably rare.

The incidence of skin perforation or slough after subcutaneous mastectomy and augmentation was 16.4 per cent but only 2 per cent after simple augmentation. DeCholnoky did not break down these figures into those occurring following immediate or delayed implantation; however, it is reasonable to assume that the incidence is much less after delayed implantation. The size of the implant is also important, particularly in subcutaneous mastectomy. The smaller the size of the implant, the less likely the chance of slough.

Shrinkage and hardening of implants were common in sponge implants and in fat or dermis-fat implants. Fat necrosis or total absorption occurred between two and ten years after dermis-fat grafts. The modern silicone sac implants are much less likely to shrink, although a certain degree of unnatural firmness must be expected in about 40 per cent of patients either unilaterally or bilaterally.

One of the disadvantages of all types of prostheses is that displacement of one or both prostheses or "buckling" of the capsule can occur. Again it is wiser to use the smaller implants whenever possible. It is equally important that a suitably sized and located subcutaneous pocket be fashioned. Even after such precautions, contraction of the fibrous capsule that forms around the implant is common and remains the chief problem following mammary augmentation with any type of prosthesis.

It seems likely that the problem will be solved

by improvement of surgical technique or modification of implant design. While further studies of wound healing may well provide the answer, helpful techniques have been advocated in the meantime to minimize the problem. Silver (1972) left the capsule intact and reinserted the implant beneath the formed fibrous capsule. Dempsey and Latham (1968) advocated placing the implants beneath the pectoralis major muscle as a method of concealing the ridges and folds of the implant. They reported 14 cases of subpectoral implants with good results. The Ashley prosthesis seems to reduce or eliminate this problem, seen in the Cronin prosthesis, because of the outer porous capsule which achieves some degree of fixation with the surrounding tissue. The balloon prostheses do not become fixed to the pectoralis fascia or the breast and therefore may tend to sag or become ptotic with the passage of time.

Open capsulotomy had been the traditional, but not always effective, method of dealing with the contracted capsule. However, the recent report of Baker, Bartels and Douglas (1976) of the closed compression technique for rupturing the capsule seems to offer a promising solution to the problem. According to their report, external manual pressure by the heel of the hands on the firm breast results in rupturing of the capsule by pressure exerted by the prosthesis. However, care must be exercised to ensure complete rupturing of the capsule circumferentially. The closed capsulotomy technique may be repeated at intervals if necessary, as the capsule begins to contract again. The technique has the advantage of being simple and is performed on an ambulatory basis. Mild sedation may be required. With the patient in the supine position, pressure is exerted with the surgeon's hands first horizontally and, following initial rupture, vertically. This sequence prevents displacement of the implant through a small incomplete tear in the capsule. The surgeon should use the heel of the hands and not thumb pressure, since a "gamekeeper's thumb" can result from excessive pressure. The patient should be observed carefully for a few hours in the postoperative period for occult hemorrhage, although this complication is rare. Some surgeons recommend self-massage by the patient on a daily basis to maintain the rupture.

Compression capsulotomy is in extensive use at this time. Long-term follow-up will determine the efficacy of this technique.

Deflation of one or both prostheses in the inflatable types can occur. Inadvertent puncture wounds during implantation, faulty valves, or wear and tear with eventual weakening and rupture of the capsule along the seam are thought to be the principal causes. Further technical improvement in the product will probably solve this vexing problem.

It is more difficult to attain a natural result in "flat-chested" women than in those with some fat or breast parenchyma which acts as padding; however, most surgeons agree that it is preferable to use smaller sized implants rather than the larger ones to achieve a natural result without palpable edges or postoperative ptosis of the implants.

As pointed out by Goulian and Conway (1969), care should be exercised in placing implants in breasts that are ptotic. Implantation only results in further ptosis or a bizarre deformity in which the implants adhere to the chest wall at a high level, and the breasts hang downward below it.

Pain in one or both breasts is rare but does occur and can be prolonged. Such pain rarely persists, requiring replacement of the implants. The cause of pain is obscure but may be the result of occult infection or pressure on sensory nerve branches.

Keloid formation or scar hypertrophy may require re-excision, radiation therapy, or intralesional steroid therapy. The treatment of true keloids is equally disappointing here as elsewhere.

The question of possible enhancement of a carcinoma potential in breast tissue by prosthetic implants seems reasonably settled by the reports of Hoopes, Edgerton and Shelley (1967) and DeCholnoky (1970). These authors reported sufficient data to rule out mammary implants as a significant causative agent in the development of breast cancer.

## SUBCUTANEOUS MASTECTOMY WITH RECONSTRUCTION

Certain diseases of the breast which are actually benign may, in some instances, be considered premalignant or sufficiently debilitating to require ablation of the glandular tissue and reconstruction. Authoritative sources disagree as to exactly what pathologic conditions of the breast may be considered premalignant, and the present methods of diagnosis of breast cancer are not sufficiently exact to provide comfort for the surgeon or for patients with such problems as progressive fibrocystic disease. Mammography has proved to be a valuable tool for increasing the accuracy of the diagnosis of breast malignancy. However, the absence of a positive finding in mammography does not always rule out carcinoma. Bader, Pellettiere, and Curtin (1970) studied a total of 529 consecutive breast biopsies in a large Chicago hospital. Sixty per cent of these biopsies were benign, while 40 per cent were malignant. Of the malignant tumors, only four were noninvasive. A high percentage of patients in the fourth decade and beyond of the group studied had multiple intraductal papillomas and/or ductal hyperplasia with atypia. They designated this group as having a "high risk" potential.

Preliminary findings by the same authors in a combined microscopic and computer analysis of 110 consecutive cases of multiple papillomas indicated that this group of women has a rate of incidence of carcinoma 12 to 13 times greater than normal for their respective age groups. Patients having large intraductal hyperplasia with microscopic atypia demonstrate a significantly higher potential for malignancy than those with well-differentiated papilloma. The authors recommend that, because of the serious malignant potential of this group, a bilateral adenomammectomy be done in patients with severe atypical papillomatosis.

Pennisi and associates (1971) emphasized the importance of prophylactic subcutaneous mastectomy. They reported two patients in whom they encountered occult breast cancers during this procedure.

Subcutaneous mastectomy with removal of almost all of the glandular parenchyma has been advocated for the past ten years or more in a variety of breast lesions (Freeman, 1962, 1969; Kelly and associates, 1966; Zbylski and Parsons, 1966; Fredericks, 1968). The usual technique of subcutaneous mastectomy (Freeman, 1969) does not remove all of the breast tissue, a fact confirmed in a study by Goldman and Goldwyn (1973). A small button of ductal and breast tissue remains attached to the nipple and areola, and often a remnant of gland is left at the end of the tail of the breast. The malignant potential is therefore decreased in direct proportion to the amount of tissue removed, and systematic examinations for the recurrence of pathologic lesions are facilitated by focusing attention on these remnants. A somewhat more extensive procedure is recommended by Bader, Pellettiere, and Curtin (1970), in which the fascia of the pectoralis muscle is elevated and resected in block with the breast tissue, as well as the basilar portions of the nipples, and sometimes the entire central portion of the nipple, if indicated by microscopic diagnosis. They also made an effort to resect almost all of the subcutaneous fat to eliminate the superficial lymphatics, thereby creating very thin skin flaps.

The occurrence of mammary carcinoma in two patients who had undergone subcutaneous mastectomy and replacement was reported by Bowers and Radlauer (1969). Unquestionably, additional cases will be found because of the high risk potential of the patients elected for this procedure. However, with more extensive dissection, as advocated by Bader, Pellettiere, and Curtin (1970), there is more likelihood of excising all glandular tissue and less likelihood of the subsequent development of malignancy in the breast remnants. However, the extended technique is also more deforming in nature, particularly when the central nipple core is resected. The decision as to whether a subcutaneous mastectomy or a total adenomammectomy should be performed rests with the diagnosis. Unquestionably, when severe papillomatosis of the breast or intraductal hyperplasia with atypia is a prominent feature, the more radical operation seems indicated.

The incidence of breast carcinoma is approximately 40 per 100,000 women over the age of 25, representing approximately 20,000 deaths in the United States alone. Peak ages are 45 to 50 years, at which time there is an increased frequency with a positive family history; a second peak age group would be approximately 65 years of age, with a low incidence of positive family history. Following menopause the incidence of benign breast lesions decreases sharply, so that palpable tumors of the breast following menopause are highly suspect.

Total ablation of the breast, including its skin envelope, nipple, and areola, for benign or suspected premalignant disease is indefensible. Such surgery results in severe deformity and has serious psychologic sequelae in the young woman. The development of modern prostheses for subcutaneous implantation has made subcutaneous mastectomy with reconstruction an acceptable alternative to simple mastectomy. The following indications have been proposed by various surgeons interested in this problem as constituting indications for subcutaneous mastectomy with prosthetic reconstruction: (1) severe or progressive fibrocystic disease (usually accompanied by frequent biopsies); (2) intractable mastodynia; (3) extensive intraductal papillomatosis; (4) a high incidence of familial breast cancer; (5) unilateral breast malignancy in a young woman; (6) a suspicious or positive mammogram without gross clinical findings; (7) lobular carcinoma in situ (bilateral in 35 per cent); (8) multiple fibroadenomas; (9) giant duct ectasia; (10) parenchymatous irregularities resulting from infection, surgical trauma, or previous biopsies.

While some surgeons advocate excision of the gland and immediate prosthetic replacement in selected cases, the experience of most surgeons indicates that the procedure is best done in two stages. The first stage consists of excision of the gland and mastopexy of redundant skin, if required. The second stage is best delayed for several weeks or months and consists of mammary augmentation with implant.

An alternative method is a one-stage procedure consisting of glandular excision and mammary reconstruction with dermis flaps. This technique is applicable to large or pendulous breasts (Goulian and McDivitt, 1972).

In an attempt to reduce the amount of residual breast tissue usually left under the nipple-areola complex and to prevent sloughing of the flaps with exposure of the implant following a subcutaneous mastectomy, Horton and associates (1974) and Rubin (1976) designed techniques in which the nipples and areolae were amputated and replaced as free grafts on the apices of the reconstructed breasts. In addition, dermis flaps were constructed and placed beneath the covering thin flap, thus providing added bulk between the implant and suture line.

The complications following subcutaneous mastectomy and reconstruction with a Silastic prosthesis were reported by Kelly, Jacobson, Fox, and Jenny (1966), Freeman (1967), and Grossman (1973). The complications are essentially those associated with implant surgery, but with an increased incidence of necrosis and circulatory embarrassment of the skin flaps.

Subcutaneous mastectomy with reconstruction has gained wide acceptance by plastic and general surgeons as a reasonable method of prophylaxis in the high risk patient.

## DEVELOPMENTAL ANOMALIES IN THE FEMALE BREAST

A number of conditions are included in this category, including polymastia and polythelia. Some authorities consider virginal hypertrophy to be a congenital abnormality. Bilateral micromastia more likely represents failure of development of the breast rather than a true congenital anomaly. However, unilateral micromastia, particularly when associated with contralateral macromastia, is probably a congenital anomaly.

Asymmetry is extremely common. However, significant asymmetry, especially unilateral micromastia, is rare. The treatment of this distressing deformity was summarized by Rees and Dupuis (1968), Horton and associates (1970), and Radlauer and Bowers (1971). Breast reconstruction may require insertion of an implant in the small side and reduction of the opposite side (Fig. 89–25) or asymmetrical augmentation of both. If contralateral reduction is not indicated, it may be exceedingly difficult to achieve near symmetry of size or shape. The inflatable balloon type of prosthesis may well find its best application in treating such problems.

Unilateral hypomastia should not be confused with amastia or athelia. Trier (1965) gave an

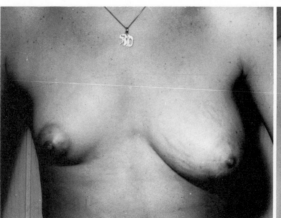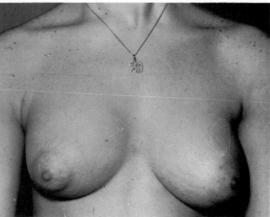

**FIGURE 89–25.**    Correction of right-sided hypomastia by augmentation with a Cronin prosthesis. The inflatable balloon type of prosthesis might prove more suitable in this type of deformity. Often it is also necessary to perform a reduction on the contralateral breast. (From Rees, T. D., and Dupuis, C. C.: Unilateral mammary hypoplasia. Plast. Reconstr. Surg., *41*:307, 1968. Copyright © 1968, The Williams & Wilkins Company, Baltimore.)

excellent review of this subject and reported on amastia, which he properly defined as absence of the mammary gland, nipple, and occasionally the pectoralis major muscle.

*Polythelia*, a descriptive term for accessory or supernumerary nipples, occurs in about 1 per cent of both male and female individuals. Supernumerary nipples are most commonly found about 5 to 6.5 cm below the normal nipple but located slightly more medially, toward the midline. Mammary tissue is usually absent in significant amounts in supernumerary nipples. Accessory nipples can be found anywhere along the course of the embryonic milk line. In the adult, this line extends from the axilla to the inguinal region, beginning laterally in the axilla and coursing medially as it approaches the inguinal region.

Supernumerary nipples are rarely of consequence. Excision is indicated, particularly when there is accessory mammary tissue associated with the nipple, since it is believed by some authorities that supernumerary nipples and glands are more apt to undergo malignant dedifferentiation with age (Copeland and Geschickter, 1950).

*Polymastia* is a term for supernumerary mammary glands. The aberrant glands are situated laterally and may vary in size from small to large, very often undergoing normal lactation. The commonest form of this anomaly is the axillary breast, which is often bilateral. Aberrant axillary tissue, particularly without nipple formation, is thought to be subject to malignant change. Aberrant breast tissue can also contain any of the usual types of breast disease, either benign or malignant. It is thought by some that aberrant mammary glands may represent a reversion to ancestral characteristics, since in general they follow the form of lower animals. It is not uncommon to find aberrant nipples or mammary tissue in association with asymmetry of the breasts or with mammary hypertrophy.

## GYNECOMASTIA

Gynecomastia or hypertrophy of breast tissue in adolescent males is a relatively common occurrence. A minimal degree of hypertrophy of mammary tissue is a normal phenomenon in the male breast during adolescence. Usually involution occurs before the age of 21 years. Mammary enlargement in the adult male may be due to excess adipose tissue or a combination of adipose and mammary tissues. Often a small discrete mass composed of periductal connective tissue surrounding mammary ducts and containing hyperplastic epithelium is found in the adult male.

In some instances, gynecomastia in late adolescence and in the adult male is associated with endocrine disorders, particularly with benign or malignant tumors of the adrenal gland. Testicular tumors, particularly chorionepithelioma, are frequently found in association with gynecomastia, and it may also occur in teratomas and other interstitial cell tumors. The exact hormonal influence on the breast tissue is obscure.

Klinefelter's syndrome includes gynecomastia in association with testicular atrophy with hyalinization of the testicular tubules; spermatogenesis is absent, and absent or markedly diminished cells of Leydig are also characteristic of this syndrome.

In a report by Nydick and associates (1961), 1890 normal boys in a summer camp were studied. The over-all incidence of gynecomastia was 38.7 per cent in Caucasians and 28.9 per cent in Negroes. Most gynecomastia occurred in the 14 to 14½ year age group. The condition was found to persist through two seasons in 27.1 per cent of the cases and for three seasons in 7.7 per cent.

Treatment of this condition varies; however, a conservative attitude should be adopted, since this is often a normal phenomenon of puberty which will disappear in one to two years. In the event gynecomastia is excessive or is prolonged after a two-year period, therapy is indicated. Young males so afflicted are frequently victimized by classmates, and the occurrence of this deformity at a critical emotional period of an adolescent's life may result in lasting emotional scars if it is not properly treated.

Simon, Hoffman, and Kahn (1973) provided a classification of gynecomastia which should prove useful in reporting surgical results.

In general, endocrine therapy has been disappointing in these cases. Simple surgical excision with preservation of the nipple and areolar structures is the simplest and most direct method of treatment. Even though the breast tissue may be of considerable size, it is extremely rare that excision cannot be accomplished through the classic periareolar incision (Fig. 89–26) described by Webster (1946).

When large amounts of breast tissue in the male are resected through a periareolar incision, a vacuum catheter suction technique, utilizing separate stab wounds, is of considerable value in reducing the incidence of postoperative hematoma and the collection of serum.

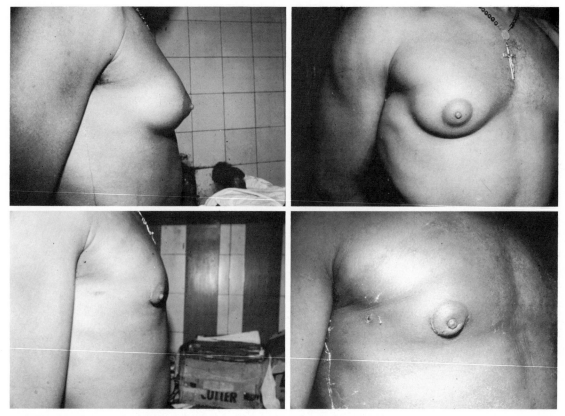

**FIGURE 89–26.** Excision of gynecomastia in a 17 year old male utilizing the periareolar incision of Webster. Very large amounts of tissue can be resected through this relatively small incision with an excellent cosmetic result.

Most authorities do not feel that persistence of mammary tissue in the male can be considered a premalignant condition. Karsner (1946) found no instances of malignancy of the breast in his review of the pathology of 284 cases of gynecomastia in servicemen.

## THE CANCER QUESTION IN MAMMAPLASTY

The question of a possible causal relationship between plastic operations on the breast and the development of mammary cancer is of considerable interest. As both reduction and augmentation operations become more common, this question assumes greater importance. The mammary gland is generally recognized as the primary site of 10 per cent of all cancers (Pack and Livingston, 1950), a high incidence. With breast cancer as common as this, it is inevitable that occasionally a tumor will be discovered either before, during, or after mammaplasty.

The world literature reveals a paucity of accurate statistics to shed light on this problem.

Maliniac (1959) reported a case of breast carcinoma discovered following a mammary reduction with free nipple transplantation. He incriminated free nipple transplantation as the catalyst in activating a malignant potential within the gland by interfering with ductile egress. Because of his belief, Maliniac reserved the free nipple transplantation technique for use only when total glandular ablation is performed.

Crikelair and Malton (1959) discovered an occult intraductal carcinoma on routine tissue block examination of resected glandular tissue following a mammary reduction operation. These authors failed to find a single well-documented case of breast malignancy following mammaplasty in the literature. They rightly stressed the value of routine microscopic pathologic examination of breast tissue removed during breast plastic operations and emphasized the importance of labeling the tissue as to whether it comes from the right or left side. Quite by coincidence, in the case reported by them, a free nipple transplantation was done on the side on which the carcinoma was discovered and a nipple transposition on the opposite side.

The paucity of accurate statistics prompted a questionnaire survey by Snyderman and Lizardo (1960). These investigators compiled statistics from 5008 reduction mammaplasties of various types. Carcinoma was discovered in five cases on preoperative examination. In five others, carcinoma was found on frozen section during the procedure. Cancer was reported by routine pathologic tissue block studies on nine cases postoperatively. These authors did not break down their findings on breast reduction operations in regard to free nipple transplantation or nipple transposition operations. Three carcinomas were discovered during the operative procedure in 2516 augmentation mammaplasties. In four others, carcinoma was discovered by routine tissue studies in the postoperative period. Questionnaires from four surgeons reported cases of carcinoma discovered at prolonged intervals after mammaplasty. In this total questionnaire study of 9172 breast plastic operations, there was an overall incidence of carcinoma in 30 patients or 0.3 per cent.

Harris (1961) circulated questionnaires to all certified plastic surgeons in the United States and received reports on 16,660 patients who had undergone augmentation mammaplasty of one form or another with alloplastic implants. At the time of his survey, there were no known cases of carcinoma in patients following augmentation mammaplasty.

An extensive review of the possible relationship of mammary augmentation and breast cancer was conducted by Hoopes, Edgerton, and Shelley (1967) and by DeCholnoky (1970).

Hoopes and his associates estimated that breast augmentation had been done in over 40,000 patients. They reported six patients, one of their own and five case reports supplied to them by other surgeons, in whom carcinoma had been diagnosed after augmentation mammaplasty. These augmentations were by various materials and techniques, which included polyvinyl sponge, silicone sponge, RTV Silastic, Cronin implants, Pangman implants, and silicone fluid injections. They were either implanted or, as in the case of the RTV and fluid silicone, injected. These were the only six patients with carcinoma that the authors were able to document, despite the thousands of operations performed and the expected 5½ per cent incidence of carcinoma of the breast in women in the general population. They pointed out that, on the basis of this general incidence, approximately 2000 out of the projected 40,000 patients with augmentation mammaplasty should be expected to develop carcinoma of the breast during their lifetimes. Certainly they fully expected to be able to discover more than six cases. Four of the patients reported by them had histologic sections available for study. Of these, two were intraductal carcinomas in young women, and two others were infiltrating lobular carcinomas. Three of the six cases proved to be of a multicentric nature. They concluded that "... the contention that a causal relationship may exist between breast implantation and the subsequent development of mammary cancer cannot be answered definitively at this time." They agreed with most investigators that there is also no current evidence to support the view that the prosthetic materials now in use in surgery enhance the potential for malignant degeneration of human breast tissue.

DeCholnoky (1970) undertook a worldwide survey in an attempt to clarify this question. He estimated that, as of late 1969, augmentation mammaplasty had been performed on an estimated 50,000 patients. In response to his questionnaire, 265 qualified plastic surgeons reported 10,941 operations, of which 80 per cent were performed in the second and third decades. The materials used in these operations were, as might be expected, of many types. His questionnaire was primarily designed to elucidate the complications of augmentation mammaplasty; however, his data on tumor formation were most interesting. Only one additional case of carcinoma was reported to add to those previously reported by Harris (1961) and Hoopes and associates (1967). DeCholnoky also estimated that an expected incidence of carcinoma among mammary augmentation patients should be expected to reach between 2000 and 3000; however, the additional case reported to him brought the total of known cases to seven. Extensive interrogation of general surgeons with considerable experience in breast cancer failed to identify additional cases of breast carcinoma in patients with augmentation. DeCholnoky emphasized the advisability of performing routine breast biopsies on patients undergoing breast augmentation, a premise also advocated by Hoopes and his coworkers.

A small percentage of the cases reported to him (1.3 per cent) were augmented by silicone injections. Many of these developed benign "silicone" cysts which subsequently became absorbed.

Twenty-three cases of benign tumor formation subsequent to augmentation were reported in the total series. Three of these were fibroadenomas, and 20 were variants of fibrocystic disease.

Certainly, from the statistics available at this time, it is not possible to establish a direct relationship between plastic surgical operations on the breast and the development of malignant tumors.

The routine use of mammography prior to breast reduction surgery, particularly in the older age group, is definitely indicated, even though it must be realized that a negative mammogram does not exclude the presence of occult malignancy. Follow-up mammograms would seem to be a wise procedure in patients with strong family histories of breast cancer. Xeroradiography and thermography of the breast also promise to be useful as diagnostic modalities and follow-up techniques after breast surgical procedures.

It is worth emphasizing that a small cancer in a very large breast must attain considerable size, or metastasize, before it is discovered. This fact would support the concept that breast reduction surgery can, in some instances, be helpful in the prevention or early detection of occult malignancy.

# Reconstruction of the Female Breast After Radical Mastectomy

## H. HÖHLER, M.D.

Radical mastectomy is a disfiguring operation that is associated with considerable mental strain for the affected woman. Many women who have lost a breast through surgery feel that in addition to suffering considerable emotional stress they have been robbed of their femininity.

In a psychological study of women who had undergone breast amputation, Renneker and Cutler (1952) equated the mental and psychological trauma of amputation of the breast with that of amputation of the penis in the male. Older women generally accepted the loss of a breast with less emotional distress. In the older age group, the breast is of minor sexual and functional importance, and with some exceptions, older women were content with wearing a prosthetic replacement.

If a woman, especially of the younger age group, is told by the surgeon that the tissue to be removed from her breast has to be examined pathologically and that she could expect a radical mastectomy in case the examination discloses a malignancy, the woman fears not only loss of her life but also mutilation of her body. If, however, the surgeon can offer the patient the prospect of an acceptable reconstruction of the breast, this would provide great consolation to her even before the operation. Many women, if they knew of the possibility of breast reconstruction, would probably seek consultation at an earlier stage rather than when the tumor progressed to a stage in which the prospects of a cure had been greatly diminished.

Breast cancer is the leading cause of death from cancer in females. In the United States, approximately 70,000 new cases are reported yearly, and as many as 31,000 women die yearly of the disease (Perras, 1976).

With the recent introduction of education and self-examination programs and newer diagnostic techniques (mammography, xerography, and thermography), it is possible that breast lesions will be detected at an earlier stage and smaller size and will be more amenable to breast reconstruction following ablation of the tumor.

The type of surgical resection of the tumor varies widely: *radical mastectomy* (Halsted, 1894), in which the breast, areola-nipple complex, pectoralis major and minor muscles, and axillary lymphatic tissue are resected; *modified radical mastectomy,* in which the muscles are preserved; *simple mastectomy,* which is limited to the breast and areola-nipple complex; and *tumorectomy* or excision of only the tumor. In the United States, *extended radical mastectomy* has been popularized by Urban (1951) and combines a radical mastectomy with resection of the chest wall in the internal mammary area. Radiation therapy, resulting in large fields of radiation damage on the chest wall, is often used in association with the above techniques. The more extensive resections leave surface defects that are covered by split-thickness skin grafts.

The problems facing the plastic surgeon are related directly to the extent of surgical resection. As emphasized by Millard (1976), the results of breast reconstruction following a simple mastectomy are superior because more skin and subcutaneous coverage are preserved than after a radical mastectomy, which is usually associated with a healed skin graft and absence of adequately vascularized soft tissue over the chest wall.

In recent years, a greater number of tumor surgeons have adopted more conservative ablative techniques, and the horizontal breast incision has also gained in popularity over the classic vertical breast incision. These factors facilitate breast reconstruction, since they not only preserve the overlying soft tissue but also result in better recipient sites for local transposition flaps. Despite these trends, the plastic surgeon must remember that *the eradication of the tumor remains the primary consideration.*

**The Post-Mastectomy Defect.** The chest wall defect confronting the plastic surgeon following ablative surgery depends on the anatomical extent of the resection:

1. the loss of the breast eminence.
2. the residual skin and subcutaneous tissue may be deficient, scarred, and tight with an inadequate blood supply; there may be a residual skin graft overlying the ribs.

3. an infraclavicular concavity resulting from the excision of the pectoral muscles.
4. the absence of the normal sweep of the pectoralis muscle across the axilla.

**Indications.** While no criticism has been expressed with respect to reconstruction of the breast after trauma or after thermal or radiation burns, reconstruction after radical mastectomy has been subject to heavy criticism. The possibility of recurrence or the development of cancer in the other breast can never be excluded. It has also been stated that reconstruction could camouflage chest wall recurrence, although the prognosis is excellent (76 per cent at 10 years) if no lymph node metastases have developed (Haagensen, 1971). It is the opinion of the author that one should consider reconstruction with women who have a favorable prognosis (Columbia Clinical Classification, Stage A; Table 89–2) and are relatively young.

Cronin and associates (1977) felt that the presence of "several positive axillary nodes" was not a contraindication to breast reconstruction. They were of the opinion that even if the patient succumbed to the disease, it was not sufficient reason to deny her the satisfaction of a breast reconstruction. However, reconstruction was definitely contraindicated in the presence of an inflammatory breast carcinoma or large, aggressive lesions with either questionable local surgical control or extensive axillary involvement.

**Timing of Reconstruction.** Improved diagnostic techniques (mammography, thermography, xerography) provide a means of detecting cancer at an early stage, i.e., before lymph node

TABLE 89–2. *The Columbia Clinical Classification*

Stage A. No skin edema, ulceration, or solid fixation of tumor to chest wall. Axillary nodes not clinically involved.

Stage B. No skin edema, ulceration, or solid fixation tumor to chest wall. Clinically involved nodes, but less than 2.5 cm in transverse diameter and not fixed to overlying skin or deeper structures of axilla.

Stage C. Any one of five grave signs of advanced breast carcinoma:
1. Edema of skin of limited extent (involving less than one-third of the skin over the breast).
2. Skin ulceration.
3. Solid fixation of tumor to chest wall.
4. Massive involvement of axillary lymph nodes (measuring 2.5 cm or more in transverse diameter).
5. Fixation of the axillary nodes to the overlying skin or deeper structures of axilla.

Stage D. All other patients with more advanced breast carcinoma, including:
1. A combination of any two or more of the five grave signs listed under Stage C.
2. Extensive edema of skin (involving more than one-third of the skin over the breast).
3. Satellite skin nodules.
4. The inflammatory type of carcinoma.
5. Clinically involved supraclavicular lymph nodes.
6. Internal mammary metastases as evidenced by a parasternal tumor.
7. Edema of the arm.
8. Distant metastases.

metastases have developed. These patients are candidates for early reconstruction, which may be started after one year if there are no signs of recurrence. In all other cases, one should allow a 5-year period to elapse before initiating reconstruction, with the realization, however, that 10-year follow-up statistics are more definitive (Haagensen, 1974). In the personal series of Haagensen (1971), recurrence (in all stages) developed with approximately the same frequency during each of the first five years following radical mastectomy; during the sixth through tenth years, the rate of recurrence steadily declined.

If, however, the patient insists on an earlier attempt at reconstruction despite the chance of recurrence and development of metastases, she must be thoroughly informed about the dangers and risks involved. Before starting reconstruction, chest roentgenograms and radioactive scans of the liver, spleen, and bones should be made to ensure that the patient does not harbor occult metastases.

## TYPES OF RECONSTRUCTIVE PROCEDURES

Following simple mastectomy or "tumorectomy," especially when a transverse incision has been used, it is possible at times to achieve an acceptable breast reconstruction by the insertion of a breast implant beneath the residual skin and soft tissues. Snyderman and Guthrie (1971) recommended that six months should elapse to allow the skin and scar to soften, following which a silicone implant can be inserted through a low horizontal incision. Z-plasties can be done to redirect surgical scars traversing the submammary fold. Such a technique following a radical mastectomy, however, is associated with an unacceptable rate of skin necrosis and erosion, fibrous capsule formation around the implant, malposition of the implant, and flattening of the underlying ribs (Freeman, 1976). The esthetic result is generally poor.

The requirements for the successful recon-

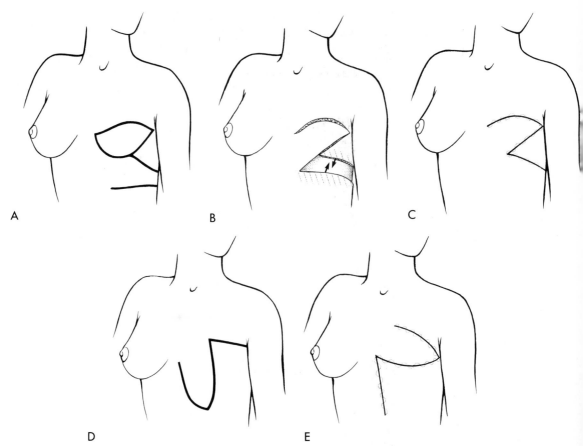

**FIGURE 89–27.** Local skin flaps. *A,* Site of ablative defect and adjacent (horizontal) flap donor area. *B,* Following transposition of the skin flap, the donor area is closed primarily. Note that undermining facilitates closure of the donor site. *C,* Following approximation of all wounds with a continuous intradermal suture. *D, E,* Example of a superiorly based vertical skin flap elevated from the upper abdomen.

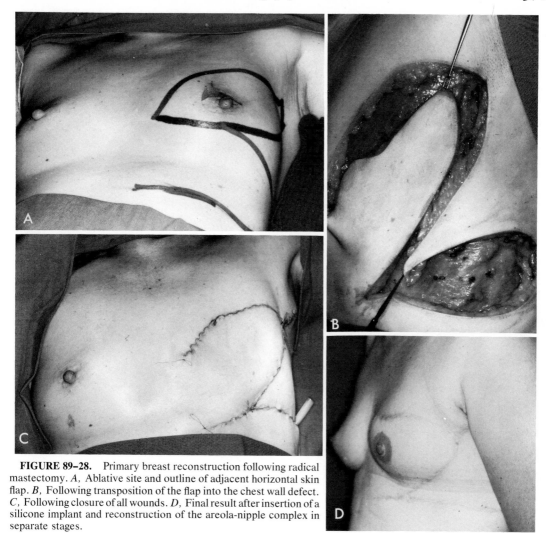

**FIGURE 89–28.** Primary breast reconstruction following radical mastectomy. *A,* Ablative site and outline of adjacent horizontal skin flap. *B,* Following transposition of the flap into the chest wall defect. *C,* Following closure of all wounds. *D,* Final result after insertion of a silicone implant and reconstruction of the areola-nipple complex in separate stages.

struction of the female breast after radical mastectomy are (Höhler, 1973, 1976):

1. replacement of the missing skin.
2. replacement of the absent glandular, fatty, and muscular tissue.
3. reconstruction of the areola-nipple complex.
4. restoration of the symmetry of the upper half of the thorax and the breast itself.

Almost all methods previously described assume that the remaining breast is to be used for the reconstruction, i.e., that it is sufficiently large and movable to make two breasts out of one (Gillies and Millard, 1957). Breast sharing procedures are often convincing in theory, but in practice the results are far from satisfactory. In addition, the relatively high incidence of or potential for malignant disease in the contralateral breast renders it unacceptable as a donor site (Urban, 1970).

Refinements in operating techniques during the last two years have made it possible to reconstruct a breast after radical mastectomy in a few stages, i.e., one or two procedures. The author's technique (Höhler, 1976) has brought about improved results so that not only breast-like mounds but esthetically acceptable breasts are reconstructed.

### Replacement of the Missing Skin

**Local Skin Flaps.** Local skin flaps are transferred from the surrounding tissue. Depending on the direction of the scar (transverse or vertical), local flaps can be elevated either from the side of the thorax in a horizontal direction (Figs. 89–27, *A* to *C* and 89–28) or from the upper abdomen in a vertical plane (Figs. 89–27, *D, E* and 89–29).

Cronin and associates (1977) have reported

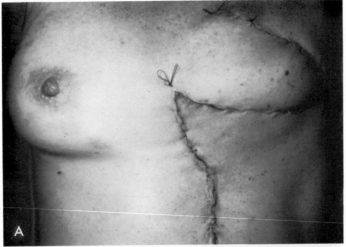

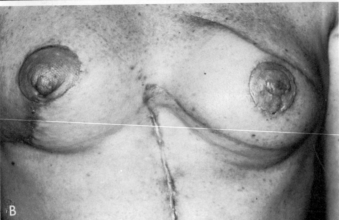

**FIGURE 89–29.** Reconstruction of the breast following radical mastectomy with a vertically oriented skin flap. *A,* Appearance following transposition of a superiorly based upper abdominal flap. *B,* Following insertion of a silicone implant, reduction of the contralateral breast, and reconstruction of the areola-nipple complex by partition of the contralateral areola-nipple (see Fig. 89–35).

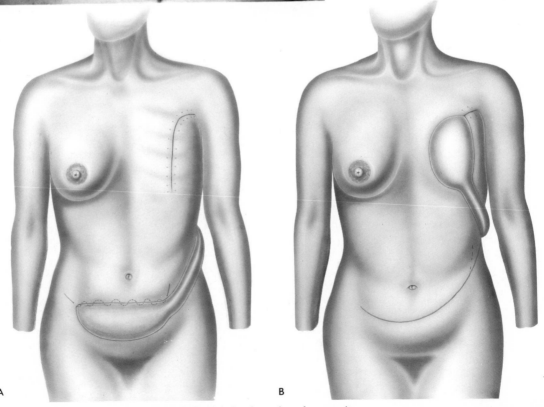

A

B

**FIGURE 89–30.** *See legend on the opposite page.*

their experience with a multiply delayed, transverse thoraco-epigastric flap. At the time of transfer to the vertical defect in the chest wall, the distal end of the flap is de-epithelized and also used to augment the infraclavicular concavity. Transposition of the flap is done two weeks after the last delay; the breast implant is inserted in a subsequent stage.

**Distant Skin Flaps.**    Gillies was a pioneer in breast reconstruction, and as early as 1942 advocated abdominal flaps based on the flanks, incorporating the umbilicus for reconstruction of the nipple (Millard, 1976).

Distant skin flaps are used only under the following situations:

1. if the patient is extremely thin and there-

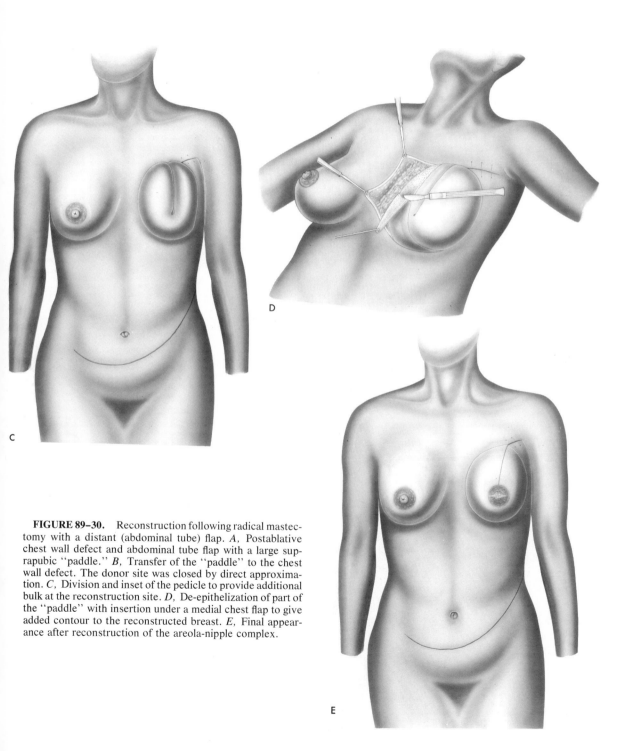

**FIGURE 89–30.**    Reconstruction following radical mastectomy with a distant (abdominal tube) flap. *A,* Postablative chest wall defect and abdominal tube flap with a large suprapubic "paddle." *B,* Transfer of the "paddle" to the chest wall defect. The donor site was closed by direct approximation. *C,* Division and inset of the pedicle to provide additional bulk at the reconstruction site. *D,* De-epithelization of part of the "paddle" with insertion under a medial chest flap to give added contour to the reconstructed breast. *E,* Final appearance after reconstruction of the areola-nipple complex.

fore no skin is available from the area adjacent to the amputation scar;

2. if the amputation defect is covered by a skin graft, or if the skin over the defect or the surrounding area has been damaged by radiation to an extent that it can no longer serve as a donor site for a local skin flap.

The author prefers to elevate a laterally based abdominal tube flap (Fig. 89–30, *A*) with a large paddle just superior to the pubis in the area of the abdominal dermolipectomy. After transfer to the recipient site (Fig. 89–30, *B*), the pedicle is also incorporated into the recipient site (Fig. 89–30, *C*) in a later stage. Part of the tube is later de-epithelized and used for additional augmentation of the reconstructed breast (Fig. 89–30, *D*). The disadvantage of the technique (Fig. 89–30, *E*) is the number of procedures and length of time involved in the reconstruction.

### Replacement of the Absent Glandular and Adipose Tissue and Muscle

**Autograft.** With a distant skin flap a "pancake" is designed on one end (see Fig. 89–30, *A*). Not only the "pancake" but also the pedicle, after de-epithelization, will be used for the replacement of the missing glandular tissue (Millard, 1976).

For the augmentation of the axillary or subclavicular deformity, the author prefers dermis-fat grafts removed from the remaining breast in the course of a reduction mammaplasty so that it corresponds in size and configuration to the newly reconstructed breast. In a similar manner, the remaining skin of the reduced breast can also serve as a full-thickness skin graft to replace any

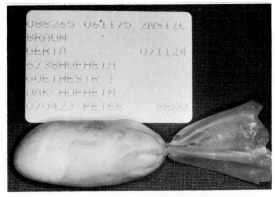

**FIGURE 89–32.** Preservation of the areola-nipple in a sterile, saline-impregnated compress in an airtight container (glove-finger) stored in a conventional refrigerator at 4°C.

areas of radiation-damaged skin in the axilla. As mentioned earlier, Cronin and associates (1977) used the distal, de-epithelized portion of the thoraco-epigastric skin flap for correction of the subclavicular concavity.

**Inorganic Implants.** Silastic implants (Cronin and Gerow, 1964) are currently the technique of choice in replacing the missing glandular, adipose tissue and muscle. The contour-form type of prosthesis has not proved to be successful because in the course of follow-up it has been observed that the constant pressure exerted by the implant tends to reduce the overlying glandular and subcutaneous tissue. Prostheses with Dacron patches are no longer used because the implants are fixed to the chest wall, and the skin, with advancing age, tends to hang inferiorly over the fixed prominence. Round and moderate-sized implants with a low profile are preferred. If

*Text continued on page 3720*

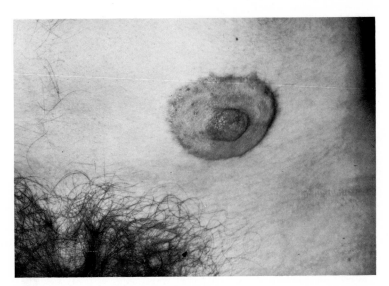

**FIGURE 89–31.** Storage of the areola-nipple as a full-thickness graft on the lower abdomen.

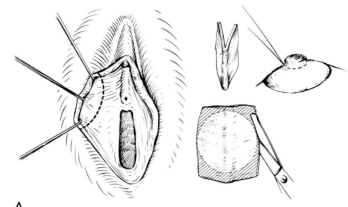

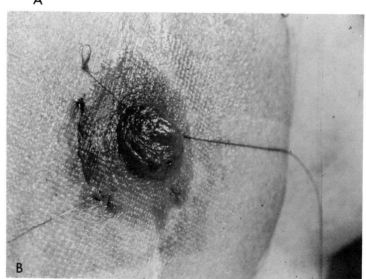

**FIGURE 89–33.** *A*, Technique of removal of labia minora graft. Note the insertion of a pursestring suture to achieve nipple prominence. *B*, Appearance following insertion of the pursestring suture.

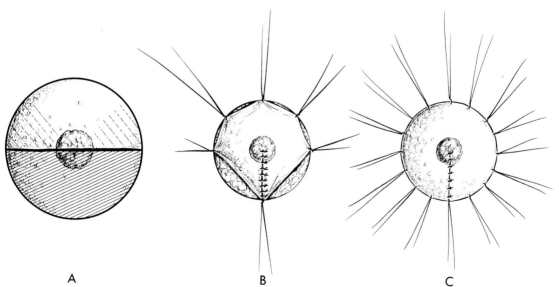

**FIGURE 89–34.** Partition of the contralateral areola-nipple complex. *A*, The lower half is resected as a full-thickness graft. The upper half is partially undermined and rotated to complete a 360° arc. *B*, Suturing of the graft on the de-epithelized recipient site. *C*, The sutures are kept long to be incorporated into a bolus dressing.

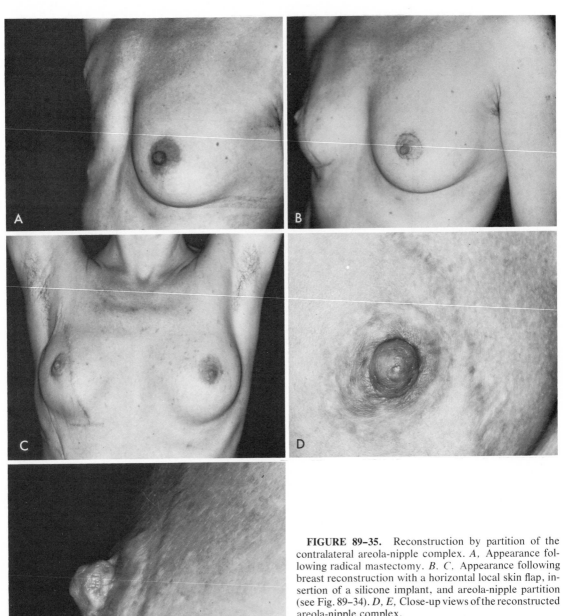

**FIGURE 89–35.** Reconstruction by partition of the contralateral areola-nipple complex. *A,* Appearance following radical mastectomy. *B. C.* Appearance following breast reconstruction with a horizontal local skin flap, insertion of a silicone implant, and areola-nipple partition (see Fig. 89–34). *D, E,* Close-up views of the reconstructed areola-nipple complex.

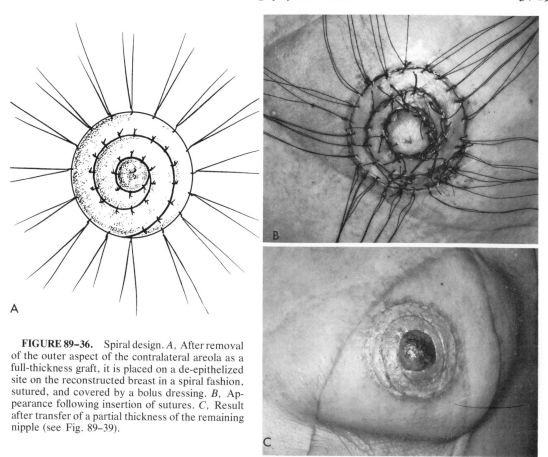

**FIGURE 89-36.** Spiral design. *A,* After removal of the outer aspect of the contralateral areola as a full-thickness graft, it is placed on a de-epithelized site on the reconstructed breast in a spiral fashion, sutured, and covered by a bolus dressing. *B,* Appearance following insertion of sutures. *C,* Result after transfer of a partial thickness of the remaining nipple (see Fig. 89-39).

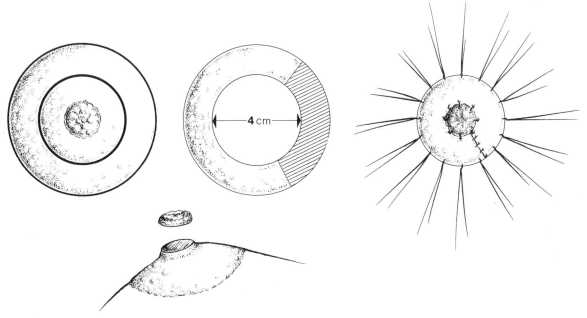

**FIGURE 89-37.** Circle design. An outer ring is removed from the areola, preserving an areola at least 4 cm in diameter; the shaded area is discarded. The full-thickness areola graft is sutured on a de-epithelized bed. A partial-thickness nipple graft provides nipple projection.

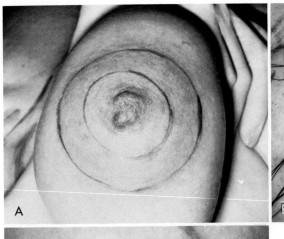

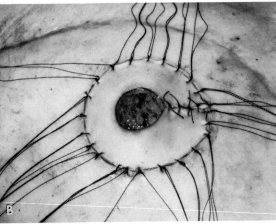

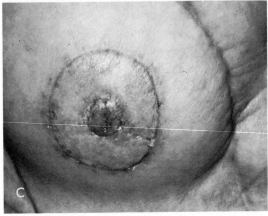

**FIGURE 89–38.** Circle design. *A,* Preoperative markings on the donor breast. *B,* Suturing of the full-thickness areola graft. *C,* Final result obtained by the technique illustrated in Figure 89–37.

the amputated gland is placed on a flat surface, one can see that it has a low profile and is round in the majority of cases.

The pocket for the implant should be made much larger than seems necessary. As early as the first postoperative day, the implant should be moved around within the cavity. Every tissue responds to the presence of a foreign body with the formation of a fibrous capsule. There is, however, also capsule formation if the implant is moved in a relatively large cavity, but the recipient site is so large that the comparatively small implant remains soft.

### Reconstruction of the Areola-Nipple Complex

**Preservation of the Areola.** Preservation of the areola, if at all possible, is always superior to any other method of substituting for or reconstructing the original areola.

Beginning in 1969, the author (Höhler, 1973) began a technique of removing the nipple as a full-thickness graft and transplanting it to the lower abdomen (Fig. 89–31). It remained "banked" for many months in this area in a certain "waiting-position" until irradiation and

reconstruction of the breast had been concluded. It was then removed as a full-thickness graft from the abdomen and transferred to a deepithelized site on the newly formed breast.

The nipple should always be preserved in this way, if possible, to be used in later reconstruction of the breast. Even if it is not used again because of recurrent disease, it provides moral support, since the patient retains hope that a reconstruction is possible and is planned.

In 1972, the investigations by Boulten and Haukohly in Germany, who reported that in 90 per cent or more of patients with carcinoma of the breast the nipple is not involved, were questioned in a report by Zippel and associates (1972). They reported that in 35 per cent of mammary carcinoma specimens examined, tumor could be demonstrated in the region of the areola-nipple complex. If the distance and size of the primary tumor were also considered, the nipple was more rarely affected by carcinoma when the primary tumor was located at a distance of more than 5 cm from the nipple and was less than 1 cm in diameter.

In the author's series, a tumor was found in the nipple in only 8.5 per cent of the specimens. Parry and Wolfort (1976) also reported that the

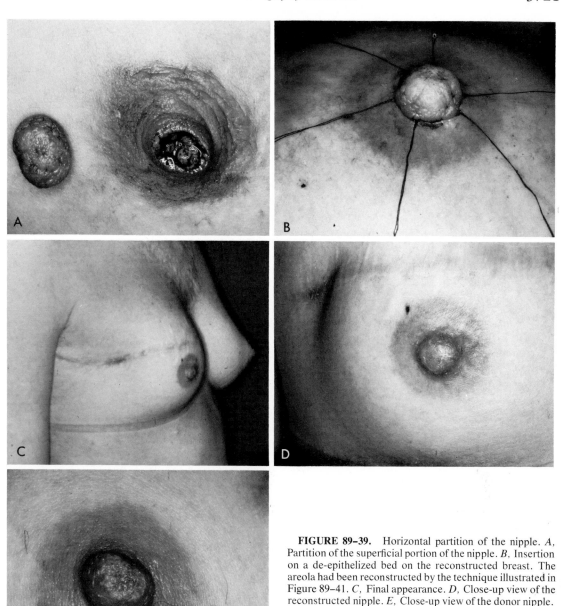

**FIGURE 89–39.** Horizontal partition of the nipple. *A,* Partition of the superficial portion of the nipple. *B,* Insertion on a de-epithelized bed on the reconstructed breast. The areola had been reconstructed by the technique illustrated in Figure 89–41. *C,* Final appearance. *D,* Close-up view of the reconstructed nipple. *E,* Close-up view of the donor nipple.

nipple was involved in only 8 per cent of resected breast specimens.

To exclude the danger of malignant tissue being transplanted, the author has modified his method in the following way: the areola-nipple complex, removed under aseptic conditions, is kept in a sterile, saline-impregnated compress in an airtight container (e.g., a glove-finger) at a temperature of 4°C in a conventional refrigerator (Fig. 89–32) until the pathologist has established whether the tissue under the nipple is free of

tumor involvement. The sections are taken from a paraffin-block (*not* "frozen sections"). The nipple can be preserved for up to one week in the refrigerator and can then be transferred as a full-thickness graft in the manner previously described.

**Labia Minora Grafts.** A semicircle of labia minora (Adams, 1949) is excised and horizontally split as shown in Figure 89–33, *A*. It is transferred as a full-thickness graft to a pre-

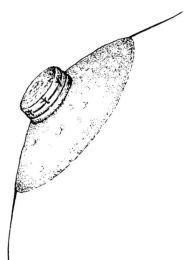

**FIGURE 89–40.** Formation of a nipple by serial application of split-thickness skin grafts removed from the rima ani at the coccygeal level.

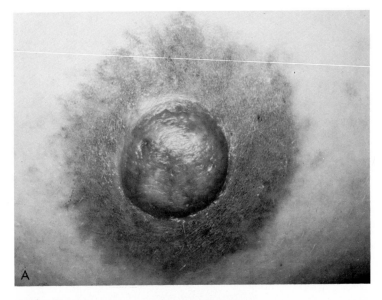

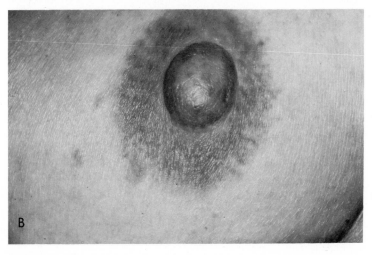

**FIGURE 89–41.** Loss of tattoo pigment and fading of simulated areola. *A*, Immediately following tattooing. *B*, One year later. Note degree of fading.

determined and de-epithelized site on the breast eminence. In order to achieve nipple prominence, a pursestring suture is inserted in the desired site of the nipple, followed by fixation with a bolus pressure dressing (see Fig. 89–33, *B*). The suture is left in place for two weeks.

**Partition of the Contralateral Areola-Nipple.** The remaining nipple and areola are transversely divided. The ends of the donor half are undermined, and in this way there results a half nipple with a smaller areola (see Figs. 89–34 and 89–35). The other half is transplanted after de-epithelization of the breast recipient site and is held in position by a bolus-type dressing (Wexler and Oneal, 1973).

In the case of a large areola, an incision is made around the areola, and the outer ring is removed and used, in either a spiral (Fig. 89–36) or circle design (Figs. 89–37 and 89–38), on the contralateral side. Cronin and associates (1977) have described a variation, termed "the conjoined spirals method."

**Formation of the Nipple by Horizontal Partition of the Remaining Nipple.** In order to achieve nipple prominence, the top of the remaining nipple is horizontally removed and transferred as a split-thickness graft to the other side (Fig. 89–39) and fixed with a bolus pressure dressing (Millard, 1972).

**Formation of the Nipple by Serial Application of Split-thickness Grafts.** Nipple projection is achieved by serial transplantation, at intervals of four weeks, of split-thickness grafts in sandwich-like fashion (Fig. 89–40). The grafts may be taken from the rima ani at approximately the coccygeal level to provide the natural red-brown color. The reconstructed nipple is of rather sturdy texture, maintains its prominence, and does not sink into the subcutaneous tissue.

**Simulating the Areola by Tattooing.** An excellent method to simulate the areola is tattooing, especially if it is done by a professional. However, the selected color should always be darker than desired, since in the course of a year it loses its intensity because of absorption of the pigment by macrophages (Fig. 89–41).

### The Contralateral Remaining Breast

As emphasized by Cronin and associates (1977), surgical procedure may be required on the contralateral breast:

1. Reduction mammaplasty or mastopexy if the remaining breast is large and ptotic.
2. Subcutaneous mastectomy in high-risk patients (see page 3704).
3. Simple mastectomy to achieve breast symmetry.
4. Augmentation mammaplasty if the remaining breast is small.

### REFERENCES

Adams, W. M.: Free transplantation of the nipples and areolae. Surgery, *15*:186, 1944.

Adams, W. M.: Free composite grafts of the nipples in mammaryplasty. South. Surg., *13*:715, 1947.

Adams, W. M.: Labial transplant for correction of loss of the nipple. Plast. Reconstr. Surg., *4*:295, 1949.

Arion, H. G.: Retromammary prosthesis. C. R. Soc. Fr. Gynécol., No. 5, May, 1965.

Ashley, F. L.: A new type of breast prosthesis. Plast. Reconstr. Surg., *45*:421, 1970.

Ashley, F. L.: Further studies on the natural-Y breast prosthesis. Plast. Reconstr. Surg., *49*:414, 1972.

Auber, V.: Hypertrophie mammaire de la puberté, résection partielle restauratrice. Arch. Franco-Belges Chir., *3*:287, 1923.

Aufricht, G.: Mammaplasty for pendulous breasts. Empiric and geometric planning. Plast. Reconstr. Surg., *4*:13, 1949.

Axhausen, G.: Ueber Mammaplastik. Med. Klin., *22*:976, 1926.

Bader, K., Pellettiere, E., and Curtin, J. W.: Definitive surgical therapy for the "pre-malignant" or equivocal breast lesion. Plast. Reconstr. Surg., *46*:120, 1970.

Baker, J. L., Bartels, R. J., and Douglas, W. M.: Closed compression technique for rupturing a contracted capsule around a breast implant. Plast. Reconstr. Surg., *58*:137, 1976.

Bames, H. O.: Reduction of massive breast hypertrophy. Plast. Reconstr. Surg., *3*:560, 1948.

Bames, H. O.: Breast malformations and a new approach to the problem of small breasts. Plast. Reconstr. Surg., *5*:499, 1950.

Bames, H. O.: Augmentation mammaplasty by lipo-transplant. Plast. Reconstr. Surg., *11*:404, 1953.

Beare, R.: Reduction mammaplasty. Presented at the Fourth International Congress of Plastic Surgery, Rome, 1967.

Berson, M.: Derma-fat transplants used in building up the breasts. Surgery, *15*:451, 1945.

Biesenberger, H.: Blutversorgung und zirkuläre Umschnedung des Warzenhofes. Zentralbl. Chir., *55*:2385, 1928.

Biesenberger, H.: Deformitaten und kosmetische Operationen der weiblichen Brust. Wien, Verlag W. Maudrich, 1931.

Boo-Chai, K.: The complications of augmentation mammaplasty by silicone injection. Br. J. Plast. Surg., *22*:28, 1969.

Boulten, S. M., and Haukohly, R. S.: Personal communication, 1972.

Bowers, D. G., Jr., and Radlauer, C. B.: Breast cancer after prophylactic subcutaneous mastectomies and reconstruction with Silastic prostheses. Plast. Reconstr. Surg., *44*:541, 1969.

Broadbent, T. R., and Woolf, R. M.: Augmentation mammaplasty. Plast. Reconstr. Surg., *40*:517, 1967.

Chaplin, C. H.: Loss of both breasts from injections of silicone (with additive). Plast. Reconstr. Surg., *44*:447, 1969.

Cheatle, G. L., and Cutler, M.: Tumor of the Breast. Philadelphia, J. B. Lippincott Co., 1931.

Conway, H.: Mammaplasty: Analysis of 110 consecutive cases with end results. Plast. Reconstr. Surg., *10*:303, 1952.

Conway, H., and Dietz, G. H.: Augmentation mammaplasty. Surg. Gynecol. Obstet., *114*:573, 1962.

Conway, H., and Goulian, D.: Experience with an injectable Silastic RTV as a subcutaneous prosthetic material. Plast. Reconstr. Surg., *32*:294, 1963.

Conway, H., and Smith, J.: Breast plastic surgery: Reduction mammaplasty, mastopexy, augmentation mammaplasty and mammary construction. Plast. Reconstr. Surg., *21*:8, 1958.

Copeland, M. M., and Geschickter, C. F.: Diagnosis and treatment of premalignant lesions of the breast. Surg. Clin. North Am., *30*:1717, 1950.

Crikelair, G. F., and Malton, D.: Mammaplasty and occult breast malignancy: Case report. Plast. Reconstr. Surg., *23*:601, 1959.

Cronin, T. D., and Gerow, F.: Augmentation mammaplasty: a new "natural feel" prosthesis. *In* Transactions Third International Congress Plastic Surgery. Excerpta Medica, Amsterdam, 1964, pp. 41–49.

Cronin, T. D., Upton, J., and McDonough, J. M.: Reconstruction of the breast after mastectomy. Plast. Reconstr. Surg., *59*:1, 1977.

Czerny, V.: Plastischer Ersatz der Brustdruse durch ein Lipom. Zentralbl. Chir., *27*:72, 1895.

Dartigues, L.: Procédé de suspension et mastopéxie par voie axillotomique. Bull. Soc. Méd. Paris, Feb. 23, 1924.

Dartigues, L.: État actuel de la chirurgie esthétique mammaire. Monde Méd., *38*:75, 1928.

deCastro Correia, P., and Zani, R.: Masseter muscle rotation in the treatment of inferior facial paralysis. Plast. Reconstr. Surg., *52*:370, 1973.

DeCholnoky, T.: Augmentation mammaplasty. Survey of complications of 10,941 patients by 265 surgeons. Plast. Reconstr. Surg., *45*:573, 1970.

Dehner, J.: Mastopexie zur Beseitgung der Hangebrust. Münch. Med. Wochenschr., *36*:1878, 1908.

Dempsey, W. C., and Latham, W. D.: Subpectoral implants in augmentation mammaplasty, Plast. Reconstr. Surg., *42*:515, 1968.

Dufourmentel, L.: La mastopéxie par déplacement sous-cutané avec transposition du mamelon. Bull. Mém. Soc. Chir. Paris, March 20, 1927.

Dufourmentel, C., and Mouly, R.: Plastie mammaire par la méthode oblique. Ann. Chir. Plast., *6*:1, 1961.

Dufourmentel, C., and Mouly, R.: Developments récents de la plastie mammaire par le méthode oblique latérale. Ann. Chir. Plast., *10*:227, 1965.

Dufourmentel, C., and Mouly, R.: Modification of "periwinkleshell" operation for small ptotic breast. Plast. Reconstr. Surg., *41*:523, 1968.

Dukes, C. E., and Mitchley, M. I.: Polyvinyl sponge implants: Experimental and clinical observations. Br. J. Plast. Surg., *15*:225, 1962.

Durstan, W.: Sudden and excessive swelling of a woman's breasts. Phil. Trans. R. Soc., London, 4th Ed., 78, 1669 (cited by Thorek, 1942).

Edgerton, M. T., and McClary, A. R.: Augmentation mammaplasty. Plast. Reconstr. Surg., *21*:279, 1958.

Edgerton, M. T., Meyer, E., and Jacobson, W. E.: Augmentation mammaplasty. II. Further surgical and psychiatric evaluation. Plast. Reconstr. Surg., *27*:279, 1961.

Edwards, B. F.: Teflon silicone breast implants. Plast. Reconstr. Surg., *32*:519, 1963.

Ewing, J.: Neoplastic Diseases. Philadelphia, W. B. Saunders Company, 1940.

Felix, E. R., Sethi, S. M., Ransdell, A. M., and Lissner, A. B.: Strömbeck mammaplasty with free nipple grafts. Plast. Reconstr. Surg., *45*:47, 1970.

Fredericks, S.: Personal communication, 1968.

Freeman, B. S.: Subcutaneous mastectomy for benign breast lesions with immediate or delayed prosthetic replacement. Plast. Reconstr. Surg., *30*:676, 1962.

Freeman, B. S.: Complications of subcutaneous mastectomy with prosthetic replacement, immediate or delayed. South. Med. J., *60*:1277, 1967.

Freeman, B. S.: Technique of subcutaneous mastectomy with replacement: Immediate and delayed. Br. J. Plast. Surg., *22*:161, 1969.

Freeman, B. S.: Experiences in reconstruction of the breast after mastectomy. Clin. Plast. Surg., *3*:277, 1976.

Gersuny, R.: Cited by Thorek (1942).

Geschickter, C. F.: Diseases of the Breast. Philadelphia, J. B. Lippincott Company, 1943.

Gillies, H., and McIndoe, A. H.: The technique of mammaplasty in conditions of hypertrophy of the breast. Surg. Gynecol. Obstet., *68*:658, 1939.

Gillies, H., and Millard, D. R.: The Principles and Art of Plastic Surgery. Boston, Little, Brown & Company, 1957, pp. 175–179.

Girard, C.: Ueber Mastoptose und Mastopexie. Verh. Dtsch. Ges. Chir., Beilage, Zentralbl. Chir., *31*:70, 1910.

Goldman, L. D., and Goldwyn, R. B.: Some anatomical considerations of subcutaneous mastectomy. Plast. Reconstr. Surg., *51*:501, 1973.

Gonzalez-Ulloa, M.: Correction of hypertrophy of the breast by means of exogenous material. Plast. Reconstr. Surg., *25*:15, 1960.

Goulian, D., and Conway, H.: Correction of the moderately ptotic breast, a warning. Plast. Reconstr. Surg., *43*:478, 1969.

Goulian, D., and McDivitt, R. W.: Subcutaneous mastectomy with immediate reconstruction of the breasts using the dermal mastopexy technique. Plast. Reconstr. Surg., *50*:211, 1972.

Grindlay, J. H., and Clagett, O. T.: Plastic sponge prosthesis for use after pneumonectomy. Proc. Staff Meet. Mayo Clinic, *24*:538, 1949.

Grindlay, J. H., and Waugh, J. M.: Plastic sponge which acts as framework for living tissues. A.M.A. Arch. Surg., *63*:288, 1951.

Grossman, A. R.: The current status of augmentation mammaplasty. Plast. Reconstr. Surg., *52*:1, 1973.

Guinard, A.: Cited by Morestin (1903).

Gupta, S. C.: A critical review of contemporary procedures for mammary reduction. Br. J. Plast. Surg., *18*:328, 1965.

Gurdin, M., and Carlin, G. A.: Complications of breast implantations. Plast. Reconstr. Surg., *40*:530, 1967.

Haagensen, C. D.: Diseases of the Breast. 2nd Ed. Philadelphia, W. B. Saunders Company, 1971.

Haagensen, C. D.: The choice of treatment of operable carcinoma in breast cancer. Surgery, *76*:685, 1974.

Halsted, W. S.: Results of operation for cure of cancer of breast performed at Johns Hopkins Hospital from June 1889 to January 1894. Am. Surg., *20*:497, 1894.

Harris, H. I.: Survey of breast implants from the point of view of carcinogenesis. Plast. Reconstr. Surg., *28*:81, 1961.

Höhler, H.: Reconstruction after mastectomy. *In* Symposium on Neoplastic and Reconstructive Problems of the Female Breast. Saint Louis, The C. V. Mosby Company, 1973.

Höhler, H.: Further progress in the technique of reconstruction of the female breast after radical mastectomy. Presented at the annual meeting of the American Society for Plastic and Reconstructive Surgery, Boston, 1976.

Hoopes, J. E., and Jabaley, M. D.: Reduction mammaplasty: Amputation and augmentation. Plast. Reconstr. Surg., *44*:441, 1969.

Hoopes, J. E., Edgerton, M. T., and Shelley, W.: Organic synthetics for augmentation mammaplasty: Their relation to breast cancer. Plast. Reconstr. Surg., *39*:263, 1967.

Horton, C. E., Adamson, J. E., Mladick, R., and Taddeo, R. J.: The unilateral hypoplastic breast. Br. J. Plast. Surg., *23*:161, 1970.

Horton, C. E., Adamson, J. E., Mladick, R. A., and Carraway, J. H.: Simple mastectomy with immediate reconstruction. Plast. Reconstr. Surg., *53*:42, 1974.

Jenny, H.: Personal communication, 1969.

Joseph, J.: Zur Operation der hypertrophischen Hangebrust. Dtsch. Med. Wochenschr., *51*:1103, 1925.

Kahn, S., Hoffman, S., and Simon, B. E.: Correction of non-hypertrophic ptosis of the breasts. Plast. Reconstr. Surg., *41*:244, 1968.

Karsner, H. T.: Gynecomastia. Am. J. Pathol., *22*:235, 1946.

Kausch, W.: Die Operation der Mammahypertrophie. Zentralbl. Chir., *43*:713, 1916.

Kelly, A. P., Jacobson, H. S., Fox, J. I., and Jenny, H.: Complications of subcutaneous mastectomy and replacement by the Cronin Silastic mammary prosthesis. Plast. Reconstr. Surg., *37*:438, 1966.

Kraske, H.: Die Operation der atrophischen und hypertrophischen Hangebrust. Münch. Med. Wochenschr., *60*:672, 1923.

Lewis, J. R., Jr.: The augmentation mammaplasty with special reference to alloplastic materials. Plast. Reconstr. Surg., *35*:51, 1965.

Longacre, J. J.: The use of local pedicle flaps for reconstruction of the breast after sub-total or total extirpation of the mammary gland and for the correction of distortion and atrophy of the breast due to excessive scar. Plast. Reconstr. Surg., *2*:380, 1953.

Longacre, J. J.: Correction of the hypoplastic breast with special reference to reconstruction of the "nipple type breast" with local dermo-fat pedicle flaps. Plast. Reconstr. Surg., *14*:431, 1954.

Longacre, J. J.: Surgical reconstruction of the flat discoid breast. Plast. Reconstr. Surg., *17*:358, 1956.

Longacre, J. J.: Breast reconstruction with local derma and fat pedicle flaps. Plast. Reconstr. Surg., *24*:563, 1959.

Lotsch, F.: Uber Hängebrustplastik. Zentralbl. Chir., *50*:1241, 1923.

McIndoe, A. H., and Rees, T. D.: Mammaplasty: Indications, technique and complications. Br. J. Plast. Surg., *10*:307, 1958.

McKissock, P. K.: Reduction mammaplasty with a vertical dermal flap. Plast. Reconstr. Surg., *49*:245, 1972.

Maliniac, J.: Breast Deformities and Their Repair. New York, Grune & Stratton, 1950.

Maliniac, J.: Use of pedicle dermo-fat flap in mammaplasty. Plast. Reconstr. Surg., *12*:110, 1953.

Maliniac, J.: Harmful fallacies in mammaplasty. Personal communication. Abstract, International Congress of Plastic Surgery, London, 1959.

Marino, H.: Glandular mastectomy: Immediate reconstruction. Plast. Reconstr. Surg., *10*:204, 1952.

Marino, H.: La Mama. Buenos Aires, Editorial Cientifica Argentina, 1957.

May, H.: Breast plasty in the female. Plast. Reconstr. Surg., *17*:351, 1956.

May, H.: Reconstructive and Reparative Surgery. 2nd Ed. Philadelphia, F. A. Davis Company, 1958.

Michel and Pousson: De la mastopexie. Bull. Mém. Soc. Chir. Paris, *23*:507, 1897 (quoted by Thorek, 1942).

Millard, D. R.: Nipple and areola reconstruction by split-skin graft from the normal side. Plast. Reconstr. Surg., *50*:350, 1972.

Millard, D. R.: Breast reconstruction after radical mastectomy. Plast. Reconstr. Surg., *58*:283, 1976.

Moore, A. M., and Brown, J. B.: Investigations of polyvinyl compounds for use as subcutaneous prostheses (polyvinyl sponge, Ivalon). Plast. Reconstr. Surg., *10*:453, 1952.

Morestin, H.: De l'ablation esthétique des tumeurs du sein. Bull. Mém. Soc. Chir. Paris, *29*:562, 1903.

Morestin, H.: Bilateral mammary hypertrophy corrected by discoid resection. Bull. Mém. Soc. Chir. Paris, *33*:201, 1907.

Mornard, P.: Mastopexie esthétique par transplantation du mamelon. Pratique Chirurgicale Illustrée (Pauchet). Paris, G. Doin et Cie, 1926.

Mutou, Y.: Augmentation mammaplasty with the Akiyama prosthesis. Br. J. Plast. Surg., *23*:58, 1970.

Noël, A.: Aesthetische Chirurgie der weiblichen Brust. Ein neues Verfahren zur Korektur der Hangebrust. Med. Welt, *2*:51, 1928.

Nosanchuk, J. S.: Silicone granuloma in breast. Arch. Surg., *97*:583, 1968.

Nydick, M., Bustos, J., Dale, J. H., and Rawson, R. W.: Gynecomastia in adolescent boys. J.A.M.A., *178*:109, 1961.

O'Conor, C. M.: Glandular excision with immediate mammary reconstruction. Plast. Reconstr. Surg., *33*:57, 1964.

Oppenheimer, B. S., Oppenheimer, E. T., and Stout, A. P.: Sarcomas induced in rodents by embedding various plastic films. Proc. Soc. Exp. Biol. Med., *79*:366, 1952.

Pack, G. T., and Livingston, E. M.: Treatment of Cancer and Allied Diseases. Vol. 1. New York, Paul B. Hoeber, 1940.

Pangman, W. J., and Wallace, R. M.: The use of plastic prosthesis in breast plastic and other soft tissue surgery. Read before 6th Congress of Pan-Pacific Surgical Association, October 7, 1954.

Pangman, W. J., and Wallace, R. M.: Personal communication, 1961.

Parry, R. G., and Wolfort, F. G.: Nipple involvement in carcinoma of the breast. Presented at the annual meeting of the American Society for Plastic and Reconstructive Surgery, Boston, 1976.

Passot, R.: La correction esthétique du prolapsus mammaire par le procédé de la transposition du mamelon. Presse Méd., *33*:317, 1925.

Penn, J.: Breast reduction. Br. J. Plast. Surg., *7*:357, 1955.

Penn, J.: Breast reduction. II. Transactions of International Society of Plastic Surgeons, 2nd Congress, London, 1959. Edinburgh, E & S Livingstone, Ltd., 1960.

Pennisi, V. R., Klabunde, E. J., and Pletsch, M. E.: The location of the nipple in breast reconstruction. Plast. Reconstr. Surg., *43*:612, 1969.

Pennisi, V. R., Capozzi, A., Walsh, J., and Christensen, N.: Obscure breast carcinoma encountered in subcutaneous mastectomies. Plast. Reconstr. Surg., *47*:17, 1971.

Perras, C.: The creation of a twin breast following radical mastectomy. A report on 50 consecutive cases, 1959–1975. Clin. Plast. Surg., *3*:265, 1976.

Pickrell, K.: An evaluation of Etheron as an augmentation material in plastic and reconstructive surgery. A long-term clinical and experimental study. Presented at the annual meeting of the American Society of Plastic & Reconstructive Surgery, Hawaii, October, 1962.

Pitanguy, I.: Breast hypertrophy. Transactions of International Society of Plastic Surgeons, 2nd Congress, London, 1959. Edinburgh, E & S Livingstone, Ltd., 1960.

Pitanguy, I.: Personal communication, 1961.

Pitanguy, I.: Surgical treatment of breast hypertrophy. Br. J. Plast. Surg., *20*:78, 1967.

Pitanguy, I., and Torres, E. T.: Histopathological aspects of mammary gland tissue in cases of plastic surgery of breast. Br. J. Plast. Surg., *17*:297, 1964.

Radlauer, C. B., and Bowers, D. G.: Treatment of severe breast asymmetry. Plast. Reconstr. Surg., *47*:347, 1971.

Ragnell, A.: Operative correction of hypertrophy and ptosis of the female breast. Acta Chir. Scand., *94*:113, 1946.

Ragnell, A.: Further experience of preservation of lactation capacity and nipple sensitivity in breast reduction. Transactions of International Society of Plastic Surgeons, 1st Congress, Sweden, 1955. Baltimore, The Williams & Wilkins Company, 1957.

Rees, T. D.: An historical review of mammaplasty. Trans. Fifth Internatl. Congr. Plast. Reconstr. Surg. Australia, Butterworths, Feb., 1971, pp. 1167–73.

Rees, T. D., and Dupuis, C. C.: Unilateral mammary hypoplasia. Plast. Reconstr. Surg., *41*:307, 1968.

Rees, T. D., and Flagg, S.: Untoward results and complications following breast reduction mammaplasty. *In* Goldwyn, R. M. (Ed.): The Unfavorable Result in Plastic Surgery: Avoidance and Treatment. Boston, Little, Brown and Company, 1972.

Rees, T. D., and Rhoads, W.: The treatment of mammary hypertrophy and ptosis. N.Y. State J. Med., *70*:20, 1970.

Rees, T. D., Guy, C. L., and Coburn, R. J.: The use of inflatable breast implants. Plast. Reconstr. Surg., *52*:609, 1973.

Regnault, P.: The hypoplastic and ptotic breast. A combined operation with prosthetic augmentation. Plast. Reconstr. Surg., *37*:31, 1966.

Regnault, P.: Indications for breast augmentation. Plast. Reconstr. Surg., *40*:534, 1967.

Renneker, R., and Cutler, M.: Psychological problems of adjustment to cancer of the breast. J.A.M.A., *148*:833, 1952.

Rubin, L. R.: The cushioned augmentation repair after a subcutaneous mastectomy. Plast. Reconstr. Surg., *57*: 23, 1976.

Silver, H. I.: Treating the complications of augmentation mammaplasty. Plast. Reconstr. Surg., *49*:637, 1972.

Simon, B. E., Hoffman, S., and Kahn, S.: Classification and surgical correction of gynecomastia. Plast. Reconstr. Surg., *51*:48, 1973.

Skoog, T.: A technique of breast reduction, transposition of the nipples on a cutaneous vascular pedicle. Acta Chir. Scand., *126*:453, 1963.

Snyderman, R. K., and Guthrie, R. H.: Reconstruction of the female breast following radical mastectomy. Plast. Reconstr. Surg., *47*:565, 1971.

Snyderman, R. K., and Lizardo, J. G.: Statistical study of malignancies found before, during or after routine breast plastic operations. Plast. Reconstr. Surg., *25*:253, 1960.

Strömbeck, J. G.: Mammaplasty: Report of a new technique based on the two-pedicle procedure. Br. J. Plast. Surg., *13*:79, 1960.

Strömbeck, J. G.: Macromastia in women and its surgical treatment. Acta Chir. Scand., Suppl. 341, 1964.

Strömbeck, J. G.: Reduction mammaplasty. *In* Grabb, W., and Smith, J. W. (Eds.): Plastic Surgery. A Concise Guide to Clinical Practice. Boston, Little, Brown and Company, 1968, pp. 821–835.

Tabari, K.: Augmentation mammaplasty with Simaplast implant. Plast. Reconstr. Surg., *44*:468, 1969.

Tamerin, J. A.: A mammaplastic procedure. Plast. Reconstr. Surg., *7*:288, 1951.

Thomas, T. G.: On the removal of benign tumours of the mamma without mutilation of the organ. N.Y. Med. J. Obstet. Rev., 1882, p. 337.

Thorek, M.: Possibilities in the reconstruction of the human form. N.Y. Med. J. Rec., *116*:572, 1922.

Thorek, M.: Plastic Surgery of the Breast and Abdominal Wall. Springfield, Illinois, Charles C Thomas, Publisher, 1942.

Thorek, M.: Plastic reconstruction of the breast and free transplantation of the nipple. J. Internatl. Coll. Surg., *9*:194, 1946.

Trier, W. C.: Complete breast absence. Plast. Reconstr. Surg., *36*:430, 1965.

Urban, J. A.: Radical excision of the chest wall for mammary cancer. Cancer, *4*:1263, 1951.

Urban, J. A.: Bilateral breast cancer. *In* Breast Cancer, Early and Late. Chicago, Year Book Medical Publishers Inc., 1970, pp. 263–270.

Velpeau, A. A. L. M.: Traité des maladies du sein et de la région mammaire. Paris, V. Masson, 1854.

Verchère, F.: Mastopexie latérale contre la mastoptose hypertrophique. Méd. Mod., *9*:340, 1898.

Villandre: Cited by Dartigues, L.: Arch. Franco-Belges Chir., *28*:325, 1925.

Warren, S.: Relation of "chronic mastitis" to carcinoma of breast. Surg. Gynecol. Obstet., *71*:257, 1940.

Watson, J.: Some observations on free fat grafts, with reference to their use in mammaplasty. Br. J. Plast. Surg., *12*:263, 1959.

Watson, J.: Personal communication. 1970.

Watson, J.: Personal communication, 1975.

Webster, J. P.: Mastectomy for gynecomastia through a semicircular intra-areola incision. Ann. Surg., *124*:557, 1946.

Wexler, M. R., and Oneal, R. M.: Areola sharing to reconstruct the absent nipple. Plast. Reconstr. Surg., *51*:176, 1973.

Wiener, D. L., Adrien, E. A., Aiache, E., Silver, L., and Tittiranonda, F.: A single dermal pedicle for nipple transposition in subcutaneous mastectomy, reduction mammaplasty, or mastopexy. Plast. Reconstr. Surg., *51*:115, 1973.

Williams, J. E.: Experiences with a large series of Silastic breast implants. Plast. Reconstr. Surg., *49*:253, 1972.

Wise, R. J.: A preliminary report on a method of planning the mammaplasty. Plast. Reconstr. Surg., *17*:367, 1956.

Wise, R. J., Gannon, J. P., and Hill, J. R.: Further experience with reduction mammaplasty. Plast. Reconstr. Surg., *32*:12, 1963.

Zbylski, J. R., and Parsons, R. W.: A method of adenectomy and breast reconstruction for benign disease. Plast. Reconstr. Surg., *37*:38, 1966.

Zippel, H. H., Citoler, P., and Olivari, N.: Zur Frage der konservativen Chirurgie beim Mamma-Carcinom. Presented at the Third Annual Meeting, Vereinigung der Deutschen Plastischen Chirurgen, Köln, 1972.

# CHAPTER 90

# RECONSTRUCTIVE SURGERY OF THE ABDOMINAL WALL

SHERRELL J. ASTON, M.D.,
AND KENNETH L. PICKRELL, M.D.

---

Spina Bifida
*John C. Mustardé, F.R.C.S., and*
*Wallace M. Dennison, M.D., F.R.C.S.*

The abdominal wall protects and surrounds the contents of the abdominal cavity and participates in a great variety of functions, such as posture, standing, walking, and bending. Other functions such as lifting, straining during urination, defecation, and the labor of childbirth require an increase in intra-abdominal pressure. In addition, the abdominal wall aids in vomiting and coughing and supports normal respiration. To the extent that the integrity of the abdominal wall is maintained, normal activities take place unnoticed and are automatic. Defects, tumors, injuries, and infection interfere with the function of the abdominal wall and require diagnosis and appropriate therapy. Thus, an intimate knowledge of the anatomy of the abdominal wall and its nerve and blood supply is of special clinical concern to the reconstructive surgeon.

Dermolipectomies of the abdominal wall are discussed in Chapter 92.

## ANATOMY OF THE ANTERIOR ABDOMINAL WALL

The anterior abdominal wall is roughly diamond-shaped. It is limited above by the lower rib margins and the xiphoid, and below by Poupart's ligaments and the pelvic brim. It varies in appearance according to the sex, weight, and age of the individual, being of slightly convex contour in the average or normal person. In the very thin individual it appears scaphoid, and in the obese person the convexity may be increased to a considerable extent so that the wall becomes pendulous, the lower portion overhanging in an apronlike fashion (see Fig. 90–1). The protuberant and pendulous abdomen is the result of subcutaneous and intra-abdominal accumulations of fat with associated relaxation of the abdominal wall.

**Landmarks.** The *umbilicus* is located below the midpoint between the xiphoid process and the symphysis pubis. It is situated over the disc between the third and fourth vertebrae and about 2 to 4 cm above the line joining the crests of the ilia. Its position may vary considerably with the type of individual. The *vitelline duct*, a fetal structure which passes through the umbilicus to the small intestine, is usually absent in the adult. If the proximal portion remains intact, it is known as a *Meckel's diverticulum*, an appendage 2.5 to 7.5 cm long and about 60 cm from the ileocecal valve. If the duct persists in its entirety, a fistula will result which discharges feculent material from the small bowel into the umbilical pit. Hernias involving the umbilicus usually contain properitoneal fat.

The *linea alba* extends from the xiphoid to the symphysis and is formed by the union of the aponeuroses of the abdominal muscles. In its upper portion it is about 0.5 cm wide, whereas below the umbilicus it becomes narrower and less distinct. Its fibers run transversely, longitudinally, and obliquely. Above the umbilicus some of the fibers enter the subcutaneous tissue and skin, producing a slightly depressed groove. Occasionally there are weak points between the transverse fibers through which properitoneal fat may herniate—*epigastric hernias*. They usually occur above the umbilicus.

The *lineae semilunares* form the lateral boundaries of the rectus muscles. They assume a slight lateral curve and extend from the pubic spines to the cartilages of the ninth ribs. They are formed by the union of the aponeuroses of the abdominal muscles as they join to form the sheaths of the rectus muscles. The upper extremity of the right semilunaris indicates the location of the fundus of the gallbladder. *McBurney's point* is located at the junction of the right semilunaris with a line drawn from the right iliac spine to the umbilicus.

The *lineae transversae* or transverse inscriptions are fibrous bands or grooves in the rectus muscles which are apparent on the abdomens of thin, muscular individuals. They are firmly adherent to the anterior sheath of the rectus muscles; posteriorly, the muscle is free of the sheath.

**Layers of the Abdominal Wall.** The anterior abdominal wall is composed of the following layers: skin, superficial fascia, muscles and their aponeuroses, properitoneal fat, transversalis fascia, and peritoneum. The skin is lax and not adherent, except at the linea alba and the umbilicus. When stretched by subcutaneous fat or by intra-abdominal tumors, including pregnancy, it may present faint white or purplish lines, the *lineae albicantes*. The superficial fascia consists of a superficial fatty layer, *Camper's fascia*, and a deeper membranous layer, *Scarpa's fascia*. The latter is attached to the medial half of Poupart's ligament, and more laterally it is continuous with the fascia lata of the thigh.

**Muscles of the Abdominal Wall.** The *external oblique,* the most superficial of the three muscles in the lateral aspect of the wall, arises from the lower eight ribs, where it interdigitates with the serratus anterior and the latissimus dorsi. Its fibers fan out, extending upward and medially to be inserted into the anterior half of the iliac crest posteriorly, and by means of its broad aponeurosis into the symphysis, the linea alba, and the xiphoid. The lower fibers of the aponeurosis are thickened to form the inguinal ligament (Poupart's), which passes between the anterior-superior iliac spines and the spine of the pubis. Just above and lateral to the pubic spine, the fibers of the aponeurosis are divided to form the external inguinal ring.

The *internal oblique* muscle lies beneath the external oblique and arises from the lumbodorsal fascia, the anterior two-thirds of the iliac crest, and the lateral two-thirds of the inguinal ligament. Its fibers radiate in a fanlike manner and pass upward and medially. The lower fibers join those of the transversus muscle to form the conjoined tendon, which is inserted into the crest and spine of the pubis and the ileopectineal line. The more superior fibers are inserted by a broad aponeurosis into the linea alba and the cartilages of the seventh, eighth, and ninth ribs. The lower border of the internal oblique arches over the inguinal canal and during contraction and shortening of these fibers aids in preventing herniations by pressure against the canal.

The *transversus* muscle is located deep to the internal oblique and arises from the lower six ribs, the lumbodorsal fascia, the anterior two-thirds of the iliac crest, and the lateral third of the inguinal ligament. It is inserted by an aponeurosis into the linea alba and by the conjoined tendon into the pubic spine and ileopectineal line.

The *rectus abdominis* muscles are long broad muscles lying longitudinally in the medial aspect of the abdominal wall. Each arises from the front of the symphysis and the pubic crest and inserts into the xiphoid and the cartilages of the fifth, sixth, and seventh ribs. Each is enclosed in its rectus sheath. The *pyramidalis* is a small triangular muscle superficial to the rectus muscle, arising from the front of the pubis and inserting into the linea alba about halfway between the symphysis and the umbilicus. The *rectus sheath* is a fibrous envelope which encloses each muscle. The anterior layer is formed by the aponeurosis of the external oblique, together with the anterior half of the internal oblique aponeurosis. The posterior layer of the split aponeurosis of the internal oblique muscle passes beneath the rectus to form the posterior layer of the sheath with the aponeurosis of the transversus muscle. All components join in the middle to form the linea alba. Behind the lower fourth of the rectus muscle the posterior layer of the sheath is absent. The inferior boundary of the sheath is called the *linea semicircularis* or *fold of Douglas*. The deep epigastric artery ascends anterior to this fold.

The *transversalis fascia* is the fascial lining of the abdominal cavity. It covers the deep surface of the transversus muscle and is separated from the peritoneum by extraperitoneal fat. Internal to this is the parietal peritoneum or serous lining of the anterior abdominal wall.

**Circulation of the Abdominal Wall.** The *arteries* of the abdominal wall are superficial and deep. The superficial arteries ascend from the femoral artery and cross toward the umbilicus. The superficial circumflex iliac artery passes laterally toward the iliac spine. This vessel has gained considerable importance since the advent of microvascular free flap transfer (see Chapters 6 and 14). The superior epigastric artery is deep; it is a branch of the internal mammary artery, which descends by piercing the posterior sheath of the rectus and enters the substance of the rectus muscle. The deep epigastric artery is a branch of the external iliac artery. It ascends in an oblique medial direction between the transversalis fascia and peritoneum and enters the rectus muscle by passing in front of the fold of Douglas. It anastomoses with the superior epigastric artery. The deep circumflex iliac artery also arises from the external iliac artery and passes laterally toward the anterior spine of the ilium between the transversalis fascia and peritoneum.

The *superficial veins* which drain the upper abdomen are the superior epigastric, the intercostals, and the axillary. The lower abdomen is drained by the superior epigastric and the superficial circumflex iliac veins, which flow into the inferior vena cava. The *deep veins* accompany the deep arteries and are similarly termed. Enlarged veins around the umbilicus are called *caput medusae*.

The *superficial lymph* drainage of the abdominal wall is into the axillary nodes. The deeper lymphatics drain into the mediastinal nodes and into those along the iliac arteries.

**Nerves.** The nerve supply of the abdominal wall is from the sixth to the twelfth thoracic nerves and the iliohypogastric and ilioinguinal nerves. The nerves supply cutaneous and muscular branches. In visceral disease the abdominal wall may contain areas of referred cutaneous pain. It has been shown that the areas of cutaneous hyperesthesia are identical with those areas that receive sensory fibers from the spinal segment to which the afferent sympathetic fibers pass. Thus, the involved organ may be identified by the site of the referred pain in some instances.

## ABDOMINAL INCISIONS

Some guidance in the proper planning of abdominal incisions, the prevention of postoperative hernias, and the best methods of repair may be gleaned from the foregoing review of anatomy. The persistently high percentage of postoperative tissue derangements, scars, and hernias which follow conventional types of abdominal incisions are witness and proof of the fact that some interrelationship exists between the making of conventional forms of abdominal incisions and their proper closure.

The standard abdominal incision is usually based upon the ease of physical access to intra-abdominal lesions. It may be and is frequently inconsistent with anatomical and physiologic conditions inherent in the abdominal wall. This is one of the three major reasons for the relative frequency of postoperative hernias, the other two being inadequate suturing or splinting and infection. Placing abdominal incisions in a physiologic manner to guard against the pulling of sutures and the disruption of the wound is one of the cardinal principles of surgery. Sutures hold best when and where they pull across tissue fibers. This can be accomplished only by making the incision so that it runs parallel to the tissue fibers. Insofar as this applies to the skin of the abdomen, a knowledge of the lines of minimal tension is essential (see Chapter 1).

One of the objections raised by the transverse abdominal incision is the argument that it cuts across abdominal muscles, but as a matter of fact this involves only one abdominal muscle, the rectus. In resuturing it, the muscle sutures hold poorly, pull out or through easily, and result in muscle diastasis. However, little or no attention is given to the fact that most vertical abdominal incisions, though sparing the recti physically, invalidate them physiologically by cutting the nerve supply. A paralyzed muscle is a functionally dead muscle. Any incision that cuts across the nerve supply of a muscle, even though the muscle heals, results in paralysis, lack of union, and eventual diastasis. Any incision that cuts across the main blood supply of a muscle results in delayed or absent healing with necrosis and retraction and so establishes a tissue void which may ultimately lead to postoperative herniation. Of even greater importance is the meticulous repair of the investing fascia, because fascia is a strong binding tissue which provides satisfactory purchase for the sutures.

The *upper abdominal wall* is tense, firm, and strong, owing to the costal attachment of the muscles and the fascia; the lateral pull of the muscles is the result of the distribution of the fascial fibers. This is one of the main reasons for the difficulty in closing upper abdominal paramedian incisions. When such incisions or closures open spontaneously following operation, it will usually be found that the defect in the musculature runs in a transverse or horizontal direction. This is strictly in accordance with the normal lines of tension of the fasciae of the upper abdomen.

The aggregate of the lines of tension in the *lower abdominal wall* is for the most part in an oblique direction. Because of the lack of the prominent lineae transversae in the lower abdomen, as contrasted with the upper abdomen, the linea alba is much weaker. The rectus muscles, not having the support of the transverse fibrous intersections, are more likely to bulge and separate after surgery or injury. However, in the lowermost portion of the abdomen, the rectus muscles and their investments are supported by the pyramidalis muscles and their fibrous fusion with the linea alba and by the reflections of the inguinal ligaments.

The making of any abdominal incision and its concomitant repair should follow the established surgical principles and the anatomical facts that have been previously outlined. The foregoing may be summarized by saying that, in a given restricted portion of the abdominal wall, an incision made contrary to the lines of tension of its components and closing such an incision by simple direct approximation results in a course of healing characterized by postoperative complication, because the intra-abdominal contents are thrust against the site of repair in the upright position. These considerations become doubly important in view of the contemporary tendency toward early ambulation of patients.

Since any incision is a mechanical cellular injury to tissues (Hartwell, 1955), it should avoid gross anatomical insult and injury to the part. If an incision contrary to the structural integrity of the part cannot be avoided or prevented, the only solution to the problem lies in careful reconstructive closure of the defect, even though this may necessitate more than simple mechanical approximation of the tissues. The ideal abdominal incision is not always possible, and frequently it is impractical because of technical considerations. Some part or level of almost every extensive incision is contrary to the anatomical peculiarities of a part. This portion of the incision and repair should receive qualitative attention in the closure.

## HERNIAS OF THE ABDOMINAL WALL

Protrusion of a portion of the abdominal contents into or through a cleft or weak spot in the abdominal wall is one of the commonest of surgical abnormalities (see Fig. 90–1).

The term hernia is probably derived from the Greek Σρυοσ, meaning a branch. It is probable that the Greek school of surgery in Rome, during the first centuries of the Christian era, practiced incision and some form of ligation of the inguinal hernial sac. In the Middle Ages the brutal firebrand and caustics were employed. The external limits of the hernia were apparently outlined with the patient in the standing position; then after he was laid upon his back and the sac emptied, the hot iron or stone was applied over its entire extent. When dissection was introduced during the sixteenth century by Vesalius and his followers, more rational methods began to appear. There was the "punctum aureum," the object of which was to pass a golden wire about the sac, twisting it tightly enough to prevent the intestine from passing through. This was later referred to as the "golden stitch" or "royal stitch."

During the eighteenth century great advances were made, especially in the anatomy of the inguinal and femoral canals, by Gimbernat, Camper, Cooper, Scarpa, and others. Cooper's work (1825) on the anatomy of hernias of the inguinal region is still current and classic. Bassini (1889) published his method of reconstructing the inguinal canal, after ligating and cutting away the sac at its neck, and four years later, in 1893, Halsted transplanted the cord anterior to

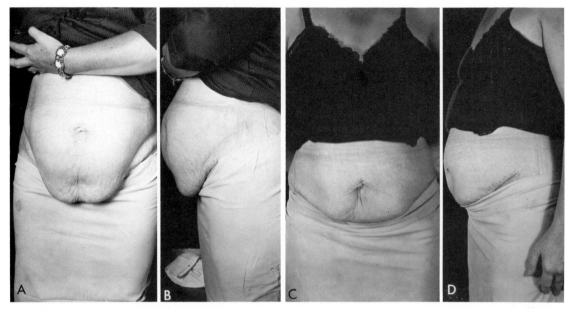

**FIGURE 90–1.** *A, B,* "Abdominal apron" with ventral hernia in a 41 year old multiparous housewife. Through a hammock incision that extended from the iliac spines to the crest of the pubis, the cutaneous abdominal wall and heavy panniculus were freed from the fascia of the external oblique superiorly to the umbilical hiatus. An imbrication repair of the large ventral hernia was performed using silk sutures. The heavy abdominal flap was drawn downward, an excess of more than 20 cm was discarded, and the wound was repaired in layers. *C, D,* Postoperative photographs four months following surgery.

the muscular and tendinous layers. Today the repair of simple hernias is one of the most satisfactory operations in surgery, and since it is adequately covered in detail in the standard surgical texts, it will not be dealt with further.

## RECONSTRUCTION OF ACQUIRED ABDOMINAL WALL DEFECTS

Defects of the abdominal wall are most commonly the result of tumor resection, radiotherapy, postoperative incisional hernia formation, massive infection, and trauma.

The more common primary abdominal wall tumors are lipomas, fibromas, neurofibromas, fibrosarcomas, and desmoids (fascial fibromas). Lipomas occasionally undergo malignant degeneration. Neurofibromas associated with von Recklinghausen's disease may likewise undergo malignant degeneration. Malignant primary abdominal wall tumors are actually quite rare. The more common types result from seeding or invasion of the abdominal wall from a primary bowel or bladder carcinoma. Transitional cell carcinoma of the bladder is well known in this regard. Radionecrosis of the abdominal wall fol-

lowing radiation therapy for such tumors is less frequent since the introduction of modern radiotherapy techniques but is still occasionally seen by the plastic surgeon (Fig. 90–2).

Postoperative incisional hernias may be related to improper surgical technique, poor tissue quality accompanying a generalized metabolic disorder, and particularly respiratory tract disorders resulting in excessive stress on the abdominal wall suture line.

Massive infections of the abdominal wall requiring surgical resection occur most frequently following gastrointestinal tract operations and may be associated with fistulas of the gastrointestinal tract. Clostridial myonecrosis is the most severe form of abdominal wall infection. Chronic infections such as tuberculosis or actinomycosis, while rare, can occur.

Massive trauma of the abdominal wall in the civilian population is most often caused by shotgun wounds. The military surgeon frequently treats not only gunshot wounds but also blast and explosion injuries. Seat belt avulsion of the abdominal wall musculature is a relatively new injury which is occasionally seen following high speed vehicular accidents.

Although the etiology of the abdominal wall

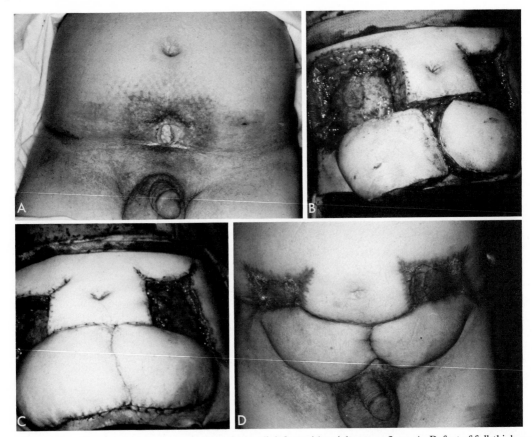

**FIGURE 90–2.** Closure of a radionecrotic abdominal wall defect with axial-pattern flaps. *A*, Defect of full-thickness of the abdominal wall. Patient had received radiation therapy for transitional cell carcinoma of the bladder 11 years earlier. The open defect had been present for approximately four months. *B*, Transposition flaps based on the superficial epigastric vessels. The flaps had been delayed three weeks earlier. *C*, Flaps sutured in position. Donor sites reduced in size by advancing and closing the superior corners. The remainder of the donor sites prior to application of split-thickness skin grafts. *D*, Healed flaps and grafted donor sites two months postoperatively. (Courtesy of Joseph G. McCarthy, M.D., Institute of Reconstructive Plastic Surgery.)

defect plays a significant role in the planning of the reconstruction, the main goals are similar: to reestablish the integrity and support of the fascial components and to provide skin coverage.

**Musculofascial Flaps.** Farr (1922) used a flap of muscle and fascia from the lower thorax to close upper abdominal defects. Wangensteen (1934) described closure of large musculofascial defects of the abdominal wall by using the iliotibial tract of fascia lata as a flap. The fascia, suspended by the tensor fasciae femoris muscle with its nerve and blood supply intact, can provide closure of abdominal wall defects below the umbilicus. However, Wangensteen (1946) pointed out that even in patients with long femurs, the longest iliotibial tract of fascia is usually too short for tension-free repair of defects beneath the costal margin.

Therefore, a large upper abdominal defect may be reconstructed with a musculofascial flap of anterior rectus sheath and part of the external oblique muscle and aponeurosis. The lower abdominal musculofascial donor site is then repaired with the iliotibial tract (Fig. 90–3). Bruck (1956) employed Wangensteen's technique in reconstructing the abdominal wall in a 3½ year old female following resection of the third recurrence of a fibrosarcoma. The bladder was sutured to a defect in the peritoneum, the musculofascial layer was closed with a fascia lata flap from the ipsilateral side, and a large skin defect was covered by a flap from the opposite lower extremity.

Lesnick and Davids (1953) described a technique of establishing integrity of the anterior abdominal wall using a musculofascial flap from one area of the abdominal wall to close a defect in another area (Fig. 90–4). A defect created by

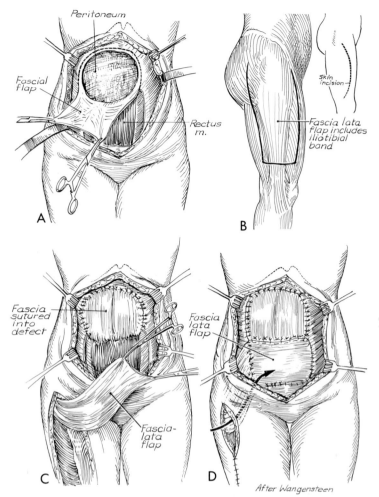

**FIGURE 90–3.** *A*, Large upper abdominal defect measuring 18 × 24 cm. Musculofascial flap of the entire anterior rectus sheath beneath the umbilicus and part of the external oblique aponeurosis and right external oblique muscle. *B*, Iliotibial tract and lateral extension of fascia lata outlined as flap. *C*, Fascial flap from the lower abdomen transferred into the defect. A fascia lata flap is mobilized. *D*, The fascia lata flap is sutured into the lower abdominal wall donor site. (After Wangensteen, O. H.: Large defects of the abdominal wall employing the iliotibial tract of fascia lata as a pedicled flap. Surg. Gynecol. Obstet., 59:766, 1934.)

excision of the lower half of the rectus muscle and rectus sheath was reconstructed with a flap of the external oblique muscle and aponeurosis detached from its costal origin and iliac insertion and transferred on its attachment to the anterior rectus sheath as a hinge.

Hershey and Butcher (1964) reported one-stage closure of large full-thickness defects of the abdominal and thoracic walls using flaps of external oblique and anterior rectus muscle fascia accompanied by the overlying skin and fat. Such flaps are broadly based laterally and posteriorly and may be made to extend across the midline (Fig. 90–5). Elevation of the flaps into the axilla or lumbar region can be done, main-

taining adequate blood supply and obviating the need for flap delay. However, Bekheit (1965) noted partial loss of such full-thickness flaps of skin and underlying muscle, which thus slowed wound healing. Although disruption or herniation does not usually occur following the elevation of full-thickness flaps, the donor or recipient site may subsequently bulge, necessitating the wearing of an abdominal support.

Gerber (1965) utilized a variation of Halsted's (1903) modification of Bloodgood's (1898) operation for repairing large inguinal hernias in order to restore abdominal wall integrity following the resection of desmoid tumors (Fig. 90–6). The anterior rectus fascia was reflected to close one

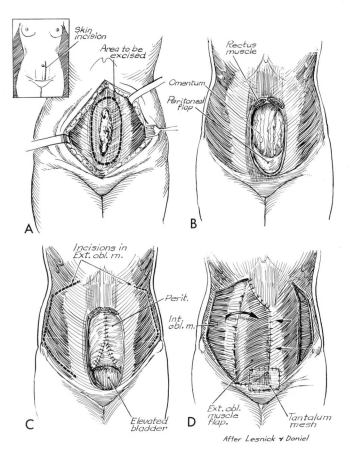

**FIGURE 90–4.** *A,* Skin incision, tumor of abdominal wall, and surrounding margin to be excised. *B,* Left rectus muscle and sheath completely excised down to pubis. A portion of the left external oblique has also been excised, as well as most of the right rectus muscle and sheath. *C,* Peritoneum has been closed by mobilizing lateral flaps of peritoneum and by mobilizing the bladder and displacing it upward. The lines of incisions in the external oblique are indicated. *D,* Musculofascial defect closed with tantalum wire mesh. (After Lesnick, G. N., and Davids, A. M.: Repair of surgical abdominal wall defect with pedicled musculofascial flap. Ann. Surg., *137*:569, 1953.)

**FIGURE 90–5.** *A,* Large anterior wall defect following resection of the upper abdominal wall, lower sternum, and medial portion of the ribs. Incisions for flap rotation and advancement outlined. *B,* Breast flaps elevated and advanced medially and inferiorly a short distance. Musculocutaneous flap containing the remaining left anterior rectus sheath and external oblique muscle rotated to close the major portion of the defect. The musculocutaneous donor site is covered with split-thickness skin graft. (After Hershey, F. B., and Butcher, H. P.: Repair of defects after partial resection of the abdominal wall. Am. J. Surg., *107*:586, 1964.)

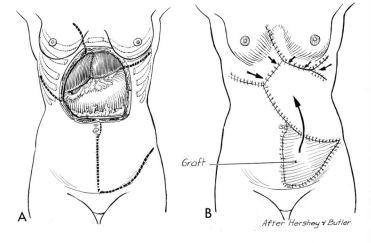

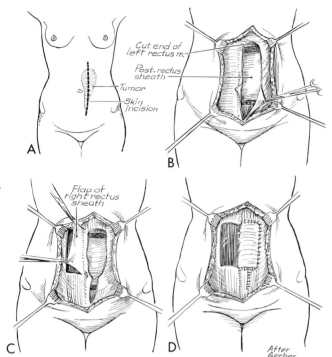

**FIGURE 90–6.** *A,* Skin incision and underlying tumor. *B,* Defect produced by excision of the tumor, left anterior rectus sheath, and left rectus muscle. *C, D,* Right anterior rectus fascia flap elevated, rotated, and sutured into position. (After Gerber, A.: Plastic repair following the removal of large desmoid tumors of the abdominal wall. Calif. Med., *95*:178, 1961.)

defect produced by resection of the contralateral rectus muscles and anterior fascia.

Ye, Devine and Kirklin (1953) reported a patient in whom a recurrent desmoid of the left lower quadrant of the abdominal wall was excised, producing a defect 10 × 10 cm. The peritoneum was closed, and tantalum mesh was sutured into the defect for abdominal support. A flap from the right upper quadrant, previously prepared and carried on the right wrist, was used to cover the tantalum mesh. A few weeks later the wrist was separated and the flap set into place. The abdominal wall remained competent through a six-month period of follow-up.

Morgan and Zbylski (1972) used an open jump flap carried from the contralateral side of the abdomen and flank on the forearm to reconstruct a full-thickness abdominal wall defect which had previously been covered with a split-thickness skin graft following radical resection for clostridial myonecrosis (Fig. 90–7). Five delays were performed prior to setting the flap into the arm. Three additional delays were performed prior to transferring the flap to the abdominal wall.

**Fascial Grafts.** Gallie (1932) reported excellent results in repairing large abdominal wall in-

**FIGURE 90–7.** *A,* Large ventral hernia covered by a split-thickness skin graft. Open jump flap set into arm carrier after five previous flap delays. *B,* Flap sutured to margin of defect after three more delays. Flap donor site covered by a split-thickness skin graft. (After Morgan, S. C., and Zbylski, J. R.: Repair of massive soft tissue defects by open jump flaps. Plast. Reconstr. Surg., *50*:265, 1972. Copyright © 1972, The Williams & Wilkins Company, Baltimore.)

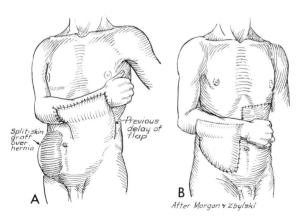

cisional hernias using a patch graft of fascia lata with the ends of the patch split into quarter-inch strips and woven into the wound margins. Two such patches sutured together with a fascial band were suggested for large defects.

McPeak and Miller (1960) noted that fascia lata was readily available and easily obtained. Because a minimal foreign body reaction, strong enough to maintain the viscera within the abdominal cavity, resulted, there was a smooth and glistening surface similar to peritoneum, therefore reducing the chance of adhesions and intestinal obstruction. Thus, fascia lata grafts were strongly advocated to repair abdominal wall defects following tumor resection (Fig. 90–8). Likewise, fascia was favored over prosthetic materials, as recurrent tumors and especially fibrous and fascial tumors may grow along the latticework of prostheses, making it difficult to differentiate recurrence of tumor from a fibrous scar reaction surrounding the prosthesis. In addition, the various metallic prostheses may interfere with postoperative radiation therapy, making it difficult to determine the amount of radiation delivered to the intra-abdominal contents; at the same time, a greater dose than desired is possibly delivered to tissues superficial to the prosthesis.

On occasion, wounds in children may be too large to close with autogenous fascia, and the use of fascia allografts is indicated. Rehn (1911) documented experimentally that transplanted fascia allografts would survive at least over a six-month period. Stephenson (1953) reported the repair of abdominal muscular agenesis in a 3 year old patient utilizing fascia lata from the mother. Functionally the repair was intact, with palpable fascial bands providing support to the abdominal wall 13 months follow-ing transplantation. The transplantation of fascia is discussed in Chapter 9.

Sewell and Koth (1955) studied freeze-dried fascia xenografts and noted that they should not be used to reconstruct abdominal wall defects. The xenografts stimulated excessive foreign tissue reaction which developed around the fascia grafts, and at the same time there was failure of ingrowth and replacement of the fascia by the host's fibroblasts. Koontz and Kimberly (1961) documented that, in dogs, electron beam–irradiated ox fascia and lyophilized dura underwent graft resorption following transplantation in a manner similar to most allografts and xenografts. Their lack of usefulness for abdominal wall repair is therefore obvious.

**De-epithelized Skin Flaps.** De-epithelized skin flaps were described by Poulard (1918) to correct scar craters, in a manner similar to the technique of reduction mammaplasty of Strömbeck (1960), the surgical treatment of lymphedema of Thompson (1962), and that described by Engdahl (1968) in reducing the extension of scars. Medgyesi (1972) described dermal skin flaps both as fascia substitutes and as a means of supporting fascial defects closed under tension (Fig. 90–9). The obvious primary advantage of flaps over free transplants is that they carry their own blood supply, making survival more certain. One of Medgyesi's three patients in whom the technique was used as a fascia substitute developed considerable bulging at the operative site, but a recurrent hernia did not develop. Studies of the fate of skin placed in a subcutaneous position in this manner showed that epithelium, hair follicles, and sebaceous glands disappear, but sweat glands are preserved (Thompson, 1960) (see also Chapter 7).

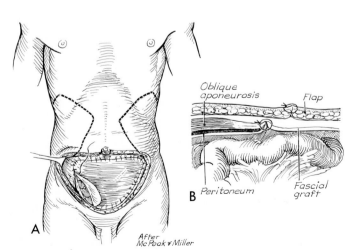

**FIGURE 90–8.** *A,* Lower abdominal defect with fascia sutured to the margins. Large thoracoepigastric flaps outlined. *B,* Transverse section showing fascia lata graft in place and under cover of flaps rotated medially and inferiorly. (After McPeak, C. J., and Miller, T. R.: Abdominal replacement. Surgery, 47:944, 1960.)

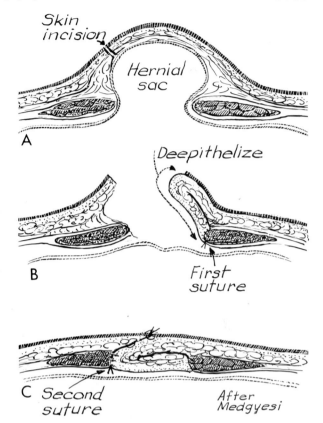

**FIGURE 90–9.** *A,* Eccentric skin incision over hernia sac provides more excess skin for shaping the flap. *B,* Hernia reduced and peritoneum closed. Skin flap has been de-epithelized and inverted so that the shaved area covers the fascial defect. The first suture approximates the fascial edge to the free edge of the shaved skin flap. *C,* Flap sutured in position. At the junction of the skin and shaved flap, an incision may be made but not allowed to penetrate the full dermis. This permits approximation of the skin edges. (After Medgyesi, S.: The repair of large incisional hernias with pedicle skin flaps. Scand. J. Plast. Reconstr. Surg., 6:69, 1972.)

**Skin Grafts.** Ferraro (1927) experimentally buried skin of unspecified size and thickness into cuts in various abdominal organs. The growth of autogenous skin implanted inside the liver, spleen, and kidney was noted, while skin allografts disintegrated. Butcher (1946) reported that full-thickness skin autografts lying loosely within the peritoneal cavity would survive, but growth of hair was retarded, and the glandular structures underwent atrophy. Horton and associates (1953) studied in dogs the behavior of split-thickness skin and dermal grafts in the peritoneal cavity and found that they grew well in the abdominal cavity on both the parietal and visceral peritoneum. Mladick and associates (1969) successfully treated a patient whose abdominal wall and peritoneum had been resected three weeks earlier, to combat clostridial myonecrosis, by the application of split-thickness skin grafts. Millard, Pigott, and Zies (1969) investigated skin grafting of full-thickness defects of the abdominal wall of the rat and dog. Grafts slightly smaller than the defect could be used, and the grafts were partially excised as the wound contracted.

Welch (1951) studied the use of allografts in the treatment of omphaloceles and found that lyophilized corium allografts are rapidly absorbed after transplantation. However, the grafts are not rejected if they are prepared in Merthiolate prior to lyophilization. When allografts are treated with Merthiolate, they become nonviable or static and fail to produce significant immunologic reaction. Such grafts actually assume a supportive biomechanical function by acting as a framework for fibroblast ingrowth, collagen deposition, and formation of a firm replacement of the anterior abdominal wall (Prpic, Belamaric, Sardesai, Walt, and Zamick, 1973). Prpic and associates (1974) used dermis autografts prepared in Merthiolate prior to lyophilization to repair surgically created full-thickness abdominal wall defects in rats.

Although the application of skin grafts is a relatively simple method for the closing of abdominal wall defects, the associated problem of lack of wall support is obvious. When the skin grafts are adherent to the surface of the gastrointestinal tract, the potential for massive adhesion formation is present. Subsequent surgery under such conditions is obviously treacherous.

### Prosthetic Support

METAL PROSTHESES. Metallic prostheses are mainly of historic interest, having been replaced by various synthetics. Silver wire was used by Witzel (1900) for hernia repair. Goepel (1900), Meyer (1902), and Bartlett (1903) employed silver wire net. Wounds closed in this manner were rigid and prone to infection. Tantalum mesh became popular in the 1940's, as it was pliable and could be used successfully in the presence of infection (Throckmorton, 1948; Bussabarger, Dumouchel, and Ivy, 1950; Crile and King, 1951). Ye, Devine, and Kirklin (1953), Cokkinis and Bromwich (1954), and Cantrell and Haller (1960) used tantalum in hernia repairs and reconstruction following resection of tumors of the abdominal wall. The dense fibrous reaction stimulated by the mesh was felt to be advantageous in the repair of large defects (Koontz and Kimberly, 1950; Flynn, Brant, and Nelson, 1951). However, tantalum mesh began to lose favor with reports of "work fracture" with fragmentation of the mesh, resulting in a weakened repair and associated pain in some patients (Pearce and Entine, 1952; McPeak and Miller, 1960).

PLASTIC PROSTHESES. Numerous plastic materials have been considered, investigated, and used in the repair of abdominal wound defects: nylon, Orlon, Teflon, Dacron, Marlex, and Mersilene. Marlex, a polyethylene derivative, has become one of the most popular synthetics. It was shown experimentally by Usher and Wallace (1958) to be well-tolerated by tissues and to produce relatively little foreign body reaction.

Marlex net has been widely employed for reconstruction of postexcisional defects secondary to tumors, trauma, and massive infections with myonecrosis. Marlex provides adequate support and high resistance to infection (Usher, 1954; Usher and Wallace, 1958; Usher and Gannon, 1959; Schmitt and Grinnon, 1967). Markgraf (1972) reported the successful closure of infected abdominal wound dehiscence in three patients by suturing Marlex mesh to the edges of the wound and allowing several weeks to elapse before obtaining skin coverage by undermining and approximating the wound margins. The immediate wound cover with Marlex, or with any synthetic, in this fashion accomplishes several goals: (1) coverage of the viscera; (2) exteriorization of the necrotic wound margins, permitting effective drainage; (3) lessening of intra-abdominal pressure, causing less stasis in the vena cava; (4) increased capacity for the distended viscera and freer diaphragmatic excursions.

Various methods of skin closure can be used with Marlex. Military surgeons in Vietnam placed Marlex mesh within the abdominal cavity, sutured it to the peritoneum and posterior fascia of grossly infected abdominal war wounds, and allowed several days for the ingrowth of granulation tissue over the Marlex. Subsequently split-thickness skin grafts were applied to the granulation tissue (Schmitt and Grinnon, 1967; Schmitt, Patterson, and Armstrong, 1967). However, when Marlex was placed in this fashion, it was necessary to prevent corrugation and irregularities of the mesh, mechanical factors which could delay the formation of granulation tissue and ultimate wound coverage by a skin graft.

Mansberger, Kang, Beebe, and LeFlore (1973) reported the repair of massive acute abdominal wall defects by a series of planned operations. First, the peritoneal defect was closed by Silastic sheeting, with physiologic wet dressings placed on the surface of the sheeting. An endogenous membrane "new peritoneum" formed under the sheeting. Because of the inertness of the plastic sheeting, the new peritoneum formed without adhesions to the abdominal viscera. The plastic sheeting was removed at three to four weeks, and the endogenous membrane and granulating wound were covered with full-thickness skin flaps or a full-thickness skin graft. Six to eight weeks later the flaps were elevated, and Marlex was used to repair the fascial defect.

Wilson and Rayner (1974) used Mersilene net, a Dacron mesh, to repair large full-thickness postincisional defects of the abdominal wall. Mersilene mesh becomes firmly infiltrated with fibrous tissue, remains flexible, and is minimally degenerative. The Mersilene net must be inserted under tension, and this is achieved by suturing the net to the intra-abdominal periphery of the wound and then pulling it outward and suturing it to the external fascial sheath. Recent studies in rats (Rayner, 1974) suggest that when sutures pass through the full thickness of the abdominal wall, as in suturing the Mersilene mesh, the point of entry of each suture acts as a minute ischemic stimulus to the intraperitoneal viscera and thus promotes a site of adhesion formation (Fig. 90–10, *A*). An "onlay technique" of avoiding peritoneal suturing and tissue ischemia is suggested as a preferable alternative (Fig. 90–10, *B*).

Rayner (1974) demonstrated that reperitonealization of the prosthetic net surface occurs simultaneously with the conversion of the fibrous coagulum that initially surrounds the net to fibrous tissue. The abdominal cavity is truly sealed by the coagulum from 24 hours onward. At 96 hours the coagulum has been converted into a cellular, loosely woven, fibrous

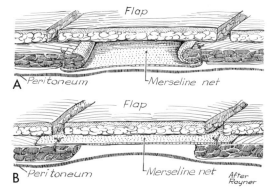

**FIGURE 90-10.** *A,* Intraperitoneal placement of synthetic mesh with sutures passing through the full-thickness of the abdominal wall, producing an ischemic stimulus to adhesion formation. *B,* Onlay technique of securing the synthetic in order to avoid intraperitoneal suturing. (After Rayner, C. R. W.: Repair of full-thickness defects of the abdominal wall in rats avoiding visceral adhesions. Br. J. Plast. Surg., 27:130, 1974.)

tissue, and the cavity surface of the net is uniformly covered with mesothelium which, by histologic examination, shows a true peritoneal layer. These findings confirm those of Ellis (1971) on the speed of reperitonealization.

**Gas Gangrene of the Abdominal Wall.** Although rare, clostridial myonecrosis of the abdominal wall is a devastating and highly lethal postoperative complication that requires prompt diagnosis and wide surgical debridement of all involved layers of the abdominal wall.

The clinical picture is characterized by wound swelling, tenderness, profuse serosanguineous drainage, and minimal wound discoloration changing to deep red or magenta within a few hours. A small amount of gas with some crepitation, and toxemia out of proportion to the temperature elevation with tachycardia, hypotension, agitation, and delirium may be observed. Although bacteriologic wound examination usually reveals a number of aerobic and anaerobic organisms, at least one species of Clostridium, usually *Clostridium welchii*, is recovered and frequently *Clostridium oedematiens* and *Clostridium septicum* are also recovered. The organisms produce nearly a dozen exotoxins, the most important of which is lecithinase. Nonlethal toxins, among which are collagenase and hyaluronidase, play an important role in the pathogenicity of the organism. The main differential diagnosis is between anaerobic clostridial cellulitis and clostridial myonecrosis. The differentiating factor is the relationship of gas to toxemia (Schwartz, 1969).

A wound containing a large amount of gas associated with mild toxemia is usually not gas gangrene. However, little or no gas associated with severe toxemia probably represents gas gangrene (clostridial myonecrosis).

Fear of not being able to close the abdominal wall defect should not limit the extent of the resection when a diagnosis of clostridial myonecrosis has been made. An area of residual infection may result in continued spread of the pathologic process or may serve as a source of fatal sepsis. Although oxygen administered at hyperbaric pressure, massive doses of antibiotics, and other adjunctive measures may help to decrease the extent of excision that is needed to control the clostridial infection, a massive forfeiture of skin, muscle, fascia, and peritoneum is usually necessary (Brummelkamp, Hogendijik, and Boerema, 1961; Sanders, 1963).

Reconstructive surgeons vary in their approach to closure of the massive defect usually produced in controlling this infection.

Mladick, Pickrell, Royer, McCraw, and Brown (1969) described resection of the entire anterior abdominal wall, the exposed viscera being allowed to form granulation tissue; full-thickness skin grafts were successfully applied three weeks later. McNally, Price, and MacDonald (1968) closed a defect with Marlex mesh, but they removed the prosthesis before applying skin grafts.

Morgan, Morain, and Eraklis (1971) reported a massive anterior abdominal wall resection including all of the right-sided muscles from the costal margin to the symphysis pubis and the entire left rectus muscle. The peritoneum was left in place and reinforced with Mersilene mesh. One month after resection, windows were cut from the Mersilene, and split-thickness skin grafts were applied on the granulation tissue arising from the visceral peritoneum of the underlying organs. Several grafting procedures were required in order to obtain complete wound closure. The authors' rationale for leaving the peritoneum intact was that it would act as a barrier to bacterial invasion of the abdominal cavity for approximately seven days before becoming necrotic. The authors prefer to resect the peritoneum when infected, as it is certain to slough, provide a nidus of infection, and delay skin graft or flap coverage of the wound. Gastrointestinal decompression and intravenous hyperalimentation can be of benefit in such patients when the viscera are exposed and split-thickness skin grafts are applied directly to their surface.

Eng, Casson, Berman, and Slattery (1973) re-

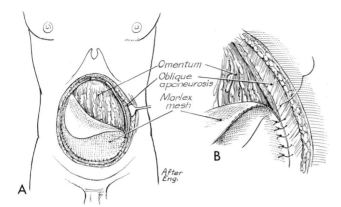

**FIGURE 90–11.** Greater omentum placed between the synthetic mesh and abdominal viscera to reduce the formation of adhesions to the mesh and to provide rapid growth of granulation tissue through the mesh. Mesh is sutured to the abdominal muscular aponeurosis rather than through the peritoneum. (After Eng, K., Casson, P., Berman, I. R., and Slattery, L. R.: Clostridial myonecrosis of the abdominal wall. Resection and prosthetic replacement. Am. J. Surg., *125*:368, 1973.)

ported a case of full-thickness resection of the anterior abdominal wall for clostridial myonecrosis, which entailed suturing the greater omentum to the edges of the parietal peritoneum and covering the omentum with Marlex mesh, which was sutured to the external oblique aponeurosis between the remainder of the abdominal wall fascia and subcutaneous tissue. By the third postoperative day there was almost complete ingrowth of granulation tissue from the omentum through the Marlex. Split-thickness skin grafts were applied to the wound on the eighth

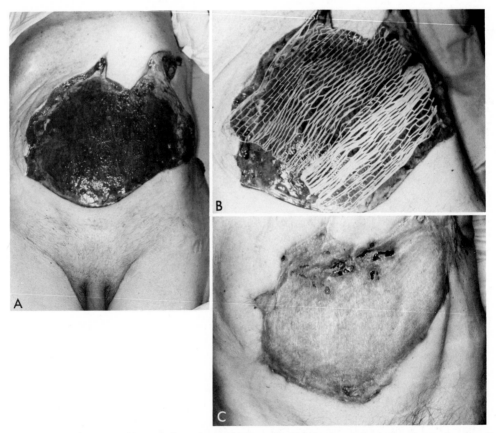

**FIGURE 90–12.** Patient treated by technique shown in Figure 90–11 following abdominal wall resection for clostridial myonecrosis. *A,* Wound on eighth day following suturing of greater omentum to the cut edge of parietal peritoneum and Marlex mesh to the external oblique aponeurosis. Granulation tissue has grown through the mesh and completely covers it. *B,* Meshed split-thickness skin graft applied to granulation tissue. *C,* Wound healing well eight weeks following application of skin grafts. (Courtesy of Phillip Casson, F.R.C.S., Institute of Reconstructive Plastic Surgery.)

postoperative day. At reoperation seven months later, few intra-abdominal adhesions were found. The latter finding was related in part to the interposition of the greater omentum between the viscera and anterior abdominal wall and prosthesis (Figs. 90–11 and 90–12).

## DEFICIENCIES AND DEFECTS OF THE ABDOMINAL WALL

Agenesis and hypoplasia in one or several of the muscular layers of the abdominal wall interfere with respiration, coughing, defecation, and urination. Congenital defects are commonly present where vessels or other structures penetrate the transversalis fascia. When the opening permits structures other than those normally present to leave the abdominal cavity, the defect is pathologic and results in herniation requiring surgical correction. The common sites of congenital defects are the internal abdominal ring, the esophageal hiatus, and the pelvic orifices through which the rectum, vagina, and urethra pass. Some of these latter abnormalities will be discussed in a later section.

### Gastroschisis and Omphalocele

Congenital and acquired defects of the umbilical area are manifold and are related to its important embryonic roles as a conduit for blood and as a temporary extracoelomic reservoir for the midgut. Many of the defects are small and require only conservative care and observation. However, of lesser incidence but of far greater importance are other anomalous conditions which demand careful attention and often corrective surgical procedures in order to restore function to a level compatible with life, if not to improve the appearance of the area.

Gastroschisis and omphalocele are congenital defects of the anterior abdominal wall with different anatomical deficits and embryologic failures but with much in common in regard to surgical treatment.

**Embryology.**   During the third week of embryonic life, closure of the body of the embryo is produced by a circumferential folding of four folds which are the condensation of embryonic mesenchyma. The four folds—cephalic, caudal, and two lateral—have somatic and splanchnic layers. The somatic layers of the cephalic,

caudal, and two lateral folds form the thoracic wall, epigastric wall, hypogastric wall, and lateral abdominal walls, respectively (Lewis, Kraeger, and Danis, 1973). The apex of the folds forms the future umbilical ring. Failure of differentiation of the mesenchyma forming the somatopleure of the lateral abdominal wall and resorption of the ectoderm adjacent to the somatopleure lead to a paraumbilical full-thickness defect in the anterior abdominal wall (Duhamel, 1963; Izant, Brown , and Rothmann, 1966; Lewis, Kraeger, and Danis, 1973). The midgut occupies the peritoneal cavity until the resorption appears.

An omphalocele (Fig. 90–13) is a perpetuation of the state existing at the 6th to 12th weeks of intrauterine life (12 to 40 mm), during which time the entire midgut passes from the abdominal cavity into the base of the yolk sac via the omphalomesenteric tract. The umbilical cord is inserted into this sac of peritoneum-amnion. Normally, accelerated linear growth of bowel occurs during the extracoelomic phase, as well as counterclockwise rotation through 270 degrees around the superior mesenteric vascular axis, prior to an orderly reduction of the bowel into the abdominal cavity. Failure of reduction of bowel and, therefore, continued extracoelomic displacement of the viscera result in an omphalocele. With large defects, the liver and spleen may accompany the bowel outside the abdominal cavity.

An omphalocele is not a true hernia, since it has no peritoneum lining its sac, and its contents have never been truly located within the abdomen. The cause of failure of reduction of the contents into the abdominal cavity is unknown. It may be related to failure of development of the abdominal wall, or it may be due to the presence of an abnormally small coelomic space which is inadequate to receive the viscera. The omphalocele sac containing the abdominal viscera may rupture prenatally or postnatally.

A hematoma or a cystic accumulation of Wharton's jelly in the base of the umbilical cord might be confused with a small omphalocele. However, the sac is usually considerably larger. It averaged 6 to 8 cm in size in a series of 19 patients (Soper and Green, 1961). The sac is usually thin and translucent immediately after delivery; however, within several hours it becomes lusterless and opaque, indicating dehydration and possible impending necrosis. Since the blood supply is poor, fissures are likely to develop, and this may be a sign of impending rupture. Sac rupture is a grave complication associated with a mortality rate of nearly 100 per

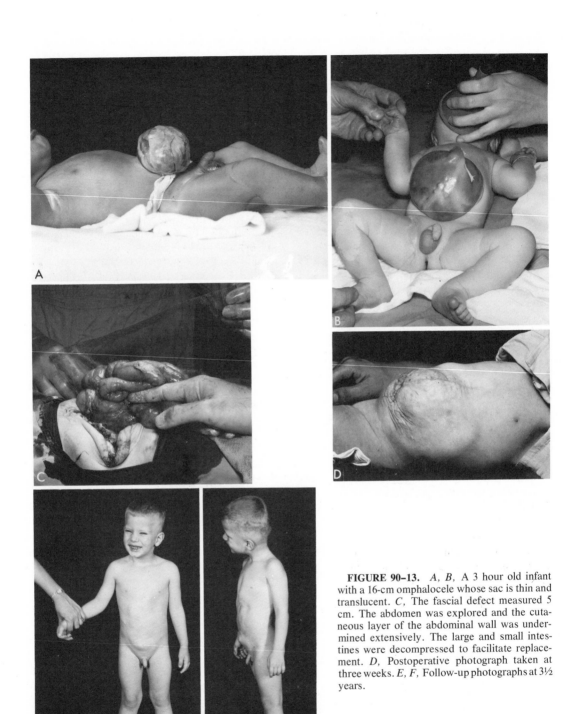

**FIGURE 90–13.** *A, B,* A 3 hour old infant with a 16-cm omphalocele whose sac is thin and translucent. *C,* The fascial defect measured 5 cm. The abdomen was explored and the cutaneous layer of the abdominal wall was undermined extensively. The large and small intestines were decompressed to facilitate replacement. *D,* Postoperative photograph taken at three weeks. *E, F,* Follow-up photographs at 3½ years.

cent (Mahour, Weitzman, and Rosenkrantz, 1973).

Gastroschisis (Fig. 90–14) is a full-thickness defect of the abdominal wall which occurs lateral to the insertion of the umbilical cord. Gastroschisis differs from an omphalocele in that there is lack of a covering sac or its remnant, the abdominal wall defect is lateral to the umbilicus, and there is a normal umbilical cord insertion (Moore and Stokes, 1953). Almost all patients with gastroschisis have in common nonrotation of the bowel, an abnormally short midgut, and a small peritoneal cavity (Hollabaugh and Boles, 1973). Nonrotation predisposes to volvulus and vascular infarction of the intestine.

Moore (1963) classified omphalocele into an *antenatal type,* in which the evisceration occurs early in pregnancy, the eviscerated intestines being distended, thickened, rigid, and covered with a gelatinous matrix, and a *perinatal type,* the evisceration presumably occurring late in pregnancy and possibly being induced by uterine contraction, with the bowel maintaining its elasticity and a minimal surface exudate.

In patients with gastroschisis or ruptured omphalocele of long duration, the eviscerated mass of bowel is thick, edematous, matted together, and covered with a fibrogelatinous membrane. Peristalsis is usually absent. However, most omphaloceles which rupture do so at or near term, and the bowel is not thick and matted (Wayne and Burrington, 1973).

**Preoperative Management.**    An infant born with an omphalocele or gastroschisis constitutes a surgical emergency. The major causes of mortality in patients with omphalocele and gastroschisis have been sepsis, increased intraabdominal pressure postoperatively, respiratory insufficiency, the catabolic state associated with prolonged intestinal ileus, and other associated congenital anomalies (Fig. 90–15) (Aitken, 1963; Rickham, 1963; Smith and Leix, 1966; Simpson and Lynn, 1968; Firor, 1971).

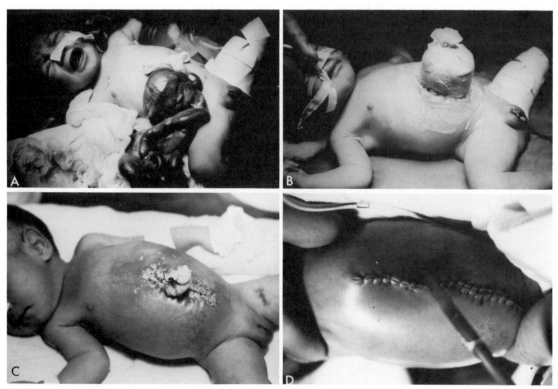

**FIGURE 90–14.**    *A,* A 4 hour old infant with a 4-cm gastroschisis defect. The stomach and almost all of the intestinal tract protruded through the defect with the umbilical cord at its left edge. The intestines were shortened, malrotated, dilated, edematous, and purple. *B,* The abdominal cavity was too small to accommodate the gastrointestinal tract. A polyester mesh sack (Mersilene) lined with silicone rubber (Silastic) sheeting was sutured to the freshened edges of the defect. *C,* Beginning on the second postoperative day, a suture was tied approximately 1 cm proximal to the suture at the apex of the sack. This was continued every other day until the sack height was obliterated. Side-to-side plication sutures progressively narrowed the horizontal dimension of the defect. *D,* At 2 weeks of age, the abdominal defect was closed in layers, and a gastrostomy tube was placed. (Figs. 90–14, 90–16 and 90–17 courtesy of Dr. W. K. T. Shim.)

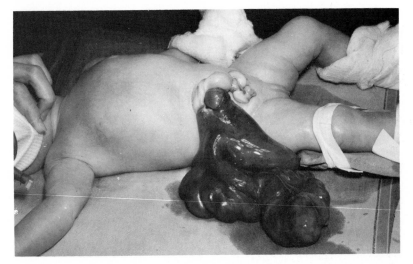

**FIGURE 90-15.** Antenatal rupture of an omphalocele sac with volvulus of exteriorized intestine. The infant was brought to the hospital four hours after birth. Postmortem examination disclosed dextroposition of the aorta, cor triloculare with common ventricle, and a small left atrium.

As outlined by Gross (1948, 1953), Soper and Green (1961), Wayne and Burrington (1973), and Mahour, Weitzman, and Rosenkrantz (1973), eviscerated organs or an intact sac should be covered with gauze sponges soaked in sterile saline or placed under a plastic bag to avoid heat, fluid, and electrolyte loss.

Preoperative management includes careful fluid volume control, parenteral administration of antibiotics, gastrointestinal intubation to prevent gastric distention and respiratory complications, preservation of body heat, blood gas determinations, and control of acid-base balance. Evacuation of meconium with rectal irrigations plays a significant role in reducing the mortality associated with these defects.

Postoperative mechanical respiratory assistance, when necessary, intravenous hyperalimentation until peristalsis returns, and tube feedings are major adjuncts in obtaining improved survival rates.

Roentgenograms of the abdomen and chest should be obtained, since they may show other malformations. The infant's blood should be typed and crossmatched for transfusion, and a venous cutdown should be performed in order to establish a relatively large caliber intravenous route for fluid administration.

Death rates, which were previously 70 to 80 per cent, have been reduced to 25 to 35 per cent (Lewis, Kraeger, and Danis, 1973; Hollabaugh and Boles, 1973; Wayne and Burrington, 1973).

**Surgical Correction.** The selection of the proper method of closure of each patient is difficult. Small defects are managed in a manner similar to that used for large umbilical hernias. The viscera are returned to the abdominal cavity, and the fascia and skin are closed in layers.

Major associated anomalies are not uncommon with gastroschisis and omphalocele and include intestinal atresia, malrotation, and volvulus, which may result in significant morbidity and mortality. Intestinal atresias occur in 20 to 25 per cent of patients (Moore and Stokes, 1953; Schuster, 1967; Allen and Wreen, 1969; Hollabaugh and Boles, 1973; Lewis, Kraeger, and Danis, 1973). Such associated anomalies are ample reason for abdominal exploration and surgical correction (Gross, 1953; Grob, 1963; Aitken, 1963; Bill, 1969; Mahour, Weitzman, and Rosenkrantz, 1973), although one-stage closure or nonoperative management of large intact omphaloceles has been advocated (Drescher, 1963; Grob, 1963; Soave, 1963; Dorogi, 1964).

Failure to diagnose associated anomalies may result in severe complications and death following surgical closure of the abdominal wall defect (Cordero, Touloukian, and Pickett, 1969).

Soper and Green (1961) advocated a one-stage operation as the procedure of choice except when the fascial defect is too large to permit coaptation of its edges. If the sac contents are small and the coelomic cavity is large enough to receive the viscera without undue tension, the sac should be excised and closure of the wound layers accomplished with interrupted, nonabsorbable suture material. Depending upon the orientation of the defect, closure may be in a horizontal or vertical plane. The three umbilical vessels and the urachus should be individually divided and ligated at the periphery of the operative field. Careful inspection of the alimentary tract for associated anomalies is important, even at the expense of enlarging the fascial defect, which may be too small to allow such investigation through its natural confines. However, a one-stage operation is not safe when either the coelomic space is abnormally small or the eviscerated structures are so large that reduction is accomplished only under tension. These factors result in elevation of intra-abdominal pressure and predispose to potentially fatal complications: intestinal kinking with obstruction, elevation of the diaphragm producing respiratory embarrassment, and compression of the inferior vena cava which may reduce venous return to the heart.

Operation may be performed in one or two stages, depending upon the ease with which the eviscerated structures can be reduced. Gross (1948) reported a two-stage method: the first stage consists of mobilizing the abdominal wall skin and subcutaneous tissues from the abdominal muscle fascia until sufficient coverage has been obtained to cover the intact amniotic sac. Several months later, when the mass can be reduced with ease, the sac is excised, and the abdominal wall is closed in layers (Fig. 90–16).

As emphasized by Soper and Green (1961), this method of management does not allow detection of coincidental alimentary tract abnor-

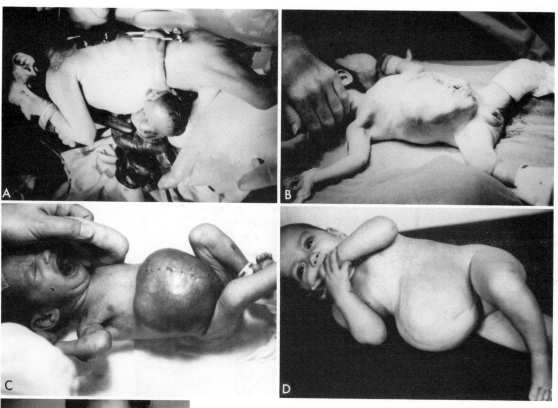

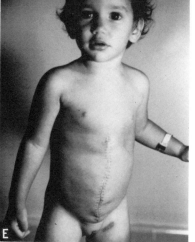

**FIGURE 90–16.** Gastroschisis treated by first-stage skin closure and second-stage fascial closure (method of Gross). *A*, Umbilical cord is located at the left edge of the gastroschisis defect. Almost all of the intestine and stomach and a portion of the liver protrude from the defect. The intestines were purple, matted, and hard. *B*, Skin flaps were elevated and approximated over the abdominal contents. *C*, At 2 weeks of age, the skin is tense, purplish, and shiny. *D*, At 6 months of age, the patient is healthy, but a large ventral hernia is present. *E*, The ventral hernia was repaired, and the rectus muscles were approximated with a prosthesis at 18 months of age.

malities at the time of the initial operation; another extensive operation may be required during a period when diagnosis may be extremely difficult and the risks of delay or a second operation exceedingly high. Soper and Green (1961) presented an alternative to Gross's first-stage operation. The sac is excised to allow exploratory laparotomy and correction of whatever associated anomalies may exist. If the sharpness or narrowness of the fascial ring is such as to compromise circulation to the herniated viscera, relaxing incisions can be made. The skin is mobilized and closed directly over the viscera. The subsequent management is the same as that presented by Gross.

Early operative management should be performed in most cases of gastroschisis and omphalocele, with nonoperative management being reserved for the poor-risk premature patient or patients with other severe congenital anomalies (Mahour, Weitzman, and Rosenkrantz, 1973).

**Closure.** If primary closure produces significant abdominal cavity reduction, a staged procedure is indicated if a high chance of mortality is to be avoided. In some patients, flank-relaxing incisions and wide undermining may be sufficient to prevent increase in intra-abdominal pressure and skin flap necrosis (see Fig. 90–16). Manual stretching of the abdominal wall occasionally provides the necessary increase in the abdominal cavity to accommodate the bowel and allow closure without tension (Izant, Brown, and Rothmann, 1966).

Resection of normal bowel, liver, or spleen to allow primary closure is not indicated (Meltzer, 1956; Buchanan and Cain, 1956). Removal of the thick fibrinous peel from the surface of the bowel prolongs surgical time and increases bleeding and mortality (Moore and Stokes, 1953; Rickham, 1963).

Silon (Silastic-coated Dacron), polyethylene, and Teflon sheets sutured to the edges of the fascial defects reduce the complications of primary skin flap closure and provide an alternate method of staged abdominal wall reconstruction (Mahour, Weitzman, and Rosenkrantz, 1973).

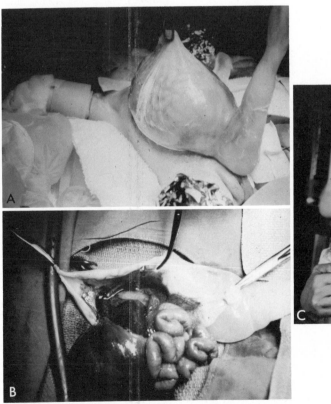
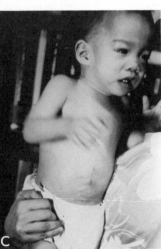

**FIGURE 90–17.** Omphalocele treated by the prosthetic silo technique similar to that shown in Figure 90–14 *B, C. A,* Huge omphalocele measuring 15 × 20 cm with a fascial defect of 6 cm in an otherwise normal full term female. *B,* Omphalocele opened showing intestines and almost the entire liver protruding through the defect. *C,* The child at 1 year of age with normal development following prosthetic silo technique closure.

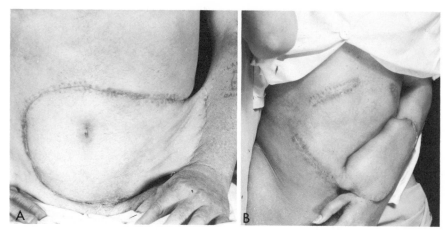

**FIGURE 90–18.**    The greater part of the abdominal wall may be transferred to a distant area; however, the pedicle should be broad and extensive. The successful transfer of a flap depends upon the adequacy of the circulation to the distal end of the flap. Delay procedures are performed to enhance the circulation. *A,* The abdominal flap has been delayed completely prior to successful transfer. *B,* The abdominothoracic flap has been partially delayed.

The silo technique using a plastic pouch provides gradual return of the viscera into the abdominal cavity as the abdominal wall relaxes and the peritoneal cavity enlarges (see Figs. 90–14 and 90–17). It is surprising how rapidly the abdomen may accommodate the viscera (Shim, 1971).

Fonkalsrud (1975) raised a word of caution about the survival rate obtained using the various prostheses as part of the abdominal wall closure. His survival rate, using a two-stage closure, at the UCLA Medical Center over the past ten years was 94 per cent. Skin closure is initially followed by fascial closure after adequate growth and development have occurred.

Attention to meticulous sterile technique is absolutely necessary in managing patients with omphalocele or gastroschisis, particularly those treated in stages using prosthetic materials.

## THE ABDOMEN AS A DONOR SITE FOR SKIN FLAPS

The surgeon's full responsibility to his patient has not been fulfilled with the removal of a lesion or an abnormality unless the final result is acceptable from both the fuctional and the esthetic standpoints (Pickrell, 1954). The patient is enti-

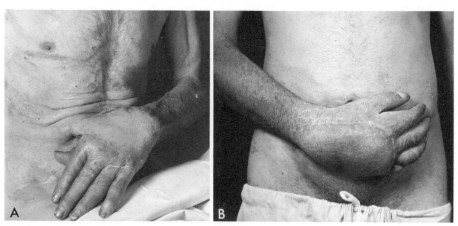

**FIGURE 90–19.**    *A,* A superior pedicle, direct transfer flap to the dorsum of the hand. *B,* An inferior pedicle, direct transfer flap to the hand.

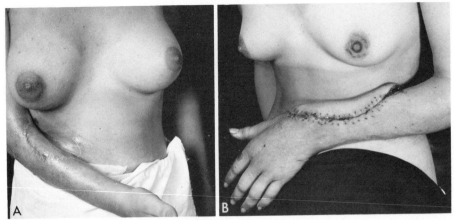

**FIGURE 90–20.**    The abdomen is an ideal donor area for direct or immediate transfer flaps to resurface areas of avulsion and scar, as shown in *A,* or fresh injury, as shown in *B.* When the breast is large or pendulous, its undersurface makes an ideal donor area, for in many instances it can be closed primarily without deformity.

tled to the best cosmetic result commensurate with a satisfactory functional result. When it is not possible to repair the defect with local tissues or a skin graft, the use of a flap is mandatory; in such cases, skin flaps are procedures of necessity.

A great variety of flaps may be constructed from the abdominal wall. Since the general principles in the planning, formation, and transfer of various types of flaps have already been dis-

cussed (see Chapter 6), this particular section will be brief and selective. The examples offered (Figs. 90–18 through 90–21) have been found to be acceptable and sufficiently representative that no attempt will be made to include all that might be offered by way of alternatives. The microvascular free flap is described in detail in Chapters 6 and 14. Axial pattern flaps include those based on the superficial epigastric and superficial circumflex iliac vessels.

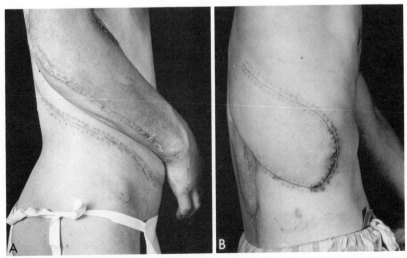

**FIGURE 90–21.**    The flank is also an ideal donor area for direct transfer flaps to resurface a forearm, as shown in *A.* Since the circulation of the distal end of the flap, shown in *B,* was precarious, it was replaced in its bed and was successfully transferred in ten days.

# Spina Bifida

## JOHN C. MUSTARDÉ, F.R.C.S., AND WALLACE M. DENNISON, M.D., F.R.C.S.

There are few malformations in which the lesion may involve as many systems in the body as does spina bifida cystica. The term "spina bifida" is applied to a developmental gap in the vertebral column through which the contents of the spinal canal may protrude. Except in its simplest form (spina bifida occulta), it is usually a grave anomaly and is commonly associated with maldevelopment of the spinal cord and paralysis of the lower limbs (motor and sensory), with trophic and vasomotor changes in the skin and paralysis of the sphincters. There may be multiple developmental errors, and many patients die at or soon after birth.

The incidence in the general population is approximately 1 in 800 births. Having had one child with overt spina bifida, parents should be warned that the chance of the malformation appearing in any later child is approximately 1 in 25. After the birth of a second child with spina bifida, the risk of recurrence increases to 1 in 10.

### EMBRYOLOGY

Early in intrauterine life the neural groove appears as a longitudinal furrow in the ectoderm on the dorsal surface of the embryo. The edges of the furrow unite to form a tube from which the nervous system is developed. The tube becomes separated from the surface by mesoderm; on the ventral side the vertebral bodies develop around the notocord. The developing vertebral arches fuse first in the thoracic region, and fusion subsequently proceeds up and down the midline. Failure of fusion gives rise to spina bifida, which is frequently associated with maldevelopment of the spinal cord and membranes.

### SPINA BIFIDA OCCULTA

This is a common anomaly which is usually of no significance and is often accidentally discovered by radiography. Frequently only one vertebra (lumbar or sacral) is affected, and there is no protrusion of cord or membranes. A local patch of hair, a nevus, a lipoma, or a small circular or ovoid area of atrophic or parchment-like skin in the lumbosacral region is suggestive of an under-

This material was previously published as two chapters in Mustardé, J. C. (Ed.): Plastic Surgery in Infancy and Childhood. Edinburgh, Churchill Livingstone, 1971. Reproduced by permission of the publisher.

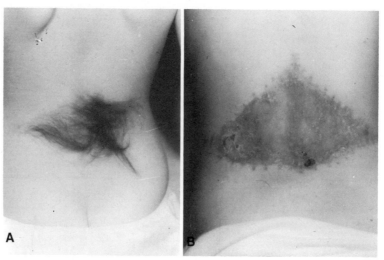

**FIGURE 90–22.** Spina bifida occulta. *A*, Preoperative view. Note tuft of hair. *B*, Appearance following excision and application of a split-thickness skin graft.

lying bone deficiency (Fig. 90–22). The condition rarely gives rise to symptoms in childhood. Minor anomalies in spinal fusion seldom, if ever, have any causal relation to enuresis. In later childhood and adolescence, neurologic signs may appear, owing to increasing tension produced at the site of the defect by disproportionate growth of the vertebral column and spinal cord. Local skin lesions may require excision for cosmetic reasons.

## SPINA BIFIDA CYSTICA

While the terms "meningocele", "myelomeningocele" (meningomyelocele), "syringomyelocele," and "myelocele" have been used, it is convenient to group all of the lesions under the broad term of "spina bifida cystica." In the rather uncommon meningocele, there is no nerve involvement; in all of the lesions, there is myelodysplasia in varying degrees with associated paralysis.

**Meningocele.** There is a herniation of the meningeal coverings through a gap in the vertebral arches which presents as a midline swelling in the back, most commonly in the lumbosacral region (Fig. 90–23, *A*) but occasionally in the cervical or thoracic region (Fig. 90–23, *B*). Rarely the defect presents to one or the other side of the midline. The meningocele is usually covered completely by normal skin, or the covering may consist of a thin and translucent layer which readily ulcerates and ruptures. No individual meningeal layers can be distinguished in this covering. The swelling is cystic and may become more tense when the child cries. A meningocele may be translucent, or it may be associated with an excess of lipomatous or angiomatous tissue.

Although the pathologist may report ectopic nerve elements in the excision specimen, there is no myelodysplasia and no paralysis. Meningocele constitutes about 14 per cent of all cases of spina bifida cystica.

**Meningomyelocele.** While the swelling may resemble the less common pure meningocele, in this anomaly there are always nerve elements in the sac (Fig. 90–24). These elements vary from normal or ectopic nerves and ectopic spinal cord to the cauda equina or the cord itself. The swelling may be entirely cystic, or there may be solid elements. If cerebrospinal fluid is aspirated and replaced by air, a lateral radiograph may demonstrate the nerve elements coursing across

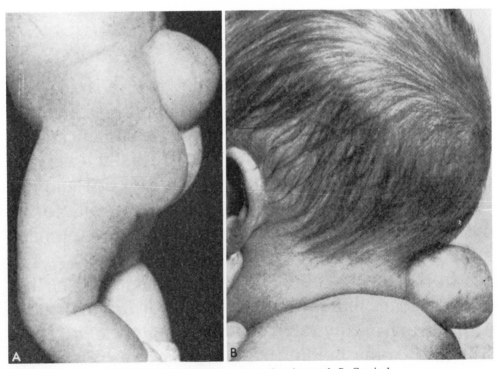

**FIGURE 90–23.** Meningocele. *A*, Lumbosacral. *B*, Cervical.

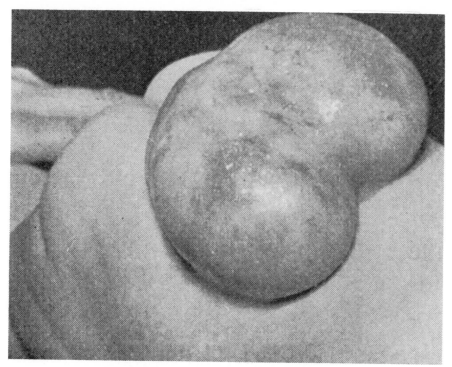

**FIGURE 90–24.** Meningomyelocele (lumbosacral).

the sac. Lumbosacral meningomyelocele is usually associated with motor and sensory paralysis of the lower limbs and paralysis of the bladder and rectum; trophic ulcers develop readily. There may be associated clubfoot, usually talipes equinovarus. Evident hydrocephalus may be present at birth, or it may develop later. This form of hydrocephalus is commonly associated with the Arnold-Chiari malformation, in which a cone of medulla and cerebellum is prolonged downward through the foramen magnum.

**Syringomyelocele.** In this rare anomaly the presenting features are similar to those of meningomyelocele, but the central canal of the cord is greatly dilated. The condition is only of embryologic interest.

**Myelocele.** In this disorder arrest of development has occurred before closure of the neural groove (Fig. 90–25), and the infant presents with a raw elliptical area from which the open cord discharges cerebrospinal fluid. At one time this condition was rarely compatible with life. Many babies were stillborn; others died within a few days from infection of the cord and

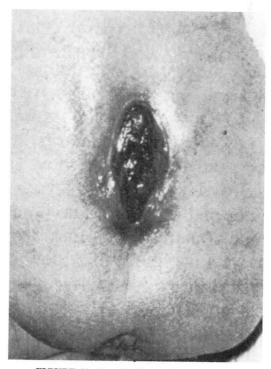

**FIGURE 90–25.** Myelocele (lumbosacral).

meninges. Since the introduction of chemotherapy, epithelization commences, and after a few days, a cystic swelling resembling meningomyelocele is present.

## DIFFERENTIAL DIAGNOSIS

The only conditions which may give rise to difficulty in the differential diagnosis are posterior enteric remnants and sacrococcygeal teratoma. Lipomas are rare tumors in infancy and childhood, but they do occur in the lumbosacral region, usually to one side of the midline. Such lipomas are almost invariably associated with spina bifida.

## MEDICAL MANAGEMENT

In 1957 in the Royal Hospital for Sick Children, Glasgow, it was estimated that 90 per cent of babies born with spina bifida cystica died of meningitis, progressive hydrocephalus, or the complications of paraplegia. About 4 per cent lived as permanent invalids in wheelchairs, and 2 per cent were able to lead an independent life after multiple orthopedic procedures. Only 1 baby in 50 grew up to lead a normal life. Today ventriculoperitoneal drainage has been replaced by ventriculoatrial shunting procedures, and the prognosis in hydrocephalus is greatly improved. Advances in chemotherapy have resulted in the control of meningeal infection. The authors were compelled to reassess their orthopedic procedures for dealing with paralysis and deformity and have made considerable progress in making incontinent children both healthy and socially acceptable by various forms of urinary diversion and regulation of bowel habit.

Before treatment is undertaken, an attempt is made to explain to the parents what surgery has to offer their child. Except in patients with spina bifida occulta, the prognosis is always guarded.

There is an early mortality of almost 40 per cent. In a simple meningocele with adequate skin covering, operation is not performed until after the infant is 3 months old. In 86 per cent of patients with spina bifida cystica (meningomyelocele, syringomyelocele, and myelocele), operation is performed within the first 24 hours of life not only to save life but also to prevent deterioration in function. Many of the infants (more than 60 per cent) survive, and by early operation the disability is decreased. It is often possible to close the spinal defect in layers. Hemangiomatous staining of the skin is common in all types of spina bifida, and after operation the hemangiomatous area may temporarily become more extensive. Over a period of years it has been found that the incidence of progressive hydrocephalus is about 50 per cent, both in patients subjected to early operation and in those on whom operation is delayed.

Occasionally, babies with a serious spinal defect (e.g., myelocele) are born with active lower limbs, and yet within a few hours after birth there is complete paralysis of the legs and sphincters. This terrifyingly rapid deterioration is due to desiccation of the cord rather than to infection or the formation of granulation tissue. As soon as possible after birth, the exposed cord is protected and kept moist with sterile isotonic saline solution or cast vinyl film until the arrival of a neurologic or surgical pediatric unit. Even during operation, the spinal cord is kept moist with saline, as it can be subjected to further drying from the heat of the operating room and from the overhead operating light.

When the back is closed, the patient is reviewed in consultation with pediatric orthopedic colleagues. The common limb deformities are paralytic clubfoot and paralytic dislocation of the hips. By manipulation, the use of calipers, and stabilizing operations, every effort is made to render the child ambulant as early as possible.

It is important to determine early if the neuropathic bladder can empty freely by evaluation with excretory urography and micturating cystography. Corrective surgery of a meningocele or meningomyelocele will never improve bladder function and may even make the situation worse.

Urinary infection is controlled by chemotherapy, and excessive leakage may be avoided by keeping the volume of urine in the bladder as small as possible. The mother, and later the child, is taught to empty the bladder at regular intervals by manual pressure. By school age a boy can usually manage a portable urinal, but this apparatus is rarely successful in the female. In the female it may be justifiable to divert the urine using a free ileal or colonic loop. This type of surgery is not without risk. Postoperatively, blood-urea tests should be supplemented by estimations of serum chloride, plasma bicarbonate, and phosphate. On a few occasions the authors have known girls to gain reasonable urinary control when they reach puberty, but often at the expense of increased residual urine.

Important as it is to achieve urinary continence, preservation of renal function is of even greater importance. Patients with spina bifida who survive the early hazards of meningitis and hydrocephalus commonly die of renal failure. Recurrent infection may be suppressed by continuous chemotherapy.

Colostomy is seldom required for bowel incontinence. By the intelligent use of laxatives and suppositories, if necessary, supported by a fairly short period of hospital or other suitable institutional treatment, bowel habits are usually rendered socially acceptable. Despite early closure of the spinal defect and the success of ventriculoatrial drainage, there is still a relatively high mortality from meningitis and infection of the urinary tract. All but 14 per cent of the children are paraplegic, and many require repeated readmission to the hospital for a variety of problems, including the development of pressure sores.

## THE SURGICAL TREATMENT OF SPINA BIFIDA

**Spina Bifida Occulta.** No treatment is required for the bifid spine or spines, but the overlying triangle of hair-bearing skin is a social embarrassment and should be removed. This can be done by excision and direct closure in a few patients, but in the majority a moderately thick split-thickness skin graft may be required (see Fig. 90–22, *B*) to provide coverage. Late signs of neurologic involvement in the lower limbs or urinary bladder may indicate the need for exploration of the spinal cord and release of restricting bands or a short ligamentum denticulatum.

**Meningocele.** True meningoceles containing no neural tissue are comparatively rare (Fig. 90–26, *A*) and generally involve only one or at most two bifid spines; they may occasionally arise from the occipital region of the skull. Treatment is comparatively simple and, while not an emergency procedure, should be performed as soon as possible in the thin-walled variety to avoid the risk of rupture of the covering layers. It consists of dissection of the neck of the meningocele (Fig. 90–26, *B*) to allow the skin-covered meningeal sac to be removed and the spinal defect to be covered by plicated flaps of lumbodorsal fascia from either side. No difficulty should be experienced in closing the skin wounds by direct approximation (Fig. 90–26, *C*).

**Meningomyelocele.** Most cystic spinal swellings are not true meningoceles but contain a varying amount of neural tissue. Despite the large size, they may present on the surface (Fig. 90–27, *A*); they generally arise, like the true meningoceles, from a single bifid spine (rarely two or more). On occasion, rupture has occurred by birth, with cerebrospinal fluid leaking freely, and the lesions must be closed as rapidly as possible to prevent the onset of meningeal infection. The risk of rupture is always present in the early stages in thin-walled cysts, and they should be considered semi-emergency problems unless the skin covering is obviously adequate. Operation involves opening the sac of the cyst to identify the neural tissue, which will be found emerging from the gap in the spinal canal and running out toward the surface layers (Fig. 90–27, *B*). As in simple meningoceles, the neck of the meningeal sac is carefully dissected by incising around the meningocele and extending the incision into the fatty layer which surrounds the neck of the sac. In very large meningomyeloceles, some of the true skin around the base of the swelling may be preserved, but this makes dissection of the neck of the sac more difficult. As much of the neural tissue as possible should be saved. It is quite probable that a large proportion of it is nonfunctional, undifferentiated tissue, but this is difficult to determine at the time of surgery. The neural tissue should be securely covered by a layer of meninges, and if need be, a laminectomy is carried out on the vertebral arch immediately above in order to accommodate the bulk of the neural tissue and meningeal covering. The remainder of the meninges and skin is discarded.

Flaps of lumbodorsal fascia are transferred from each side to provide strong cover, and the skin is closed primarily. Even when a relatively enormous meningomyelocele is present, there is usually no difficulty in obtaining skin closure (Fig. 90–27, *C*), although a rotation flap may occasionally be required.

**Myelocele.** Myeloceles are flat and noncystic, with bifid spines lying opened out at 180 degrees, but cystic swellings may exist on either side of the plaque of exposed neural tissue even at birth (Fig. 90–28); such lesions are sometimes referred to as meningomyeloceles. The exposed neural tissue is extremely sensitive for the first few hours after birth and, if touched in any way, gives rise to a massive reflex reaction in the lower limbs with increase in spasm of the muscles. The reflex is quickly lost, and the limbs lose any power of movement they may have had in a

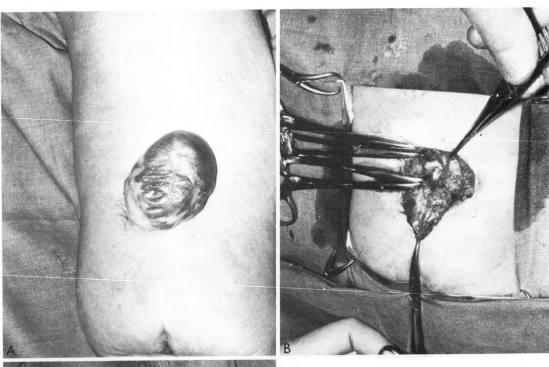

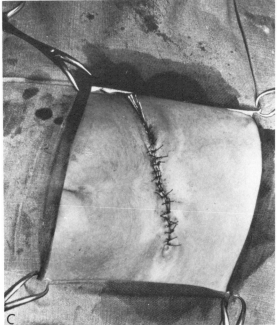

**FIGURE 90–26.** Meningocele (lumbosacral). *A*, Preoperative appearance. *B*, Involvement of only a single spine; note the narrow meningeal pedicle. *C*, Closure of skin by direct approximation.

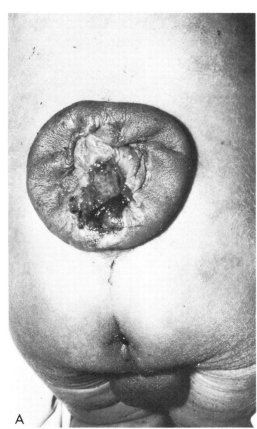

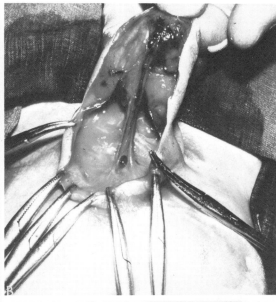

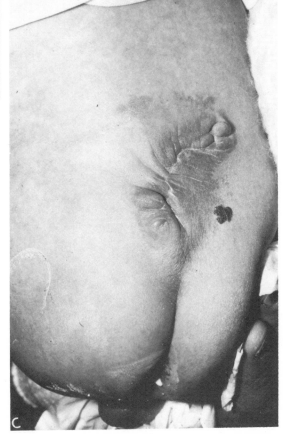

**FIGURE 90–27.** Meningomyelocele. *A*, Large lumbosacral meningomyelocele (ruptured). *B*, Narrow stalk of neural tissue passing from the spinal cord to the skin of the sac. *C*, Skin closure by direct approximation.

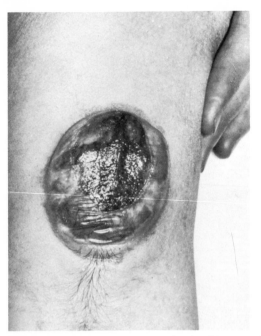

**FIGURE 90–28.** Lumbosacral myelocele with exposed neural tissue.

matter of a few hours, so that operation on these babies is one of the most pressing of all neonatal emergencies.

In cases of extensive and severe spina bifida (see Fig. 90–28) in which the cord is grossly involved and the neural tissue is present on the surface as a red, raw area, the problem of repairing the actual neural tube and its immediate coverings usually presents little technical difficulty (Fig. 90–29, *A, B*). The abundance of meningeal lining from the cystic tumor around the cord tissue provides adequate material, which can be rotated as a flap on each side to cover the neural tissue. The real difficulty is to produce a strong covering layer for the reconstructed cord and meninges, which will be adequate for practical purposes and yet be simple and safe to obtain.

In the severe type of case, not only are the spines bifid but also the bifid processes are turned outward to lie horizontally. The lumbodorsal fascia is usually restricted to two comparatively narrow strips on the lateral side of the tips of the widely separated processes; when mobilized, these narrow strips of fascia are inadequate to stretch across the defect in the spine to form a protective covering.

In addition, the problem of provision of skin cover over the neural tube and its meningeal coverings is sometimes almost insurmountable, especially if seven or eight spines are affected. Widespread undermining and flap rotation (Paterson, 1959), although they may sometimes permit the transfer of skin and subcutaneous tissue over the area, are often followed by wound breakdown and necrosis of tissue because of tightness of the suture line and interference with the vascular supply of the skin.

Moreover, if one is able to obtain a sound covering layer of skin for the neural tissues, the reformed cord is left vulnerable and ill-protected; in most cases, it is lying on the summit of an abnormally convex spine (Nash, 1963).

It became apparent to the authors that all of the problems enumerated above might be overcome if the whole of the lateral mass of spinous processes and spinal muscles could be turned in to form a new spinal canal, with a bony skeleton inside and muscle tissue on the outside (Fig. 90–29, *C, D*). Not only would such a structure provide adequate protection for the cord, but also the muscle on the outside would form a suitable bed on which to place a split-thickness skin graft (Mustardé, 1966).

The operative technique which has evolved has the additional merit of requiring almost no undermining of the skin; hence, apart from the elimination of necrosis of the skin, there is considerably less blood loss than it was previously possible to achieve. By injecting local anesthetic with adrenalin around the junction of the meningomyelocele and under the skin of the back (Fig. 90–30, *A*), the blood loss has been reduced to minimal proportions, and no intravenous therapy is necessary.

The technique, which is performed in the first few hours of life to prevent irrecoverable paraplegia (Sharrard, 1963; Maudsley, Rickham, and Roberts, 1967), involves excision of the thin, transparent epithelium on the surface but careful preservation of all true skin on the meningomyelocele, whether discolored or not. The meningeal layer, overlying the outwardly displaced spinous processes and lumbodorsal fascia, is incised around the periphery (Fig. 90–30, *B*) and turned in as a flap on each side so that it can be sutured in a water-tight junction over the inverted neural tissue (Fig. 90–30, *C*). If the exposed neural tissue is large in area, it can be tubed and covered by the meninges.

An incision is made vertically into the mass of the spinal muscles on either side, about 2 cm lateral to the tips of the bifid spines (Fig. 90–30, *D*). At first, the incision is made vertically to a depth of 1.5 cm, and then the knife is turned horizontally so that the muscle mass is undermined to within about 3 mm of the horizontally lying tips of the bifid spines (Fig. 90–31, *A*).

Each of the bifid spines is carefully located and fractured inward (Fig. 90–31, *B, C*), using a

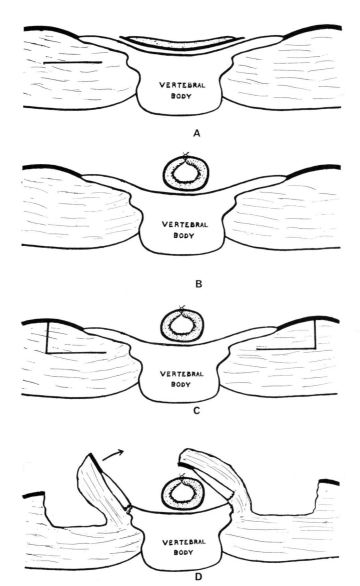

**FIGURE 90–29.** Schematic representation of steps in repair of severe spina bifida. *A,* Neural tissue opened out as a flat plaque. *B,* Neural tissue tubed and covered by meningeal layer. *C,* Lateral muscle mass incised along lines indicated. *D,* Bifid spinous processes fractured and osteomuscular flaps brought over to form new spinal canal over reformed spinal cord.

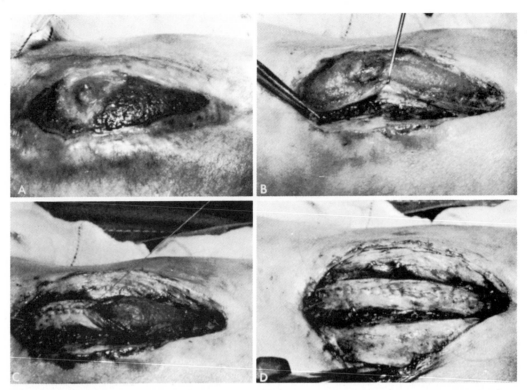

**FIGURE 90–30.** Stages in repair illustrated in Figure 90–29. *A,* Injection of dilute epinephrine solution into cutaneous margin around the defect. *B,* Separation of neural tissue and meninges from skin by sharp dissection. *C,* Closure of meningeal layer over the tubed neural tissue. *D,* Vertical incision into lateral muscle mass.

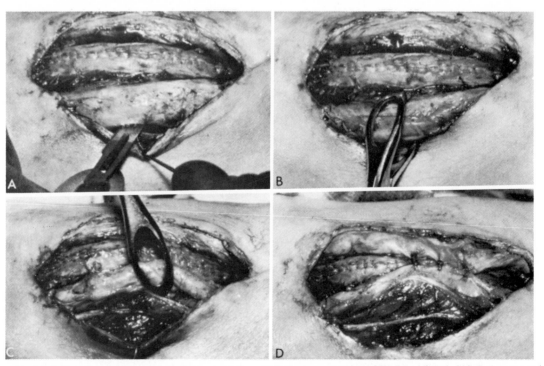

**FIGURE 90–31.** *A,* Horizontal dissection toward tips of bifid spines. *B,* Each spine is grasped by tissue forceps at its narrowest point. *C,* The spine is fractured and the osteomuscular flap is turned medially. *D,* Approximation of osteomuscular flaps in the midline.

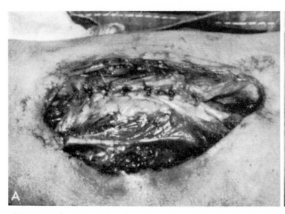
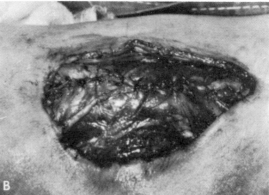

**FIGURE 90–32.** *A,* Approximation of the lumbodorsal fascia. *B,* Approximation of the spinal muscle mass over the lumbodorsal fascia.

suitable instrument such as Lane's tissue forceps; the muscle mass at each side, along with the fractured spinous processes, is brought across to meet its counterpart to form a musculo-osseous covering for the reconstructed cord (Fig. 90–31, *D*). The approximation of the lateral masses is best done in two planes: a deep lumbodorsal fascial layer (Fig. 90–32, *A*), and a superficial muscular layer (Fig. 90–32, *B*). This technique prevents the later tendency for the reconstructed spinal canal to gape open. If the sacrum is involved, the lumbodorsal fascia attached to the iliac crest is turned in, along with a thin slice of the cartilage of the crest, to provide a covering layer.

The skin of the back, and any skin which has been preserved from the lateral walls of the meningocele, is sutured to the underlying muscle *without any tension* (Fig. 90–33, *A*). It may be preferable to leave an area of muscle exposed in the center if there is the slightest tightness on the skin edges when an attempt is made to close the defect. When the skin can be easily approximated, the edges are sutured together, and a light pressure dressing is applied. If the defect cannot be completely closed without tension, a split-thickness skin graft is removed from one of the buttocks and is sutured to the edges of the defect (Fig. 90–33, *B*). The ends of the sutures are left long and tied over a pad of cotton wool or plastic sponge, and a top dressing is applied overall, adhesive plaster being used for fixation. One week later, the dressings over the skin graft are removed; the dressings over the donor site are left untouched for an additional week.

As would be expected, the exposed muscle layer readily accepts a skin graft. The end result, whether the skin has been closed directly or a graft applied, is to produce a soundly healed spine with protective bony arches and with a substantial layer of overlying soft tissue (Fig. 90–34).

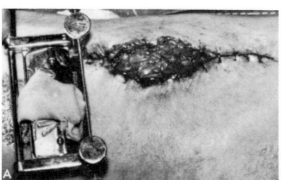
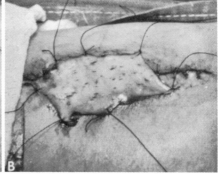

**FIGURE 90–33.** *A,* The skin flaps sutured to the underlying muscle without any tension. *B,* Application of a split-thickness skin graft to the exposed muscle.

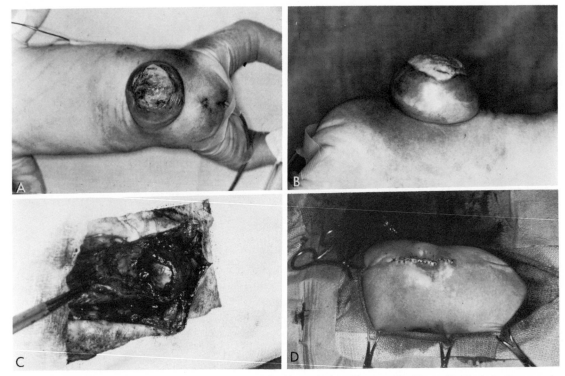

**FIGURE 90–34.** Lumbosacral meningomyelocele repaired by technique illustrated in Figure 90–29. *A, B,* Preoperative appearance. *C,* Intraoperative view. *D,* Closure of skin flaps by direct approximation.

Early closure of severe spina bifida may tend to accelerate the appearance of hydrocephalus, and some indication of the likelihood of the onset of this condition may be obtained from the presence or absence of greatly enlarged fontanelles at birth.

## REFERENCES

Aitken, J.: Exomphalos. Analysis of a 10-year series of 32 cases. Arch. Dis. Child., *38*:126, 1963.

Allen, R. G., and Wrenn, E. L., Jr.: Silon as a sac in the treatment of omphalocele and gastroschisis. J. Pediatr. Surg., *4*:3, 1969.

Bartlett, W.: An improved filigree for the repair of large defects in the abdominal wall. Ann. Surg., *38*:47, 1903.

Bassini, E.: Nuovo methodo per la cura radicale dell'ernia. Atti Congr. Ass. Med. Ital. (1887) Pavia, *2*:179, 1889.

Bekheit, F.: Repair of defects after partial resection of the abdominal wall. J. Egypt. Med. Assoc., *48*:727, 1965.

Bill, A. H., Jr.: Omphalocele. *In* Mustard, W. T., Ravitch, M. M., Synder, W. H., Jr., Welch, K. J., and Benson, C. D. (Eds.): Pediatric Surgery. Vol. 1. 2nd Ed. Chicago, Year Book Medical Publishers, 1969, p. 685.

Bloodgood, J. C.: The transplantation of the rectum muscle in certain cases of inguinal hernia in which the conjoined tendon is obliterated. Johns Hopkins Bull., *9*:96, 1898.

Bruck, H.: A method of reconstructing the whole abdominal wall. Br. J. Plast. Surg., *9*:108, 1956.

Brummelkamp, W. H., Hogendijik, J., and Boerema, I.: Treatment of anaerobic infections (clostridial myositis) by drenching the tissue with oxygen under high atmospheric pressure. Surgery, *49*:299, 1961.

Buchanan, R. W., and Cain, W. L.: A case of a complete omphalocele. Ann. Surg., *143*:552, 1956.

Bussabarger, R. A., Dumouchel, M. L., and Ivy, W. H.: Use of tantalum mesh to repair a large surgical defect in the anterior abdominal wall. J.A.M.A., *142*:984, 1950.

Butcher, E. O.: Hair growth and sebaceous glands in skin transplanted under skin and into the peritoneal cavity in the rat. Anat. Rec., *96*:101, 1946.

Cantrell, J. R., and Haller, J. A.: Peritoneal reconstruction after extensive abdominal wall resection. Surg. Gynecol. Obstet., *110*:363, 1960.

Cokkinis, A. J., and Bromwich, A. F.: Tantalum repair of very large incisional hernia. Br. J. Surg., *45*:623, 1954.

Cooper, A. P.: Lectures on the Principles and Practice of Surgery. Boston, F. Tyrell, 1825.

Cordero, L., Touloukian, R. J., and Pickett, L. K.: Staged repair of gastroschisis with Silastic sheeting. Surgery, *65*:676, 1969.

Crile, G., and King, D. E.: Successful use of tantalum mesh to repair an abdominal wall defect in the presence of massive faecal contamination. Surgery, *29*:914, 1951.

Dorogi, J.: Improved conservative treatment of exomphalos. Lancet, *2*:888, 1964.

Drescher, E.: Observations on the conservative treatment of exomphalos. Arch. Dis. Child., *38*:125, 1963.

Duhamel, B.: Embryology of exomphalos and allied malformations. Arch. Dis. Child., *38*:147, 1963.

Ellis, H.: The cause and prevention of postoperative intraperitoneal adhesions. Surg. Gynecol. Obstet., *133*:497, 1971.

Eng, K., Casson, P., Berman, I. R., and Slattery, L. R.:

Clostridial myonecrosis of the abdominal wall. Resection and prosthetic replacement. Am. J. Surg., *125*:368, 1973.

Engdahl, E.: Strengthening of scars with a buried dermal sheet. Scand. J. Plast. Surg., *2*:109, 1968.

Farr, R. E.: Closure of large hernial defects in the upper abdomen. Surg. Gynecol. Obstet., *34*:264, 1922.

Ferraro, V.: Innesti auto-ed omoplastici di pelle in orgen: e nei muscoli. Arch. Sci. Med. (Torino), *51*:149, 1927.

Firor, H. V.: Omphalocele—An appraisal of therapeutic approaches. Surgery, *69*:208, 1971.

Flynn, W. J., Brant, A. E., and Nelson, G. G.: Four and one-half year analysis of tantalum gauze used in the repair of ventral hernia. Ann. Surg., *134*:1027, 1951.

Fonkalsrud, E. W.: Personal communication, 1975.

Gallie, W. E.: Closing very large hernial openings. Ann. Surg., *96*:551, 1932.

Gerber, A.: Plastic repair following the removal of large desmoid tumors of the abdominal wall. Calif. Med., *65*:178, 1965.

Goepel, R.: Ueber die Verschliessung von Bruchpforten durch Einheilung geflochtener, fertiger Silberdrahtnetz. Verh. Dtsch. Ges. Chir., Berlin, *29*:174, 1900.

Grob, M.: Conservative treatment of exomphalos. Arch. Dis. Child., *38*:148, 1963.

Gross, R. E.: New method for surgical treatment of large omphaloceles. Surgery, *24*:277, 1948.

Gross, R. E.: The Surgery of Infancy and Childhood. Its Principles and Technique. Philadelphia, W. B. Saunders Company, 1953.

Halsted, W. S.: The radical cure of inguinal hernia in the male. Johns Hopkins Hospital Bull., *4*:17, 1893.

Halsted, W. S.: The case of the more difficult as well as the simple inguinal ruptures. Johns Hopkins Bull., *14*:203, 1903.

Hartwell, S. W.: The Mechanisms of Healing in Wounds. Springfield, Ill., Charles C Thomas, Publisher, 1955.

Hershey, F. B., and Butcher, H. P.: Repair of defects after partial resection of the abdominal wall. Am. J. Surg., *107*:586, 1964.

Hollabaugh, R. S., and Boles, E. T.: The management of gastroschisis. J. Pediatr. Surg., *8*:263, 1973.

Horton, C., Georgiade, N., Campbell, F., Masters, F., and Pickrell, K.: The behavior of split-thickness and dermal skin grafts in the peritoneal cavity. An experimental study. Plast. Reconstr. Surg., *12*:269, 1953.

Izant, R. J., Brown, F., and Rothmann, B. F.: Current embryology and treatment of gastroschisis and omphalocele. Arch. Surg., *93*:49, 1966.

Koontz, A. R., and Kimberly, R. C.: Tissue reactions to tantalum mesh and wire. Ann. Surg., *131*:666, 1950.

Koontz, A. R., and Kimberly, C. R.: Electron irradiated ox fascia and lyophilized dura mater. Arch. Surg., *82*:318, 1961.

Lesnick, G. N., and Davids, A. M.: Repair of surgical abdominal wall defect with pedicled musculofascial flap. Ann. Surg., *137*:569, 1953.

Lewis, J. E., Kraeger, R. R., and Danis, R. K.: Gastroschisis: Ten-year review. Arch. Surg., *107*:218, 1973.

McNally, J. B., Price, W. R., and MacDonald, W.: Gas gangrene of anterior abdominal wall. Am. J. Surg., *116*:779, 1968.

McPeak, C. J., and Miller, T. R.: Abdominal replacement. Surgery, *47*:944, 1960.

Mahour, G. H., Weitzman, J. J., and Rosenkrantz, J. G.: Omphalocele and gastroschisis. Ann. Surg., *177*:478, 1973.

Mansberger, A., Kang, J. S., Beebe, H. G., and Le Flore, L.: Repair of massive acute abdominal wall defects. J. Trauma, *13*:766, 1973.

Markgraf, W. H.: Abdominal wound deficiencies. A

technique for repair with Marlex mesh. Arch. Surg., *105*:728, 1972.

Maudsley, T., Rickham, P. P., and Roberts, J. R.: Long-term results of early operation on open myeloceles and encephaloceles. Br. Med. J., *1*:663, 1967.

Medgyesi, S.: The repair of large incisional hernias with pedicle skin flaps. Scand. J. Plast. Surg., *6*:69, 1972.

Meltzer, A.: Huge omphalocele ruptured *in utero*. J.A.M.A., *160*:656, 1956.

Meyer, W.: Implantation of filigree of silver wire in the cure of herniae usually considered inoperable, 1902.

Millard, D. R., Jr., Pigott, R., and Zies, P.: Free skin grafting of full-thickness defects of abdominal wall. Plast. Reconstr. Surg., *43*:569, 1969.

Mladick, R. A., Pickrell, K. L., Royer, J. R., McCraw, J., and Brown, I.: Skin graft reconstruction of a massive full-thickness abdominal wall defect. Plast. Reconstr. Surg., *43*:587, 1969.

Moore, T. C.: Gastroschisis with antenatal evisceration of intestines and urinary bladder. Ann. Surg., *158*:263, 1963.

Moore, T. C., and Stokes, G. E.: Gastroschisis. Surgery, *33*:112, 1953.

Morgan, A., Morain, W., and Eraklis, A.: Gas gangrene of the abdominal wall: Management after extensive debridement. Ann. Surg., *173*:617, 1971.

Morgan, S. C., and Zbylski, J. R.: Repair of massive soft tissue defects by open jump flaps. Plast. Reconstr. Surg., *50*:265, 1972.

Mustardé, J. C.: Meningomyelocele: The problem of skin cover. Br. J. Surg., *53*:36, 1966.

Nash, D. F. E.: Meningomyelocele: The problem of skin cover. Proc. R. Soc. Med., *56*:506, 1963.

Paterson, T. J.: The use of rotation flaps for excision of lumbar meningomyelocele. Br. J. Surg., *46*:606, 1959.

Pearce, A. E., and Entine, J. H.: Experimental studies using tantalum mesh as a full-thickness abdominal wall prosthesis. Am. J. Surg., *84*:182, 1952.

Pickrell, K. L.: Section on Plastic Surgery: Maxillofacial and Reconstructive Surgery. *In* Jonas, K. C. (Ed.): Babcock's Principles and Practice of Surgery. Philadelphia, Lea & Febiger, 1954, p. 169.

Poulard, A.: Traitement des cicatrices faciales. Presse Med., *26*:221, 1918.

Prpic, I., Belamaric, J., Sardesai, V., Walt, A. J., and Zamick, P.: Lyophilised corium grafts for repair of abdominal wall defect. Br. J. Plast. Surg., *26*:35, 1973.

Prpic, I., Belamaric, J., Rosenberg, J. C., Sardesai, V., Walt, A. J., and Zamick, P.: Use of xenograft coverage for reconstruction of abdominal wall defect. Br. J. Plast. Surg., *27*:125, 1974.

Rayner, C. R. W.: Repair of full-thickness defects of the abdominal wall in rats avoiding visceral adhesions. Br. J. Plast. Surg., *27*:130, 1974.

Rehn, E.: Verh. Dtsch. Ges. Chir., I Teil, S., *87*:390, 1911.

Rickham, P. P.: Rupture of exomphalos and gastroschisis. Arch. Dis. Child., *38*:138, 1963.

Sanders, G. B.: Gas gangrene of the abdominal wall. XX Congrès de la Société Internationale de Chirurgie, 1963.

Schmitt, H. J., Jr., and Grinnon, G. L.: Use of Marlex mesh in infected abdominal war wounds. Am. J. Surg., *113*:825, 1967.

Schmitt, H. J., Jr., Patterson, L. T., and Armstrong, R. C.: Re-operative surgery of abdominal wall wounds. Ann. Surg., *165*:173, 1967.

Schuster, S. R.: A new method for the staged repair of large omphalocele. Surg. Gynecol. Obstet., *125*:837, 1967.

Schwartz, S. I. (Ed.): Infection. *In* Principles in Surgery. New York, McGraw-Hill, 1969.

Sewell, W. H., and Koth, D. R.: Homologous and heterologous freeze-dried fascia used to repair diaphragmatic and abdominal wall defects. Surg. Forum, 6:351, 1955.

Sharrard, W. J.: Meningomyelocele: Prognosis of immediate operative closure of sac. Proc. R. Soc. Med., 56:501, 1963.

Shim, W. K. T.: Surgical treatment of gastroschisis. Arch. Surg., 102:524, 1971.

Simpson, T. E., and Lynn, H. B.: Omphalocele: Results of surgical treatment. Mayo Clin. Proc., 43:65, 1968.

Smith, W. R., and Leix, F.: Omphalocele. Am. J. Surg., 111:450, 1966.

Soave, F.: Conservative treatment of giant omphalocele. Arch. Dis. Child., 38:130, 1963.

Soper, R. T., and Green, E. W.: Omphalocele. Surg. Gynecol. Obstet., 112:501, 1961.

Stephenson, K. L.: A new approach to the treatment of abdominal muscular agenesis. Plast. Reconstr. Surg., 12:413, 1953.

Strömbeck, I. O.: Mammaplasty: Report of a new technique based on the two pedicle procedure. Br. J. Plast. Surg., 13:79, 1960.

Thompson, N.: A clinical and histological investigation into the fate of epithelial elements buried following the grafting of "shaved" skin surfaces. Br. J. Plast. Surg., 13:219, 1960.

Thompson, N.: Surgical treatment of chronic lymphoedema of the lower limb. With preliminary report of new operation. Br. J. Med., 26:1, 1962.

Throckmorton, T. D.: Tantalum gauze in the repair of hernias complicated by tissue deficiency. Surgery, 23:32, 1948.

Usher, F. C.: A new plastic prosthesis for repairing tissue defects of the chest and abdominal wall. Am. J. Surg., 97:623, 1954.

Usher, F. C., and Gannon, J. P.: Marlex mesh: A new plastic for replacing tissue defects. Experimental studies. Arch. Surg., 78:131, 1959.

Usher, F. C., and Wallace, S. A.: Tissue reactions to plastics. A.M.A. Arch. Surg., 76:99, 1958.

Wangensteen, O. H.: Large defects of the abdominal wall employing the iliotibial tract of fascia lata as a pedicled flap. Surg. Gynecol. Obstet., 59:766, 1934.

Wangensteen, O. H.: Repair of large abdominal defects by pedicled fascial flaps. Surg. Gynecol. Obstet., 82:144, 1946.

Wayne, E. R., and Burrington, J. D.: Gastroschisis: A systemic approach to management. Am. J. Dis. Child., 125:218, 1973.

Webster, J. P.: Thoracoepigastric tubed pedicles. Surg. Clin. North Am., 17:145, 1937.

Welch, K. L.: Use of homograft in the treatment of omphaloceles. Surgery, 29:100, 1951.

Wilson, J. S. P., and Rayner, C. R. W.: The repair of large full-thickness post-excisional defects of the abdominal wall. Br. J. Plast. Surg., 27:117, 1974.

Witzel, O.: Ueber den Verschluss von Bauchwunden und Bruchpforten durch versenkte Silberdrahtnets. Zentralbl. Chir., 27:257, 1900.

Ye, R. C., Devine, K. D., and Kirklin, J. W.: Extensive recurrent desmoid tumor of the abdominal wall: Radical excision followed by reconstruction of abdominal wall with plastic procedure. Report of a case. Plast. Reconstr. Surg., 12:59, 1953.

# CHAPTER 91

# THE PRESSURE SORE

Ross M. Campbell, M.D.,
and José P. Delgado, M.D.

By definition a pressure sore is generally considered to be an area of ulceration and necrosis of the skin occurring in any part of the body but usually over an underlying bony prominence which is subject to prolonged or often repeated pressure. Such areas of ulceration are also known as bedsores and decubitus ulcers.* Sir James Paget (1873) was among the first to ascribe the etiology of bedsores to pressure, saying that such sores were "the sloughing and mortification or death of a part produced by pressure," usually over bony prominences. They are a common accompaniment of prolonged confinement, whether to bed or to a wheelchair, and they are found with increased frequency in all forms of paralysis, including paraplegia, quadriplegia, and hemiplegia. They range in severity from the incipient bedsore, in which there may be simple erythema of the skin without an actual break in the epidermal surface, through all stages of destruction of tissue, including skin, fat, muscle, and bone. Because of their occurrence, rehabilitative measures may be postponed, and morbidity is often severe and prolonged; if they are uncontrolled and infection develops, death may ensue.

---

*"Decubitus" is the past participle of the Latin verb "decubare," to lie down, and should be reserved for the description of pressure ulcers which develop when the patient is recumbent. The term "pressure sore" is preferable.

## HISTORY

Although Holmes (1915) made the first serious attempt to analyze paraplegia resulting from gunshot wounds, treatment of these lesions was essentially nonsurgical until 1945. There may have been many reasons for this lag, chief among them being the fact that rehabilitation of paralyzed patients was not undertaken in an organized fashion until World War II. Since the lesions are generally of a disagreeable nature, imagination was not stimulated to find a surgical solution. Cannon, O'Leary, O'Neil, and Steinsieck (1950) stated that Scoville, at Cushing General Hospital during the war, advocated surgical closure. Lamon and Alexander (1945) are credited in the literature with the first report of the surgical closure of decubitus ulcers with protective systemic coverage by penicillin. It is likely that the introduction of antibiotics enhanced surgical courage to the extent that a surgical procedure in contaminated tissues could be done as an elective procedure. Most writers credit Davis (1938) with the idea of using flap replacement of scar epithelium in healed ulcers to provide bulky and well-padded skin coverage over bony prominences.

A significant contribution to the overall therapy, not of a surgical but of a nutritional nature, was made by Mulholland and coworkers in 1943. Through the use of amino acid and dextrose dietary supplements, which restored positive nitrogen balance in a mixed group of general surgical and paraplegic patients, relatively rapid healing of pressure sores was reported.

Other reports of the surgical treatment of pressure sores in the World War II wounded appeared in the literature. Among these were papers by Barker (1945), White, Hudson, and Kennard (1945), Gibbon and Freeman (1946), Croce, Schullinger, and Shearer (1946), Barker, Elkins, and Poer (1946), White and Hamm (1946), and Croce and Beakes (1947). Technical advances followed quickly thereafter until most surgeons began to favor the large single pedicle type of flap for resurfacing the defect.

Recommendations for the removal of bony prominences were also reported (Kostrubala and Greeley, 1947; Blocksma, Kostrubala, and Greeley, 1949). These writers recommended the removal of the tuberosity of the ischium. Conway and coworkers (1951) stated that they had increased their operative successes in ischial ulcers from 47 per cent before using ischiectomy to 81 per cent after its adoption. To counteract the enthusiasm for this method of radical bone removal, sometimes referred to as total prophylactic ischiectomy, Comarr and Bors (1958) reported an incidence of perineourethral diverticula in 46 per cent of patients with spinal cord injuries in whom the ischium had been removed as part of the operation. When bilateral total ischiectomy was performed, the incidence was 58 per cent. In this regard it should be noted that Chase (1962) urged extreme caution in radical bone excision, and Guthrie and Conway (1969) admitted that there was a high rate of perineal ulcer development following total ischiectomy.

That interest in this challenging problem has not waned is evidenced by the continuing flow of published reports. Radical measures, such as bilateral high thigh amputation with the use of residual thigh skin flaps to cover large remaining defects, have been described (Georgiade, Pickrell, and Maguire, 1956; Chase and White, 1959; Berkas, Chesler, and Sako, 1961; Spira and Hardy, 1963; Royer, Pickrell, Georgiade, Mladick, and Thorne, 1969). Continuing research into treatment includes large island flap coverage of extensive ulcers (Weeks and Brower, 1968); the use of the skin of nearly the entire lower leg skin, including the sole of the foot, by filleting and amputating in the mid-femoral area (Burkhardt, 1972); and the use of a gluteal muscle flap (Stallings, Delgado, and Converse, 1974). There is also continuing research into the causation of, and the possibility of prevention of, pressure sores.

Causation has been demonstrated by controlled investigation conducted in the laboratory with animals (rats, guinea pigs, and dogs) and with human beings; conclusions have been drawn by experimental proof (Brooks and Duncan, 1940; Groth, 1942; Husain, 1953; Kosiak, Kubicek, Olson, Danz, and Kottle, 1958; Kosiak, 1959).

Gelb (1952) estimated that there were 2000 to 2500 spinal cord injuries among U.S. troops in World War II and proportionally similar occurrences in the troops of the allies and enemy troops. Increasing civilian mechanization in industry and transportation and increasing participation in recreation cannot fail to send more and more victims to the hospital with spinal cord injuries. "The increase in morbidity of the elderly patient, chronically ill and disabled as a result of decubitus ulcer has persisted since the beginning of man and even in this era of modern medicine continues to be a frequent and serious complication seemingly accentuated by greater life expectancy with the inevitable increase in chronic illness" (Schell and Wolcott, 1966). Therefore, the spotlight of hope directed toward the reclamation of many of these sadly disabled people by workers in the field of rehabilitation, such as Rusk and his colleagues, should be of interest and inspiration to the surgical worker in the field. In addition, there has been a greater governmental interest, as well as concern on the part of voluntary social agencies. Finally, the insurance companies who bear a heavy financial burden for the care of many of the victims of accident or disease must be encouraged to support research at both the clinical and laboratory levels to the ultimate benefit of the afflicted individual, his family, and the community.

## ETIOLOGY

The single most important factor in the causation of pressure sores is excessive pressure. While other factors play a contributory role, unrelieved pressure for periods variously estimated at from 1 to 12 hours is the major etiologic agent. Landis in 1930, using a microinjection method to study capillary blood pressure, reported an average pressure of 32 mm Hg in the arteriolar limb, 20 mm Hg in the mid-capillary bed, and 12 mm Hg in the venous side. Kosiak and coworkers (1958) showed that even with 5-cm foam rubber seat cushions, the pressure on the skin under the ischial tuberosities and surrounding areas averaged in excess of 150 mm Hg. Prolonged pressure, therefore, must inevitably lead to ischemia and necrosis.

The lowering of the nutritional status, whether by infection, starvation, or inanition, plays an important role in the formation of pressure sores. Hubay, Kiehn, and Drucker (1957) felt that a disturbed metabolic state is necessary for both their formation and their chronicity. While one might agree as to chronicity, it is not essential that the metabolic state be disturbed. Pressure sores have been known to develop within a few days in healthy young adult males suddenly immobilized because of accident or disease.

Neurotrophic factors have been invoked to explain the development of pressure sores in the past, but substantiating proof has so far failed to materialize. Charcot (1879) believed that damage to trophic centers regulating nutrition resulted in development of "neurotic necrosis" when aided by local pressure, but Brown-Séquard (1853), using small paralyzed animals (transection of the cord), prevented development of ulcers by keeping the areas clean and free of pressure. However, according to Nojarova (1962), who made a study of the Russian literature, the neurotrophic factor is considered of primary importance in that country. In essence, although there is disagreement concerning the roles of the autonomic nervous system and the central nervous system, there appears to be agreement on the effect of overstimulation of the autonomic nervous system. When this occurs there is a change in local metabolism through disturbance of reflex control of skin circulation. As a result, pathologic changes occur, leading to the development of an ulcer. By interrupting or altering nerve impulse transmission, by achieving a "slowdown effect" through infiltration with a weak procaine solution, the trophic function of the nerves is allegedly restored.

At present, the authors are not prepared to accept this theory, since it is possible that other factors relating to the correct diagnosis and recovery of spinal cord or root lesions may play a more important role than procaine injections.

Munro (1940), on the other hand, believed that interruption by cord injury of the autonomic reflex arcs which control skin circulation resulted in a lessened ability of the skin to react to pressure.

**Experimental Studies.** Research into the effects of pressure has been reported by Groth (1942) and Brooks and Duncan (1940). In a series of experiments in rabbits, both paralyzed and normal, Groth subjected the shaved gluteal regions to different pressures transmitted by a simple lever device for varying periods of time. The effect on the treated areas was observed both macroscopically and microscopically. Animals of 2 to 3 kilograms were exposed to a surface pressure of 143 mm Hg for three to four hours. Macroscopic changes were seen after a few days. The changes consisted of slight swelling, redness, and small hemorrhages and progressed to well-circumscribed foci of necrosis, light grayish red to yellow gray in color, surrounded by a narrow reddish zone. At times the well-circumscribed foci were missing, and the changes appeared as distinct stripes running in the direction of the muscle fibers. No changes were apparent in the nerves and larger blood vessels of the area. On microscopic examination there were capillary hemorrhages, waxy degeneration of Zenker, vacuolation, or loss of striation, followed on the second to third day after pressure application by calcification in some of the necrotic muscle fibers. Phagocytosis, with beginning interstitial proliferation producing granulation tissue which formed a wall of demarcation around the necrotic musculature, was also observed. Seven days following the application of pressure, a collagenous ground substance developed, leading to scar formation. Even in the animals that showed no macroscopic changes, there were microscopic alterations such as described previously. As one might suspect, the longer the duration of pressure, the greater the extent of the changes.

Among the conclusions drawn by Groth were the following:

1. Pressure sores simulating those found in man can be produced experimentally.

2. Decubiti occur more frequently in flaccid paralytics than in spastics.

3. The larger the muscle mass, the greater the ability to withstand pressure.

4. The effective pressure force increases toward the smaller surface. This accounts for the greater destruction of tissue found at the base of the inverted cone, typified by the small area of skin redness or destruction overlying a bony prominence, such as the trochanter. As one progresses more deeply into the wound, a wider area of destruction is seen until the width reaches its maximum at the level of the bony prominence. This condition is frequently observed in both ischial and trochanteric ulcers and even to a lesser degree over the sacrum.

5. Generalized sepsis in an animal leads to

local infection at the site of pressure, with abscess formation, extension of inflammation, thrombosis of the larger vessels, and consequently broader distribution of tissue necrosis. However, large vessel thrombosis per se is not a cause of ulceration because of the extensive collateral circulation usually present.

Kosiak (1959), in a well-controlled experiment using healthy dogs subjected to accurately controlled pressures ranging from 100 to 550 mm Hg for periods of 1 to 12 hours, came to the same conclusion, i.e., that prolonged pressure was the direct and main cause of pressure sores. Microscopic examination of tissue obtained 24 hours after the application of 60 mm Hg pressure for only one hour showed cellular infiltration, extravasation, and hyalin degeneration. Tissue subjected to higher pressures for longer periods of time showed, in addition, muscular degeneration and venous thrombosis. He concluded that intense pressure of short duration was as injurious to tissue as lower pressures of longer duration. The tissue ischemia in both cases led to irreversible cellular changes producing ultimate necrosis and ulceration.

Kosiak disagreed with Groth in regard to the location and degree of severity of the changes, stating that they extended equally throughout the area under pressure instead of being most severe at the deepest part overlying the bony prominence. His conclusion was that skin and subcutaneous tissue act to provide a sling or suspension effect, with the result that only a fraction of the applied pressure is transmitted to the deep tissues.

Brooks and Duncan (1940) noted the development of dry gangrene in dogs' legs following the application of a tourniquet for 17 hours. Husain (1953) reported microscopic changes in rat muscle subjected to a pressure of 100 mm Hg for as little as one hour. His microscopic findings were essentially similar to those reported by Groth (1942) and Kosiak (1959).

Changes in capillary blood flow experimentally produced showed greater instability at low perfusion pressures, and these were reported by Nichol and associates (1951), who noted cessation or temporary reversal of flow at a low positive pressure. In 1951 Burton and Yamada also described the so-called transmural arterial pressure as pressure ranging from 20 to 30 mm Hg less than the mean arterial pressure, at which point there is a cessation of flow of arterial blood in the forearm of a man.

One of the earliest workers, Landis (1930), using microinjection techniques, reported that the average pressure in the arteriolar limb was 32 mm Hg and increased to 50 mm Hg during histamine flare.

McLennan, McLennan and Landis (1942), following the work of Landis, established a normal range of capillary pressure of from 16 to 33 mm Hg. It thus follows, according to Kosiak (1959), that complete tissue ischemia might be present when pressures slightly in excess of average capillary blood pressures are applied to the body, thus affirming the desirability and need for frequent changes of position.

**Clinical Aspects.**   The loss of subcutaneous fat and a diminished muscle mass are conducive to the development of undue pressure over bony prominences. Anemia, hypoproteinemia, vitamin deficiency, and lowered skin resistance, through poor personal hygiene which results in maceration of the skin surfaces, may contribute to the development of a pressure sore or ulcer. Carelessness on the part of the attendants or the patient, whereby a "brush burn" may be inflicted by rapid passage of a body part over a sheet or by traumatizing the skin against the arm of a wheel chair, may cause skin damage. The chafing of casts and brace straps and the use of too small a wheelchair or a poorly padded seat on the chair have been responsible for the development of either superficial skin breakdown or ischemia followed by tissue necrosis in the deeper layers. Even the time-honored alcohol rub followed by dusting with talcum powder has been implicated by Bateman (1956). He felt he could improve the results and save much nursing time by having pressure areas washed only twice a week, unless they were badly soiled, without soap, alcohol rub, or talcum powder. In place of powder he used a thin layer of silicone cream smeared on the skin. Ward (1963) also described the use of silicone cream.

Circulatory stasis and edema due to impairment of venous or lymphatic drainage consequent upon the loss of muscular activity (Exton-Smith and Crockett, 1957) may contribute to the devitalization of the part and can be partially corrected by either passive or active movement. Griffith (1966) suggested that early ambulation helped to preserve muscle tone, improved circulation, helped to avoid prolonged pressure at certain points, and arrested soft tissue calcification.

Rough removal of adhesive tape, poor protection of skin surfaces, burns by excessively hot water bottles or heat lamps, and the shearing forces acting on sacral and buttock skin by the simple maneuver of raising the invalid's bed to a sitting position (Reichel, 1958) are included among the many extrinsic factors contributing to ulceration.

Petersen and Bittmann (1971), in a study of a population of 517,000 Danes localized to the County of Arhus, found an incidence of 61.5 pressure sores per 100,000, with the frequency increasing steeply with advancing age. In about 50 per cent of the patients, the sores had developed during hospital stays.

Perhaps because of better habits of personal hygiene accompanied by a greater sense of personal welfare, pressure sores seem to occur less frequently in the female than in the male. Harding (1961), in an analysis of 100 rehabilitated paraplegics, reported that 78 were males and 22 were females; in his opinion, this disproportionate figure was explained by the fact that men are more naturally exposed to injury and the hazards of traffic, work, and warfare. Sanchez, Eamegdool, and Conway (1969) reported a change in etiology between 1964 and 1968, during which interval vehicular accidents rose from 25 per cent in the 1964 group of paraplegics to 37 per cent in the 1969 series. This development could change the distribution by sex, since so many automobile accidents involve both sexes. Wars presumably will always show a preponderance of male involvement.

The etiologic factors are manifold, being a combination of intrinsic and extrinsic elements, *but the principal cause is pressure, working alone or in combination.*

**Paraplegia in Relation to Pressure Sores.** Paraplegia may be caused by trauma or disease. Holdsworth (1954) has made important observations on traumatic paraplegia that might have some bearing on our understanding of the problem of ulcer development at certain sites and might influence the management of patients from the inception of the paraplegia. His study of 71 patients showed that correct nursing care, careful attention to simple bladder drainage, and proper rehabilitation measures resulted in an avoidance of all serious complications, maintenance of the general health of the patient, and a reduction in hospitalization to an average of 9 to 10 months. In these patients not one serious bedsore developed, and in reviewing his paper, one is impressed with the care exercised in the diagnostic assessment of the injury, a factor which must have been reflected in the notable results achieved.

THE TYPE AND LEVEL OF THE LESION. First, the level of the lesion must be accurately determined. Since the spinal cord ends at the lower border of L1 (Fig. 91–1), any lesion below this level is purely a root lesion, and regeneration after transection is possible, whereas in a true cord lesion, there is no potential for regeneration. The prognosis in a root paralysis is better. The initial effect of a severe injury of the spinal cord is suppression of function below the level of the lesion. This suppression may be anatomical, in whole or in part, or physiologic. In the latter case, the capability of recovery exists. The extent of recovery is directly related to the severity and extent of the anatomical division. Partial recovery of power and sensation occurs with partial division. If the cord is completely divided, the isolated segments recover local reflex activity, and the paralysis is of the upper motor neuron type, but anesthesia remains unchanged. When the anatomical division of the roots is complete, a flaccid paralysis will occur eventually.

During the period of suppression of function, it is impossible to determine the extent of the anatomical damage to the cord, and as long as the condition persists, there is uncertainty as to the possibility of recovery of any cord function. As a result, there is controversy about the initial treatment of these injuries: (1) If the cord is divided, no known form of treatment alters the prognosis. Therefore, in a complete transection of the cord, when the diagnosis is not in doubt, the patient can be started immediately on a routine of turning without fear of causing further damage. (2) If the cord is intact, there will be some recovery without treatment as long as it is protected from further injury. This means that a certain amount of immobilization is essential, a course which complicates the preventive therapy of pressure sores. (3) In partial lesions, decompression by laminectomy or cordotomy may assist recovery. If laminectomy is indicated, there should be an open operation as soon as warranted, with internal fixation allowing routine turning of the patient to be started.

During the initial period of *spinal shock*, the paralysis is flaccid in nature. As a result many of these patients are left in the supine position in which undue pressure against the bony prominences of the occiput, thorax, sacrum, and heels may be allowed to develop. At these points, pressure sores may appear rapidly unless care is used to prevent prolonged pressure. In the patient with injury without transection, some function may return after several weeks. Isolated cord segments may regain some function, and reflexes may reappear. The paralysis which was flaccid during the shock period becomes spastic or of the upper motor neuron type and may lead to the development of ulcers in quite different

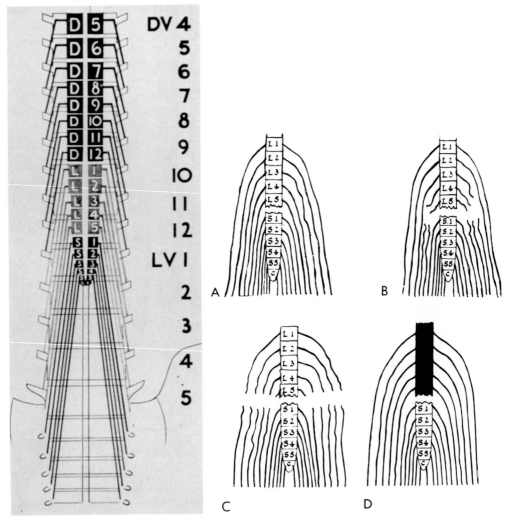

**FIGURE 91–1.** *Left,* The relationships of the vertebrae of the spinal cord and nerve roots. *Right,* Types of nerve damage. *A,* Cord divided; complete root escape. *B,* Cord divided; partial root escape. *C,* Cord and all roots divided. *D,* Cord divided; destruction of gray matter of lumbar segments. (From Holdsworth, F. W.: Traumatic paraplegia. Ann. R. Coll. Surg., *15:*281, 1954.)

sites. If the patient is still restricted to bed, he may be turned on his side, incurring the risk of developing ulcers over the greater trochanters, or there may be spastic pressure of knee rubbing against knee or internal malleolus against internal malleolus, which combined with friction and maceration may result in ulcers in these areas. If the patient has been allowed to assume a sitting position and is not carefully instructed concerning the avoidance of pressure, he may develop ischial ulcers as well as ulcers along the margins of the plantar surface of the heel and foot.

In *spinal concussion*, the initial effects are the same as in so-called spinal shock, but there is a return to normal motor and sensory function eventually. The latter shows some sign of recovery in a few hours, and Holdsworth (1954) stated

that he had never seen total motor and sensory loss following concussion. Recovery commences with the appearance of sensation or motor power or both. The return of any sensation in any segments, no matter how perverted, leads to the expectation of further recovery, and one can be certain that the cord is not transected. However, the failure of sensation to reappear or the occurrence of reflex activity of any kind other than anal or bulbocavernosus without sensory or motor activity indicates that there has been a transection of the cord.

When there is complete paralysis and anesthesia due to a root lesion that is extensive, the root should be freed of pressure and protected from further injury.

Lesions above D10 are pure cord lesions with

only a few unimportant roots involved, whereas fracture-dislocations below L1 are pure root lesions. If the cord lesion is partial and the vertebral fracture is stabilized without resorting to internal fixation, turning of the patient in bed will not be dangerous.

External fixation or splinting in a plaster bed, a treatment which had been advocated in the past, is conducive to the development of pressure sores.

THE EFFECT OF SPASTICITY. Spasticity, which not only contributes to the development of bedsores but also presents a serious surgical obstacle, has been reported as occurring in 40 per cent of the patients of Cannon, O'Leary, O'Neil and Steinsieck (1950) and in 54 per cent of the patients in the series of Pollock and coworkers (1951). The cord stump has been referred to by Scarff and Pool (1946) as a trigger zone upon which afferent stimuli from the posterior roots may fall, evoking a reflex response in the muscle masses below the lesion. Pollock and coworkers (1951), on the basis of their clinical observations, stated that the higher the cord lesion, the higher the incidence of spasticity in mass reflex, e.g., 96 per cent in the cervical region, 40 per cent in the lumbar. An understanding of the neurologic factors involved is essential because of the possible prevention of ulcers through the ability to predict the sites most likely to be involved, and because such information guides the surgical treatment of pressure sores located in regions subject to considerable movement as a result of spasticity. The subject of spasticity relief will be developed further when such forms of treatment as alcohol washes, phenol injection (Griffiith, 1966), anterior and posterior rhizotomy, and their physical and psychologic effects are described.

**Experimental Studies Dealing with the Production, Prophylaxis, and Therapy of Cord Injuries.** Investigation of the histopathology of controlled spinal cord trauma in experimental animals has shown that spreading hemorrhage produces increasingly greater degenerative changes in the cord (Wagner, Dohrmann, Taslits, Albin, and White, 1969), indicating the importance of the time factor to the effects of reversible and irreversible trauma, with progressive hemorrhagic necrosis of the spinal cord as the end result (Ducker and Assenmacher, 1969).

Ducker and Assenmacher (1969) have also defined a 300 gram-centimeter concussion-contusion applied to animal spinal cord as a reversible force, i.e., the early paralysis caused may represent contusion to the neural element with associated conduction loss. Recovery is possible because the nutritional state of the spinal cord is maintained. However, irreversible trauma occurs with a 500 gram-centimeter force, and neuronal recovery is not possible because of inadequate spinal cord nutrition.

Circulatory changes seen following the initial trauma progress over the next 48 hours with marked inflammatory response in the vessel walls, increased leakage from the vascular system, and progressive hemorrhagic necrosis of the spinal cord. Cord edema is enhanced, and the authors feel the combination leads to the development of an intramedullary hematoma. Under these circumstances the nutritional state of the spinal cord becomes irreversibly impaired, and neuronal recovery becomes an impossibility.

With these findings in mind, it follows that any factor that prevents or retards this progressively destructive mechanism must be investigated.

Steroid therapy by parenteral administration, as used by Ducker and Hamit (1969), has been shown to be of value in preventing permanent paraplegia in traumatized beagles, as compared with untreated control animals subjected to the same force and left permanently paralyzed.

Drug therapy is the subject of considerable research by Osterholm and associates (1971). The investigation, which offers the ultimate possibility of prevention or reduction of disability following cord trauma, has led to a technique of injecting alpha methyl tyrosine (A.M.T.) within 15 minutes of the infliction of trauma.

Alpha methyl tyrosine, a highly toxic drug which has a deleterious nephrotoxic effect and can lead to uremia and death, has been used only in laboratory cats. It has the effect of providing chemical protection against hemorrhagic cord injury by acting against norepinephrine, a chemical essential for spinal cord function. After cord trauma, it accumulates in concentration in the tissues and leads to additional cord destruction by vasospasm, hemorrhage, sloughing, and major tissue destruction. Hemorrhage within the cat's cord begins about one hour after trauma and increases in severity over the next few hours until beginning necrosis occurs in the fourth hour, and complete destruction results by 24 hours.

Alpha methyl tyrosine given to cats within 15 minutes of spinal trauma (500 gram-centimeter force) inhibits the destructive action of norepinephrine and prevents hemorrhagic necrosis. Approximately 75 per cent of the animals treated walked normally or with minor extremity weakness. While the nephrotoxic effects of alpha methyl tyrosine cannot be controlled in humans, other norepinephrine antagonists are currently under study and offer promise of medical control of spinal cord injuries.

## PATHOLOGY OF PRESSURE SORES

**Gross Pathology.** Although there is an inclination to think of these lesions only in terms of their chronicity, it should be realized that there is an acute phase (Fig. 91–2). This may take the form of erythema or redness, due to pressure, then pass through the stages of swelling, blistering, cyanosis, and beginning tissue necrosis. It is frequently found that the acute phase may be reversed by relief of pressure and other measures. Although the senior author recommended moderate heat to accompany the relief of pressure in the first edition of this text, Kosiak and associates (1958) feel that it should not be used because it increases the metabolic requirements in an area already impoverished with regard to blood supply and thus may lead to additional tissue ischemia.

An incipient pressure sore may be mistaken for an ischiorectal or other form of acute abscess and may be incised for drainage of pus which is not present. Instead of pus, grayish yellow necrotic fat may be exposed. This may become infected after incision, with resultant further destruction of tissue, followed by the development of a craterlike defect. Occasionally, if there is infection elsewhere in the body, organisms may settle in the traumatized area, even though the skin covering may be intact. In such cases, pus and necrotic fat may be apparent following incision of the area.

In ulcers of the chronic form, there generally is deep destruction extending from skin and fat through fascia, muscle, and synovial membrane, if adjacent to a joint, and even into the joint. Osteitis or osteomyelitis with bone destruction may be present. In the most advanced cases, dislocations and pathologic fractures are commonly present.

The ulcer of long standing that has passed through periods of repeated healing and breakdown may show considerable growth of marginal scar epithelium of a thin, shiny nature with wide surrounding zones of dense scar tissue. The granulation tissue may be pale and purulent with little or no sign of activity because of the gradual impairment of the blood supply by the progressive vascular constriction caused by the dense scarring at the base. Some chronic ulcers show evidence of arrested epithelial ingrowth from the margin, resulting in turned in, curled margins. This is especially true of deep ulcers in which it is impossible for the epithelium to line

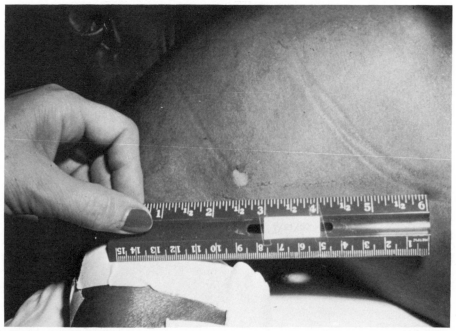

**FIGURE 91–2.**    Early pressure sore of the axillary fold region resulting from a Stryker frame.

the edges of the sides of the ulcer, owing to the failure of granulation tissue to grow upward and thus eliminate deep pockets.

The products of bacterial invasion and tissue breakdown form a foul-smelling, purulent discharge which in itself is destructive of new epithelium. The continuous discharge of proteolyzed material leads to protein deficiency, anemia, temperature fluctuation, malaise, and a general lowering of the constitutional status.

Among the infecting organisms are staphylococci, streptococci, *Pseudomonas aeruginosa, Escherichia coli, B. proteus,* and others, often in combination. The character of the purulent exudate, i.e., consistency and color, depends on the major infecting organism. Systemic administration of antibiotics, selectively matched to the infecting organism, is useful at times. However, their value is questionable in older chronic ulcers with heavy scarring and thrombosed vessels, factors which prevent access of the antibiotic to the ulcer.

The suppurative process may track great distances along fascial planes, establishing ramifying sinus tracts (Lopez and Aranha, 1974), penetrating bursae, entering joint cavities through the destruction of the joint capsule, and causing septic arthritis or joint destruction and dislocation (Fig. 91–3). Genitourinary complications, septicemia, and death may occur (Campbell, 1959).

In a retrospective autopsy study (Dalton, Hackler, and Bunts, 1965) of paraplegic patients, secondary amyloidosis was found in 40 per cent of those surviving the initial injury by at least one year. Seventy per cent of this subgroup died of renal failure secondary to renal amyloidosis. Chronic bedsores were a major factor in the development of amyloidosis in the paraplegic.

In summary, it can be stated that pressure sore ulcers may take two major forms or may represent a combination of the two. They may start as superficial lesions involving skin alone, or skin and fat, and may be treated in the early stages in a conservative fashion, because the condition is reversible if the ischemic tissue receives pressure relief and an enhanced oxygen supply. For the latter serial transfusions (Matheson and Lipschitz, 1956; Kosiak, 1959) increase the oxygen-carrying component. The use of hyperbaric oxygen has been described by Fischer (1969) in diabetic ulcers, stasis ulcers, and pressure sores of varying sizes with reported encouraging results. The second form may appear as an area of reddening of the skin with a small opening or no opening at all. Beneath the surface, however, there is widespread destruction in a cone-shaped area extending through all layers of tissue down to and even including bone.

**Histopathology.** These lesions are indistinguishable from other (nonspecific chronic) ul-

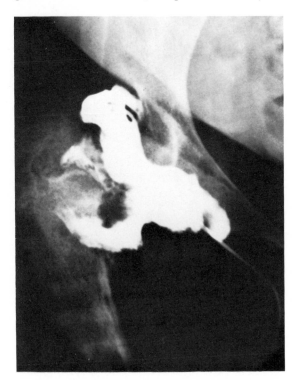

**FIGURE 91–3.** Sinogram showing communication between an ischial pressure sore and the hip joint. (Courtesy of Dr. J. G. McCarthy, Institute of Reconstructive Plastic Surgery.)

cers except in their extent. In the early stages of redness and swelling, there is vascular dilatation and interstitial edema, followed by epidermal separation, capillary clotting and hemorrhage, Zenker's waxy degeneration of muscle fibers, vacuolation, and death of tissue cells. Cellular infiltration of the affected tissues by neutrophils and lymphocytes occurs. Phagocytosis is increased, and a wall of demarcation formed by interstitial proliferation develops around the necrotic area.

Deposition of collagen in the granulation tissue at the base and margins of the ulcer may become so heavy that wound healing is seriously impaired. Thrombosis of larger vessels progresses, with the development of successively greater areas of tissue necrosis. Calcific deposits may be identified at times in necrotic muscle fibers.

## CLINICAL ASPECTS

It is helpful to attempt to assess the lesions and thus their treatment according to seven clinically distinct developmental stages (Campbell, 1959).

1. Simple skin erythema over a pressure area. This is considered reversible in most instances and will subside if pressure is relieved.

2. Redness, swelling, and induration, with occasional blistering and desquamation of epidermis. This condition may be reversible if there is immediate and prolonged relief of pressure combined with wound hygiene.

3. Skin destruction with fat exposure. If relief of pressure and wound hygiene are instituted immediately and if the area is small, there may be spontaneous epithelization. If pressure relief is inadequate or infection supervenes, destruction of tissue may be progressive.

4. Necrosis of skin and fat extending to fascia or muscle. Surgical treatment is indicated after debridement and a trial period of conservative therapy.

5. A combination of skin, fat, and muscle necrosis almost invariably requires surgical intervention at an early date.

6. Bone involvement in the form of periostitis, osteitis, or osteomyelitis. While early conservative measures of therapy, including pressure relief, wound hygiene, and debridement, are indicated, there is little hope that spontaneous healing will occur. Even if healing does occur, the covering of epithelial scar is so thin and vulnerable to minimal trauma that one should not waste time on prolonged conservative measures of therapy.

7. All of the above features plus osteomyelitis, septic arthritis, possible pathologic fracture or gross dislocation of joints, septicemia, and possible death. This state should never be reached in a modern hospital, but it is still seen from time to time, particularly in the quadriplegic patient.

**Sites of Occurrence.** Knowledge of the sites of predilection is useful from the standpoint of prophylaxis.

Yeoman and Hardy (1954), in a detailed analysis of 240 pressure sores in paraplegics, reported the following sites of involvement:

| SITE | NUMBER | PERCENTAGE |
|---|---|---|
| Ischium | 68 | 28 |
| Sacrum | 64 | 27 |
| Heel | 44 | 18 |
| Trochanter | 27 | 12 |
| External malleoli | 20 | 8 |
| Tibial crest | 10 | 4 |
| Anterosuperior spine | 5 | 2 |
| Costal margin | 2 | 1 |
| Total | 240 | 100 |

In a review of 1604 pressure sores in paraplegics, Dansereau and Conway (1964) reported the following anatomical distribution:

| | |
|---|---|
| Ischial tuberosity | 28% |
| Trochanter | 19% |
| Sacrum | 17% |
| Heel | 9% |
| Malleolus | 5% |
| Pretibial | 5% |
| Patella | 4% |
| Foot | 3% |
| Anterosuperior spine | 2.5% |
| Elbow | 1.5% |
| Miscellaneous | 6% |

Petersen and Bittman (1971), in a study of pressure sores in and around the County of Aarhus, Denmark, found that in 63 per cent of patients, they developed while in the hospital. Sacral, ischial, and trochanteric sores were the most common; 10 per cent of the sores were found in ambulatory patients; 37 per cent were in wheelchair patients, and 53 per cent in bedridden patients.

The factors determining the site of involvement are many and include the state of paralysis—whether flaccid or spastic—whether or not the patient is bedridden, and, if so, whether he is supine or prone. He may be in a wheelchair or may possibly be wearing braces, and, if so, certain sites are more subject to pressure than others. The location of the patient's bed in relation to his roommates (Gelb, 1952) or to a television set or window view may determine the site of involvement, since he may spend long hours watching the television screen or facing away from a wall and conversing with his roommates.

The early weeks after the onset of accident or disease are generally a period of flaccid paralysis and loss of vasomotor control, both being factors that contribute to tissue breakdown. The patient generally lies supine, with changes of position to the side. Thus it is to be expected that sacral ulcers may develop, followed closely in frequency by trochanteric ulcers. Along with these, calcaneal, thoracic, and even occipital sores may occur. Pressure sores involving the anterosuperior spine of the ilium, knees, tibial crests, elbows, and dorsum of the foot have a much smaller incidence, because the patient generally is not placed in the prone position, or if he is, this position is tolerated so poorly by most patients that it may be discontinued rather quickly.

If spasticity develops, the bedridden patient may develop medial condylar and medial malleolar sores with great rapidity, owing to repeated rubbing of these parts against each other through spasm. There may also be associated trochanteric and sacral ulcers.

When the patient is finally allowed to sit up in bed, new sites are subjected to pressure, notably the ischial tuberosities, where a rapid breakdown of skin and subjacent tissues may follow the assumption of this position. Guttmann (1955) and Reichel (1958) have both referred to shearing stress exerted on sacral and buttock skin by the elevation of the bed to a sitting position as a possible major cause of sacral pressure sores.

Sitting in a wheelchair may expose the thoracic or sacral regions to some pressure, but more generally the pressure is exerted against the buttocks; thus, the ischial tuberosities, where a major portion of the weight is borne, may break down. It must also be emphasized that the dependent feet, which frequently become edematous and less able to withstand the pressure of resting on a foot piece, may show tissue necrosis on the plantar and posterior aspects of the heels and the lateral margins of the toes unless adequate protection is provided.

No surface of the body is immune to the development of ulcers. They have also been observed in soft tissue areas, such as the mid-thigh, calf, upper arms, and forearms, and the situation is, of course, much worse in the quadriplegic population.

It is true, in general, that these lesions develop more quickly in the patient whose nutritional status is lowered. In long-standing ulcers the copious discharge of the products of proteolysis results in a nitrogen imbalance with a lowering of the serum proteins, anemia, and vitamin deficiency. When any or all of these situations are present, there is a reduction in both the fat and lean body mass and a reduced ability to heal traumatized areas. An extension of the processes of breakdown is encouraged, and a vicious cycle may be instituted unless steps are taken to interrupt it.

## TREATMENT

It is possible to divide treatment into two major categories: (1) systemic, and (2) local, whether conservative or surgical.

### Systemic Treatment

**Nutritional Measures.** The prime concern after relief of pressure and wound toilet is the restoration of the patient's nutritional status. The measures undertaken vary according to the chronicity of the lesion and the general physical state. Of prime importance is the administration of a high protein, high caloric, high vitamin diet. In the presence of hypoproteinemia, development of ulcers is rapid, and healing is slow. By restoring a positive nitrogen balance, the healing of damaged tissue is facilitated.

Measures correcting the nutritional imbalance must be instituted early and must show results before any but lifesaving surgery is attempted. In practice, it has been found that a daily intake of 135 gm of protein given in the form of lean meats, cheese, skimmed milk, protein hydrolysate, and amino acids is effective. Vegetable protein is important, but animal protein is preferable. It may be necessary to supplement oral feedings by the use of a nasogastric tube or by hyperalimentation.

The appetite of many of these patients is naturally poor because of their inactivity and invalidism; stimulation of the appetite is indicated. Among the simplest and most effective measures is a very old one with considerable appeal to most patients: the administration of an ounce of wine or liquor before meals.

If fat occupies too great a proportion of a patient's diet, it may be found that he is unable to ingest adequate protein. It may be wise to reduce the fat and increase the carbohydrate content of his menu.

If blenderized diets are impractical, high protein liquid diets are commercially available but are relatively more expensive and are hyperosmolar.

Intravenous hyperalimentation with a long-term, indwelling, centrally placed venous catheter is possible. Amino acid–glucose solutions are available for this purpose, and recently fat emulsions have once again become commercially available. The procedure for alimentation by this route has been standardized.

In general, it is less expensive, less complicated, and more effective to aliment the patient by the oral route whenever possible.

In the case of vitamin deficiency, some restoration will occur as a result of the dietary measures, but these are supplemented by the administration of multivitamins. A geriatric formula type of vitamin compound has been found useful in these patients.

Unless there is a serum protein level above 6 mg per 100 ml, surgery should not be undertaken except as a life-conserving measure.

The inculcation of a psychologic desire to get the operation over with and thus start a rehabilitation program with the least possible delay may be of greater value than all of the foregoing measures.

**Treatment of Anemia.** The correction of anemia goes hand in hand with the correction of the protein deficiency. A combination of diet, drugs, and blood transfusion may be required. Liver should be included as a regular item on the menu. Iron preparations, which may have an additional beneficial effect in that they reduce the frequency of loose stools, thus helping maintain cleanliness in certain affected regions, are given by mouth or injection. It may be necessary to give repeated transfusions of whole blood two or three times a week, not only preoperatively but also during and after operation. By the judicious use of these measures, an effort is made to raise the hemoglobin level to a minimum of 12 gm, although some writers prefer a level of 15 gm (Matheson and Lipschitz, 1956). At any rate, the red cell mass should be raised as high as possible preoperatively and should be maintained at this level in the postoperative period.

**Cooperation with Other Services.** Infection, either at the site of the lesion or remote from it, must be eliminated as far as possible. This point needs no further elaboration except to make a plea for greater cooperation between hospital services, especially those covering the genitourinary, neurosurgical, dermatologic, and dental areas.

It is important in the handling and rehabilitation of these patients to secure the advice and assistance of many other specialized services. The orthopedic service is consulted for advice concerning the prevention or correction of flexion contractures, the treatment of septic joint fractures, and the stabilization of joints. The rehabilitation department can assess the patient's capabilities and outline a training program designed to make him self-sufficient, in so far as it is possible, or even self-supporting. The psychologist and psychiatrist may be consulted to help solve problems associated directly or indirectly with the general situation. The social service worker may be required to render assistance in the settlement of the patient's family affairs or to enlist the aid of welfare or vocational rehabilitation agencies.

**Relief of Spasm.** The presence of spasm in close to 50 per cent of paraplegic patients must be of serious concern to all who treat these patients. Cannon and coworkers (1950) reported that spasm was serious enough to interfere with surgery in one-third of their spastic paraplegics. Consequently, it is necessary to consult the neurosurgeon when this condition exists.

When no ulcers are present, measures to correct spasm must be considered from the standpoint of prophylaxis. When there are sores, the continued spasmodic movement of the parts will in most instances prevent healing. If surgical treatment is contemplated, it is essential that the spasms be controlled and eliminated, or the surgery will fail almost without exception.

Nevertheless, any consideration of the correction of spasm must also take into account the fact that such measures as anterior rhizotomy and alcohol injection may destroy reflex sexual activity and bladder control, thus greatly reducing the patient's psychologic sense of adequacy and social acceptance. As emphasized by Chase and White (1959), paraplegics have been robbed of so many functions that preservation of sexual function is an important aspect of rehabilitation. In connection with sexual ability, Talbot (1949, 1955), Munro (1954), and Zietlin, Cottrell, and Lloyd (1957) have reported complete erection in a range of from 66 to 74 per cent of male paraplegics. Talbot reported that anterior rhizotomy destroyed reflex sexual activity in 6 out of 10 of his patients, and alcohol injection abolished erection in 28 out of 30 patients studied by Bors

(1948). This argument in fact was used by Chase and White (1959) to support the use of bilateral high-thigh amputation in paraplegics rather than subjecting these patients to neurosurgical intervention for spasm. Harding (1961) was of the opinion that intrathecal alcohol blocks and dorsal rhizotomy, which in his series yielded only temporary improvement in about half the cases, should be abandoned. He believed that procaine block, which Munro (1954) showed controlled mass reflex spasm permanently in selected patients, should be more widely used. When this fails, selective anterior rootlet rhizotomy and bilateral anterior dorsolumbosacral rhizotomy should be considered. Bors (1948) relieved spinal reflexes by peripheral obturator neurectomy combined with adductor myotomy.

The recent introduction of dantrolene sodium (Dantrium) offers hope of a chemotherapeutic way of controlling the spasticity resulting from spinal cord injury. The medication is administered in oral form and should be used with caution in patients with preexisting liver disease.

It will be realized, therefore, that the problem of spasm relief is not a simple one, there being many factors to consider. The merits and demerits of each method must be weighed carefully in the light of the overall situation. It is only after such deliberation and after discussion with the patient that a course of treatment, which is permanently damaging to his physical status, should be performed. It must be stated, however, that a hard choice must often be made, because it would be of little advantage to retain bladder and erectile function if by so doing it proved to be impossible to cover a gross ulcer that might cause the patient to be totally incapacitated and bedridden and might possibly lead to his demise.

**Relief of Pressure.** Since the first edition of this book was written, many developments in the field of pressure relief have occurred and are still being explored and developed. The expense involved in this form of therapy is a major drawback in many instances and has prevented widespread adoption.

Formerly the main method of pressure relief lay in the extensive use of bulky nonabsorbent dressings applied to the affected parts. Reference was made to springy synthetic nonabsorbent fibers, such as Acrilan and Dacron, encased in an absorbent cover of cotton. Their use was preferred to the type of flat absorbent dressings so frequently seen on the wards of many hospitals.

However, the work involved in changing the bulky dressings in a time of high labor costs, plus their overall inefficiency, led to a search for better and more efficient methods. Because these newer methods have not yet come into general use and because of the high cost involved, their adoption will likely be slow; the older methods of pressure relief are still widely utilized, and they should be reviewed.

In practice, a dressing of sterile Acrilan or Dacron fiber, built up to a thickness of 5 to 7.5 cm over a regular absorbent gauze dressing and held in place by Elastoplast or Montgomery straps, produces a light, airy, resilient dressing which diffuses heat, allows air to circulate, and does not become sodden. It may be necessary to protect the skin under the Elastoplast or the straps by painting the skin with tincture of benzoin, collodion, or some of the aerosol sprays.

There are other methods of pressure relief that have been used, namely, sheepskin (Ewing and coworkers, 1964; Nyquist and Bors, 1964) placed beneath the patient or applied to specific areas such as the foot in the form of easily removed bootees (Butterworth and Golding, 1965). This was a step forward, but laundering posed certain difficulties, as the sheepskin either disintegrated or became so hard that it did not serve its purpose. Synthetic deep-piled pads were substituted successfully and were widely used because of laundering ease.

Another substitute material is silicone gel used in a cushion or pad (Spence, Burke, and Rae, 1967). These pads provide fairly good weight distribution but are quite expensive, and some patients find them hard to use. The Jobst Hydro-float flotation pad is somewhat cheaper and fits all size wheelchairs. The cost may be further reduced by using air cushions filled with water.

The water bed was first described by Arnott in 1838 and mentioned by Paget in 1873 but more or less remained in limbo until Weinstein and Davidson (1965) published a report of an updated modern version for the prevention and treatment of decubitus ulcer. They described both a bed and a seat. Harris (1965, 1967) and Dewis, Caplan, and Pache (1968) reported favorably on the use of the bed using a plastic bladder to hold the water, which was contained in a Styrofoam form contoured to the body.

Pfandler in 1968 presented a comprehensive review of the whole subject of flotation for pressure relief, describing the principle (Archimedes), variations, and experience with its use at the University of Rochester Rehabilitation Center. A lifting device to make nursing care easier was incorporated into the contoured fiber glass bed, and the patient lies on a free-floating vinyl sheet called Staph-check, which is impregnated with a chemical formula designed to inhibit the growth of Staphylococcus organisms. The depth of the water varies from 1 foot at the shoulders to 2½ feet at the buttocks. This allows the patient to assume a sitting position while still floating freely.

Thornhill and Williams (1968) reported their experiences with the water mattress in a large city hospital. They described ten patients who had satisfactory results from several points of view: (1) all ulcers showed signs of healing; (2) no new ulcers or lesions were observed in any patient while on the water mattress; and (3) the healing time was accelerated. Dewis, Caplan, and Pache (1968) reported that the routine nursing care was continued, and only dry sterile dressings were applied to the ulcers. The patients were turned to increase their comfort and to aid pulmonary drainage. Frequent turning proved to be unnecessary, since the fluid support eliminated many of the pressure points.

Some of the commercial preparations evolved during this period were the DePuy Flote-bed manufactured by DePuy, Inc., Hydro-float manufactured by Jobst, and, of course, variations of these making use of such equipment as sports air cushions and camping mattresses filled with water in an attempt to reduce the expense. One of the great difficulties with the latter is the frequency with which leaks occur. Although they can be patched, there is considerable escape of water before the leak is discovered.

One difficulty encountered was the inability of the patient to adjust to a jiggling, constantly moving surface. Another difficulty was observed when it came to changing position, and another involved difficulty in breathing because of limited movement or limited activity. An unexpected effect in many instances was the fact that once the patient became accustomed to the bed, he also became addicted to it and resisted being moved to a regular bed.

Kosiak and coworkers (1958) made a comparison of the pressures exerted at 12 points on the thigh, ischium, and coccyx when the patient was positioned on various materials. Kosiak found that pressure on a flat board varied from 50 to 500 mm Hg. That on a wooden office seat varied from 97 to 200 mm Hg, and that on a board with a 2-inch foam rubber pad from 53 to 160 mm Hg. These findings were recorded in 11 spinal injury patients, and the highest pressures were found to be exerted over the ischia and coccyx.

When these patients sat on an alternating pressure pad at ½-inch excursion, pressures in the inflated position ranged from 100 to 275 mm Hg. In the deflated position, pressures at critical sites were about equal to or below the level of the arterial diastolic pressure in all but four sites around the ischia and coccyx. Pressure greater than capillary pressure was exerted at least half the time at all sites and constantly in four critical areas.

Weinstein and Davidson (1966) found water bed pressures of 18 mm Hg (average) against the heels, 19 mm Hg against the sacrum, and about 25 mm Hg against the trochanters when the patient was lying on his side. These pressures are below capillary pressures at heart level, which range from 20 to 30 mm Hg, so that the vicious circle of pressure producing vascular occlusion, anemia, and tissue necrosis is broken.

Baran and associates (1972), using a new mattress of a specially engineered polyurethane foam* and a regular hospital mattress, compared various site pressures in five patients and noted that the pressures differed significantly. Another study of 16 patients by the same investigators, using a different method of recording pressures and adding an additional element of recommended support (the water mattress), yielded even stronger evidence of differences in favor of the polyurethane mattress.

While considerable improvement was secured in the relief of pressure by these methods, the ultimate goal of weightlessness or total pressure relief remains elusive. The British Hover bed, following the principle of the British Hover craft in which jets of air are used to support a mass above ground or sea level, supports the body in reverse on jets of air directed upward. A disadvantage of this method is the intensely disagreeable noise produced by the powerful fans necessary to provide the supporting jets. The desiccating effect of blowing warm air over wounds is undesirable, and the fact that electrical or mechanical failure might allow the patient to slide to the hard, flat surface below is always a potential hazard.

The noise factor was also encountered at first with the latest development in flotation therapy, the air-fluidized bed developed by Artz and Hargest (1971) and others at the Medical College of South Carolina. The use of this bed is well covered in a publication called The Air Fluidized Bed, Clinical and Research Symposium, edited by Artz and Hargest (1971).

The basic principle involves supporting the body on a bed whose fluid consists of air and

---

*Medic-Ease Corporation, 62 Erdman Avenue, Princeton, N.J. 08540.

ceramic spheres. According to Artz and Hargest, the fluid is not to be confused with liquid which is wet. The principle is simple, i.e., an object of any size or shape can be supported in an air stream if the volume and pressure of the stream are sufficient. By using hundreds of millions of ceramic spheres, 74 to 125 microns in size and made of crown optical glass with no free silica present, the density of the supporting medium is increased, and the volume of air necessary to support the body is markedly decreased. The volume of air is approximately 5 per cent of that required for the British Hover bed. This results in a motor which is less powerful and much quieter than that of the Hover bed. The patient is separated from direct contact with the spheres by a sheet of square-weave monofilament polyester woven to a controlled 37-micron porosity (Hargest, 1969). This keeps the spheres in the bed, with the exception of an insignificant number of undersized spheres. The latter may cause a slight dust problem for a few days, while permitting free passage of warmed, humidified air which can be closely controlled to obtain the optimum temperature and humidity for the patient, creating an environment which inhibits bacterial growth (Sharbaugh and Hargest, 1971). The bed of spheres is approximately 12 inches deep at rest. When the blower is activated, the depth of the spheres is increased only ½ inch, and yet it provides the flotation equivalent to 17 inches of water for a 250-pound body. The body mass resting on the ceramic sphere and air bed penetrates to a distance of only 4 inches. Because of the penetration effect of the mass, there are surface pressures which are less than those obtained when the body rests on a foam mattress or a water-filled bladder. Since the polyester sheet provides no support but moves freely to contour itself to the depression, no shearing forces are developed to damage the tissues.

Body wastes and secretions, which ordinarily would be considered sources of auto- and cross-contamination, have not been a problem. Studies by Sharbaugh and Hargest (1971) have shown that sequestration and desiccation of microorganisms within the air-fluidized bed system constitute the main contributing factor in the bactericidal and fungicidal ability of the system, a factor making it of incalculable value in the hospital environment. Because of the very low pressures exerted on the body, the bed can be used for paraplegics and other decubitus-prone patients directly after surgery. Lying on skin grafts and flaps has not been harmful, and dressing changes are simple (Hofstra, 1971).

Some disadvantages are: (1) active suction is sometimes necessary to maintain urinary drainage; (2) the noise may be annoying not only to the patient but also to other patients in the same room; (3) the bed is heavy, necessitating some reinforcement at the corners; (4) it is costly.

Favorable aspects, as reported by Hofstra (1971), are: (1) patient comfort is increased; (2) the need for medication to control restlessness and to aid sleep is greatly reduced; (3) the patient shows physiologic improvement, so that his appetite is improved; (4) the skin remains dry and does not become macerated; (5) skin lesions are cleaner with promotion of accelerated healing.

The use of foam rubber rings is not satisfactory. They lead to a false sense of security on the part of the nursing staff, with a possible reduction in the frequency of position changes ordered by the doctor. In addition, while relieving pressure at one point, they may produce an annular area of pressure around this point which can lead to vascular constriction and disastrous results.

Blocks of foam rubber used as seats on wheelchairs may be either solid or cored. They afford some protection. However, they do not allow adequate circulation of air, and they tend to sag if laid on the canvas seat of the patient's chair. The sagging can be eliminated by the introduction of a piece of plywood across the canvas seat. It might be preferable to substitute as a seat pad one of the light, porous, foamed plastics in the form of a block 7.5 to 10 cm thick. These plastics have great resilience and shock absorption power and form a good protective pad beneath the ischial tuberosity for the patient who is in a wheelchair. When the patient is in a chair, he should be urged by all who see him to shift his position with great frequency until it becomes an ingrained habit. Houle (1969) evaluated a number of seat devices designed to prevent ischemia leading to ulceration. There are many types of seat cushions all aimed at the same objective, i.e., the reduction of pressure on the ischial tuberosities to the greatest degree possible.

For the bedridden patient, the foam rubber or plastic sectional mattress has properly replaced the usual types of inner springs. A more refined development is the alternating pressure mattress, which is, however, rather costly. The principle is sound, and these mattresses have proved helpful, but we consider as superior the support systems which have been previously described.

The Stryker frame proves in practice to be

somewhat less than perfect. This is largely due to the fact that the canvas surfaces of the mattress are relatively unyielding. In some instances when the patient has been left in the prone position for an excessive length of time, ulcers have developed through pressure in the anterior axillary folds (see Fig. 91–2). The fact that the patient must have an attendant come regularly to turn him places his helpless body at the mercy of attendants who may unconsciously resent a rigid time table.

The revolving bed (Circolectric)* may be helpful not only in reducing direct pressure to sensitive sites but also in helping to maintain vascular and muscular tone. The bed is particularly useful in the postoperative period in turning a patient following flap coverage of a sacral, ischial, or trochanteric defect.

Too much reliance, however, must not be placed on any automatic instrument or substitute for human care and attention. A rocking bed devised to improve circulation in paraplegics has been use-tested in the Dublin Paraplegic Center; no patients have developed pressure sores (Rusk, 1969).

It must be kept in mind that, while pressure is being relieved in the area of an ulcer, other areas must not be subjected to undue pressure, especially during the postoperative period. Therefore, special care in positioning and padding of the unaffected parts must be taken.

### Roentgenographic Studies.

If there are sinus tracts and infected bursae, it is advisable to take roentgenograms using a contrast medium instilled into the tracts (see Fig. 91–3). The devious paths of the sinus tracts can thus be identified before surgery, and their presence may be an indication for more extensive surgery. The degree of involvement revealed by the roentgenogram is often quite astounding. An ischial ulcer may show osteomyelitis of the tuberosity, but in addition, the suppurative process may track medially and anteriorly toward the pubis, especially in a patient who has been placed in the prone position. A trochanteric ulcer may show peripheral extensions around the thigh in the fascial and muscle planes. There may be extensions upward from the trochanter to the femoral neck and into the hip joint, producing a septic arthritis or pyarthrosis. A sacral decubitus may communicate with the hip joint (Lopez and Aranha, 1974). Heterotopic bone can be demonstrated in many ulcers of long standing, with some deposits reaching a large size. Although

*Manufactured by Orthopedic Frame Company, Kalamazoo, Michigan.

simple superficial periostitis is no contraindication to surgery when there is involvement of joints, the problem of treatment may be complex, and orthopedic consultation should be obtained. Resection of the femoral head may be indicated if there is a sinus tract communicating with the hip joint.

## Local Treatment

**Conservative Treatment.** Local treatment is aimed at securing a surgically clean wound. If the ulcer is not too large, it will fill in from below, and epidermal growth from the sides will produce a closed wound. However, coverage by scar epithelium is unsatisfactory because of associated vulnerability to the minimal trauma of daily activities.

Most pressure sores when first seen require surgical debridement of all of the necrotic material, whether it be skin, fat, or muscle or all three. Fragments of dead bone at the base of the wound may be found lying free, and if they are not removed they will continue to cause drainage. Fibrous septa are broken down, and unilocular or multilocular infected bursae are opened for free drainage. Devitalized fascia or tendons should be excised. Such simple surgical measures can generally be performed at the patient's bedside with only an occasional complication, such as mild bleeding. Extensive debridement should be done in the operating room, and the procedure may have to be repeated several times. The surgeon must be prepared to replace excessive blood loss by having crossmatched blood available in the operating room.

Surgical debridement is the most reliable, although some modest success with enzymatic debridement had been reported by Morrison and Casali (1957). Some patients have shown skin irritation with the prolonged use of this preparation, but the irritation disappeared when the medication was stopped and saline dressings substituted. In addition to helping clean up the wound, there was a suppression of the associated foul odor. Other enzyme preparations have been described, among them a proteolytic enzyme-antibiotic mixture which was reported to be effective in chronic leg ulcers (Spencer, 1967). Its application to pressure sores has not been reported at the time of this writing.

Frequent dressing changes are preferable, and wet-to-dry fluff gauze dressings are particularly suited to the rapid removal of necrotic material from the wound.

Irrigations of the depths of the ulcer, particularly those in the trochanteric and ischial areas, should be done daily or with each dressing change. Our preference is for a mixture of hydrogen peroxide and saline in equal parts. It is relatively bland, and the foaming action of the hydrogen peroxide provides a satisfactory mechanical flushing effect. Plain saline wet dressings and dilute acetic acid dressings have their advantages, and the use of 1.5 per cent Dakin's solution applied in the form of continuous moist dressings has shown good results (Griffith and Schultz, 1961). The surrounding skin may be protected by preparations such as a thick film of zinc oxide ointment or silicone cream to prevent maceration.

Clark and Rusk (1953) have reported positive results with the use of dried blood plasma applied locally; others have recommended the local application of antiseptic or antibiotic substances. Our own preference is for the use of simple measures known to be effective, economical, and relatively certain. If an exceedingly large ulcer surface is moderately clean, a simple split-thickness skin graft is often applied to obtain a closed wound preparatory to doing a definitive flap procedure. This helps immeasurably in preventing inordinate protein loss and in restoring the hematocrit and the nutritional balance to levels which enhance the chances for success.

Immersion in tepid water with soap suds may be instituted three to seven days before operation with beneficial effects on the wound. It is not generally necessary to pad the bottom of the tub, especially if one recalls that the weight of the totally immersed adult is reduced to about 10 to 15 pounds on the average. Nyquist (1959) recommended brine baths. Moist saline dressings alone or combined with an antibiotic, applied for 24 to 48 hours before operation, have been effective in providing a clean granulating surface with a relatively low bacterial count.

It should be emphasized that at the commencement of local therapy, cultures of the ulcer drainage should be taken, the organisms identified, and their sensitivity to various antibiotics determined. The local use or application of antibiotics is usually ineffective, but it is felt that the systemic use of an effective drug matched to the organism may prove to be of value initially. It is used as a therapeutic measure when the organism has invaded other parts of the body. However, antibiotics are of little use in the older chronic ulcers with heavy scarring and thrombosed vessels in the area of inflammation, for the simple reason that these conditions prevent access of the therapeutic agent to the ulcerated sites.

The foregoing methods of conservative therapy may result in the healing of small or medium-sized ulcers after a period of time. It is unusual for a large ulcer to resurface itself, but on occasion this has been seen. In many instances, particularly when the level of the healed surface is below that of the surrounding skin and is not subject to pressure, healing may be adequate. As a general rule, however, the quality of the new skin covering is of a low grade without sebaceous or sweat glands or well-developed dermal and subdermal layers. Such scar epithelium is generally dry and thin with a poor blood supply and must be lubricated by the application of petrolatum, cocoa butter, cold cream, lanolin, or similar preparations. Areas thus healed are more subject to breakdown on slight trauma than is normal skin because of poor vascularity and quality; healing is generally slower when there has been disruption of the continuity of such a skin surface.

With the conservative method of treatment, not only is the initial healing time lengthy, but also there may be repeated periods of morbidity due to minor trauma and tissue breakdown. Because of these factors, physicians treating pressure sores feel that relatively early surgical therapy offers the best hope in the form of earlier closure and improved ability to withstand subsequent trauma. In addition, the achievement of the overall rehabilitation of the patient is a factor of the greatest importance economically, socially, and psychologically. There is no question that only a very small percentage of pressure sores can be treated adequately by conservative therapy.

**Surgical Treatment.** The history of the surgical closure of bedsores began with the report of four cases by Davis in 1938. The importance of the excision of the underlying bony prominence was also appreciated toward the end of World War II. This surgical concept was significant for several reasons: first, it eliminated an important element of infection, since it was demonstrated by microscopic studies that changes ranging from fibrosis to osteomyelitis were present in the affected bone; second, it also provided for the elimination of the projecting bony eminence, a significant factor in the recurrence of ulcers (Kostrubala and Greeley, 1947). Also in the same year, the Plastic Surgery Service at the Bronx Veterans Administration Hospital suggested the use of split-thickness skin grafts to resurface the donor defects created by the rotation of large flaps (Conway and associates, 1951). In 1948, Bors and Comarr, in a report on the treatment of ischial ulcers, advocated covering the open bony surface with flaps of nonfunctioning muscle. In 1956 Georgiade, Pickrell, and Maguire reported bilateral high thigh amputation for "end stages" of decubiti.

The gradual evolution in the surgical treatment of pressure sore has led to the presently accepted surgical objectives: (1) excision of the ulcerated area, including the underlying bursa and the usually infected scar tissue and/or undermined skin that encircles the defect; (2) resection of any existing bony prominence; (3) resurfacing of the defect with healthy skin, including adequate subcutaneous tissue padding; (4) designing the flaps as large as possible; (5) obtaining additional padding by the use of muscle flaps if subcutaneous tissue is not adequate.

TIMING OF SURGERY. Elective reconstructive surgery should not be contemplated unless the general condition of the patient has stabilized and the ulcer shows the following signs of improvement: (1) clearance of all necrotic tissue; (2) appearance of healthy granulation tissue; (3) a tendency for the ulcer to decrease in size by diminution of the extent of the undermining and/or evidence of advancing epithelial margins.

OPERATIVE TECHNIQUES. Almost anyone who has had the opportunity to treat pressure sores will agree that the best method of covering the average defect is by using large local skin flaps. However, multiple other means of closure have been employed. Some of these other methods may have an application under special conditions and in certain individuals. The authors would like to emphasize, however, that in their experience none of the other methods approaches the adaptability and effectiveness of the large local flap.

*Skin grafts.* Split-thickness skin grafts should not be used as a definitive treatment for pressure ulcers. Because they are thin and adhere to the underlying bone, they are susceptible to minimal trauma, particularly if overlying a bony prominence.

Split-thickness skin grafts are mostly indicated in patients in whom the magnitude of the ulcer is such as to make the task of immediate flap repair impossible. In these cases temporary coverage with skin grafts is indicated to prevent the continuous loss of protein through the wound and to establish a healed wound prior to flap coverage. It will also help in many instances to reduce the size of the original defect by centripetal movement on the ulcer margins associated with graft contraction.

Another indication for the use of a split-thickness skin graft is the small superficial cutaneous defect adjacent to a large and deep pressure sore; the technique is also feasible in those cases in which the ulceration is located so that the bulk of pressure is taken up by the surrounding tissues, as in the case of a deep but small ulcer.

Finally, split-thickness skin grafts may be employed in cases in which the weight-bearing trauma will be minimal, such as in the heel ulcer of a bedridden or wheelchair-confined patient. In addition, it should be emphasized that ideal conditions for ulcer repair are not always present, and surgical compromise may be necessary, as in the patient in whom a local flap may not be available because of scarring or previous surgery.

Wesser and Kahn (1967) recommended a modification of the Hynes (1954) technique of a reversed dermis graft to cover the ulcer. In turn, the graft is covered by a thin split-thickness skin graft serving as a biological dressing during the immediate postoperative period. The dermis graft is followed four weeks later by a thick split-thickness skin graft. The total graft is considered to be 2 to 3 times thicker than the thickest split-thickness skin graft; it consists of a thick layer of dermis, a small amount of fat, and a thick split-thickness skin graft.

*Excision and closure.* The earliest method of surgical treatment of pressure sores, simple excision and closure, has some supporters (Yeoman and Hardy, 1954). It is quite appealing in certain cases of linear superficial skin lesions in which the subcutaneous tissue is not deeply involved. Under any circumstances this procedure represents, at best, a surgical compromise (Campbell and Converse, 1954; Berger, 1957) aimed solely at closing the defect. However, this type of repair is only temporary, and there will be subsequent recurrence of the ulcer because of increased tension on the suture line. In addition, with simple closure there remains an underlying bony prominence beneath an area of poorly vascularized scar tissue; the surgical scar is consequently susceptible to the noxious effects of pressure with subsequent secondary ulceration.

The authors condemn the use of stellate type closures (White, Hudson, and Kennard, 1945; Croce, Schullinger, and Shearer, 1946). The hazards to wound healing are multiplied with the increased possibility of slough of the flap tips. Moreover, the placement of many scars over a single area is a violation of one of the basic principles of reconstructive surgery.

*Tube flaps.* Tube flaps have been used with success in those patients in whom there is no available donor tissue in the vicinity of the defect. The procedure is lengthy, however, because numerous stages are involved. The possibility of complications is multiplied, and the time involved in the reconstruction may be excessive.

*Tumbler flaps.* Stenström (1956) has used a variation of the bipedicle flap in which a non-tubed skin flap is constructed and subsequently tumbled over with a rotation of 360 degrees to the recipient site. This type of flap is a modification of one originally described by Lexer in 1931.

A comparative investigation with equally sized non-tubed skin and tube flaps, based on the clearance of intracutaneously injected radioactive sodium, demonstrated that both the non-tubed skin flap and the tube flap had approximately the same circulatory capacity (Stenström, 1956).

*V-Y advancement flaps.* V-Y advancement flaps have been used with varying success. Their use should be reserved for those unusual cases in which no other available method can be employed because the resulting scars usually lie over the bony prominence and the suture lines tend to be irregular.

*Bipedicle flaps.* Bipedicle flaps have been recommended in the past for the closure of trochanteric and pretibial ulcers (Fig. 91–4). The procedure, however, has definite limitations in that the size of the defect to be closed has to be

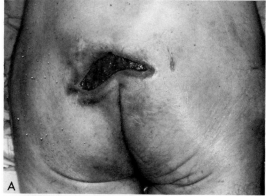
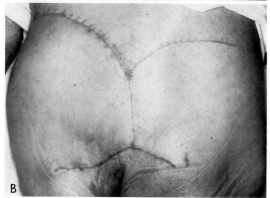

**FIGURE 91–5.** Double-rotation flaps. *A,* Large sacral defect with extensive undermining. *B,* Appearance following excision of ulcer and scar, partial sacrectomy, and coverage with distally based double-rotation flaps. Note the midline position of the resulting scar.

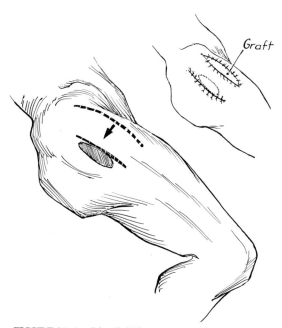

**FIGURE 91–4.** Bipedicle flap coverage of a trochanteric ulcer. The technique is inadequate for larger lesions, as mobility of the flap is limited.

relatively small, because the wider the bipedicle flap, the less mobility it will have. In addition, the amount of tension placed on the pedicles is increased with the degree of advancement required to cover larger defects; thus the viability of the flap is jeopardized. In almost all cases the secondary defect must be resurfaced with a split-thickness skin graft.

*Double rotation flaps.* As recommended by Osborne in 1955, double rotation flaps are used mainly, but not exclusively, for large sacral defects. The flaps are based distally, rotated medially, and sutured in the midline (Fig. 91–5). While they provide adequate soft tissue coverage, the resultant midline scar is a definite drawback, and the risk of secondary breakdown is increased. It is preferable to make one of the flaps as large as possible to cover the greater part of the defect and at the same time allow placement of the suture line off the midline. These flaps are combined with ostectomy of the spinous processes of the sacrum.

*Neurovascular island flaps and free flaps.* The most recent surgical advance in the treatment of pressure sores in paraplegics is the neurovascular island flap first described by Dibble in 1974. Recently this concept has been expanded by Daniel, Terzis and Cunningham (1976).

The great advantage of this method is that a sensory skin flap not only provides coverage but also restores sensation. An attempt at a neurovascular free flap transfer in a paraplegic patient resulted in failure (Daniel, Terzis and Cunningham, 1976). However, a microvascular free flap has been successfully performed to reconstruct the lower extremity of a paraplegic (Shaw, Baker and Morello, 1976).

From the preceding it may be inferred that the authors' preference is for the large, single rotation or transposition flap for the coverage of the pressure sore. There are many cases in which, owing to local conditions or because of special characteristics of the defect, alternative procedures must also be considered. However, in every instance the following established surgical principles for the treatment of pressure sores should be followed: (1) excision which is sufficiently wide to include the defect, adjacent scar, and any existing sinus tracts; (2) removal of the underlying bony prominence to minimize the possibility of recurrence; (3) provision of sufficient soft tissue coverage to cushion the area. Whenever the soft tissues are not thick enough for sufficient padding of certain areas, additional coverage with muscle flaps and other measures have been recommended.

GENERAL PRINCIPLES OF SURGICAL TREATMENT

*Preoperative preparation of the patient.* Assumption of the prone position for increasing lengths of time in the preoperative period prepares the patient for the prolonged positioning required in the postoperative phase when surgery is planned for sacral, ischial, and in some instances trochanteric ulcers. The majority of patients initially find the position disagreeable to intolerable, but they can be persuaded into assuming it. It is desirable that they do this preoperatively, so that they know what to expect following operation and become accustomed to feeding themselves in this position. It is also a training period for bowel evacuation, which may pose a problem following surgery.

*Anesthesia.* General endotracheal anesthesia is preferred to local infiltration and/or sedation alone, to avoid spasmodic reflex muscle movements. However, other surgeons find sedation alone acceptable provided an anesthesiologist is in attendance to monitor the physiologic status of the patient.

A competent anesthesiologist, supervising fluid and whole blood replacement and capable of giving ample warning to the surgeon of the beginning of shock or the development of cardiac complications, is essential to the proper functioning of the surgical team. Paraplegic patients have wide fluctuations in blood pressure and pulse rate and lack the usual compensatory physiologic (sympathetic) responses to hypovolemia. There is often considerable blood loss despite the most exacting techniques. From a psychologic standpoint also, the conscious patient may be unduly worried or concerned about chance remarks made by the surgical team, or he may become extremely restless through fear that he is lying too long in one position and may incur an additional pressure sore. Under general anesthesia these worries are eliminated, and the surgeon can devote himself totally to the problem of coverage.

*Operating room conduct and preparation.* On the morning of surgery the ulcer is cleaned and a dry dressing applied. A new indwelling Foley catheter should be introduced to prevent changes in position while the patient's mobility is restricted during the postoperative period. The catheter is allowed to drain freely into a recipient closed system container.

Once the patient is in the operating room, anesthesia is induced, and the endotracheal tube is placed while the patient is on the stretcher. The patient is positioned on the operating table, the surgeon being particularly careful to provide abundant cushioned support to the exterior bony prominences, anterior superior iliac spines, knees, tibial crests, and dorsum of the feet. The positioning of the patient is accomplished in such a way as to provide adequate exposure not only of the defect but also of the adjacent donor area.

The skin is prepared with the antiseptic solution of choice. Care is exercised to prevent the solution from running down and forming a pool on the dependent surface, possibly the groin, where signs of irritation develop in susceptible patients.

The entire area is draped to provide ample exposure, and no towel clips are used on the skin. If necessary, a few sutures may be placed for fixation of the surgical drapes.

The next step is to outline the extent of the ulceration, which is self-evident by external examination. However, in many patients there is a variable degree of undermining which may be present around the periphery of the ulcer. It is important to determine the extent of the undermining by exploring with the finger or probing with a curved clamp in all directions. By applying slight upward pressure to the clamp, its tip may be felt or seen projecting through the skin; at this point a mark is made with ink (see Fig. 91-6, *B*). In this manner a series of dots outline the extent of the undermining. This is a necessary maneuver because the above surfaces are covered by a pale, shiny granulation tissue, which is the source of serous drainage. The surface has the appearance of an endothelial type of lining. This tissue should be carefully removed either by including it with the ulcer if it is of limited extent, or by means of surface excision down to normal-appearing tissue if the undermining is extensive. If any of the tissue of the undermined area is left behind, the risk of seroma formation under the flap and its sequelae of delayed adherence or nonadherence of the flap to the undersurface is considerably increased.

*Outlining the flap.* Before the lesion is excised, planning and outlining of the flap are mandatory. Several details should be emphasized; the adjacent skin is examined for mobility and laxity and for lines of minimal tension that may allow the flap to rotate or advance in the most favorable manner (see Chapter 6).

On occasion the most desirable area for flap design cannot be utilized because of a coexisting ulcer or scarring which interferes with the proposed flap blood supply. In addition, since the problem of pressure sores is one involving many episodes, the possibility that the flap design might sacrifice a potential donor site for a subsequent ulcer should also be considered. It is imperative that the patient's future be kept in mind by making every possible effort to conserve his tissues and to avoid rendering other areas unusable by ill-placed scars. In addition, if the flap is of large dimensions, a later flap may be designed within the confines of the original if there is a recurrence.

In the event that the length of the planned flap is excessive, a delay may be necessary as a preliminary stage. After the above factors are carefully considered, a tentative outline of the flap is marked with ink (Campbell, 1959; Griffith and Schultz, 1961).

*Ulcer excision.* The extent of the excision should include all of the scarred and discolored skin. It should be emphasized that in most cases all of the undermined skin, if not too extensive, should be excised. If the undermined area is double the size of the defect, the excision is restricted to abnormal-looking skin and the glistening covering on the surfaces of the undermined area. Excision of the bursa-like wall down to healthy-looking tissue must include the core

of the ulcer, as well as the underlying bony prominence (see Fig. 91-6, *G*). The bone is removed with an osteotome, and any irregularities resulting from the osteotomy are smoothed out with a rasp. Bleeding from the bony surface is controlled either by lightly tapping with the rounded head of a chisel so as to obliterate the open spaces or by sparingly applying Gelfoam.

The bleeding from soft tissue surfaces is best controlled with the electrocautery and fine-pointed forceps for the small vessels; moderate-sized bleeding points are ligated with 4-0 catgut. For the control of rather extensive capillary oozing due to large areas of scarring and a deficient or absent vasomotor response, it is preferable to pack the cavity with a laparotomy pad soaked in warm saline solution.

At this point in the operation, a review of the excised area is undertaken to determine the completeness and adequacy of the resection. The surgeon must search for areas of undermining that may have been left behind, residual scar tissue that will prevent adequate healing, sharp bony edges, and so forth. The tentative flap outline is then planned as to size and orientation in relation to any possible changes in size or shape of the excised area.

*Elevating the flap.* The flap is elevated by sharp dissection in a plane superficial to the underlying deep fascia. Care should be exercised because the various planes of fascia, subcutaneous tissue, and muscle are often not clearly defined, particularly in a patient with paraplegia of long standing. Entrance into muscle is an unnecessary hazard that may subsequently give rise to hematoma formation. While the dissection is continued, the flap edges are held with skin hooks or silk sutures applied to the dermis. When large flaps are required, care is observed to avoid any sharp folding or angulation at any point in the flap; for this purpose the flap can be gently rested on a folded laparotomy pad or towel. Bleeding from the underside of the flap surface should be controlled with 5-0 plain catgut suture ligatures in preference to electrocoagulation. In the region of the base of the flap, special care should be exercised to avoid division of any large vessels.

It is advisable at this time to place a suction draining device along the lines of dependency before the flap is rotated into position. Once this is done, the flap is held in place with interrupted sutures of 3-0 or 4-0 plain catgut. The "creeping advancement" technique (see Fig. 91-6, *N*) not only provides a means of securing the flap in position but also has the added advantage of decreasing the possibility of a large fluid collection under the flap. These sutures should be placed in the direction of the flap vessels and should not be inserted too deeply into the flap in order to avoid injury to the nutritive vessels.

The edges of the wound are approximated with interrupted plain catgut sutures in the subcutaneous layer. In such a manner, when the monofilament nylon skin sutures are inserted, they serve mainly for skin coaptation and do not provide strength to the wound closure.

If the flap rotation and/or advancement has resulted in a secondary defect, this is covered by a split-thickness skin graft held in place by a tie-over bolus dressing; the placing of sutures at the adjacent flap margin should be avoided. The skin grafts are preferably taken from available areas above the anesthetic level.

Dressings are not employed, and the flap is left exposed. The suture lines are covered with antibiotic ointment. This technique provides a more direct way of observing any possible postoperative changes in the color and/or temperature of the flap, signs which are indicative of circulatory impairment.

*Postoperative care.* The postoperative care in the treatment of a pressure sore is of the utmost importance. Beginning from the time the patient is transferred from the operating table, care must be exercised to prevent motion or stretching of the flap area. The bed or stretcher is padded with cushions, pillows, and foam rubber pads to make the patient's position as comfortable as possible. The Milton Roy (air-fluidized) bed is unsurpassed for this purpose, because the patient can lie on his flap without harming it. With obese individuals, the effect of possible undesirable gravitational pull of pendulous tissues should be kept in mind and avoided. Undue mobility of the patient is forbidden; the patient and attendants are warned of the disruptive effects of unnecessary movements. This does not imply, by any means, that the patient has to remain completely immobile. The position can be changed from the prone slightly to the side position by the intelligent use of props inserted under the hips and chest. It is obligatory to control any residual spasms that may be present during the immediate postoperative period.

A check of the hematocrit for possible additional blood replacement is made in the recovery room and again within the first 12 hours.

Suction drainage is maintained for approximately 96 hours, at which time it is removed if there is no significant amount of drainage.

If the patient is having loose bowel movements that are soiling and contaminating the surgical area, an effort is made to constipate the

patient. The use of low residue diets and codeine is helpful. However, when the stool is formed, it is not necessary to induce constipation.

The skin sutures, unless there is evidence of skin reaction, are left in place for approximately 12 to 14 days. The prone position is maintained for approximately two weeks. The patient is then allowed to have more freedom of movement and positional changes, but weight-bearing is not permitted. After approximately six weeks the patient may be exposed to pressure on the repaired area, beginning with short periods of ten minutes and progressively increasing the time by daily increments of five to ten minutes or more. It must be emphasized to the patient in particular, as well as to the personnel involved with his care, that it is absolutely essential to establish a daily inspection routine in the morning, as well as after completion of each pressure period, of all the areas that have been subjected to pressure. If there is any evidence of skin discoloration, pressure should be immediately relieved and discontinued until all redness disappears.

In addition to the daily inspection, the patient should be instructed that it is his responsibility to make frequent changes in position, whether he is in a wheelchair or a bed. This point is absolutely essential, and it should be constantly stressed to the patients that this is a lifelong concern whenever they are subjecting any area of their bodies to pressure, especially if it has been surgically repaired.

SPECIFIC SITES OF ULCERATION AND THEIR SURGICAL MANAGEMENT

*Ischial ulcers.* This is the most common location of pressure sores. In order to obtain a satisfactory long-term result that will allow the patient to withstand the pressures of the sitting position, the basic reconstructive principles, as described earlier, should be applied (Fig. 91–6). An important part of the operation is the ischiectomy. There is, however, a point of controversy concerning the extent of the bony resection, with some advocating the so-called total prophylactic ischiectomy (Kostrubala and Greeley, 1947; Blocksma, Kostrubala, and Greeley, 1949); the authors prefer a more conservative approach, i.e., partial ischiectomy to avoid urethral diverticula and perineal ulcers. A flat or gently rounded ischial tuberosity surface is produced, which still functions as a sitting support.

When a large ischial ulcer is removed and is associated with an ostectomy, a large and deep defect may result. Several measures have been proposed to obliterate the resultant dead space.

*Text continued on page 3789*

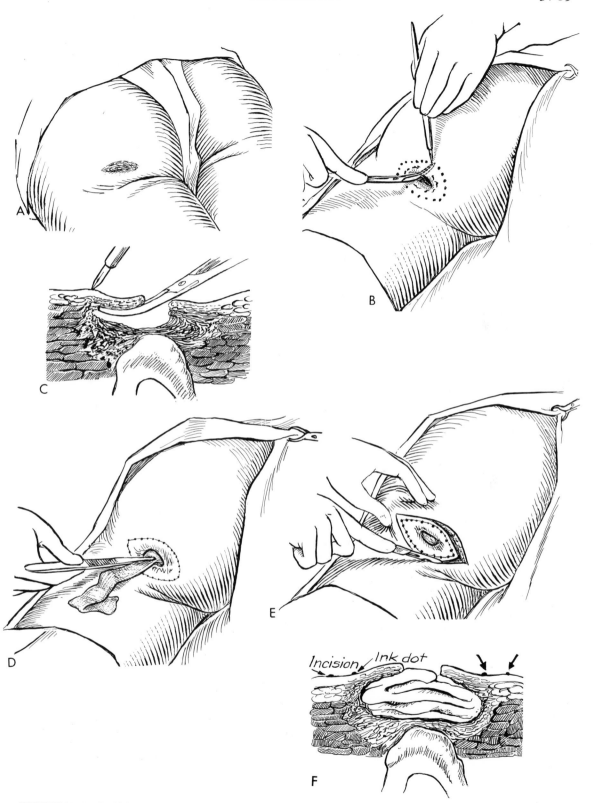

**FIGURE 91–6.** Ischial ulcer. *A* to *D,* The widest extent is shown by a hemostat and marked on the skin surface with ink. The defect is filled with Betadine-soaked packing. *E, F,* Extent of soft tissue resection.

*Legend continued on the following pages*

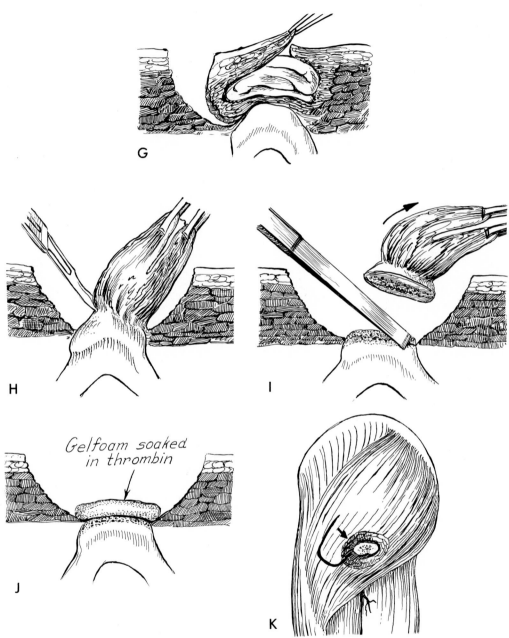

**FIGURE 91-6** *Continued.*   *G, H, I,* Partial removal of ischial tuberosity. *J,* Hemostasis is facilitated by the application of Gelfoam (soaked in thrombin) on the bony surface. *K,* A flap of gluteus muscle may be rotated into the osseous defect; alternatively, a biceps femoris muscle flap may be employed.

*Legend continued on the opposite page*

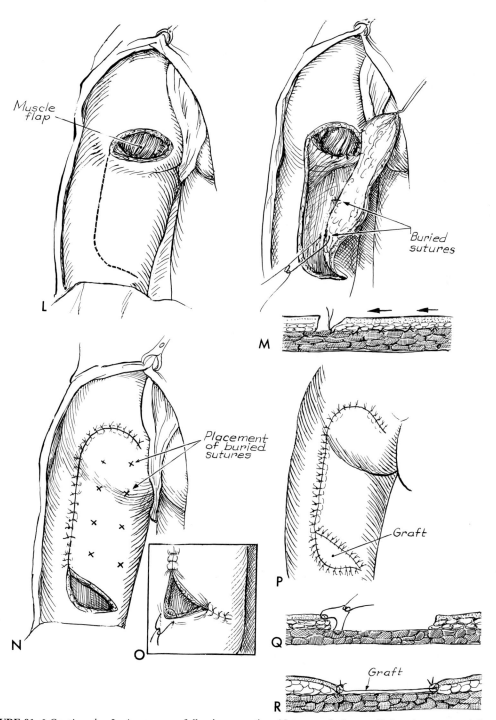

**FIGURE 91–6** *Continued.* *L,* Appearance following resection. Note muscle flap applied to the osseous defect. Large rotation flap is outlined. *M,* "Creeping" advancement of rotation flap by securing undersurface of flap to deep muscles by catgut sutures. *N,* Flap has been rotated into the defect. *O,* The donor defect closed primarily by the V-Y principle. *P, Q, R,* Technique of resurfacing donor site by a split-thickness skin graft. Note that the skin surface of the flap is sutured to the defect prior to the application of the skin graft.

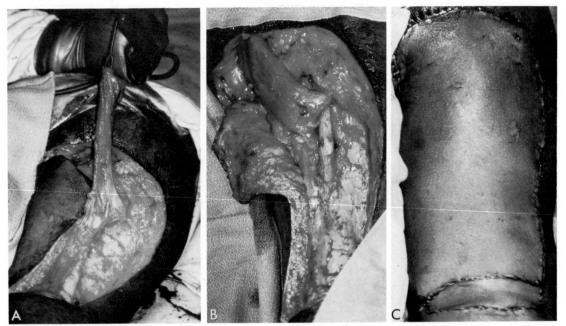

**FIGURE 91–7.** Biceps femoris muscle flap. *A,* Long head of the biceps femoris muscle dissected free and divided at its distal insertion. Note the proximal vascular pedicle at the base of the muscle. *B,* The muscle is rolled upon itself, filling the deep ischial defect. *C,* The operation is completed following rotation of the posterior thigh flap and split-thickness skin graft coverage of the donor defect.

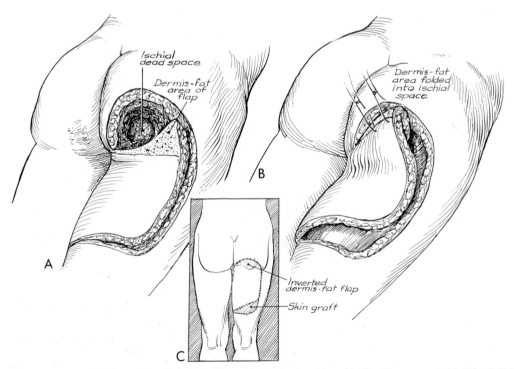

**FIGURE 91–8.** Ischial defect and medially based flap with proximal end de-epithelized by removal of 0.014 to 0.016 inch split-thickness skin graft. *B,* The de-epithelized surface folded and secured by catgut sutures to the depths of the ischial defect. *C,* Procedure completed, showing the final position of the buried dermis-fat flap. Donor defect has been resurfaced by a split-thickness skin graft. (After Tulenko.)

Blocksma and coworkers (1949) attempted to fill the defect by the "fanning out" of the obturator internus muscle and at the same time covering the cut end of the ischial bone. Another variation of the muscle flap technique that can be applied is one that uses the long head of the biceps femoris muscle, which is detached from its lower insertion and rolled upon itself to provide padding and to fill the space (Fig. 91–7). The technique of muscle flaps is discussed in Chapter 86.

Tulenko (1967) proposed a technique in which the proximal end of a large saddle flap is de-epithelized by removal of a 0.014–0.016 inch skin graft; the de-epithelized segment is folded upon itself and inserted to occupy the ischial dead space (Fig. 91–8). Tuerk (1969) has used vulvar tissue to cover a defect in the ischial region.

*Sacral ulcers.*   The conventional treatment consisting of excision of the ulcer and scar, ostectomy (coccyx and sacral crests), and the use of large rotation flaps with or without skin grafting of the donor defect usually suffices in most cases (Fig. 91–9). Superiorly based flaps are less desirable because they have a poorer blood supply and the resulting scars lie in the gluteal fold where they are exposed to pressure during sitting.

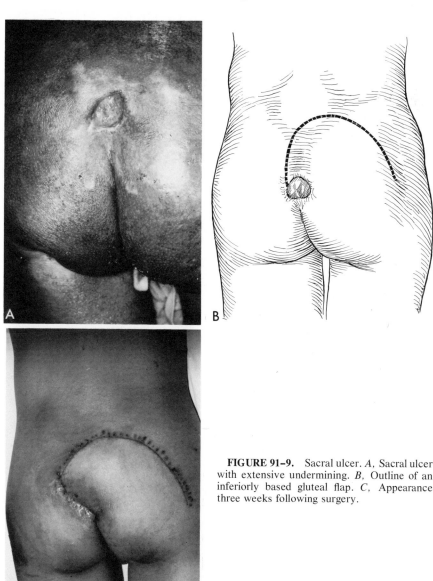

**FIGURE 91–9.**   Sacral ulcer. *A,* Sacral ulcer with extensive undermining. *B,* Outline of an inferiorly based gluteal flap. *C,* Appearance three weeks following surgery.

In the more difficult cases in which there is no available adjacent tissue, tube flaps or the tumbler flap technique may be used. In cases which are difficult because of a small-sized patient, a double rotation flap utilizing almost all of the available skin of the patient's back has been used (see Fig. 91–5).

In a patient with extensive scarring of the adjacent donor areas, a variation utilizing separate flaps from the lower dorsolumbar and gluteal areas can be considered (see Fig. 91–10).

In a patient in whom none of the above techniques can be used, a variation of the muscle flap technique originally described by Ger (1971) is indicated (see also Chapter 86). In this operation (Stallings, Delgado, and Converse, 1974), the gluteus maximus muscle is detached from its trochanteric and sacral insertions, and its neurovascular pedicle is preserved (Fig. 91–11). The flap is turned upside down and applied to the open area of the sacrum and surrounding tissues to which it is attached. The surface of the open muscle is covered with a thick split-thickness skin graft; if necessary, a simple advancement of the surrounding tissues can be obtained to decrease the size of the defect and complete the closure.

Another choice is the reverse dermis graft as used by Wesser and Kahn (1967). A thick dermis graft is applied in a reverse fashion on the sacral ulcer and covered with a thin split-thickness skin graft. The latter acts as a "biological dressing." Only a partial take of the skin graft can be expected. At a second stage four weeks later, a thick split-thickness skin graft is applied either as a sheet or as postage stamps. The coverage is approximately two to three times thicker than the thickest split-thickness skin graft. The thickness of the coverage can be augmented by serial application of the technique.

*Trochanteric ulcers.* Some trochanteric ulcers might heal without surgery, but this occurs only in those that are relatively superficial. Some trochanteric ulcers can be treated conservatively with only a 48 per cent expected rate of success. This figure must be contrasted with the much higher success rate of 86 per cent for those ulcers treated by excision of the ulcer and bursa, resection of the greater trochanter and part of the lateral femoral shaft, and coverage by a local rotation flap (Fig. 91–12) (Dansereau and Conway, 1964).

While skin grafts are still used for closure of some of these ulcers, in our opinion they should be reserved for those patients in whom adequate subcutaneous tissue is present (Dansereau and Conway, 1964). While excision and primary closure seem to be favored by some, the authors condemn this method because of the reasons already discussed, i.e., wound tension and un-

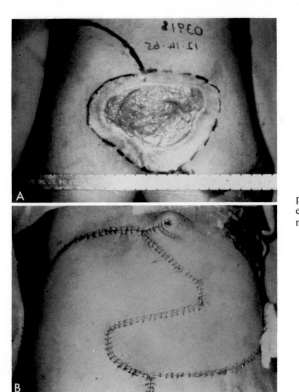

**FIGURE 91–10.** *A,* Large sacral ulcer in a small-sized patient necessitating large double-rotation flaps. *B,* Ulcer excised and the defect closed by dorsolumbar and gluteal rotation flaps.

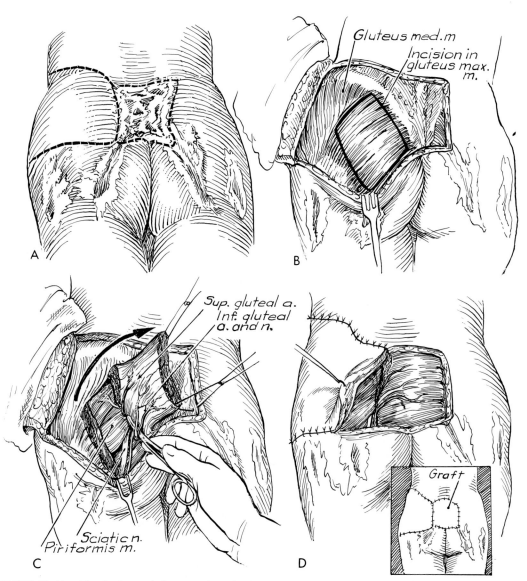

**FIGURE 91–11.** Muscle flap technique. *A,* Sacral defect. Outline of planned excision and laterally based buttock flap. *B,* Outline of gluteus maximus flap following elevation of buttock flap. *C,* Preservation of neurovascular pedicle of the gluteus maximus flap. *D,* Muscle flap rotated into defect. A split-thickness skin graft has been applied on the muscle flap. (From Stallings, J. O., Delgado, J. P., and Converse, J. M.: Turn over island flap of gluteus maximus muscle for the repair of sacral decubitus ulcer. Plast. Reconstr. Surg., *54:*52, 1974. Copyright © 1974, The Williams & Wilkins Company, Baltimore.)

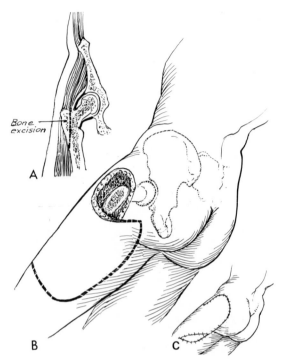

**FIGURE 91-12.** Trochanteric ulcers. *A,* Lateral view showing the line of trochanteric resection. *B,* Defect resulting from ablation of the ulcer, scar, and trochanteric prominence. *C,* Anteriorly based flap transposed into position with a split-thickness skin graft covering the donor defect.

The resurfacing of defects of this area is also discussed in Chapter 86.

*Ulcers of the scapula, iliac crest, and spine-costal margin.* These are less common sites of involvement. Most will respond to conservative therapy and/or split-thickness skin grafting coverage. In cases of ulcers of the anterior superior iliac spine, excision of the bony prominence including a portion of the iliac crest may be required.

*Elbow ulcers.* The elbow region is one of the rarest places for the development of bedsores. It is usually seen only in quadriplegics in whom prolonged prone positioning has been used. A conservative treatment of dressing changes is advisable. However, in quadriplegic patients excision and closure of the ulcer are indicated following debridement of all of the damaged tissue. If the ulcer is deep, an abdominal flap for tissue replacement might be indicated (Fig. 91–14).

*Multiple pressure sores.* It is also necessary to discuss a difficult problem which, in spite of greatly improved medical and surgical care, is still occasionally seen: the patient who develops large or, what is more frequent, multiple, almost confluent ulcers, usually of the ischial, sacral, and trochanteric areas. A similar problem is posed by the patient with multiple recurrences in whom all of the local tissue donor sites available for coverage have been exhausted. Most of

stable scar overlying the bone. In addition, the resultant scars interfere with other possible flap donor sites if other ulcers subsequently develop.

*Heel ulcers.* Heel ulcers frequently heal spontaneously, but in cases in which the size of the ulcer exceeds 3 cm in diameter, a split-thickness skin graft is the treatment of choice. This method shortens the time involved in healing; moreover, the healed skin graft is more resistant than scar epithelium to trauma.

*Knee ulcers.* Several methods of treatment are suggested, and the type of surgery may vary with the location of the ulcer and the depth of involvement.

For superficial and small ulcers, conservative treatment with split-thickness skin grafting may be sufficient. Rotation flaps, with or without patellectomy, may be adequate (Fig. 91–13) for the treatment of large and deep lesions. Muscle flaps, as discussed in Chapter 86, can also be employed.

*Pretibial and foot ulcers.* Ulcers located in this area respond fairly well to the principles of conservative treatment. If necessary, a split-thickness skin graft can be used with advantage.

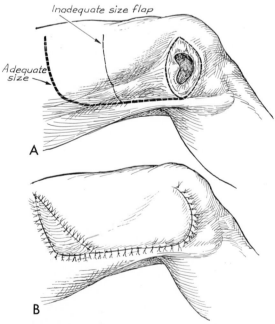

**FIGURE 91-13.** Knee ulcer. *A,* Proposed outline of the flap and area of resection. Note design of inadequately sized flap. *B,* Final appearance. Donor defect was resurfaced with a split-thickness skin graft.

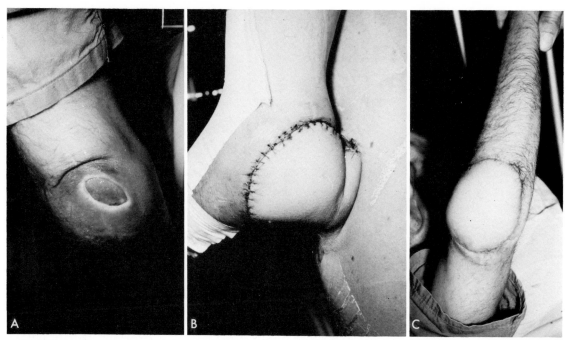

**FIGURE 91–14.** Ulcer over olecranon. *A,* Patient with large, deep olecranon ulceration. *B,* Abdominal flap in place. *C,* Final result.

these patients are totally dependent socially as well as economically. Many of them lack the motivation and insight to deal with their problem. Usually a typical clinical picture is manifest: a bedridden patient is not able to use a wheelchair because of practically fused or ankylosed hips, knees, and ankles; in addition, complicating factors, such as osteomyelitis of the femur and/or ischium, chronic flexure contractures, and pyarthrosis of the hip, may be present, aggravating the already sad condition of these unfortunate patients.

A plan of amputation with utilization of the filleted tissue of the thigh for resurfacing of the multiple involved areas has been proposed. Although Conway and coworkers (1951) reported a case of hip disarticulation for a complicated trochanteric ulcer, it was Georgiade, Pickrell and Maguire (1956) who first advocated the use of the soft tissue of the amputated thigh as a total thigh flap for patients with trochanteric ulcers complicated by pyarthrosis of the hip and osteomyelitis of the femur.

Chase and White (1959), in recommending the use of bilateral high thigh amputation for the rehabilitation of paraplegics, discussed the advantages and disadvantages of amputation. The advantages are:

1. Improvement of maneuverability. By removing the paralyzed legs, the body's center of gravity is reoriented to accomplish agile movements with the arms as the only source of power.

2. Elimination of leg ulcers, skin infections, unresponsive edema, and osteomyelitis.

3. Improved vascular response. Paraplegics have, according to Bors (1948), a deficient vasomotor control. If a large portion of the source, namely that in the legs, is eliminated, the hyperfunction demand on the remaining vascular tree is less.

4. Elimination of spasm with preservation of visceral and sexual function, unlike with rhizotomy or intrathecal injection of alcohol.

5. Use of thigh tissue for transfer to damaged areas.

6. Additional psychologic, cosmetic, and metabolic advantages.

The disadvantages of the operation should, however, be carefully evaluated:

1. Functional. The average paraplegic is said to have an approximately 80 per cent chance of walking with crutches; 30 per cent do well with braces; however, only 10 per cent make use of this type of locomotion aid.

2. Cosmetic. Absence of legs may be a disturbing sight for some patients.

3. Stabilization. Legs are needed for stabilization before upper girdle strength is developed.

4. Irreversibility. This may be a source of emotional stress.

From a 16-year accumulated experience, Royer, Pickrell, Georgiade, Mladick, and Thorne (1969) presented a comprehensive study of the use of total thigh flaps for extensive decubiti. Indications for selecting this type of operation, when standard procedures are no longer feasible, are: (a) multiple or recurrent ulcers with insufficient adjacent tissue; (b) large trochanteric ulcers complicated by pyarthrosis and/or osteomyelitis of the femur; (c) multiple ulcers associated with ankylosed hip or knee joints; (d) single ulcers too large to be covered by rotation flaps; (e) ulcers with associated pelvic osteomyelitis.

Preoperative preparation in these cases should be complete. Proper attention to blood volume and control of muscle spasm by drugs or neurosurgical techniques are important preoperative measures. Local wound care to clean the ulcer bed should be done before

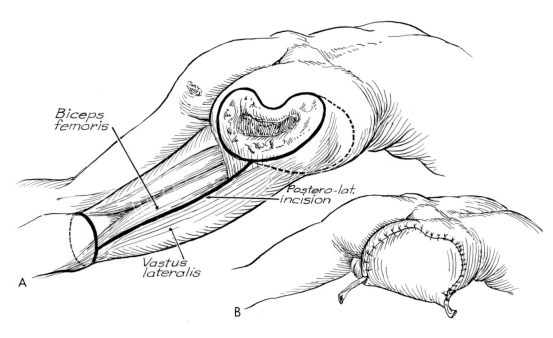

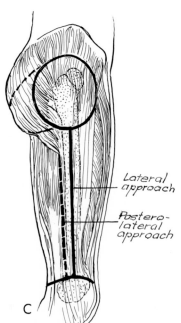

**FIGURE 91–15.** Total thigh flap, as suggested by Georgiade, Pickrell, and Maguire (1956), for large areas of compromised soft tissues and hip joint involvement. *A,* Lateral approach incision line between the biceps femoris and vastus lateralis muscles. *B,* The flap has been sutured in place after disarticulation of the extremity. *C,* The difference between the lateral and posterolateral approach.

surgery. Preoperative roentgenograms and sinograms (Lopez and Aranha, 1974) (see Fig. 91–3) are helpful in determining intra-articular involvement of the pelvis and may aid in detecting not only the presence but also the extent of osteomyelitis. Such studies also help to determine the area of bone to be removed.

Careful urologic studies are paramount in the preoperative evaluation because of the frequency of urinary complications, particularly in those with indwelling catheters. Urine cultures are obtained to identify organisms prior to treatment. Intravenous pyelograms and cystograms will demonstrate stones, ureteral reflux, or hydronephrosis. Urinary diversion by an ileal loop should be undertaken prior to surgical repair of the ulcer if the patient shows evidence of a neurogenic bladder, vesicoureteral reflux, hydronephrosis, hydroureter, or recurrent pyelonephritis.

Amputation and filleting is a formidable technical procedure, even with the use of a pneumatic tourniquet, and should be reserved for those patients with an extensive ulceration that has not responded to more conservative procedures. An estimation of the tissue required determines the length of the flap. In a case in which a total thigh

flap is required, the lower circumferential incision is made in the region of the popliteal space, as suggested by Georgiade and coworkers (1956) (Fig. 91–15). If sacral defects are to be covered, a level approximately 9 inches below the knee should be chosen (Fig. 91–16). At this point the incision is extended onto the thigh.

The type of thigh incision recommended by Georgiade, Pickrell, and Maguire (1956) and Royer and associates (1969) has a definite advantage over the incision advocated by Spira and Hardy (1963) along the posterior aspect of the thigh (see Fig. 91–16). The former (see Fig. 91–15) is made along the posterolateral aspect of the thigh, with the dissection in the relatively avascular plane of the lateral intermuscular septum, located between the vastus lateralis and the biceps femoris, and extended toward its insertion in the linea aspera. The dissection is subperiosteal up to the level of the greater trochanter, at which level the femur can be divided. If necessary, because of associated pyarthrosis, a hip disarticulation can also be accomplished at the same time. If osteomyelitis is present, extensive resection of the acetabulum and ischium may be performed. The surrounding soft tissue is used to fill the dead space.

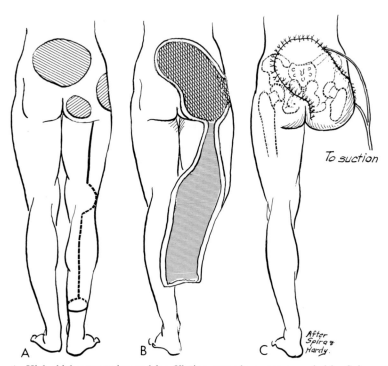

**FIGURE 91–16.** *A,* High thigh amputation and leg filleting procedure recommended by Spira and Hardy (1963) for patients with multiple or extensive ulcerations. *B,* Filleting of leg and thigh soft tissues has been completed. The ulcerated areas have been excised en bloc. *C,* Leg flap folded upon itself, covering the entire sacrotrochanteric-ischial areas.

The distal end of the flap is folded upon itself, and the opposing soft tissue and fascia are carefully approximated to obliterate all dead space. Two or more catheters are used for suction purposes.

One variation of the flap is the island leg flap described by Weeks and Brower (1968). The entire length of the soft tissue of the leg down to the level of the metatarsus is used for coverage of extensive ulcers (Fig. 91–17). The technique consists of filleting of the soft tissues from the foot, with the plane of dissection between the subcutaneous tissue and the extensor tendons anteriorly and the plantar fascia posteriorly, with preservation of the anterior tibial vessels. The filleting continues up subperiosteally to the tibia, fibula, and lower femur. The femoral vessels are mobilized through Hunter's canal to obtain a neurovascular pedicle of 8 to 10 inches in length. The vascular pedicle is passed between the posterior thigh muscles, and the flap is fitted into the defect.

In a follow-up of 41 thigh flaps performed on 28 paraplegics (Royer, Pickrell, Georgiade, Mladick, and Thorne, 1969), the most common complications were postoperative hemorrhage, infection, sinus tracts, wound dehiscence, acute pyelonephritis, and malrotation of the femoral stump. There was a total of 34 complications. It was significant that only 5 of the 28 patients (18 per cent) did not require additional surgery for recurrent ulcers or wound complications. Of the 17 survivors, only 9 were free of recurrent ulceration; of the 11 who died, only 2 were free of ulceration at the time of death. The total recurrence rate was approximately 60 per cent.

COMPLICATIONS

*Necrosis.* As with any skin flap, the most feared complication is necrosis. This may occur in a limited fashion at the most distal portion of the flap, or it might involve the major portion of the flap.

Clinical signs of circulatory impairment appear fairly early. As a first sign, within a few minutes or hours into the postoperative period, a mottled bluish discoloration may be present over the affected area, and with this, a change in the surface temperature of the flap is perceptible. These might be the only evident clinical changes; a few hours later the condition might improve, and the flap may regain its normal color and temperature.

When signs of improvement fail to appear and the area of involvement is located peripherally

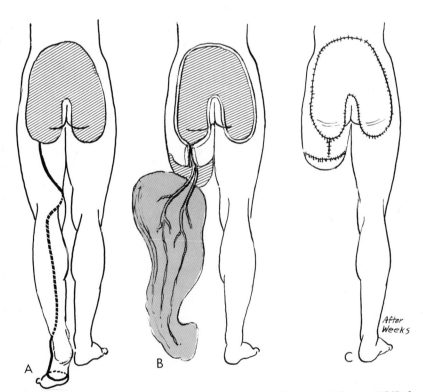

**FIGURE 91–17.** *A,* Incision outline of the operation recommended by Weeks and Brower (1968) for extensive and confluent ulcerations. *B,* Filleting of tissues with vascular pedicle, including anterior tibial and femoral vessels. *C,* Coverage of the entire sacral and ischial areas.

and/or locally, it may be because the suture line is too snug, leading to local edema. In this situation removal of some sutures may prove beneficial. In addition, restoring the flap to its donor site is sometimes necessary.

The necrosis is occasionally established but is of a relatively superficial nature, being manifested only by blistering of the epidermis. This condition is also reversible after a few days; however, when the necrosis is more advanced with involvement of the dermal layer, the small wound defect that results can frequently be closed by surgical approximation.

When it is evident that a major portion of the flap has been lost, it is advisable to proceed with the excision of the necrotic area within a week of the original procedure, followed, as soon as possible, with coverage by a split-thickness skin graft, until the time when a flap from an adjacent area can be rotated into position.

*Hematomas and seromas.* Hematomas and seromas are the most common causes of flap necrosis, prolonged wound healing, and infection. They should be immediately evacuated upon discovery because of their deleterious effect upon the flap circulation through stretching and collapse of the nutritional vessels when distention of the flap occurs owing to underlying fluid or blood accumulation. The collection can also interfere with the ingrowth of vessels to the flap from the recipient bed.

The fluid accumulation can be removed by needle aspiration and/or gentle expression of the jellylike clotted blood through a portion of the wound where the sutures have been removed. A large hematoma must be evacuated in the operating room.

*Infection.* This complication is rarely seen, but if it develops it should be treated, after appropriate bacteriologic studies, by the proper antibiotic administered systemically.

*Wound separation.* This occurs occasionally, particularly in the debilitated patient or in the flap sutured under tension. When debilitation is a factor, redoubled efforts should be made to improve the nutritional status. Wound tension generally indicates defective planning of the flap or an effort to close the donor wound without using a split-thickness skin graft when the indications were clear that such a graft should have been used (Conway and associates, 1951).

*Recurrence.* The recurrence rate following the surgical repair of bedsores is high despite continued improvement in technique. In a follow-up of 100 paraplegics, the recurrence rate was 44 per cent within four years of surgery (Harding, 1961). In the series reported by Griffith and Schultz (1961), 49 of the 73 ulcers surgically treated were recurrent; the three troublesome sites of recurrent ulceration were sacral (12), trochanteric (18), and ischial (19). The causes of recurrent ulceration were (1) residual sharp bony prominence following inadequate ostectomy; (2) overlying scar tissue because the surgical wound had healed by secondary intention; (3) application of a split-thickness skin graft over bone; (4) residual sinus tract; (5) osteomyelitis; and (6) dehiscence of a surgical wound associated with spasticity. Contributing factors were (1) poor hygiene; (2) malnutrition and anemia; (3) prolonged sitting; and (4) prolonged immobilization in bed because of medical problems.

## REFERENCES

Arnott, N.: Elements of Physics or Natural Philosophy, General and Medical. Vol. 1. Philadelphia, Lea and Blanchard, 1838, p. 499.

Artz, C. P., and Hargest, T. S.: Air-fluidized bed. *In* Artz, C. P., and Hargest, T. S. (Eds.): Clinical and Research Symposium. Medical University of South Carolina, Milton Roy Co., 1971.

Baran, E., Payandeh, A., Strax, T., Sokolow, J., and Grynbaum, B. B.: Deforming pressure measurements and a new type mattress. Paper presented at American Congress of Rehabilitation Medicine, Denver, Colorado, Aug. 20–25, 1972.

Barker, D. E.: Surgical treatment of decubitus ulcers. J.A.M.A., *129*:160, 1945.

Barker, D. E., Elkins, C. W., and Poer, D. H.: Methods of closure of decubitus ulcers in the paralyzed patient. Ann. Surg., *123*:523, 1946.

Bateman, F. J. A.: Silicone barrier cream in prevention of bedsores. Br. Med. J., *1*:554, 1956.

Berger, J. S.: Surgical treatment of decubitus ulcers. Plast. Reconstr. Surg., *20*:206, 1957.

Berkas, E. M., Chesler, M. D., and Sako, Y.: Multiple decubitus ulcer treatment by hip disarticulation and soft tissue flaps from the lower limbs. Plast. Reconstr. Surg., *27*:618, 1961.

Blocksma, R., Kostrubala, J., and Greeley, P.: The surgical repair of decubitus ulcers in paraplegics. Plast. Reconstr. Surg., *4*:123, 1949.

Bors, E.: Veterans Administration Technical Bulletin. TB 10–503, Washington, D.C., Dec. 15, 1948.

Bors, E., and Comarr, A. E.: Ischial decubitus ulcer. Surgery, *24*:680, 1948.

Brooks, B., and Duncan, G. W.: Effects of pressure on tissues. Arch. Surg. *40*:696, 1940.

Brown-Séquard, C. E.: Experimental researches applied to physiology and pathology. New York, H. Bailliere, 1853.

Burkhardt, B. R.: An alternative to the total-thigh flap for coverage of massive decubitus ulcers. Plast. Reconstr. Surg., *49*:433, 1972.

Burton, A. C., and Yamada, S.: Relation between blood pressure and flow in human forearm. J. Appl. Physiol., *4*:329, 1951.

Butterworth, R. F., and Golding, C.: A device for treating

pressure sores around the ankles. Geriatrics, *20*:413, 1965.

Campbell, R. M.: The surgical management of pressure sores. Surg. Clin. North Am., *39*:509, 1959.

Campbell, R. M., and Converse, J. M.: The saddle flap for surgical repair of ischial decubitus ulcers. Plast. Reconstr. Surg., *14*:442, 1954.

Cannon, B., O'Leary, J. J., O'Neil, J. W., and Steinsieck, R.: An approach to the treatment of pressure sores. Ann. Surg., *132*:760, 1950.

Charcot, J. M.: Lectures on the Disease of the Nervous System. Delivered at La Saltpètrière. Translated from the Second Edition by G. Sigerson. Philadelphia, Henry C. Lea, 1879.

Chase, R. A.: Personal communication, 1962.

Chase, R. A., and White, W. J.: Bilateral amputation in rehabilitation of paraplegics. Plast. Reconstr. Surg., *24*:445, 1959.

Clark, A. B., and Rusk, H. A.: Decubitus ulcers treated with dried blood plasma; preliminary report. J.A.M.A., *153*:787, 1953.

Comarr, A. E., and Bors, E.: Perineal urethral diverticulum—Complication of removal of ischium. J.A.M.A., *168*:2000, 1958.

Conway, H., Stark, R. B., Weeter, J. C., Garcia, F. A., and Kavanaugh, J. D.: Complications of decubitus ulcers in patients with paraplegia. Plast. Reconstr. Surg., *7*:117, 1951.

Croce, E. J., and Beakes, C. H. C.: The operative treatment of decubitus ulcer. New Engl. J. Med., *237*:141, 1947.

Croce, E. J., Schullinger, R. N., and Shearer, T. P.: Operative treatment of decubitus ulcer. Ann. Surg., *123*:53, 1946.

Dalton, J. J., Jr., Hackler, R. H., and Bunts, R. C.: Amyloidosis in the paraplegic; incidence and significance. J. Urol., *93*:553, 1965.

Daniel, R. K., Terzis, J. K., and Cunningham, D. M.: Sensory skin flaps for coverage of pressure sores in paraplegic patients. A preliminary report. Plast. Reconstr. Surg., *58*:317, 1976.

Dansereau, J. G., and Conway, H.: Closure of decubiti in paraplegics. Report on 2000 cases. Plast. Reconstr. Surg., *33*:474, 1964.

Davis, J. S.: Operative treatment of scars following bed sores. Surgery, *3*:1, 1938.

Dewis, L. S., Caplan, H. I., and Pache, H. L.: Treatment of decubitus ulcers by use of a water mattress. Arch. Phys. Med., *49*:290, 1968.

Dibble, D. G.: Use of a long island flap to bring sensation to the sacral area in young paraplegics. Plast. Reconstr. Surg., *54*:220, 1974.

Ducker, T. B., and Assenmacher, D.: The pathological circulation in experimental spinal cord injury. Proceedings of the Seventeenth V.A. Spinal Cord Injury Conference. Bronx, New York, Sept. 29, 30, Oct. 1, 1969, p. 10.

Ducker, T. B., and Hamit, H. F.: Experimental treatments of acute spinal cord injury. J. Neutrosurg., *30*:693, 1969.

Ewing, M. R., Garrow, C., Conn, B., Pressley, T. A., Ashley, C., and Kinsella, N. M.: Further experiences in the use of sheep skins as an aid in nursing. Med. J. Aust., *2*:139, 1964.

Exton-Smith, A. N., and Crockett, D. J.: Nature of oedema in paralyzed limbs in hemiplegic patients. Br. Med. J., *2*:1280, 1957.

Fischer, B. H.: Topical hyperbaric oxygen treatment of pressure sores and skin ulcers. Lancet, *2*:405, 1969.

Gelb, J.: Plastic surgical closure of decubitus ulcers in paraplegics as result of civilian injuries. Plast. Reconstr. Surg., *9*:525, 1952.

Georgiade, N., Pickrell, K., and Maguire, C.: Total thigh flaps for extensive decubitus ulcer. Plast. Reconstr. Surg., *17*:220, 1956.

Ger, R.: The surgical management of decubitus ulcers by muscle transposition. Surgery, *69*:106, 1971.

Gibbon, J. H., and Freeman, L. W.: The primary closure of decubitus ulcers. Ann. Surg., *124*:1148, 1946.

Griffith, B. H.: Pressure sores. *In* Gibson, T. (Ed.): Modern Trends in Plastic Surgery. 2nd Ed. London, Butterworths, 1966.

Griffith, B. H., and Schultz, R. C.: The prevention and surgical treatment of recurrent decubitus ulcers in patients with paraplegia. Plast. Reconstr. Surg., *27*:248, 1961.

Groth, K. E.: Clinical observations and experimental studies of the pathogenesis of decubitus ulcers. Acta Chir. Scand., *87* (Suppl. 76):207, 1942.

Guthrie, R. H., and Conway, H.: Surgical Management of decubiti in paraplegics. *In* Proceedings of the Seventeenth V.A. Spinal Cord Injury Conference. Bronx, New York, Sept. 29, 30, Oct. 1, 1969.

Guttmann, L.: The problem of treatment of pressure sores in spinal paraplegics. Br. J. Plast. Surg., *7*:196, 1955.

Harding, R. L.: An analysis of one hundred rehabilitated paraplegics. Plast. Reconstr. Surg., *27*:235, 1961.

Hargest, T. S.: A ceramic application in patient care. Presented at a Symposium on Use of Ceramics in Surgical Implants. January 31 to February 1, 1969. Clemson University and South Carolina State Development Board.

Harris, C.: Decubitus ulcers in the sick aged. J. Am. Geriatr. Soc., *13*:538, 1965.

Harris, C.: Flotation as an aid in the treatment of decubitus ulcers. J. Am. Geriatr. Soc., *15*:605, 1967.

Hofstra, P. C.: The air-fluidized bed for spinal injuries. *In* Artz, C. P., and Hargest, T. S. (Eds.): Clinical and Research Symposium. Medical University of South Carolina, 1971.

Holdsworth, F. W.: Traumatic paraplegia. Ann. R. Coll. Surg., *15*:281, 1954.

Holmes, G.: The Coulstonian Lectures on spinal injuries of warfare. Br. Med. J., *2*:716, 815, 855, 1915.

Houle, R. J.: Evaluation of seat devices designed to prevent ischaemic ulcer in paraplegic patients. Arch. Phys. Med., *90*:587, 1969.

Hubay, C. A., Kiehn, C. L., and Drucker, W. R.: Surgical management of decubitus ulcers in the post-traumatic patient. Am. J. Surg., *93*:705, 1957.

Husain, T.: Experimental study of some pressure effects on tissues, with reference to bed-sore problem. J. Path. Bact., *66*:347, 1953.

Hynes, W.: The skin-dermis graft as an alternative to the direct or tubed flap. Br. J. Plast. Surg., *7*:97, 1954.

Kosiak, M.: Etiology and pathology of ischemic ulcers. Arch. Phys. Med., *40*:62, 1959.

Kosiak, M., Kubicek, N. G., Olson, M., Danz, J. N., and Kottle, F. J.: Evaluation of pressure as a factor in the production of ischial ulcers. Arch. Phys. Med., *39*:623, 1958.

Kostrubala, J. C., and Greeley, P. W.: The problem of decubitus ulcers in paraplegics. Plast. Reconstr. Surg., *2*:403, 1947.

Lamon, J. G., and Alexander, E. J.: Secondary closure of decubitus ulcer with aid of penicillin. J.A.M.A., *127*:396, 1945.

Landis, E. M.: Micro-injection studies of capillary blood pressure in human skin. Heart, *15*:209, 1930.

Lexer, E.: Die gesunte wiederherstellings chirurgie. Band I. Leipzig, Johann Ambrosious Barth, 1931.

Lopez, E. M., and Aranha, G. V.: The value of sinography in the management of decubitus ulcers. Plast. Reconstr. Surg., *53*:208, 1974.

McLennan, C. E., McLennan, M. T., and Landis, E. M.: The effect of external pressure on the vascular volume of the forearm and its relation to capillary blood pressure and venous pressures. J. Clin. Invest., *21*:319, 1942.

Matheson, A. T., and Lipschitz, R.: Nature and treatment of trophic pressure sores. S. Afr. Med. J., *30*:1129, 1956.

Morrison, J. E., and Casali, J. L.: Continuous proteolytic therapy for decubitus ulcers. Am. J. Surg., *93*:446, 1957.

Mulholland, J. H., CoTui, F., Wright, A. M., Vinci, V., and Shafiroff, B.: Protein metabolism and bedsores. Ann. Surg., *118*:1015, 1943.

Munro, D.: Care of the back following spinal cord injuries: A consideration of bedsores. New Engl. J. Med., *223*:391, 1940.

Munro, D.: The rehabilitation of patients totally paralyzed below the waist, with special reference to making them ambulatory and capable of earning their own living, end result study of 445 cases. New Engl. J. Med., *250*:4, 1954.

Nichol, J., Girling, F., Jerrard, W., Claxton, E. B., and Burton, A. C.: Fundamental instability of small blood vessels and critical closing pressures in vascular beds. Am. J. Physiol., *164*:330, 1951.

Nojarova, P.: Personal communication, 1962.

Nyquist, R. H.: Brine bath treatments for decubitus ulcers. J.A.M.A., *169*:927, 1959.

Nyquist, R. H.: A protective "skin-guard" splint. Paraplegia, *3*:56, 1965.

Nyquist, R. H., and Bors, E.: Useful appliances in spastic patients following spinal cord injury. Paraplegia, *2*:120, 1964.

Osborne, R.: The treatment of pressure sores in paraplegic patients. Br. J. Plast. Surg., *8*:214, 1955.

Osterholm, J. L., Mathews, S. J., Irvin, J. D., and Angelakos, E. T.: A review of altered norepinephrine metabolism attending severe spinal injury. Results of alpha methyl tyrosine treatment and preliminary studies. Personal communication, 1971.

Paget, J.: Clinical lecture on bed-sores. Student's J. and Hosp. Gazette (London), *1*:144, 1873.

Petersen, N. C., and Bittmann, S.: The epidemiology of pressure sores. Scand. J. Plast. Surg., *5*:62, 1971.

Pfandler, M.: Flotation, displacement and decubitus ulcers. Am. J. Nursing, *68*:2351, 1968.

Pollock, L. J., Boshes, B., Finkelman, I., Chor, H., and Brown, M.: Spasticity, pseudospontaneous spasms, and other reflex activities late after injury to the spinal cord. Arch. Neurol. Psychiat., *66*:537, 1951.

Reichel, S. M.: Shearing force as a factor in decubitus ulcers in paraplegics. J.A.M.A., *166*:762, 1958.

Royer, J., Pickrell, K., Georgiade, N., Mladick, R., and Thorne, F.: Total thigh flaps for extensive decubitus ulcers. A 16 year review of 41 total thigh flaps. Plast. Reconstr. Surg., *44*:109, 1969.

Rusk, H. A.: New horizons in rehabilitation medicine. *In* Proceedings of the Seventeenth V.A. Spinal Cord Injury Conference. Bronx, New York, Sept. 29, 30, Oct. 1, 1969.

Sanchez, S., Eamegdool, S., and Conway, H.: Surgical treatment of decubitus ulcers in paraplegics. Plast. Reconstr. Surg., *43*:25, 1969.

Scarff, J. E., and Pool, J. L.: Factors causing massive spasm following transection of cord in man. J. Neurosurg., *3*:286, 1946.

Schell, V. C., and Wolcott, L. E.: The etiology and management of decubitus ulcers. Mo. Med., *63*:109, 1966.

Sharbaugh, R. J., and Hargest, T. S.: The effect of air-fluidized systems of microbial growth. Clinical and Research Symposium. Medical University of South Carolina, 1971.

Shaw, W., Baker, D., and Morello, D.: Personal communication, 1976.

Spence, W. R., Burke, R. D., and Rae, J. W., Jr.: Gel support for prevention of decubitus ulcers. Arch. Phys. Med., *48*:283, 1967.

Spencer, M. C.: Treatment of chronic skin ulcer by a proteolytic enzyme-antibiotic preparation. J. Am. Geriatr. Soc., *15*:219, 1967.

Spira, M., and Hardy, S. B.: Our experience with high thigh amputations in paraplegics. Plast. Reconstr. Surg., *31*:344, 1963.

Stallings, J. O., Delgado, J. P., and Converse, J. M.: Turn over island flap of gluteus maximus muscle for the repair of sacral decubitus ulcer. Plast. Reconstr. Surg., *54*:52, 1974.

Stenström, S.: Tumbler flaps. Acta Chir. Scand., Suppl. 213, 1956.

Talbot, H. S.: Report on sexual function in paraplegics. J. Urol., *61*:265, 1949.

Talbot, H. S.: Sexual function in paraplegics. J. Urol., *73*:91, 1955.

Thornhill, H. L., and Williams, M. L.: Experience with the water mattress in a large city hospital. Am. J. Nursing, *68*:2356, 1968.

Tuerk, M.: Foreskin and vulva as ancillary tissue sources. Panminerva Medica, *11*:2, 1969.

Tulenko, J. F.: Surgical treatment of ischial decubitus ulcers with buried derma-fat flap. Plast. Reconstr. Surg., *40*:72, 1967.

Wagner, C. W., Jr., Dohrmann, G. J., Taslits, N., Albin, M. S., and White, R. J.: Histopathology of experimental spinal cord trauma. *In* Proceedings of the Seventeenth V.A. Spinal Cord Injury Conference. Bronx, New York, Sept. 29, 30, Oct. 1, 1969.

Ward, J.: Silicone cream for pressure sores. Nursing Times, *59*:1303, 1963.

Weeks, P. M., and Brower, T. D.: Island flap coverage of extensive decubitus ulcers. Plast. Reconstr. Surg., *42*:433, 1968.

Weinstein, J. D., and Davidson, B. A.: A fluid support mattress and seat for the prevention and treatment of decubitus ulcers. Lancet, *2*:625, 1965.

Weinstein, J. D., and Davidson, B. A.: Fluid support in the prevention and treatment of decubitus ulcers. Am. J. Phys. Med., *45*:283, 1966.

Wesser, D. R., and Kahn, S.: The reversed dermis graft in the repair of decubitus ulcers. Plast. Reconstr. Surg., *40*:252, 1967.

White, J. C., and Hamm, W. G.: Primary closure of bed sores by plastic surgery. Ann. Surg., *124*:1136, 1946.

White, J. C., Hudson, H. W., and Kennard, H. E.: The treatment of bedsores by total excision with plastic closure. U.S. Naval Med. Bull., *45*:445, 1945.

Yeoman, M. P., and Hardy, A. G.: The pathology and treatment of pressure sores in paraplegics. Br. J. Plast. Surg., *7*:179, 1954.

Zeitlin, A. B., Cottrell, T. L., and Lloyd, F. A.: Sexology of the paraplegic male. Fertil. Steril., *8*:337, 1957.

# CHAPTER 92

# DERMOLIPECTOMY OF THE ABDOMINAL WALL, THIGHS, BUTTOCKS, AND UPPER EXTREMITY

Ivo Pitanguy, M.D.

In contemporary society the slim female figure is in vogue. Increased affluence, heavy ingestion of food, and diminished physical activity are responsible for the frequent request to eliminate the signs of obesity or other abnormal body contour defects. The prevention of obesity through dieting and exercising consistently gives more rewarding results than surgical resection of excess adipose tissue. In certain ethnic groups, adipose tissue may accumulate in rather conspicuous areas, however, often independent of either food intake or energy expenditure. Adipose accumulation in the abdominal wall and the lateral aspects of the thighs and buttocks is the most frequent indication for surgical dermolipectomy. These localized adiposities, with or without tissue flaccidity, can often be improved by appropriate surgical procedures. Massive loss of weight in obese individuals may be followed by loose, flabby skin hanging apronlike on the abdominal wall and thighs.

## ABDOMINAL DERMOLIPECTOMY

The abdominal wall is deformed in various pathologic conditions. Multiple pregnancies and diminution of the nervous innervation of the abdominal musculature following multiple operations may result in musculoaponeurotic flaccidity (Fig. 92–1), muscular diastasis, and hernias of the abdominal wall. Retracted surgical scars, striae, and the sequelae of previous abdominal dermolipectomies can complicate the clinical picture.

**History.** The first dermolipectomies of the abdominal wall were performed by surgeons who were repairing massive umbilical hernias. The dermolipectomy facilitated the herniorrhaphy and relieved the patient of a pendulous abdomen. In his thesis (1960), Voloir alluded to a case report of an abdominal wall lipectomy by

3800

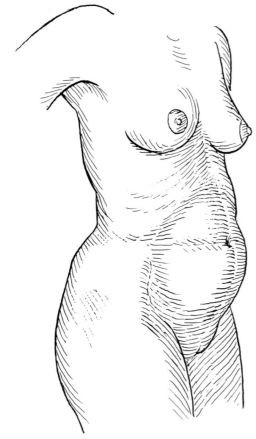

**FIGURE 92–1.** Abdominal adiposity associated with flaccidity of the aponeurotic muscle layer of the abdominal wall.

Demars and Marx (1890) in France. Kelly (1899) called attention to the dermolipectomy in the United States. Case reports subsequently became more numerous in Europe, especially in France and Germany. At the French Congress of Surgery in 1905, Gaudet and Morestin reported transverse closure of the umbilicus in the repair of large hernias in conjunction with resection of excess skin and fat with preservation of the umbilicus. Desjardins (1911) resected a composite of skin and fat weighing 22.4 kg through a vertical elliptical incision. In 1911 Amedée Morestin, the younger brother of Hippolyte Morestin, published five cases of dermolipectomy performed through transverse elliptical incisions. In Germany, Weinhold (1909) recommended a midline type of excision. Jolly (1911) favored a low transverse elliptical excision; Schepelmann (1918) preferred a vertical midline excision extending from the xyphoid to the pubis.

Consequently, in the evolution of the technique of dermolipectomy of the abdominal wall,

three methods have been advocated: (a) vertical midline resection, (b) transverse resection, and (c) a combination of the vertical and transverse methods.

The classic lipectomy incisions are shown in Figure 92–2. They include those of Kelly (1899, 1910), Weinhold (1909), Babcock (1916, 1939), Schepelmann (1918, 1924), Küster (1926), Flesch-Thebesius and Wheisheimer (1931), Thorek (1924), Pick (1949), Barsky (1950), Galtier (1955), and Gonzalez-Ulloa (1960). Castanares and Goethel (1967) published a modification of the classic techniques in which they combined the vertical and transverse excisions with little or no undermining, which greatly reduced the operating time. Grazer (1973) reviewed his technique in 44 abdominoplasties and recommended a low transverse incision with a vertical limb extending to the old umbilicus. Fischl (1973) felt that, in patients with excess skin and striae in the absence of an abdominal apron, a vertical abdominoplasty, which removes an ellipse of skin, is preferable. Schwartz (1974) advocated elevating the fat apron by suspension by towel clips to a rubber tube stretched between the metal posts used for gynecologic stirrups. Heavy interrupted sutures were then passed through the base of the suspended apron, and in this way excessive blood loss was prevented. Regnault (1975) reported a lower transverse incision in the shape of a W.

**Surgical Principles.** The incision should be as short as possible; it may be lengthened to accommodate lateral bulging and thus correct any discrepancy in length between the upper and lower skin margins. The incision should be directed slightly downward toward the lateral aspect of the trunk, in order to confine the scar to the area normally covered by a bikini-type bathing suit. The rapidly diminishing size of swimming apparel is an increasing surgical challenge.

Extensive undermining in the supra-aponeurotic plane provides exposure of the entire abdominal wall and permits reinforcement of any defects of the musculoaponeurotic wall. These maneuvers are responsible for slimming of the waist and contouring of the abdominal wall. Excessive tension of skin that has not been undermined cannot achieve these goals.

Preoperative marking of the total amount of lipocutaneous tissue to be resected not only is of little technical help but also may be deceptive. Markings of the projected line of resection should be made only after the flap has been completely undermined.

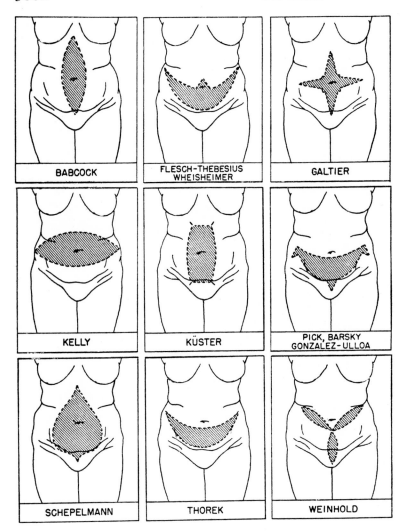

BABCOCK

FLESCH-THEBESIUS WHEISHEIMER

GALTIER

KELLY

KÜSTER

PICK, BARSKY GONZALEZ-ULLOA

SCHEPELMANN

THOREK

WEINHOLD

**FIGURE 92–2.** Incisions used in dermolipectomy and plastic reconstruction of the anterior abdominal wall. (From Pickrell, K. L.: Excess adipose tissue in the abdominal wall. *In* Converse, J. M. (Ed.): Reconstructive Plastic Surgery. Philadelphia, W. B. Saunders Company, 1964, p. 1951.)

In order to ensure adherence of the flap to its bed and to prevent serosanguineous collections, a plaster of Paris dressing, spread over the abdomen and evenly distributed by the weight of a sandbag, is employed in lieu of suction drainage. The plaster dressing, which is left in place for one or two postoperative days, minimizes local pain without hindering diaphragmatic excursions. However, a sudden increase of the intra-abdominal pressure consequent to the musculoaponeurotic reinforcement may hamper respiratory movements in patients with chronic pulmonary pathology. Such patients should be evaluated preoperatively and pulmonary function studies performed.

**Surgical Technique of the Author.**    The median line of the abdomen is drawn with a marking pen (Fig. 92–3), and a stay suture is inserted at the caudal pole (superior border of the pubis).

The superior anterior iliac spines are marked (Fig. 92–4, *A*). The incision line, drawn along the superior limit of the pubic hair, crosses the inguinal fold and continues horizontally until it transects a vertical projection from the iliac spine. In patients with very large abdomens, it may be necessary to extend the incision laterally, with a slight curve downward to compensate for excessive tissue along the superior margin and to avoid unduly long visible scars (Fig. 92–4, *B*).

When the undermining of the flap in the supra-aponeurotic plane (Fig. 92–5) reaches the umbilicus, the flap is divided along the median line of the abdomen, and the umbilicus is circumcised. The dissection proceeds to the costal margin; the umbilicus remains attached by its pedicle, which must be sufficiently wide to assure an adequate vascular supply.

Reinforcement and correction of the musculo-

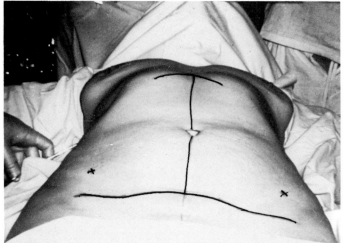

**FIGURE 92–3.** The median line of the abdomen and the incision line along the superior limit of the pubic hair have been drawn.

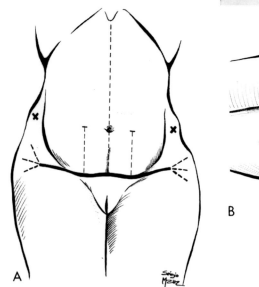

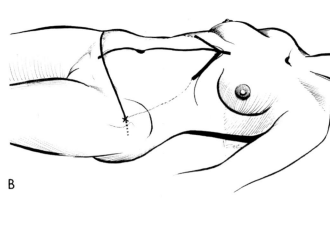

**FIGURE 92–4.** *A*, Frontal view showing the marks (x) over the anterior superior iliac spines. The dotted lines indicate the possible lateral extensions of the incision line. *B*, Lateral view showing the median line of the abdomen and the superior limits of the dissection at the costal margin.

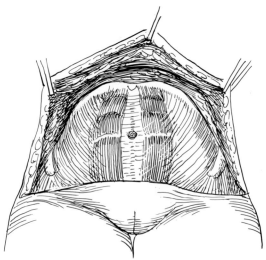

**FIGURE 92–5.** The flap has been undermined in the supra-aponeurotic plane.

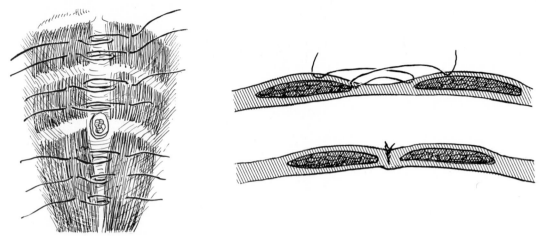

**FIGURE 92–6.** Reinforcement of the aponeurotic layer (closed method).

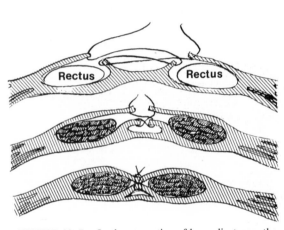

**FIGURE 92–7.** In the correction of large diastases, the aponeurosis is incised prior to surgical reinforcement (open method).

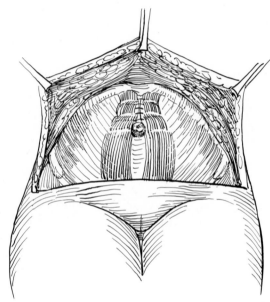

**FIGURE 92–8.** The flap has been elevated, and reinforcement is begun at the xiphoid area.

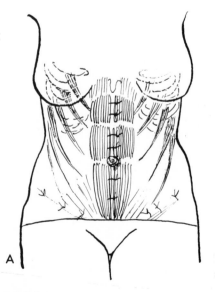

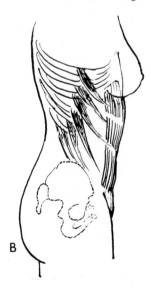

**FIGURE 92–9.** *A,* Frontal view showing the completed musculoaponeurotic reinforcement. *B,* Lateral view.

aponeurotic layers of the abdominal wall (Fig. 92–6) are commenced close to the xyphoid process to avoid bulging of the upper abdomen and are extended to the pubic region; excessive tension must be avoided. Opening of the aponeurosis is not obligatory and is usually reserved for correction of very large diastases and hernias (Fig. 92–7, 92–8, and 92–9).

The operating table is adjusted so that the waist is flexed and the flap is pulled inferiorly and medially in order to estimate the amount of tissue to be excised (Fig. 92–10). Avoidance of undue tension ensures adequate blood supply to

*Text continued on page 3809*

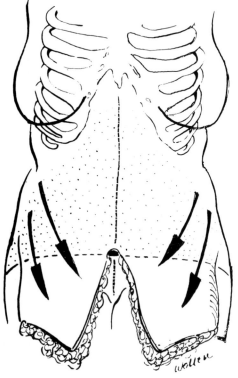

**FIGURE 92–10.** The flaps are advanced in an inferior and medial direction, as indicated by the arrows.

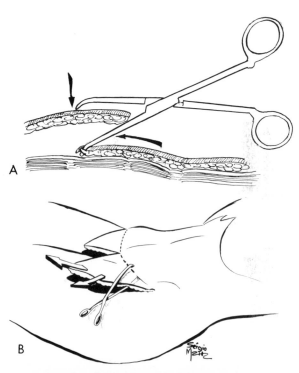

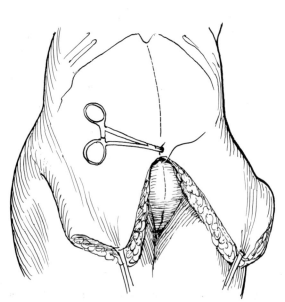

**FIGURE 92–11.** A temporary stay suture is inserted in the midline at the planned level of excision.

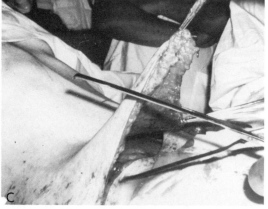

**FIGURE 92–12.** Forceps designed by the author to determine the line of resection of the flap. *A,* The superior limb marks the projected line with methylene blue, while the inferior part is employed for countertraction. *B,* The inferior limb of the forceps is applied for countertraction. *C,* After the flap has been advanced in an inferomedial direction, the forceps is closed to mark the planned line of resection of the flap.

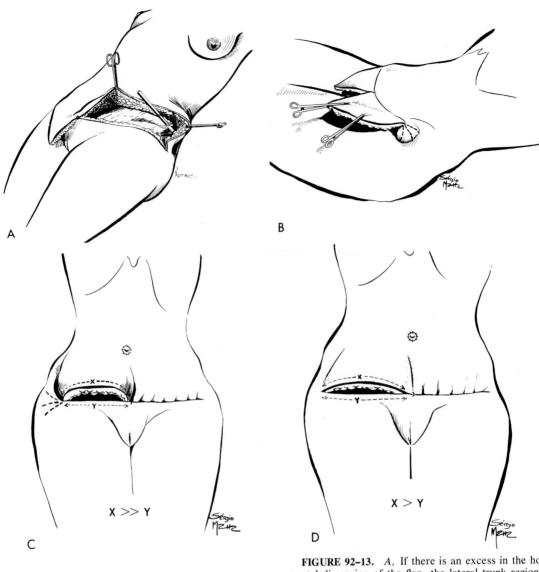

A

B

C

X >> Y

D

X > Y

**FIGURE 92–13.** *A,* If there is an excess in the horizontal dimension of the flap, the lateral trunk region is further undermined. *B,* Dotted lines indicate possible lateral extensions of the incision line to avoid dog-ears in patients with gross deformities. *C,* The horizontal excess of the flap is indicated by X. *D,* X is only slightly greater than Y because of a lateral extension of the incision line.

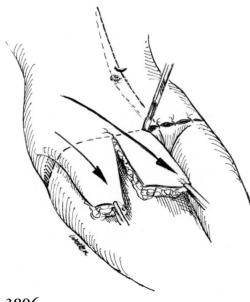

**FIGURE 92–14.** Vertical incisions of the distal portion of the flap facilitate the planned resection. Arrows indicate the direction of the pull of the flap at the time of excision.

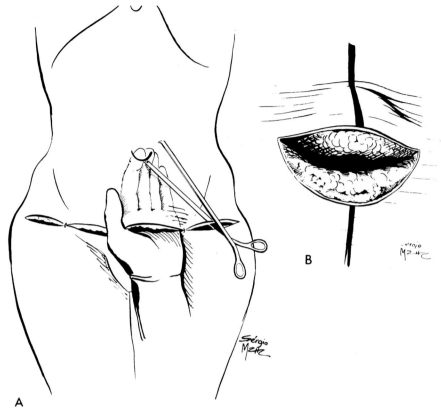

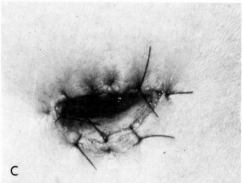

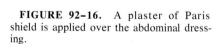

**FIGURE 92–15.** *A,* A curvilinear incision is made in the flap overlying the pedicle of the umbilicus. *B,* The shape of the incision transecting the median line of the abdomen. *C,* The pedicle has been sutured to the fenestration in the flap. There is a resulting natural, semilunar appearance.

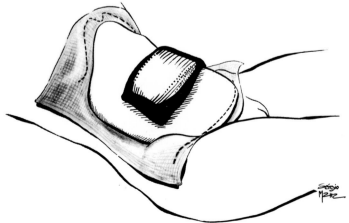

**FIGURE 92–16.** A plaster of Paris shield is applied over the abdominal dressing.

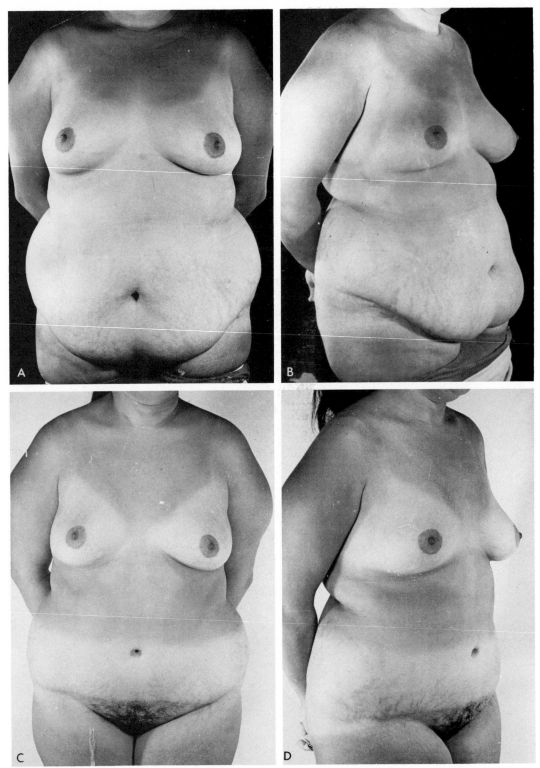

**FIGURE 92–17.** *A,* Preoperative frontal view of a female patient with adiposity and flaccidity of the abdominal wall. *B,* Preoperative profile. *C,* Postoperative frontal view following the author's technique. *D,* Postoperative profile.

the distal aspect of the flap. A temporary suture is placed in the midline between the two skin edges at the planned level of excision (Fig. 92–11). The planned resection of skin and adipose tissue is outlined, using a special forceps (Fig. 92–12).

The excess portion of the abdominal flap is excised after traction is applied in an inferior and medial direction. Any discrepancy resulting from an excess in the horizontal dimension of the flap (Fig. 92–13, *A* to *D*) is corrected or decreased by extending the incision laterally. Vertical cuts into the flap (Fig. 92–14) facilitate resection of the distal portion of the flap.

The navel is reattached to the dermis-fat flap through a curved incision with superior concavity (Fig. 92–15, *A*, *B*). When traction is applied to the flap, the umbilicus, which has contracted upon itself, expands and assumes a natural, semilunar appearance (Fig. 92–15, *C*).

As described previously, a plaster of Paris shield applied over a well-padded dressing and maintained in position with elastic bandages

**TABLE 92–1.** *Indications for Abdominal Dermolipectomy*

| | | |
|---|---|---|
| Flaccidity | 280 | 52% |
| Postsurgical scars | 198 | 35% |
| Multiple pregnancies | 91 | 17% |
| Muscular diastasis | 17 | 3% |
| Umbilical hernias | 34 | 6% |
| Sequelae of abdominoplasty performed by other surgeons | 34 | 6% |

distributes the weight of the overlying sandbags (Fig. 92–16). This helps to achieve adherence of the flap to the bed and also to avoid a serosanguineous collection. One must emphasize the fact that excessive traction or insufficient undermining of the flap may prevent satisfactory results. Tension can be alleviated by positioning the patient in a semi-Fowler position during the procedure and by slowly extending the position during the postoperative period.

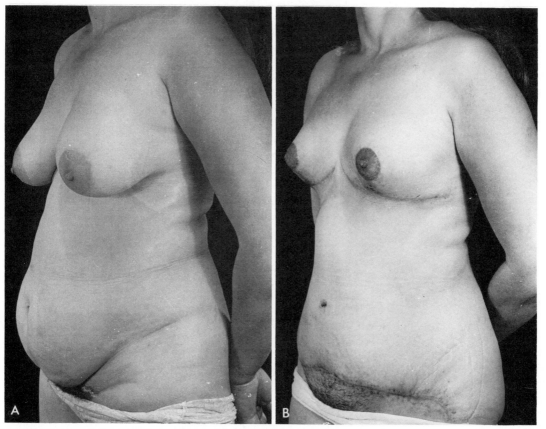

**FIGURE 92–18.** *A*, Preoperative appearance of a patient with macromastia and abdominal adiposity. *B*, Appearance following reduction mammaplasty and abdominoplasty. Note prominence of surgical scars in the early postoperative period.

**Results.**    A study of 539 consecutive abdominoplasties performed by the above technique between 1953 and 1974 was completed. Table 92–1 analyzes the indications for surgery. Over half of the patients underwent corrective surgery for flaccidity of the abdominal wall. Abdominal surgical scars, the "washboard abdomen" following multiple pregnancies, muscular diastases, umbilical hernias, and problems associated with previously performed abdominoplasties were other surgical indications.

The age of the patients is outlined in Table 92–2. Most of the patients were in the age group from 25 to 49 years, and this reflected the age for child-bearing and gynecologic procedures.

In the series there were 77 complications

TABLE 92–2.    *Age of Patients Undergoing Abdominal Dermolipectomy*

| YEAR | NUMBER OF CASES | PER CENT |
|------|-----------------|----------|
| Until 20 | 3 | 0.5 |
| 20–24 | 24 | 4.4 |
| 25–29 | 70 | 12.9 |
| 30–34 | 85 | 15.9 |
| 35–39 | 112 | 20.7 |
| 40–44 | 65 | 12.2 |
| 45–49 | 82 | 15.2 |
| 50–54 | 38 | 7.05 |
| 55–59 | 28 | 5.3 |
| 60–64 | 20 | 3.7 |
| 65–69 | 7 | 1.2 |
| 70– | 5 | 0.9 |
| | Total: 539 | |

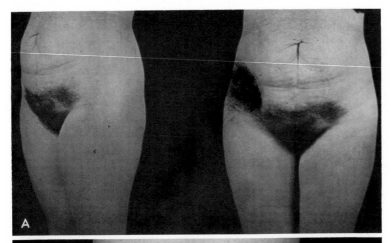
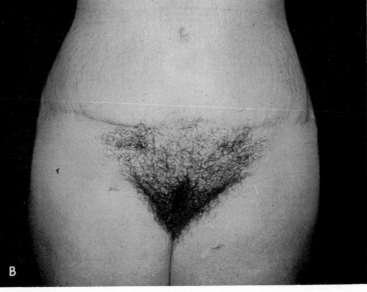

**FIGURE 92–19.** *A*, Abdominal flaccidity associated with a depressed lower midline scar. *B*, Result obtained by the author's technique.

TABLE 92–3. *Study of the Complications in Abdominal Dermolipectomy Performed Between the Years 1953 and 1974*

| | | |
|---|---|---|
| Serosanguineous collections (required drainage) | 14 | 2.5% |
| Serosanguineous collections (no drainage) | 18 | 3.3% |
| Hypertrophic scars | 20 | 3.7% |
| Dehiscence of sutures | 2 | 0.3% |
| Small area of sloughing not requiring additional surgery | 8 | 1.4% |
| Area of sloughing requiring additional surgery | 2 | 0.3% |
| Poor appearance of scar and body contour | 2 | 0.3% |
| Residual adiposity in the epigastrium (vertical incision because of other scars) | 2 | 0.3% |
| Temporary postoperative emotional disorders | 2 | 0.3% |
| Suture reaction | 5 | 0.9% |
| Minor slough of umbilical scar associated with umbilical hernias | 2 | 0.3% |

(Table 92–3). Serosanguineous collections occurred in 32 patients, 14 of whom required surgical drainage. Twenty patients had hypertrophic or cosmetically unacceptable scars. There was some degree of flap necrosis in ten patients, but only two required corrective surgery.

Patients who have undergone corrective surgery by the author's technique are shown in Figures 92–17 to 92–21.

## DERMOLIPECTOMY OF THE THIGHS AND BUTTOCKS

The accumulation of localized adipose tissue on the lateroposterior aspect of the thighs and buttocks produces an esthetically ungraceful appearance known as trochanteric lipodystrophy or the "riding breeches" deformity. In addition to the bulging area of adiposity, a depression is often noted on the posterior lateral aspect of the buttocks. A similar deformity is frequently apparent on the inner side of the thighs, usually accompanied by flaccidity of the skin and subcutaneous tissue. Drooping of the buttocks secondary to musculocutaneous flaccidity due to aging is another type of deformity.

**Author's Technique for Correction of Trochanteric Lipodystrophy.** The localized adiposity along the lateral side of the thighs may be accompanied by a depression (Fig. 92–22). The fusiform area of skin and subcutaneous fat to be resected is marked while the patient is standing. The lateral extremity of the planned excision extends upward toward the anterior superior iliac spine. The superior margin should include the posterolateral depression (see Fig. 92–22, *A*, *B*). As the fusiform wedge of skin and subcutaneous fat is excised (Fig. 92–23, *A*), the convexity of the posterior buttock is maintained by beveling the edges so that the lower flap can be advanced under the upper flap. A small amount of undermining (Fig. 92–23, *B*) creates superior and inferior flaps and facilitates the

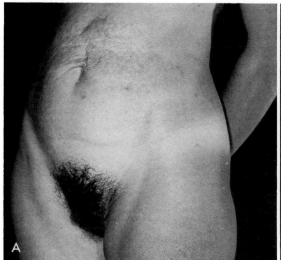 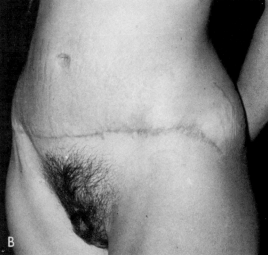

**FIGURE 92–20.** *A*, Appearance of the abdominal wall following multiple pregnancies ("washboard abdomen"). *B*, Postoperative appearance following abdominal dermolipectomy by the author's technique.

above flap advancement. The inferior flap is then rotated in a superior direction toward the midline (Fig. 92–24). The flaps are approximated (Fig. 92–25), and any posterolateral depression should be corrected.

The results obtained by this technique are illustrated in Figures 92–26 and 92–27.

**Technique for Correction of the Flaccidity of the Anterior Femoral and Medial Thigh Region.** This deformity is frequently associated with trochanteric lipodystrophy and can be corrected at the same operative session. The posterior incision is extended medially along the medial aspect of the thigh in the direction of the inguinal crease (Fig. 92–28). Elevation and rotation of the thigh is directed medially with posterior anchorage (Figs. 92–29 and 92–30). The rotation facilitates closure by permitting approximation without tension at the medial aspect of the thigh. In more pronounced cases, it may be necessary to undermine the area (Fig. 92–31).

*Text continued on page 3818*

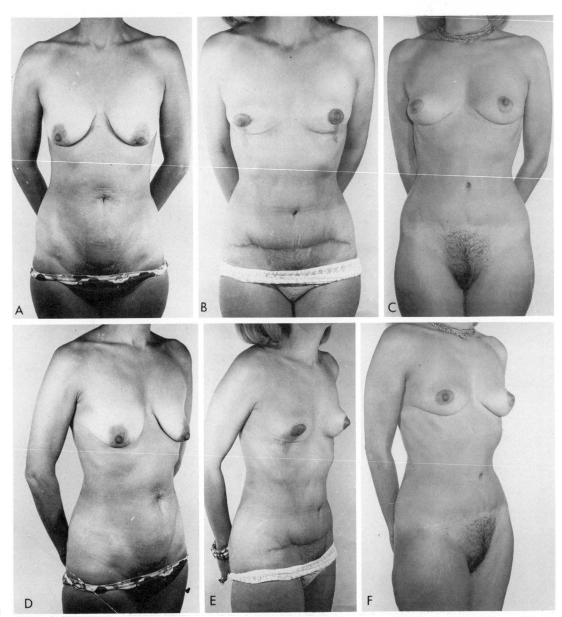

**FIGURE 92–21.**  *A*, Postpregnancy abdominal flaccidity associated with ptosis of the breasts. *B*, Immediately following abdominoplasty and mastopexy. *C*, Appearance four years following surgery. Note the improvement in the appearance of the scars. *D*, Preoperative oblique view. *E*, Immediate postoperative result. Note the lateral extent of the abdominal incision. *F*, Four years following surgery.

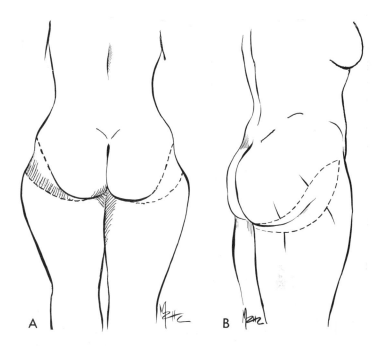

**FIGURE 92–22.** Posterior view of the planned area of excision of skin and subcutaneous fat. Note the posterolateral depressions included in the resection. *B,* Incisions extend superiorly and laterally toward the anterior superior iliac spine.

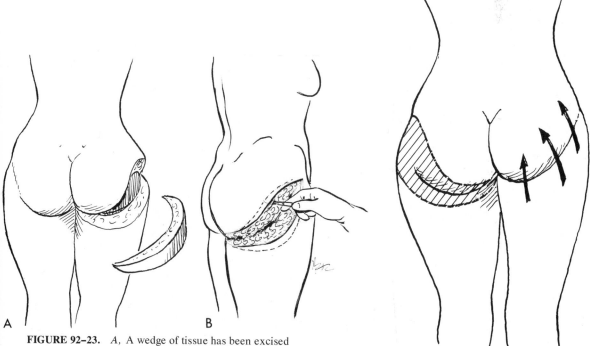

**FIGURE 92–23.** *A,* A wedge of tissue has been excised and the edges of the incision beveled. *B,* Undermining of the edges for a small distance facilitates advancement of the lower flap to reestablish the natural convexity of the buttock.

**FIGURE 92–24.** The arrows indicate the direction of the lower flap advancement.

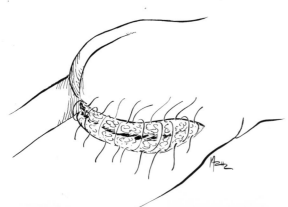

**FIGURE 92–25.** Approximation of the wound edges.

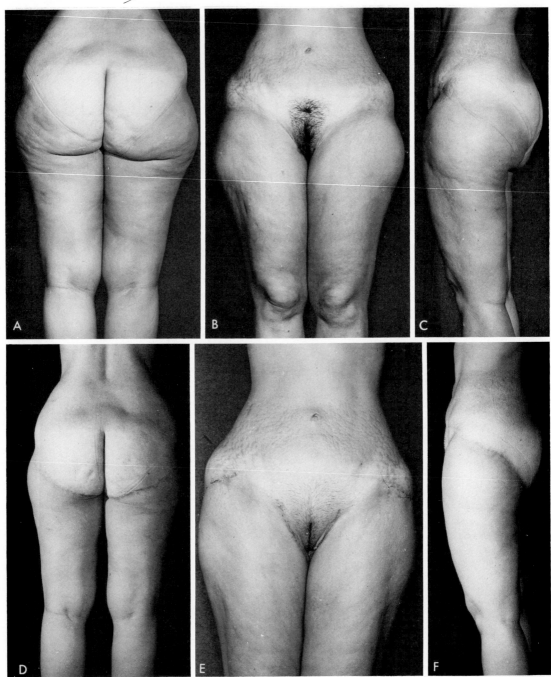

**FIGURE 92–26.** *See legend on the opposite page.*

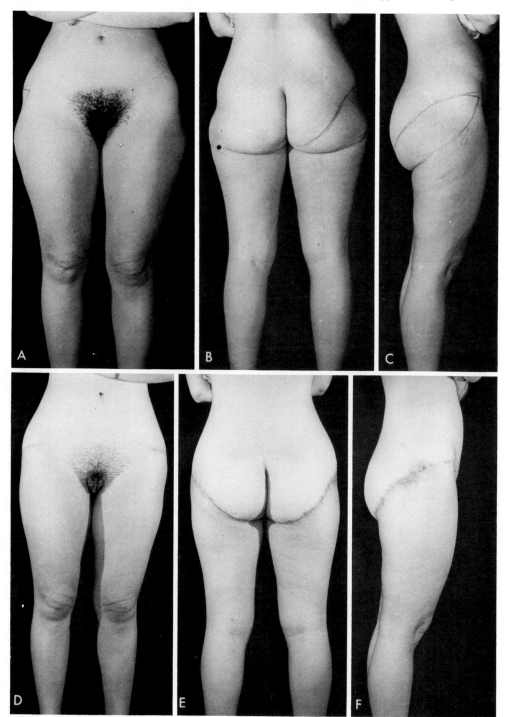

**FIGURE 92–27.** *A*, Preoperative frontal view of a patient with trochanteric lipodystrophy. *B*, Posterior view showing the upper limit of the planned resection. *C*, Preoperative profile showing the outline of the planned excision. *D*, Postoperative frontal view following correction by the author's technique. *E*, Postoperative posterior view. *F*, Postoperative profile.

**FIGURE 92–26.** *A*, Posterior view of a patient with trochanteric lipodystrophy. *B*, Preoperative frontal view. *C*, Preoperative profile. *D*, Postoperative posterior view following the author's technique. *E*, Postoperative frontal view. *F*, Postoperative profile.

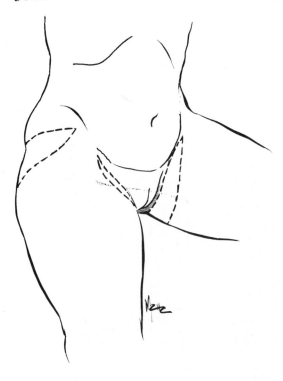

**FIGURE 92–28.** If the medial thigh deformity is associated with trochanteric lipodystrophy, the medial pole of the fusiform strip is extended into the inguinal crease.

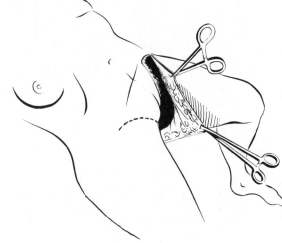

**FIGURE 92–29.** Limited undermining to create an inferior flap may be necessary.

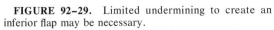

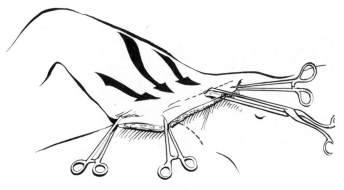

**FIGURE 92–30.** The flap is advanced medially and superiorly, and an appropriate amount of skin and subcutaneous tissue is resected.

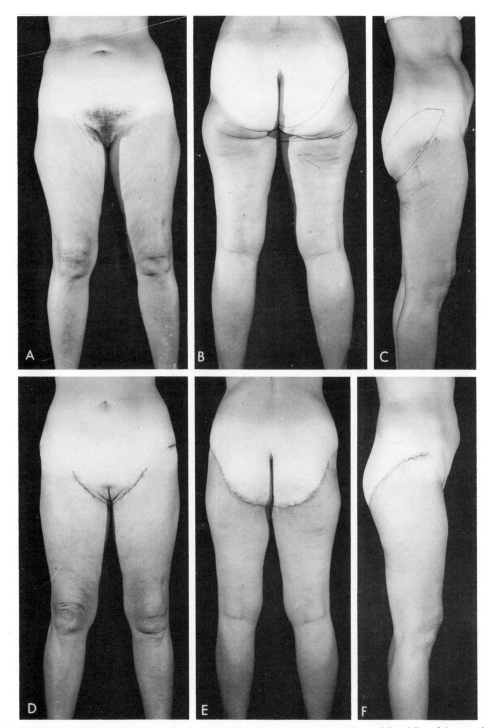

**FIGURE 92–31.** *A,* Preoperative view of a patient with trochanteric lipodystrophy and flaccidity of the anterior femoral and medial thigh regions. Note the extension of the planned resection into the inguinal crease. *B,* Posterior view with outline of the planned excision. *C,* Preoperative profile. *D,* Postoperative frontal view following the author's technique. *E,* Postoperative posterior view. *F,* Postoperative profile.

TABLE 92–4. *Indications for Dermolipectomy of the Thighs and Buttocks*

| | | |
|---|---|---|
| Trochanteric lipodystrophy | 55 | 57.4% |
| Flaccidity of the anterior femoral and medial thigh region | 21 | 21.8% |
| Drooping buttocks | 14 | 14.5% |
| Gluteal hypertrophy | 1 | 1.0% |
| Sequelae of previous lipectomies | 5 | 5.3% |
| Total: | 96 | |

**Technique for Correction of Drooping Buttocks.** In cases of drooping buttocks due to musculocutaneous weakness and to flaccidity, the resection is restricted to the posterior aspect and consists only of skin and a thin layer of subcutaneous tissue. The closure is accomplished in two planes, after rotation of the flap upward and outward, remodeling, and upward traction on the buttocks (Fig. 92–32 and 92–33).

**Results.** A review of 70 consecutive patients who have undergone crural dermolipectomies has been completed. Analysis of the series according to the indications for surgery is shown in Table 92–4. Patients with generalized lipodystrophy, in general, are poor candidates for

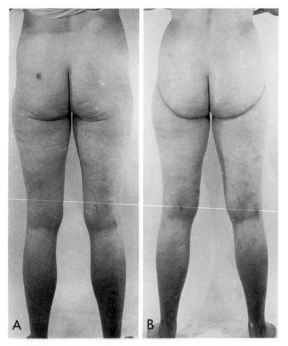

**FIGURE 92–32.** *A,* Preoperative posterior view of a patient with hanging buttocks. *B,* Postoperative appearance.

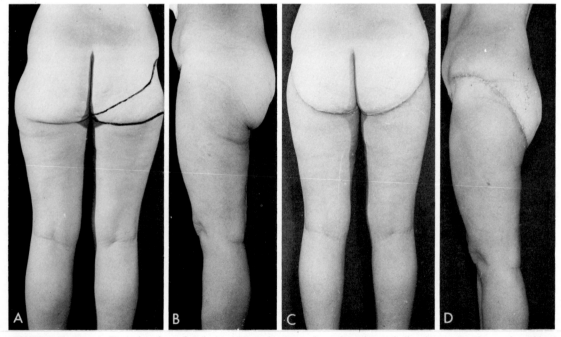

**FIGURE 92–33.** *A,* Posterior view of patient with hanging buttocks and trochanteric lipodystrophy. Correction of both deformities is achieved at the same procedure. *B,* Preoperative profile. *C,* Postoperative posterior appearance. *D,* Postoperative profile.

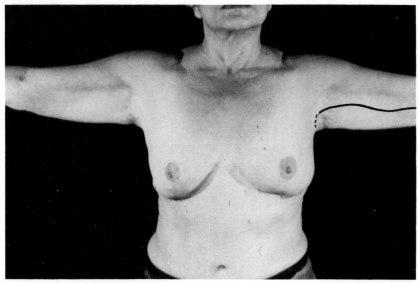

**FIGURE 92–34.** The incision is outlined with the patient in a standing position and the arms fully abducted in order to show the projection of the inner aspect of the biceps muscle, usually where the area of redundant skin begins.

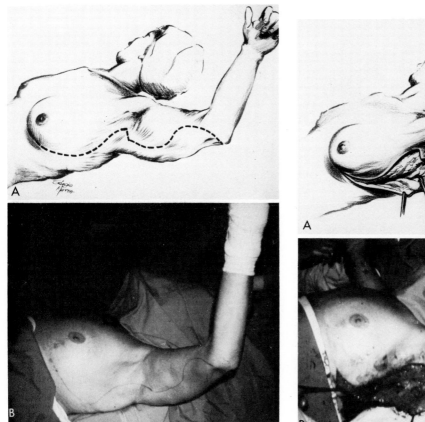

**FIGURE 92–35.** The incision extends from the infra-mammary sulcus toward the elbow, allowing a break in the axillary region.

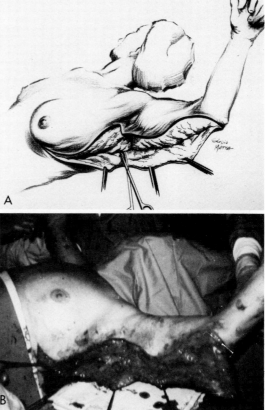

**FIGURE 92–36.** The incision has been made and the flaps have been undermined.

corrective surgery. Occasionally such a patient may be accepted for surgery provided the palliative character of the procedure and the relatively high risk of recurrence are carefully explained to the patient.

## DERMOLIPECTOMY OF THE UPPER EXTREMITY

It is essential to preplan by determining the incision line with the patient in a standing position and the arms extended so as to show the osteomuscular topographic projection. The redundant portion of skin usually follows a sinuous line along the medial side of the arms, approximately coinciding with the inner margin of the biceps muscle (Fig. 92–34). This line is extended laterally and toward the elbow, so as to indicate the amount of resection of flaccid and redundant skin (Fig. 92–35). In the proximal direction, the line is extended through the axilla, where it is interrupted to avoid a resultant retractile scar (Lewis, 1973). Continuing it, one designs an inci-

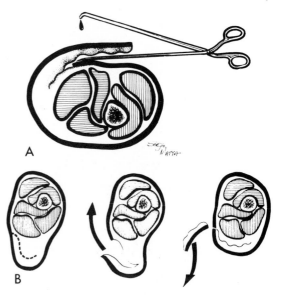

**FIGURE 92–37.** *A,* Cross-sectional view of the arm showing the traction, countertraction, and demarcation of the area that will be resected. *B,* Sequence of views showing the extent of undermining through the subcutaneous tissue and the subsequent traction and resection of the flap.

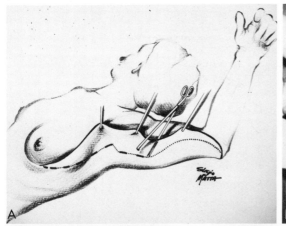

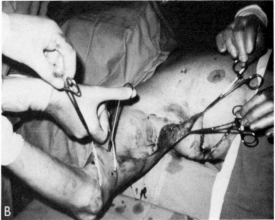

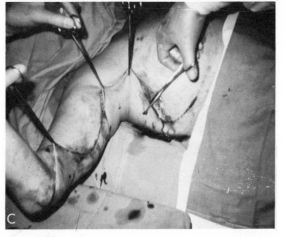

**FIGURE 92–38.** *A, B,* Traction and countertraction of the flap and delineation of the area that will be excised using the Pitanguy forceps. *C,* Outlining the area of excision in the lateral region of the thorax.

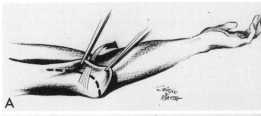

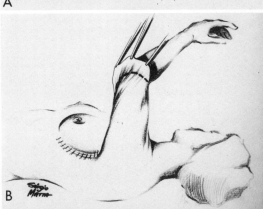

**FIGURE 92–39.** Traction in the region of the elbow is directed equally on all sides.

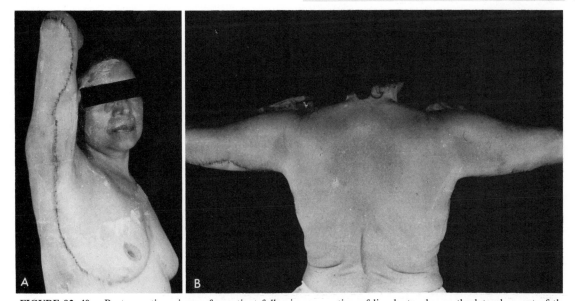

**FIGURE 92–40.** Postoperative views of a patient following correction of lipodystrophy on the lateral aspect of the thorax, inner side of the arm, and elbow ten days after surgery.

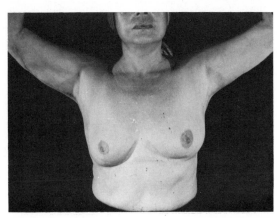

**FIGURE 92–41.** Postoperative view of a patient four weeks after surgical correction.

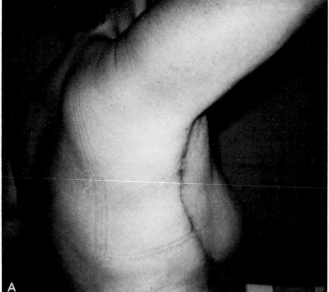
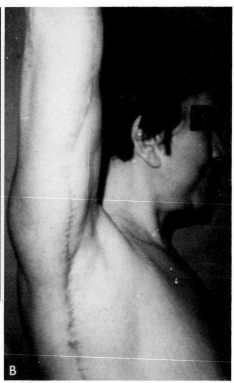

**FIGURE 92–42.** Late postoperative view showing a scar of satisfactory quality without a contracted component.

sion that goes from the posterior axillary line to the inframammary sulcus; this will be the surgical approach to correct the flaccidity on the lateral aspect of the thorax.

The dissection is carried anteroposteriorly, elevating flaps of sufficient length for the desired resection (Fig. 92–36). The area to be resected is outlined with Pitanguy forceps (Pitanguy and coworkers, 1974). Countertraction is provided at the anterior border of the incision, and the flap is advanced to a position that will furnish the desired result. The wound is closed without any tension to avoid a cosmetically unacceptable scar (Figs. 92–37 and 92–38).

When traction is applied to the skin of the elbow region, it should be directed equally on all sides (Fig. 92–39). When the deformity is localized exclusively on the arm, the extensions of the incision to the elbow or to the lateral region of the thorax can be eliminated.

Closure of the wound is made in four layers: deep subcutaneous tissue (adipose tissue), subdermal, intradermal, and skin. The first three layers are sutured with self-absorbing material, and the skin is closed with interrupted 5–0 nylon sutures. A semicompressive dressing is covered by an adhesive elastic bandage. Results are shown in Figures 92–40 and 92–41.

Other techniques employ a longitudinal incision along the inner side of the arm, resulting in a linear scar which is more visible and esthetically less acceptable. The sinuous incision, extending to the lateral region of the thorax, yields a superior cosmetic result (Fig. 92–42).

## REFERENCES

Babcock, W. W.: The correction of the obese and relaxed abdominal wall with especial reference to the use of buried silver chain. Am. J. Obstet. Gynecol., *74*:596, 1916.

Babcock, W. W.: Plastic reconstruction of the female breasts and abdomen. Am. J. Surg., *43*:269, 1939.

Barsky, A. J.: Principles and Practice of Plastic Surgery. Baltimore, The Williams & Wilkins Company, 1950.

Castanares, S., and Goethel, J. A.: Abdominal lipectomy; a modification in technique. Plast. Reconstr. Surg., *40*:379, 1967.

Desjardins, P.: Résection de la couche adi d'obesité extrème (lipectomie). Rapport par Dartigues. Paris Chirurg., *3*:466, 1911.

Fischl, R. A.: Vertical abdominoplasty. Plast. Reconstr. Surg., *51*:139, 1973.

Flesch-Thebesius, M., and Wheisheimer, K.: Die Operation des Hängebauches. Chirurg, *3*:841, 1931.

Galtier, M.: Traitement chirurgical des obésités de la paroi abdominale avec ptose. Mém. Acad. Chir., *81*:12, 341, 1955.

Gonzalez-Ulloa, M.: Belt lipectomy. Br. J. Plast. Surg., *13*:179, 1960.

Grazer, F. M.: Abdominoplasty. Plast. Reconstr. Surg., *51*:617, 1973.

Jolly, R.: Die Operation des Fettbauches. Berl. Klin. Wochenschr., *29*:1317, 1911.

Kelly, H. A.: Report of gynecological cases. Johns Hopkins Med. J., *10*:197, 1899.

Kelly, H. A.: Excision of the fat of the abdominal wall—lipectomy. Surg. Gynecol. Obstet., *10*:229, 1910.

Küster, H.: Operation bei Hängebrust und Hängeleib. Monatsschr. Geburtsh. Gynäk., *73*:316, 1926.

Lewis, J. R., Jr.: Atlas of Aesthetic Plastic Surgery. Boston, Little, Brown & Company, 1973, pp. 271–276.

Morestin, A.: La restauration de la paroi abdominale par résection etendue des téguments et de la graisse sous-cutanée et le plissement des aponévroses superficielles envisagé comme complément de la cure radicale des hernies ombilicales. Thèse, Paris, 1911.

Pick, J. F.: Surgery of Repair: Principles, Problems, Procedures. Abdomen (Abdereplasty). Vol. 2, Chapter 24, p. 435. Philadelphia, J. B. Lippincott Company, 1949.

Pickrell, K. L.: Excess adipose tissue in the abdominal wall. *In* Converse, J. M. (Ed.): Reconstructive Plastic Surgery. Philadelphia, W. B. Saunders Company, 1964, p. 1951.

Pitanguy, I., Yobar, A. A., Pires, C. E., and Matta, S. R.: Aspectos atuais das lipectomias abdominais. Bol. Cir. Plast. Rev. Bras. Cirurgia, *19*:149, 1974.

Regnault, P.: Abdominoplasty by the W technique. Plast. Reconstr. Surg., *55*:265, 1975.

Schepelmann, E.: Ueber Bauchdeckenplastik mit besonderes Berucksichtigung des Hängebauches. Beitr. Klin. Chir., *111*:372, 1918; Zentralbl. Gynäk., *48*:2289, 1924.

Schwartz, A. W.: A technique for excision of abdominal fat. Br. J. Plast. Surg., *27*:44, 1974.

Thorek, M.: Plastic Surgery of the Breast and Abdominal Wall. Springfield, Ill., Charles C Thomas, Publisher, 1924.

Voloir, P.: Opérations plastiques sus-aponévrotiques sur la paroi abdominale antérieure. Thèse, Paris, 1960.

Weinhold, S.: Bauchdeckenplastik. Zentralbl. Gynäk., *38*:1332, 1909.

*Part Six*

# THE GENITOURINARY SYSTEM

# CHAPTER 93

# EMBRYOLOGY OF THE GENITOURINARY SYSTEM

CLIFFORD C. SNYDER, M.D.,
DOUGLAS S. DAHL, M.D.,
AND EARL Z. BROWNE, JR., M.D.

Daring investigations by experimental embryologists of early genitourinary developmental anatomy in the human are alluring, but their results are at best circumstantial. Dissected morphology comparatively observed is subject to diverse opinions and interpretations. Scientists who devote a lifetime to this study remain mystified as to the origin and the mode of development of specific germ cell organizations which establish an adult anlage.

One of many problems is the temporary existence of a specific embryonic structure that appears for a few days and then vanishes without ever becoming functional (Patten, 1953; Arey, 1966). Another unsolved mystery is why the fetal testis is a designator of sex assignment. The findings of other investigators have been confirmed by showing that the female rabbit can develop an entire feminine genital system after removal of the fetal ovaries (Jost, 1958). Conversely, castration of the male rabbit fetus eliminates masculine characteristics. The entire genital system is feminized as the animal simulates the ovariectomized female fetus. If testicular castration is surgically or radiologically performed within the first four weeks of fetal life in rabbits, masculinity is prevented. However, later castration does not inhibit male organogenesis.

These are only two examples of many embryologic complexities. It is also necessary to note that many interpretations are derived from experiments with lower animals and adapted to the human fetus, a comparison not entirely authentic. Finally, the nomenclature used by one investigator may describe a specific primordial development which is the same as that of another investigator who insists on a different term, confusing the subject and the reader (Paul and Kanagasuntheram, 1956).

## EARLY EMBRYOLOGIC DEVELOPMENT

Although the urinary and genital tracts are physiologically dissimilar, they are closely related both embryologically and anatomically. Both arise from a common mesodermal ridge and maintain a critical and intimate relationship throughout embryologic development. The urinary component of this system is made up of organs concerned with the formation and excre-

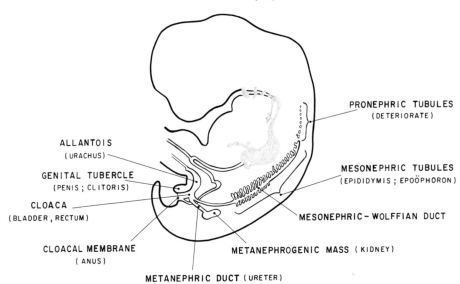

**FIGURE 93–1.**   The normal human embryo between the fourth and sixth weeks of fetal life. Although the genital tubercle has made its appearance and is identifiable, the genitalia of the two sexes are identical at this stage of development.

tion of urine, while the genital component is associated with sexual reproduction.

The development of this polyfunctional mechanism is equally complex. It originates from three embryonic structures, all of which exist only temporarily. The earliest of these three transitory structures develops during the second week after fertilization and is called the *pronephros*. It is soon replaced by the *mesonephros,* which in turn atrophies between the twelfth and fourteenth weeks to undergo metamorphosis into the third rudimentary structure, the *metanephros*. This is regarded as the renal secretory anlage and is not destined to function as a permanent organ. The collecting and secreting system of the mature kidney develops from the metanephros (Jordan and Kindred, 1942; Hamilton, Boyd, and Mossman, 1962). These three rudimentary structures, which disappear in the human, persist as functional units in some lower animals and in birds (Arey, 1954).

As the pronephric tubules degenerate, the mesonephric tubules grow and bulge ventrad into the coelom (Fig. 93–1). These bulges expand into an elevation to be named the *urogenital ridge* (Simkins, 1932). Both systems, urinary and reproductive, develop from this mesodermal ridge (Boving, 1965; Witchi, 1948). The ridge grows rapidly and divides into a lateral mesonephric ridge, which is destined to form the urinary components of the system, and a medial genital ridge, which is the undifferentiated gonad of the reproductive portion. The urogenital ridge

deepens in its center to produce a groove from which a pair of *müllerian ducts* appears. Medial to these ducts another pair takes form, called the *wolffian* ducts. All of these ducts empty into a common dilated cavity, the *cloaca* (Pohlman, 1911). At this early stage the cloaca is separated from the outside environment by a most important thin tissue called the *cloacal membrane* (Fig. 93–1). The destiny of the lower genitourinary and the gastrointestinal tracts is dependent upon the developmental course of the cloaca and its membrane. If the membrane fails to rupture, an anal atresia or imperforate anus results (Dalcq, 1938; Campbell, 1956). Complex features of genitourinary embryology often lead to deformities involving both systems. One third of all patients with genital malformations in the authors' series have associated urinary tract anomalies.

## EMBRYOLOGY OF URINARY TRACT ANOMALIES

**The Kidney.**   Genitourinary organogenesis begins when a small mesodermal elevation appears on the cephalodorsal aspect of the coelomic cavity about the second week after fertilization. This area is known as the *pronephros* and develops several pairs of transversely oriented tubules. These tubules never function and actually disappear in two weeks. However, the tubules have attached ducts which extend caudally in the embryo, and these persist to become known as the *mesonephric* or *wolffian ducts* (see Fig. 93–1). During this period another minute structure is developing from a thickening of the same coelomic area and becomes the *mesonephros*. The latter is destined to develop into the sex gonad (Fig. 93–2). The mesonephros also has tubules which grow into long, twisting structures and cause expansion of the urogenital ridge into the coelomic cavity. These tubules will eventually be the epididymis of the testicle or the epoophoron of the ovary. The expanding urogenital ridges spread apart to allow a longitudinal groove to form between them (Spaulding, 1921; Glenister, 1958).

The entire cluster of mesonephric tubules is attached to the mesonephric or wolffian duct, which plays a critical role in forming the ultimate kidney, as well as the male reproductive system. When the embryo is four weeks old, a solid bud of tissue begins to protrude from the wolffian duct near its junction with the cloaca. This ureteral bud elongates into a metanephrogenic mass (see Fig. 93–1), which is induced to become the kidney. The ureteral bud divides and subdivides into branches to be converted into a renal pelvis, calyces, papillary ducts, and collecting tubules (Langman, 1963). The nephrons later appear in association with a terminal branch of the ureter.

Errors in wolffian duct formation and ureteral malbudding account for many specific anomalies. Agenesis of the wolffian duct produces unilateral absence of the kidney, ureter, vas deferens, and epididymis. Polybudding of the wolffian duct results in total ureteral duplication and triplication. Incomplete duplication of a ureter or a renal pelvis is a consequence of premature branching of the ureteral stalk. Inhibition of ureteral budding at the level of the collecting tubules is considered the cause of a form of polycystic renal disease. As soon as the metanephrogenic mass and the ureteral stalk coalesce, the developing kidney begins its migration cranially, rotating as it ascends and thus orienting the renal pelvis from its ventral to a final medial position (see Figs. 93–1 and 93–2). Factors interfering with migration or rotation contribute to such disturbances as pelvic ectopia, cake kidney, crossed renal ectopia, and the horseshoe kidney. In time, the ureteral orifices and the wolffian ducts separate, and the terminations of the latter become the male ejaculatory ducts and seminal vesicles. In the female, vestigial wolffian remnants persist and occasionally produce clinically significant large cysts and tumors.

**The Cloaca.** Normal cloacal evolution is essential for the development of the lower urinary tract, the genitalia, and the infraumbilical abdominal wall. Figure 93–1 depicts the status of the cloaca in the six week old embryo. The dilated hind gut is seen to form a common chamber which extends ventrally into the allantois and caudally into the tailgut. The wolffian ducts enter the chamber laterally, and communication with the urinary tract is established. The anterior wall of the cloaca becomes fused with the ventral abdominal ectoderm, forming the cloacal membrane, which occupies a relatively large area of the ventral abdominal wall. A primitive streak of mesoderm surrounding the cloacal membrane is initially responsible for the

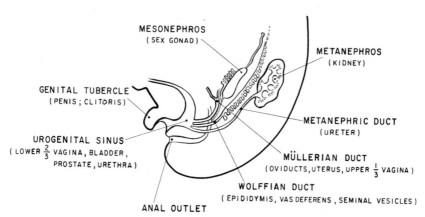

**FIGURE 93–2.**　The human embryo between the eighth and tenth weeks of fetal life. Note the relative organogenesis. The primitive kidney is "ascending" and the gonads are "descending" as a result of the straightening of the fetal body.

genital tubercle and anal hillock and ultimately gives rise to the abdominal musculature. Separation of the rectum from the bladder is accomplished by a thickening of the urorectal septum and by a medial migration of the mesenchymal perineal mound. As the genital swellings enlarge around the cloacal membrane, the cloacal structure gradually sinks, moves slowly caudad, and then naturally ruptures. Completion of a solid perineal body confirms the creation of a dorsal anal outlet and a ventral urogenital sinus.

During the period that the hindgut is establishing a normal external outlet, the cloaca is internally dilating and will eventually form a considerable portion of the urinary bladder. The bladder is developed by the sixth week of fetal life. A rather common congenital anomaly of this organic receptacle is *exstrophy of the bladder*. Exstrophy of the urinary bladder is a dramatic result of a developmental error at this stage of embryologic development. Exstrophy means "turning inside out," and therefore the term has been used to signify the condition in which the inside of the bladder is exposed on the abdominal wall without an anterior covering. Moreover, the bladder actually turns inside out when intra-abdominal pressure is exerted. A review of the developmental anatomy of bladder exstrophy indicates that there has been a continuing interest for the past century in the genesis of this anomaly. Simon (1852) described exstrophy of the bladder as a condition in which there is an absence of the lower abdominal wall, as well as of the anterior wall of the bladder. In a paper concerning the treatment of this anomaly, Maydl (1894) suggested that there was an actual absence of bladder wall. Today there is considerable question regarding this suggestion, and there are those who regard the anomaly as a cleft which can be easily closed (Snyder, 1958; Campbell, 1963).

Connelly (1901) collected the many theories that had been advanced as to the causes of bladder exstrophy and placed them into three categories. The first category, called mechanical, included such hypotheses as a short umbilical cord which caused changes in embryonal development, an upward extension of the cloacal cleft which resulted in an absence of the anterior abdominal wall, and constriction of the genitourinary tract comparable to hydrocephalus and syringomyelocele. The second category was designated as pathologic and included the possibility of inflammatory and degenerative processes which produced an ulceration and necrosis of the abdominal wall. The third category, arrested development, presented such factors as cloacal membrane adhesions, mesodermal deficiencies, and a persistent open blastophore. Connelly (1901) stated that such anomalies as epispadias, exstrophy of the bladder, umbilical hernia, cleft lip, and cleft palate occurred during the first four weeks of embryonic life.

Von Geldern (1924) was one of the first investigators to attempt to reproduce the deformity. He subjected frog eggs to 0.6 per cent sodium chloride solution and was able to produce various arrests in the development of the neural plate, including a cleft in the neural tube which in turn resulted in numerous anomalies. Muecke (1964) has proved by embryologic studies that persistence of the cloacal membrane produces cloacal exstrophy in the chick, a condition homologous to human bladder exstrophy in which the bladder develops a flat, irregular plate of mucosa-covered smooth muscle contiguous with the abdominal wall. In human exstrophy, the anterior abdominal wall muscles are separated by the vesicle plate. The ureteral orifices emerge to the exterior within the exteriorized bladder, and the posterior urethra is everted, forming an epispadias. The pubic bones, which develop in the anterior abdominal wall mesenchyme, are widely separated. The penis in the male and the clitoris in the female are bifid. Isolated epispadias in the male and subsymphyseal epispadias in the female are lesser degrees of the same deformity and are accompanied by diastasis pubis.

Many other theories have been advanced but never proved, and these are discussed by such authors as Fraser and Fainstat (1951), Patten and Barry (1952), Neel and Schull (1951), and Paul and Kanagasuntheram (1956). A likely hypothesis is that the paired primordia of the genital tubercle are displaced too far caudally, causing failure of convergence in the midline and thus failure to reinforce the ventral body wall (Patten, 1953). Since the bladder is an abdominal organ, during its embryonic stage it lies exposed in this area, and such a cleft would eventuate in exstrophy of the bladder. Once the separation of the ventral cloaca from the dorsally positioned rectum is complete, the ventral cloaca continues its closure and is primordial to the urethral canal, the bladder, the penile shaft or vaginal canal, and the glans or clitoris. As the bladder enlarges, the abdominal wall and the pubis develop in the ventral mesenchymes. The allantois normally atrophies and becomes the urachus. If this natural sequence of development encounters complications, umbilical fistulas, cysts, and even sinuses between the umbilicus and the bladder may result. The ureteral buds become completely detached from the wolffian ducts, merge with the bladder floor, and contribute to the lateral portions of the trigone. The ureters usually completely penetrate the bladder wall and course obliquely for 1.5 to 2.0 cm beneath the mucosa. The submucosal tunnel serves a valvular function by preventing reflux of urine from the bladder into the ureter and protecting the ureter from the higher intravesical pressures. Defective intravesical tunnels are a common anomaly, and the resulting vesicoureteral reflux is the most common cause of ascending pyelonephritis.

Failure of the ureteral bud to blend with the bladder at the proper location results in the relatively common condition of ureteral ectopia. More often associated with complete duplication of the ureters, the ectopic orifice lies caudad to the orthotopic orifice and drains the cranial portion of the ipsilateral kidney. Females are more commonly affected than males, and ectopic ureters have been found to terminate on the perineum, vagina, and multiple sites of the urethra. Most of the ectopic ureters in males terminate in the prostatic urethra or join the seminal vesicle.

## EMBRYOLOGY OF GENITAL TRACT ANOMALIES

The sex of the embryo cannot be determined by observation of the external genitalia until the eighth to tenth week. The genital primordia are present but are merely masses of indifferent or so-called "sexless" tissues. Differences in development of the wolffian and müllerian ducts, the urogenital ridge and sinus, and the cloacal tubercle are responsible for the differentiation into male and female sexes. In the male, the müllerian ducts atrophy, but the wolffian ducts continue to develop and form part of the epididymis, the ductus deferens, and the ejaculatory ducts (Williams, 1968). In the female, the wolffian ducts atrophy, whereas the müllerian ducts grow to form the uterus, oviducts, and vagina. The fused distal ends of the müllerian ducts make contact and coalesce with the urogenital sinus. This forms the uterine cavity and vagina (see Fig. 93–2).

In some animals the fusion of the müllerian ducts does not continue cephalad, and this results in paired uteri or a bicornuate uterus. Various other degrees of this anomaly in the human female result in such anomalies as atresia of the uterus, double vagina, or absence of the vagina. The uterine (fallopian) tubes are derivatives of the upper portion of the müllerian ducts. There are various types of hermaphroditism which may result from faulty development in this region, and these are discussed in Chapter 100.

At the beginning of the sixth week, a conical prominence appears between the umbilical cord and the tail (Figs. 93–1, 93–2, and 93–3) and is known as the *genital tubercle*. On its caudal slope is a median groove, and laterally there are two folds. During the seventh week, the genital tubercle elongates and forms the *phallus* and an expanded end which becomes the glans. These are the primordia of the *penis* if the embryo is a male, and of the *clitoris* if it is a female (Federman, 1967). If the genital tubercle fails to form because of mesodermal agenesis or dysgenesis, the penis does not develop (Richart and Benirschke, 1960; Carter, Isa, Hashem and Raasch, 1968). The anterior portion of the cloacal membrane (Fig. 93–3), the *urogenital membrane,* ruptures and opens to the surface as a sinus. Meanwhile, a pair of elevated folds, called the *genital folds,* develop on each side of the urogenital sinus. If the genital folds fail to unite over the urogenital sinus, the most common urethral congenital anomaly, *hypospadias,* results, and this may be of various degrees of severity. During this same period of development, a second pair of lateral folds appears, called the *genital swellings.* In the severest type of hypospadias, the penoscrotal variety, both the genital folds and the genital swellings fail to unite. If the urethral groove remains and completely divides the penile shaft,

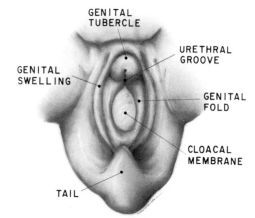

**FIGURE 93–3.** Composite drawing of a series of human embryos illustrating the primordial organic development of the external genitalia into recognizable structures, which are yet undifferentiated as to sex.

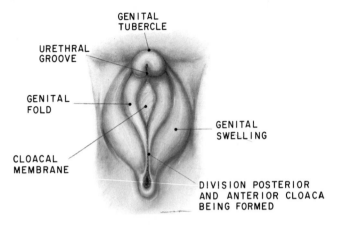

GENITAL
TUBERCLE

URETHRAL
GROOVE

GENITAL
FOLD

GENITAL
SWELLING

CLOACAL
MEMBRANE

DIVISION POSTERIOR
AND ANTERIOR CLOACA
BEING FORMED

**FIGURE 93–4.**   Composite drawing depicting cloacal evolution at the stage of division of the anterior receptacle from the primitive anorectal system. The genital swellings are beginning to bulge as either a scrotum or labia majora.

an uncommon anomaly known as a *double penis* develops. The authors have repaired a double penis with Z-plasties. Campbell (1951) has described other cases. As the urethra forms there is a redundant fold of epithelium that develops at the base of the glans and covers the penile tip, the *prepuce* or foreskin. This fold of skin fuses at the ventral aspect of the base of the glans and remains tethered as the *frenulum*.

If the embryo is to be a normal male, the paired folds close and form the penile urethra with a deeply pigmented median raphé; if they remain separated, the labia minora of the female are formed. The thicker and more lateral genital swellings become the scrotum of the male and the labia majora of the female (Figs. 93–3 to 93–8). The stages of development of the external genitalia in the female are less extensive than those observed in the male. The phallus bends slightly forward and forms the clitoris. The genital folds never coalesce in the midline but form the *labia minora*. The genital swellings develop into the labia majora. The lower portion of the urogenital sinus becomes the vaginal introitus or orifice (see Fig. 93–8).

The primitive bladder is primordial to the male bladder and the prostatic urethra to the ejaculatory ducts. In the female it forms the bladder and the proximal two-thirds of the urethra. The bladder trigone is formed from the mesonephric ducts.

In the condition known as *epispadias*, the urethra opens on the upper surface of the penis. This is a rare anomaly and usually exists in its severest form with exstrophy of the bladder. In the female the urethra is incompletely covered dorsally and is accompanied by a bifid clitoris. The newborn may become continent in the mild forms or incontinent in the severe types. The disorder is thought to be due to a failure of the

mesenchyme to develop caudal to the cloacal membrane. The urogenital sinus remains open in the male, and therefore the infraumbilical musculature is also undeveloped (see Chapter 96).

The undifferentiated gonads start as growths on the anterior surface of the mesonephros, the *germinal or genital ridge*. The male gonads descend as a result of a straightening of the embryo body rather than an actual descent into the scrotum (Gruenwald, 1943; Wyndham, 1943). Their final position is in the genital swellings, which become fused to form the scrotum. The testicular vessels and nerves elongate to make the testicular descent possible. The origins of these vessels remain high in the posterior abdomen. At least one testicle should be housed in the cooler atmosphere of the scrotum, because the warm abdominal cavity is harmful to the seminiferous tubules. The migra-

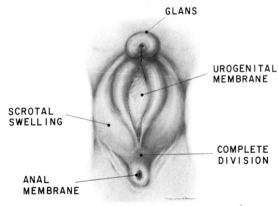

GLANS

UROGENITAL
MEMBRANE

SCROTAL
SWELLING

COMPLETE
DIVISION

ANAL
MEMBRANE

**FIGURE 93–5.**   Composite drawing demonstrating complete separation of the anterior urogenital membrane from the anal outlet. The genital swellings are still bifid and resemble a primordial scrotal sac. The phallus has not demonstrated whether it is to be a penile shaft or a clitoris.

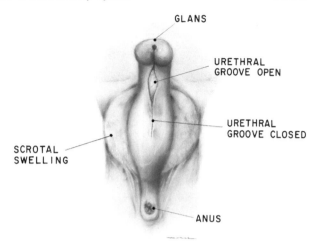

GLANS

URETHRAL
GROOVE OPEN

URETHRAL
GROOVE CLOSED

SCROTAL
SWELLING

ANUS

**FIGURE 93–6.** Composite drawing showing a growing male penile shaft with a developing urethral canal. If maturation is disturbed, the urethral groove may remain open with development of the most common urethral congenital anomaly—hypospadias.

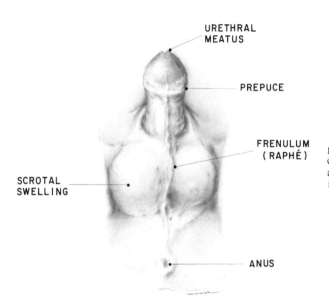

URETHRAL
MEATUS

PREPUCE

FRENULUM
(RAPHÉ)

SCROTAL
SWELLING

ANUS

**FIGURE 93–7.** Development of the male external genitalia has been successfully completed. The masculine phallus is bioptyped from the genital tubercle anlage. The scrotum developed from the coalesced genital swellings with a completed midline raphé.

**FIGURE 93–8.** Feminization of the external genitalia has been achieved from the determined embryologic rudiments as labeled.

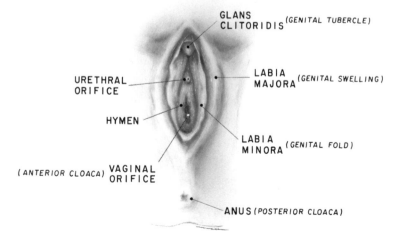

GLANS
CLITORIDIS (GENITAL TUBERCLE)

LABIA
MAJORA (GENITAL SWELLING)

URETHRAL
ORIFICE

HYMEN

LABIA
MINORA (GENITAL FOLD)

(ANTERIOR CLOACA) VAGINAL
ORIFICE

ANUS (POSTERIOR CLOACA)

tion is usually completed by the eighth intrauterine month. If the migration does not develop and the gonads remain intra-abdominal, the male becomes sterile. Ectopia of the male gonad is commonly known as *undescended testicle* or *cryptorchidism*. The germinal ridge also contains epithelial cells which proliferate to form the spermatogenic cells of the testes and the graafian follicles of the ovary. The prostate gland is derived from the urethral epithelium, and its homologue in the female is Skene's ducts (Hinman, 1935). The ovaries, during the third month, descend to the pelvic brim. Their final resting position is on the posterior surface of the broad ligament. The round ligament attaches the ovary to the uterus and prevents descent of the gonads into the labia majora.

## REFERENCES

Arey, L. B.: Developmental Anatomy. 6th Ed. Philadelphia, W. B. Saunders Company, 1954, p. 3.

Arey, L. B.: Developmental Anatomy. 7th Ed. Philadelphia, W. B. Saunders Company, 1966, p. 295.

Boving, B. G.: Anatomy of reproduction. *In* Greenhill, J. P. (Ed.): Obstetrics. 13th Ed. Philadelphia, W. B. Saunders Company, 1965, p. 26.

Campbell, M. F.: Clinical Pediatric Urology. Philadelphia, W. B. Saunders Company, 1951.

Campbell, M. F.: Indications for urologic examination in infants and children. Med. Rec. Ann. (Houston), 50:267, 1956.

Campbell, M. F.: Urology. 2nd Ed. Philadelphia, W. B. Saunders Company, 1963.

Carter, J. P., Isa, N. N., Hashem, N., and Raasch, Jr., F. O.: Congenital absence of the penis: A case report. J. Urol., 99:766, 1968.

Connelly, F. G.: Exstrophy of the bladder. J.A.M.A., 36:637, 1901.

Dalcq, A. M.: Form and Causality in Early Development. London, Cambridge University Press, 1938.

Federman, D. D.: Abnormal Sexual Development. Philadelphia, W. B. Saunders Company, 1967, p. 5.

Fraser, F. D., and Fainstat, T. D.: Causes of congenital defects. Am. J. Dis. Child., 82:593, 1951.

Geldern, C. E. Von: Etiology of exstrophy of the bladder. Arch. Surg., 8:61, 1924.

Glenister, T. W. A.: A correlation of the normal and abnormal development of the penile urethra and of the infraumbilical abdominal wall. Br. J. Urol., 30:117, 1958.

Gruenwald, P.: The normal changes in the position of the embryonic kidney. Anat. Rec., 85:163, 1943.

Hamilton, W. J., Boyd, J. D., and Mossman, H. W.: Human Embryology. 3rd Ed. Baltimore, The Williams & Wilkins Company, 1962.

Hinman, F.: Principles and Practice of Urology. Philadelphia, W. B. Saunders Company, 1935.

Jordan, H. E., and Kindred, J. E.: A Textbook of Embryology. 4th Ed. New York, D. Appleton-Century Company, 1942.

Jost, A.: Embryonic sexual differentiation. *In* Jones, H. W., and Scott, W. W. (Eds.): Hermaphrodism, Genital Anomalies and Related Endocrine Disorders. Baltimore, The Williams & Wilkins Company, 1958, p. 15.

Langman, J.: Medical Embryology. Baltimore, The Williams & Wilkins Company, 1963, p. 120.

Marshall, B. F., and Muecke, E. C.: Variations in exstrophy of the bladder. J. Urol., 88:766, 1962.

Maydl, K.: Ueber die Radikaltherapie der Blasenektopie. Wien Med. Wochenschr., 44:25, 1894.

Muecke, E. C.: The role of the cloacal membrane in exstrophy. The first successful experimental study. J. Urol., 92:659, 1964.

Neel, J. V., and Schull, W.: Human Heredity. Chicago, University of Chicago Press, 1954.

Patten, B. M.: Human Embryology. 2nd Ed. Philadelphia, The Blakiston Company, 1953, p. 549.

Patten, B. M., and Barry, A.: The genesis of exstrophy of the bladder and epispadias. Am. J. Anat., 90:35, 1952.

Paul, M., and Kanagasuntheram, R.: The congenital anomalies of the lower urinary tract. Br. J. Urol., 28:64, 1956.

Pohlman, A. G.: The development of the cloaca in human embryos. Am. J. Anat., 12:1, 1911.

Richart, R., and Benirschke, K.: Penile agenesis. Arch. Pathol., 70:137, 1960.

Simkins, C. S.: Development of the human ovary from birth to sexual maturity. Am. J. Anat., 51:465, 1932.

Simon, J.: Ectopia vesicae. Lancet, 2:568, 1852.

Snyder, C. C.: A new therapeutic concept of the exstrophied bladder. Plast. Reconstr. Surg., 22:1, 1958.

Spaulding, M. H.: The development of the external genitalia in the human embryo. *In* Contributions to Embryology, No. 61, Vol. 13. Washington, D.C., Carnegie Institution of Washington, 1921.

Williams, R. H.: Textbook of Endocrinology. Philadelphia, W. B. Saunders Company, 1968, p. 451.

Witchi, E.: Migration of germ cells of human embryos from the yolk sac to the primitive gonadal folds. Contrib. Embryol., 32:67, 1948.

Wyndham, N. R.: A morphological study of testicular descent. J. Anat., 77:179, 1943.

# CHAPTER 94

# HYPOSPADIAS: SOME HISTORICAL ASPECTS AND THE EVOLUTION OF TECHNIQUES OF TREATMENT

## DONALD WOOD-SMITH, F.R.C.S.E.

The problems confronting the surgeon in the reconstructive surgery of hypospadias are two-fold: correction of the penis and reconstruction of the urethra. Correction of the penile deformity is achieved by elimination of the chordee. The repair of the urethra may be done by (1) use of local tissues in the form of various flaps including tubed flaps, (2) skin grafts, or (3) miscellaneous other methods. The surgical technique for the correction of hypospadias is discussed in Chapter 95.

A brief historical review of various methods employed in the past, which have led to the development of present-day methods, follows. Duplay published the first important paper on the subject of hypospadias in the Archives Générales de Médecine in 1874. He gave credit to Anger for presenting to the Société de Chirurgie in 1874 a report of the first successful repair of hypospadias. This repair was accomplished by a technique based on that described by Thiersch (1874) for the repair of epispadias (Fig. 94–1). Duplay then described his version of the Thiersch technique, relating in detail his method of repair.

Since this time numerous operations have appeared, all claiming originality on various aspects of technique. Backus and DeFelice (1960) found over 150 "original" techniques; a profusion of papers describing modifications and results exists in the literature.

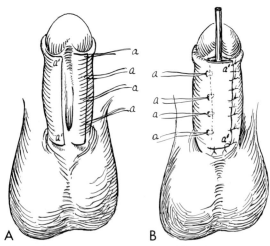

**FIGURE 94–1.** Procedure of M. Théophile Anger. (Redrawn from Duplay, S.: Archives Générales de Médecine, Vol. 23, 1874.)

## CORRECTION OF THE CHORDEE

Petit in 1837 described in his *Oeuvres Complètes* the pathology of the chordee, following a dissection in the cadaver. However, Mettauer must receive credit for publishing in 1842 the first case of surgical division of a chordee.

Duplay in 1874, describing the correction of chordee, made a transverse incision distal to the hypospadiac opening, resecting a segment of the fibrous chordee, and closed the incision longitudinally after the manner of Heineke-Mikulicz (Fig. 94–2).

In 1926 Edmunds described a two-stage procedure. The first stage consists of incising the base of the frenulum dorsally to produce a bipedicle flap of frenulum (Fig. 94–3, *A*). In the second stage, the bipedicle flap is divided centrally, and the incisions are extended from the base of the bipedicle flaps ventrally around the base of the corona and continued proximally to a point immediately distal to the hypospadiac opening. The fibrous chordee is removed, and the flap is opened and applied to the ventral surface of the penis (Fig. 94–3, *B, C, D*).

Blair, Brown, and Hamm in 1933 described a one-stage procedure achieving a result similar to that obtained by the Edmunds procedure. Byars (1964) modified the procedure, and it is described in the following chapter.

Nesbit (1941), in the belief that the longitudinal scar on the roof of the new urethra would interfere with healing of the urethroplasty, made a circular incision immediately posterior and parallel to the corona; the whole foreskin was peeled back to the hypospadiac opening. The rudimentary corpus spongiosum was removed,

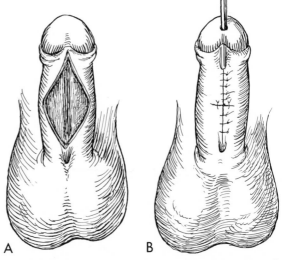

**FIGURE 94–2.** *A*, Transverse incision and resection of chordee. *B*, Closure of the incision longitudinally after the manner of Heineke-Mikulicz. (Redrawn from Duplay, 1874.)

and the skin was replaced and incised transversally on its dorsal aspect. The glans was drawn through the newly formed opening and sutured to its margins. The ventral defect was closed in a transverse manner (Fig. 94–4).

## RECONSTRUCTION OF THE URETHRA

**Use of Local Tissues.** Dieffenbach, in 1837, unsuccessfully pioneered the reconstruction of the urethra by raising a fold of skin along either

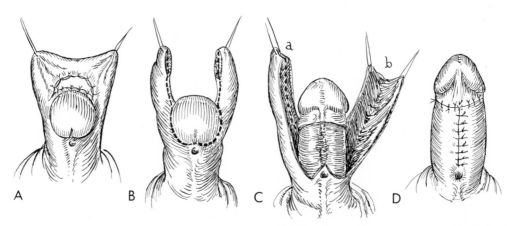

**FIGURE 94–3.** The Edmunds operation for correction of the penile deformity and chordee. A six-week wait is allowed between stages *A* and *B*. In the second stage the flap is divided centrally, and after excision of the fibrous chordee the penis is straightened and the opened out flaps applied to its ventral surface. (Redrawn from Edmunds, A.: Pseudo-hermaphrodism in hypospadias. Lancet, *1*:323, 327, 1926.)

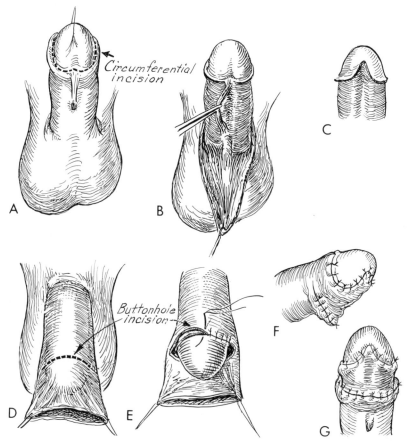

**FIGURE 94–4.** The Nesbit procedure. *A,* Coronal incision. *B,* Resection of fibrous chordee with peeling back of the penile skin to the hypospadiac opening. *C,* The denuded penile shaft. *D, E,* The glans is brought through and sutured to the edges of a buttonhole incision on the dorsum of the penile skin. *F, G,* The original prepuce opening is closed in a transverse fashion. (Redrawn from Nesbit, R.: Plastic procedure for correction of hypospadias. J. Urol., *45*:699, 1941.)

side of the proposed urethra, suturing the edges together after incising along the apices of the folds. After relaxing incisions were made on the lateral aspects of the penis, the two edges were united over the reconstructed urethra. His efforts in this direction were notably unsuccessful, and it remained for Anger (1874), utilizing Thiersch's method of epispadias repair, to perform the first successful cure of hypospadias.

Duplay (1874b, 1880) employed a buried skin strip in his reconstruction of the glanular urethra, making either a single central and two lateral incisions or two lateral incisions combined with two smaller central incisions, and suturing the edges together over the central mucosal strip with a sound in place (Fig. 94–5). This is similar to the method described by Thiersch (1869) to form a glanular urethra during reconstruction for epispadias. Thiersch made two lateral incisions, isolating a central skin strip, and approximated the edges of the incisions over the skin strip forming the glanular urethra (Fig. 94–6).

This is the first recorded example of the use of the buried skin strip method described by Denis Browne in the reconstruction of the urethra. Duplay's first stage consisted of the formation of the glanular urethra and the correction of the chordee by the previously described method. In the second stage, in a manner similar to that of Dieffenbach, parallel incisions were made on the ventral surface of the penis,

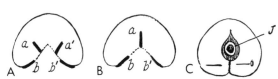

**FIGURE 94–5.** Duplay's method of reconstruction of the glanular urethra. *A,* Two lateral incisions are made, and the edges b and b′ are united over the intervening mucosa. *B,* An alternate method. A single central incision is made, and the two points b and b′ are united. *C,* Final result with sound in place. (Redrawn from Duplay, 1874.)

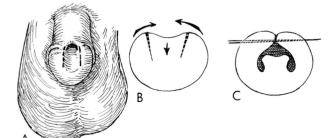

**FIGURE 94–6.** Thiersch's operation for glanular hypospadias. *A*, *B*, Two lateral incisions are made. *C*, Skin and subcutaneous tissue edges are united over the buried strip of glanular epithelium. (Redrawn from Davis, J. S.: Plastic Surgery. Philadelphia, P. Blakiston Son & Company, 1919.)

extending from the hypospadiac opening to the glanular urethra. The central skin flap was raised at its periphery and a catheter inserted into the hypospadiac opening and through the glanular urethra. The central skin flap was wrapped around the catheter. Two lateral skin flaps were raised, advanced medially, and sutured together over the newly formed urethral tube by fine sutures (Fig. 94–7). This was aided by the tension-relieving sutures (described in Duplay's paper in 1880). Duplay referred vaguely to the use of relaxing incisions on the dorsal and lateral aspects of the penis but did not consider this an essential part of the procedure (Fig. 94–8).

Rochet, in 1899, utilized a tubed flap taken from the scrotum, the flap originating immediately posterior to the hypospadiac opening and drawn distally along the body of the penis to exit at the glans. The advantage claimed for this flap was the elimination of fistulas between the old and the new urethra. A catheter was left in the urethra for an initial period of

eight days. This otherwise excellent method suffered from the distinct disadvantage of inclusion of hair-bearing skin within the urethral canal and obstruction caused by the accumulation of calcareous deposits on the hairs (Fig. 94–9).

Davis (1940, 1955) modified this method by the use of a tubed flap from the dorsum of the penis to form a new urethra. Broadbent, Woolf, and Toksu (1961) have further refined this method of repair (Fig. 94–10).

Bucknall (1907) described a procedure similar in concept to Rochet's and suffering from a similar disadvantage. The penis is drawn over the abdomen and the scrotum drawn caudally; parallel lines of incision are made from the corona of the penis to the region of the hypospadiac opening and for an equal distance on the anterior aspect of the scrotum. The skin on both edges of the incisions is raised, the penis is then flexed to the scrotum, and the central strip of skin is tubed around a catheter by suturing the opposing skin edges. The opposing skin edges of

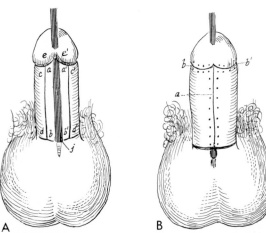

**FIGURE 94–7.** Duplay's method of reconstruction of hypospadias. Lateral flaps outlined in *A* are mobilized and united over the newly formed cutaneous urethral tube wrapped about a catheter. (Redrawn from Duplay, 1874.)

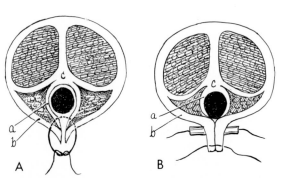

**FIGURE 94–8.** *A*, Duplay's original method of closure of the skin flap over the newly formed urethral canal. *B*, Duplay's later method of closure of the skin flap over the newly formed canal with "stop sutures." (Redrawn from the original, *A* in 1874 and *B* in 1880.)

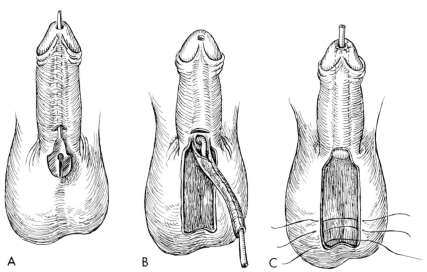

**FIGURE 94-9.** *A,* Rochet's procedure. A new tunnel is formed through a short transverse incision just distal to the hypospadiac opening. *B,* A new tubed flap is raised from the central scrotum and wrapped around a catheter. *C,* The newly formed flap is drawn through the canal and sutured to the new meatus. The secondary defect is closed by direct approximation. (Redrawn from Davis, J. S.: Plastic Surgery. Philadelphia, P. Blakiston Son & Company, 1919.)

penis and scrotum are also approximated by sutures. The catheter is removed after four days, and after three to four weeks the penis is freed from the scrotum, the skin edges being united across the newly formed urethral tube. The scrotal defect is closed by direct approximation (Fig. 94–11).

Ombrédanne (1911) introduced a method similar in principle to that of Bucknall: a flap is raised in a direction proximal to the hypospadiac opening and rotated distally so that its most proximal point lies at the glans. Proximal to the hypospadiac opening the defect is closed by direct approximation of the skin edges. Distal to the hypospadiac opening, the defect is closed by buttonholing the frenulum dorsally. The glans is passed through the defect and sutured to the wound edges; the frenulum is rotated posteriorly to cover the raw area; the two lateral pedicles are later divided (Fig. 94–12). The disadvantage

**FIGURE 94-10.** Penoscrotal hypospadias with associated chordee. *A,* Incision carried distally onto the preputial skin. *B,* The mobilized skin strip is tubed about the hypospadiac opening. The chordee is corrected at this stage after reflecting the ventral skin. *C,* The new urethra is threaded through a gutter in the glans. *D,* If the skin closure is tight, a dorsal slit is made and the defect grafted, preferably with excess prepuce skin. (Redrawn from Broadbent, T. R., Woolf, R. M., and Toksu, E.: Hypospadias. One-stage repair. Plast. Reconstr. Surg., 27:154, 1961.)

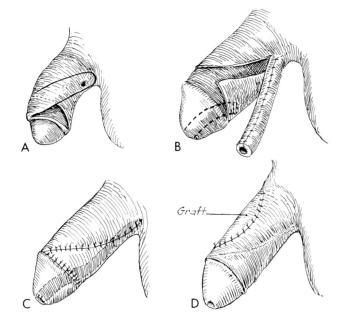

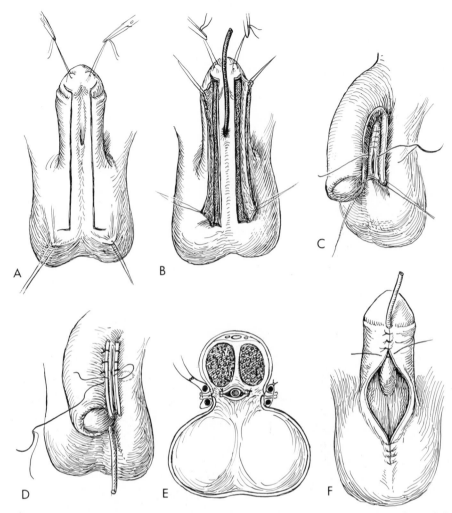

**FIGURE 94–11.** Bucknall's procedure. *A,* Parallel incisions are made along the ventral surface of the penis and scrotum. *B,* The skin flaps are raised laterally. *C,* The opposing skin edges of the penis and scrotum are united to form a new urethral tube about a catheter. *D, E,* Union of the penile and scrotal skin about the newly formed urethral tube. *F,* After three to four weeks, the penis is freed and the skin edges are united across the new urethral tube; the secondary scrotal defect is closed. (Redrawn from Jones, H. W., and Scott, W. W.: Hermaphroditism, Genital Anomalies and Related Endocrine Disorders. Baltimore, The Williams & Wilkins Company, 1958.)

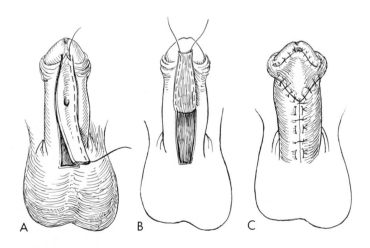

**FIGURE 94–12.** The method of Ombrédanne. *A,* Incisions are made parallel to the urethra and its anterior prolongation and a flap is raised proximally. *B,* The proximal flap is rotated distally and the skin edges approximated. *C,* The frenulum is buttonholed dorsally; the glans is drawn through and the frenulum sutured to the ventral surface of the glans to cover the ventral aspect of the new urethral tube. (Redrawn from Caucci, A., and Caucci, N.: La nostra experienza sulla cura dell'hypospadia. Minerva Chir., *8*:7, 1958.)

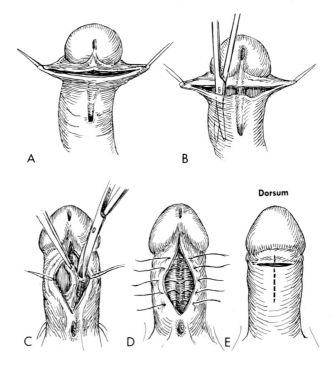

**FIGURE 94–13.** Denis Browne's procedure —first stage. *A, B,* Correction of the chordee by a transverse frenulum incision and raising of the ventral penile skin. *C,* Excision of the fibrous chordee. *D,* Skin edges are united in a longitudinal direction. *E,* A longitudinal dorsal incision is made and allowed to spread widely to relieve ventral tension. (Redrawn from Browne, D.: Observations on the treatment of hypospadias. Trans. Internatl. Soc. Plastic Surgeons, 2nd Congress, 1959. Edinburgh, E. & S. Livingstone, 1960.)

of this procedure is the formation of a pouch-like urethra with poor terminal control of micturition.

Denis Browne (1946, 1949, 1950) published a different approach to the repair of hypospadias. The first stage of the operation, performed preferably at 18 months of age, consists in correction of the chordee and a meatotomy; a dorsal relaxation incision is made and allowed to spread widely (Fig. 94–13). This procedure is regarded as an essential part of the technique, and although aggravating the hypospadias, it allows the penis to develop normally; at four to five years of age, prior to starting school, the second stage urethroplasty is performed (Fig. 94–14).

The second stage, the urethroplasty, is immediately preceded by a perineal urethrostomy with a self-retaining (Malecot) catheter passed into the bladder. A strip of skin is outlined from

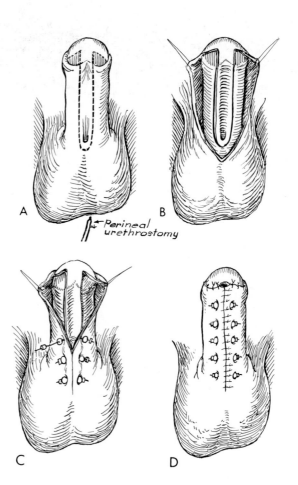

**FIGURE 94–14.** D. Browne's method—second stage, the urethroplasty. *A,* Perineal urethrostomy with a self-retaining catheter in place; incisions outlined. *B,* Lateral skin flaps are raised with wide undermining over a central skin strip connecting the urethral orifice and the glans. *C,* After a dorsal relaxing incision, tension-relieving sutures fixed with glass beads held by aluminum buttons are placed in position. *D,* Procedure completed by fine interrupted sutures. (Redrawn from Browne, D.: Operation for hypospadias. Postgrad. Med. J., *25*:367, 1949.)

the urethral orifice to the corona of the glans, the adjacent skin is widely undermined, and a small triangular area is excised from either side of the glans. After wide undermining and a dorsal relaxing incision, the skin flaps are joined over the skin strip by fine catgut sutures. Tension-relieving sutures, fixed with glass beads and held in position by aluminum buttons, are added. A major point is that the two opposing surfaces are not brought into intimate contact by the tension-relieving sutures. The defect produced by the dorsal relaxing incision is allowed to heal by spontaneous epithelization. The tension-relaxing sutures are removed after one week and the catheter on the tenth day. The perineal fistula usually heals within a few days after removal of the catheter.

The differences in techniques between the Denis Browne repair and that of Duplay are immediately obvious on comparison of Figures 94–15 and 94–8, *B*, both reproduced from the authors' original papers. However, Duplay in 1880 wrote, ". . . although the catheter is not really covered I have been able to convince myself that there are no ill effects upon the new canal."

**Use of Skin Grafts.**   Nové-Josserand, in 1897, first described the use of a skin graft to form a new urethra. In his original technique, a transverse incision 2 mm long is made immediately distal to the hypospadiac opening, and a bistoury is passed through the loose subcutaneous tissues to the glans penis. A split-thickness skin graft approximately 2 cm wide is obtained, wrapped around a sound, and passed through a cannula lying in the tract. The probe is left in place for seven days, then withdrawn. Daily catheterization is performed for a period of approximately seven months. The illustrations are from Nové-Josserand's last article published in 1919 (Fig. 94–16).

The frequent stricture and fistula formations following this method caused its rapid fall into disrepute, until it was revived by McIndoe in 1937 with several modifications.

McIndoe (1948) overcame the tendency toward contracture and subsequent stricture formation by requiring that the patient wear a dilator in the canal for a minimum period of six months following surgery. Only after this time was the urethra anastomosed to the hypospadiac opening, after temporary diversion of the urinary stream by perineal urethrostomy. Young and Benjamin (1948, 1949) described a similar method.

The details of reconstruction of the urethra with a full-thickness skin graft are given in Chapter 95.

Many types of grafts, both autografts and allografts, have been utilized in various attempted methods of reconstruction of the urethra. Notable among these is that of Schmieden, who in 1909 transplanted the ureter with unsuccessful results. Axhausen (1918) and McGuire (1927) transplanted the appendix, both as an allograft and an autograft, without success. Legueu in 1921 unsuccessfully used the ureter as an autograft.

Marshall and Spellman (1955) reported free grafts of bladder mucosa with only one failure but noted frequent stricture formation.

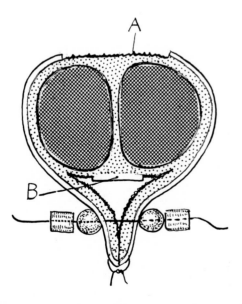

FIGURE 94–15.   The completed Denis Browne operation redrawn from his original article, illustrating (*A*) the widely spread dorsal skin and (*B*) the flat strip of buried epithelium. Note that the tension-relieving sutures do not bring the opposing surfaces of the flaps into intimate contact.

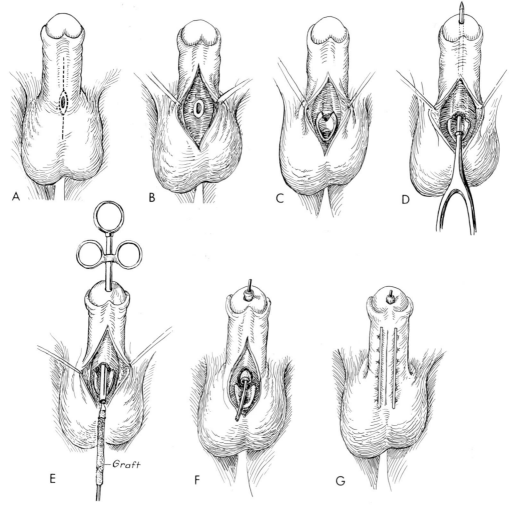

**FIGURE 94–16.** The method of Nové-Josserand. *A,* The skin incision is outlined. *B, C,* Skin flaps are raised about the hypospadiac opening. *D,* A cannula is passed to the glans. *E,* The catheter wrapped in a split-thickness graft is drawn through the cannula to exit at the glans. *F,* The proximal end of the cannula is passed into the posterior urethra. *G,* The completed procedure. (Redrawn from Nové-Josserand, G.: Des hypospadias étendus par la tunellisation avec greffe dermo-épidermique. J. Urol., *8:*449, 1919.)

## REFERENCES

Anger, T.: Quoted by Duplay, S.: De l'hypospadias périnéo-scrotal et de son traitement chirurgical. Presentation at the Société de Chirurgie, Paris, 1874.

Anger, T.: Hypospadias péno-scrotal, compliqué de cordure de verge; redressement du pénis et urétroplastie par inclusion cutanée; guérison. Rap. d. Guyon. Bull. Soc. Chir. Paris, *1:*179, 1875.

Axhausen, G.: Prognosis of transplantation of the appendix in hypospadias. Berl. Klin. Wochenschr., *55:*1065, 1918.

Backus, L. H., and DeFelice, C. A.: Hypospadias then and now. Plast. Reconstr. Surg., *25:*146, 1960.

Blair, V. P., Brown, J. B., and Hamm, W. G.: The correction of scrotal hypospadias and epispadias. Surg. Gynecol. Obstet., *57:*646, 1933.

Broadbent, T. R., Woolf, R. M., and Toksu, E.: Hypospadias. One-stage repair. Plast. Reconstr. Surg., *27:*154, 1961.

Browne, D.: An operation for hypospadias. Lancet, *1:*141, 1946.

Browne, D.: Operation for hypospadias. Postgrad. Med. J., *25:*367, 1949.

Browne, D.: Hypospadias. *In* Maingot, R. (Ed.): Techniques in British Surgery. Philadelphia, W. B. Saunders Company, 1950, p. 412.

Browne, D.: Observations on the treatment of hypospadias. Trans. Internatl. Soc. Plast. Surg., 2nd Congress, 1959. Edinburgh, E. & S. Livingstone, Ltd., 1960.

Bucknall, R. T. H.: A new operation for penile hypospadias. Lancet, *2:*887, 1907.

Byars, L. T.: Hypospadias and epispadias. *In* Converse, J. M. (Ed.): Reconstructive Plastic Surgery. Philadelphia, W. B. Saunders Company, 1964.

Caucci, A., and Caucci, N.: La nostra experienza sulla cura dell'hypospadia. Minerva Chir., *8*:7, 1958.

Davis, D. M.: The pedicle tube graft in the surgical treatment of hypospadias in the male. Surg. Gynecol. Obstet., *71*:790, 1940.

Davis, D. M.: Results of pedicle tube-flap method in hypospadias. J. Urol., *73*:343, 1955.

Davis, J. S.: Plastic Surgery. Philadelphia, P. Blakiston Son & Co., 1919.

Dieffenbach, J. F.: Guérison des fentes congénitales de la verge. I. De l'hypospadias. Gaz. Hebd. Méd., *5*:156, 1837.

Duplay, S.: De l'hypospadias périnéo-scrotal et de son traitement chirurgical. Arch. Gén. Méd., *23*:513, 1874a.

Duplay, S.: Nouvelle méthode opératoire applicable au traitement de l'hypospadias périnéo-scrotal. Arch. Gén. Méd., *23*:657, 1874b.

Duplay, S.: Sur le traitement chirurgical de l'hypospadias et l'épispadias. Arch. Gén. Méd., *5*:257, 1880.

Edmunds, A.: An operation for hypospadias. Lancet, *1*:447, 1913.

Edmunds, A.: Pseudo-hermaphrodism in hypospadias. Lancet, *1*:323, 327, 1926.

Jones, H. W., and Scott, W. W.: Hermaphrodism, Genital Anomalies and Related Endocrine Disorders. Baltimore, The Williams & Wilkins Company, 1958.

McGuire, S.: Use of the vermiform appendix in the formation of a urethra in hypospadias. Ann. Surg., *85*:391, 1927.

McIndoe, A. H.: An operation to cure adult hypospadias. Br. Med. J., *1*:385, 1937a.

McIndoe, A. H.: Treatment of hypospadias. Am. J. Surg., *38*:176, 1937b.

McIndoe, A. H.: Deformity of the male urethra. Br. J. Plast. Surg., *1*:29, 1948.

Marshall, V. F., and Spellman, R. M.: Reconstruction of the urethra in hypospadias using the vesicle mucosal grafts. J. Urol., *73*:335, 1955.

Mettauer, J. P.: Practical observations on those malformations of the urethra termed "hypospadias" and "epispadias." Am. J. Med. Sci., *4*:43, 1842.

Nesbit, R.: Plastic procedure for correction of hypospadias. J. Urol., *45*:699, 1941.

Nové-Josserand, G.: Traitement de l'hypospadias; nouvelle méthode. Lyon Med., *85*:198, 1897.

Nové-Josserand, G.: Des hypospadias étendus par la tunellisation avec greffe dermo-épidermique. J. Urol., *8*:449, 1919.

Ombrédanne, L.: Hypospadias pénien chez l'enfant. Bull. Mém. Soc. Chir. Paris, *37*:1076, 1911.

Petit, J. L.: Oeuvres Complètes. Edition 1837, p. 717.

Rochet, B.: Nouveau procédé pour refaire le canal pénien dans l'hypospadias. Gaz. Hebd. Méd. Chir., *4*:673, 1899.

Thiersch, K.: Ueber die Enstehungsweise und operative Behandlung der Epispadie. Arch. Heilk., *10*:20, 1869.

Thiersch, K.: Ueber die feineren anatomischen Veränderungen bei Aufheilung von Haut auf Granulationen. Verh. Dtsch. Ges. Chir., Third Congress, 1874, pp. 67–75.

Young, F., and Benjamin, J. A.: Repair of hypospadias with free inlay skin grafts. Surg. Gynecol, Obstet., *86*:439, 1948.

Young, F., and Benjamin, J. A.: Pre-school age repair of hypospadias with free inlay skin grafts. Surgery, *26*:384, 1949.

# CHAPTER 95

# HYPOSPADIAS

## Charles E. Horton, M.D., and Charles J. Devine, Jr., M.D.

Hypospadias is a congenital deformity in which the urethral meatus is located on the ventral surface of the penis proximal to its normal position at the tip of the glans. The deformity is caused by premature involution of the interstitial cells of the developing testes with cessation of androgen production and consequent incomplete masculinization of the external genitalia (Devine, 1970). Depending upon the extent of development at the time when the condition occurs, the abnormal meatus may be located at any point from the perineum to the corona.

### PATHOLOGIC ANATOMY

The glans is typically flattened with a shallow groove on the ventral surface. The ventral portion of the prepuce is absent, so the dorsal preputial skin appears excessively long, producing a hooded appearance to the penis. When the meatus is in the region of the scrotum or perineum, the scrotum will be bifid, having a groove of hairless skin between the two halves. The ventral penile skin distal to the meatus is thin, and the subcutaneous structures—dartos fascia, Buck's fascia, and corpus spongiosum—are absent, being replaced by a fan-shaped band of dense fibrous tissue, which causes a ventral curvature of the penis called chordee. The

proximal termination of this band surrounds the urethral meatus. Distally it inserts into the ventral aspect of the glans penis, extending from one edge of the hooded prepuce to the other (Fig. 95-1). Fortunately, these types occur much less frequently than do the lesser degrees of hypospadias. In more severe situations, it may be difficult to determine the sex of the newborn patient by inspection of the genitalia alone (Horton and Devine, 1972).

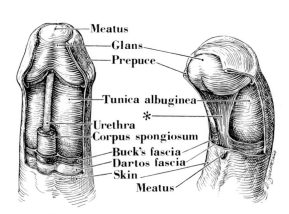

**NORMAL**          **HYPOSPADIAS**

**FIGURE 95-1.** Anatomy of the normal penis and that in hypospadias. The fan-shaped band of fibrous tissue marked with an asterisk is the structure which holds the penis in chordee.

3845

## INCIDENCE

A low familial incidence of hypospadias has been reported and has also been observed by the authors. Most cases occur sporadically. Genetic studies have shown no characteristic chromosomal defect. Hypospadias, one of the most common congenital anomalies, occurs approximately once in every 300 male births. Undescended testes and renal anomalies are more frequent in individuals with hypospadias than in the general population. Each affected patient should have an intravenous pyelogram and sex chromatin study. Cystoscopy and cysto-urethrography should be done if there is any history suggestive of voiding difficulties, and these techniques should also be used in the more severe degrees of hypospadias to rule out müllerian duct remnants.

## HISTORY

Heliodorus and Antilius, Greek surgeons who lived during the first century A.D., first mentioned treatment for hypospadias, consisting of amputation of the penis distal to the meatus; the tip of the stump was formed into the shape of a glans with a glowing cautery. Galen (circa 200 A.D.) and Paulus of Agentia (circa 400 A.D.) mentioned the condition and recommended similar therapy (Rogers, 1973).

The first successful hypospadias repair in the United States was probably done by Mettauer of Virginia in 1836, who described the fibrous tissue which causes the chordee and recommended that it be "liberated" to straighten the penis prior to reconstruction. Since that time, over 200 surgical procedures have been described for the repair of hypospadias (see Chapter 94). Many of the great pioneers of surgery have made contributions to the repair of hypospadias: Paré (1510), Dupuytren (1831), Dieffenbach (1837), Gross (1864), Thiersch (1869), Anger (1874), Duplay (1880), Nové-Josserand (1897), Mayo (1901), Davis (1919), Ombrédanne (1923), Blair and Brown (1933), and Young (1937).

## EMBRYOLOGY

The embryology of the genitourinary system is discussed in Chapter 93, but a resumé follows. At about the second week of development, the embryo consists of a two-layered disc with a midline groove (the primitive streak) near its caudal end. A third cell layer (the mesoderm) begins to proliferate, and mesodermal cells migrate peripherally, separating the outer layer (ectoderm) from the inner (endoderm). Caudal to the primitive streak, the ectoderm and endoderm remain fused and form the cloacal membrane, as mesodermal cells pile up around it to form the cloacal ridges. Owing to rapid and uneven growth, the embryo buckles, forming the head and tail folds, the cloacal membrane and ridges becoming part of the ventral wall of the embryo. The cloacal folds continue to grow, and a mound (the genital tubercle) is formed cranial to the membrane. A midline groove persists in the tubercle and extends to its tip, where an epithelial tag is formed. The tubercle lengthens, carrying the urethral groove with it.

By six to seven weeks, the hindgut is divided into ventral (urogenital) and dorsal (rectal) portions by an endoderm-lined fold (the urorectal septum) which meets the cloacal membrane, dividing it into the urogenital and anal membranes. Rupture of these membranes forms the urogenital ostium and the anus. The appearance of the external genitalia at this stage is essentially similar for both sexes.

At approximately the fifth week of fetal development, the primordial germ cells, which have formed in the wall of the yolk sac close to the allantois, migrate into the germinal ridge, initiating differentiation of the gonads. The Y chromosome of the male germ cells causes this tissue to become a testis. The interstitial cells of Leydig become especially notable during the fourth to fifth month of development but have almost disappeared by the eighth month.

In the absence of testes, the external genitalia grow into a normal configuration. The genital tubercle becomes the clitoris, the urogenital folds become the labia minora, and the labio-scrotal swellings, which later appear, enlarge to form the labia majora. In the male, under the influence of a substance secreted by the developing testis, the genital tubercle grows rapidly and assumes a more cylindrical shape until it is recognizable as a phallus. At its distal end a definite groove appears to delineate the glans. The urethral groove deepens from the urogenital ostium far out onto the shaft, and the lateral edges (the urethral folds) become prominent. At the end of three months, the original urogenital ostium closes, and tubing of the urethra progresses distally with the urogenital ostium advancing before it. The seam remains as a prominent median raphé.

As the urethra forms, mesenchyme coalesces

around the deepening groove and becomes the corpus spongiosum and the covering fascias. Closure of the urethra continues to the developing glans penis, where the urogenital ostium is present as a diamond-shaped opening at the corona. The glans enlarges, and its urethral groove deepens. The glans closes over the groove, but its edges do not fuse at this stage; the deep epithelial-lined tract remains open and is filled with desquamated epithelial cells.

At about the third month, a roll of skin arises on either side of the urethral opening. This ridge gradually extends to encircle the shaft of the penis and grows out to cover the corona. This skin forms the prepuce which extends to sheath the glans. As the prepuce grows, the edges of the glans seal the glanular urethra until the urethral meatus reaches its final location at the site of the former epithelial tag. The deep epithelial tract in the glans now forms the fossa navicularis (Devine, 1958).

## HYPOSPADIAS WITH AND WITHOUT CHORDEE

Hypospadias can occur without chordee, and chordee can occur without hypospadias. The latter is more frequent than the former and has been present in 30 of the approximately 500 cases the authors have treated. In these cases the urethral meatus emerges at the tip of the penis; however, severe chordee is present. The prepuce appears normal and is not deficient on the ventral surface. This type of case must be differentiated from very minor degrees of hypospadias in which the urethral meatus emerges near but not at the exact tip of the penis. The prepuce is deficient ventrally. These cases represent minor variants of hypospadias and should not be diagnosed as chordee without hypospadias. When the meatus is subglandular and no chordee is evident, treatment should be deferred for three to four years after birth to make certain that chordee does not occur with growth. If, at age four, no chordee is noted, it is safe to circumcise the child. Many of these cases will require only a meatotomy.

**Chordee Without Hypospadias.** Three distinct types of chordee without hypospadias can be recognized, and these represent deficient development of the structures surrounding the urethra (Devine and Horton, 1973). In type I the urethra is present as a thin membrane tube beneath the skin. In type II the urethra and the corpus spongiosum have formed. In both of these types, chordee is caused by a fibrous band lying deep and lateral to the urethra. In type III Buck's fascia is also present, and the fibrous tissue is found lateral to the urethra and superficial to Buck's fascia (Fig. 95–2). In all of these types, the urethral meatus is at the tip of the glans, and the prepuce is normal.

If the fibrous tissue can be excised without damage to the urethra, chordee without hypospadias can be repaired without urethroplasty.

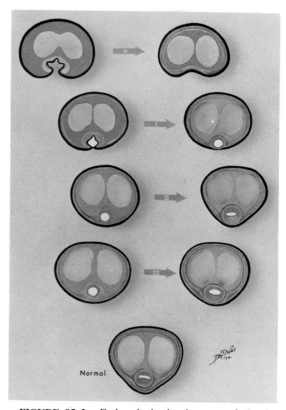

**FIGURE 95–2.** Embryologic development of chordee without hypospadias. Hypospadias and chordee without hypospadias are aspects of a congenital defect and occur when development of the urethra is halted by failure of the evocator substance elaborated by the testis. The figures on the left demonstrate closure of the urethral tube and sequential envelopment by consolidated mesenchyme. The figures on the right demonstrate hypospadias and the three forms of chordee without hypospadias that result from cessation at corresponding stages on left. Types of chordee without hypospadias are labeled on arrows: H. hypospadias. Chordee-causing tissue derives from the mesenchymal anlage of the corpus spongiosum, Buck's fascia, and dartos fascia. Urethra is not present. I, type I. Urethra is present. Chordee-causing tissue derives from the anlage of the corpus spongiosum, Buck's fascia, and dartos fascia. II, type II. Urethra and corpus spongiosum are present. Chordee-causing tissue derives from the anlage of Buck's fascia and dartos fascia. III, type III. Urethra, corpus spongiosum, and Buck's fascia are normal. Chordee-causing tissue is derived from the anlage of the dartos fascia. (From Devine, C. J., Jr., and Horton, C. E.: Chordee without hypospadias. J. Urol., *110*:264, 1973. Copyright 1973, The Williams & Wilkins Company, Baltimore.)

In type I, the urethra should be left attached to the skin while the corpora cavernosa are cleaned of fibrous tissue. The urethra will then stretch with the skin to fit the straightened penis. Special care will be necessary to protect the urethra, as it consists of an extremely thin layer of tissue. In type II, the urethra and the corpus spongiosum must be separated from both the skin and the corpora cavernosa. Removal of the fibrous tissue will usually allow sufficient elongation of the existing urethra. Sometimes, however, the dissection will have to be carried proximally into the normal structures to allow adequate mobilization. In type III, removal of the fibrous tissue from beneath the skin allows the penis to straighten, as structures deep to the fibrous tissue are normal.

While there may be a condition of "congenital short urethra," the authors have not encountered it in our series of cases. All of our patients had chordee due to abnormal fibrous tissue deposited lateral to and beneath the urethra. In our experience, when the abnormal fibrous tissue is totally resected, the urethra stretches adequately, and the penis elongates naturally without chordee. Occasionally, if the ventral skin surface is deficient, Z-plasty or a preputial transfer must be performed to achieve adequate lengthening of the ventral skin.

Should the condition "congenital short urethra" occur and release of the abnormal scar tissue proves to be inadequate, the urethra is divided in the midshaft area and a full-thickness preputial skin graft tube repairs the urethral defect. If the urethral meatus is not in its normal position on the glans penis or if the prepuce is hooded, a urethroplasty is necessary.

**Hypospadias Without Chordee.** Occasionally hypospadias occurs without chordee; however, examination of these patients during an erection may reveal chordee which needs correction. If the meatus is located proximal on the shaft to a degree that impairs urination or procreation, urethroplasty is indicated. A glanular V-flap simplifies construction of the urethra to the tip of the glans; therefore, for psychologic reasons, in many cases the more distal lesions should be repaired.

## MODERN TECHNIQUES FOR REPAIR OF HYPOSPADIAS

Certain principles of reconstruction must be adhered to for successful surgery. The chordee must be corrected and the penis straightened prior to construction of the new urethra. All of the fibrous tissue causing chordee must be resected so that there will be no residual or recurrent chordee after healing has occurred. The urethra should be constructed from hairless skin and must be elastic, of normal caliber without stricture or diverticulum, and extend to the tip of the penis with a meatus which produces a controllable stream of urine.

Many successful techniques for repair of hypospadias are being used by various surgeons. For many years it was felt that urethroplasty must not be combined with resection of tissue causing chordee, because if the chordee recurred after reconstruction of the urethra, the new urethra would have to be sacrificed in subsequent corrections. Consequently, the majority of surgeons preferred to repair hypospadias in two or more stages.

The most popular multiple-staged repair among plastic surgeons has been the Byars modification of the Thiersch-Duplay operation. Duplay (1874) first corrected the chordee and straightened the penis (see Chapter 94). Excess preputial tissue was transferred from the dorsum of the penis to the ventral surface. Byars (1951) modified the operation by splitting the prepuce in the midline and bringing the preputial flaps as far distally on the ventral surface of the penis as possible. This provided an excess of tissue for later reconstruction of the urethra. After an interval of at least six months, a central strip of skin was tubed on the ventral surface of the penis, and the tubed strip of skin was extended as far distally as possible. Byars covered the new urethra by undermining the lateral skin edges and approximating them in the midline with a multilayered closure (Fig. 95–3). In his earlier reports, Byars did not perform an anastomosis of the new urethra with the old urethra at the second stage of surgery. He allowed the new urethra to heal spontaneously, and at a third stage he closed the fistula which existed between the two areas. In his later reports, the new urethra was anastomosed to the old urethra at the second stage. Byars obtained primary healing in a higher percentage of cases than had previously been reported. This technique is still yielding excellent results in those cases in which multistaged repairs are necessary. However, the meatus cannot be brought to the exact tip of the penis; in addition, the spatulate shape of the glans is not changed.

The Denis Browne (1949) operation has been popular with urologists since first being reported

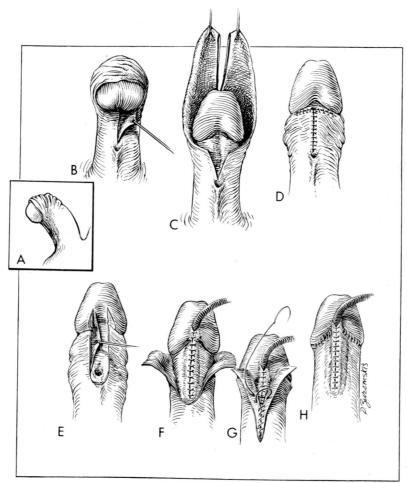

**FIGURE 95–3.** Technique of Thiersch-Duplay as modified by Byars. *A,* Penis with chordee. *B,* Midline incision from the urethral meatus to the corona and around the penis proximal to the glans. *C,* Tissue causing chordee is resected. An incision is made in the midline of the unfolded prepuce. *D,* Flaps of preputial skin transferred to the ventrum. *E,* At a second stage, a central strip is isolated to form the urethra. The tissues beneath this flap will be loose enough to allow it to form a tube without extensive undermining. *F,* The tube having been formed, a circumcising incision is completed, and the lateral flaps of skin are widely mobilized. *G,* The edges of the flaps can be brought together with multiple layers of closure "in depth." *H,* The skin edges are approximated.

approximately 30 years ago. The chordee is corrected and the penis is straightened at the first stage of surgery; urethroplasty is not attempted for at least six months. Browne utilized the fact that a buried strip of skin will grow to form a tube (Browne, 1953). At the second stage of surgery, parallel incisions are made on the ventral surface of the penis, extending from the meatus to the end of the penis. These incisions isolate a midline strip of skin, the width of which depends upon the desired caliber of the new urethra. The lateral skin is then widely undermined and approximated in the midline to cover the buried strip of skin. A dorsal relaxing incision allows the lateral skin to approximate without tension. Browne recommended the use of an indwelling catheter and glass beads on the wire sutures closing the skin, which allow later release of tension if major swelling and edema occur postoperatively (Fig. 95–4). A perineal urethrostomy is used to divert the urine from the repair. Although the technique is basically sound, many operators have noted a high incidence of fistula and stricture formation. The procedure also leaves the abnormal spatulate-shaped glans uncorrected, with resultant

difficulty in construction of the urethra to the tip of the glans. The operation is recommended for the expert surgeon; however, an exceptionally high rate of complications may occur if the surgeon is not thoroughly familiar with the technique.

Culp (1959) has modified the Cecil (1955) operation and has achieved excellent results with this technique of hypospadias repair. Chordee is released at the first stage of surgery. After a proper interval for healing, a urethra is constructed by tubing a central strip of skin on the ventral surface of the penis, using the technique originally described by Thiersch and Duplay and covering the raw surface by burying the penis in a pocket developed in the scrotum. The penile skin edges and subcutaneous tissues over the urethral repair are meticulously approximated to the appropriate scrotal layers by multiple sutures. The scrotal-penile anastomosis is later separated, leaving abundant scrotal skin on the penis to cover the ventral surface (Fig. 95–5).

Wehrbein (1943) and Smith (1955) also used scrotal skin to cover the ventral surface of the penis at a second stage of surgery. They constructed a tube from scrotal skin at the first

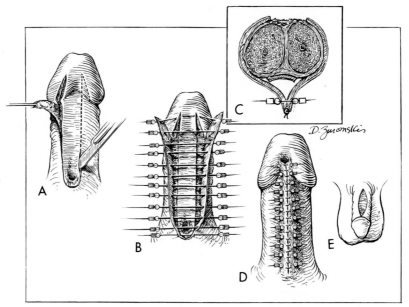

**FIGURE 95–4.**    Technique of Denis Browne. *A,* After the chordee is released and a suitable time is allowed for healing to occur, an incision outlining a strip of skin is made around the urethral meatus out to the glans penis. The edges of skin should not be undermined but should be left attached securely to the shaft of the penis. The strip need not be as broad as the one used to form a tube in the Thiersch-Duplay type of urethroplasty. Lateral flaps are then widely mobilized so that they can be closed easily over the skin strip. *B,* Wire sutures placed through and through remove tension from the suture line. *C,* Cross section of the completed repair. Skin edges are approximated by silk or absorbable sutures. The tension-relieving wire sutures deep to this layer are secured by metal stops, with a glass bead between the stop and the skin edge. Should edema develop, pressure can be taken from the suture line by crushing and removing the glass beads. *D,* The completed repair. *E,* The incision on the dorsum of the penis relieving tension on the suture line. The incision should not cross the junction between the penis and the abdominal skin.

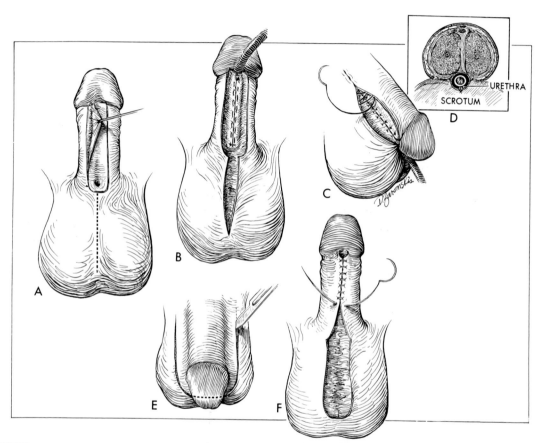

**FIGURE 95–5.** Technique of Cecil-Culp. *A,* After preliminary straightening of the penis, a U-shaped incision is made around the meatus and extended to the glans. The wider tube should be used as in the Thiersch-Duplay urethroplasty, and the tube will form without excessive undermining. An incision is continued into the scrotum from the proximal end of the U-shaped incision for a distance equal to the length of the penis. *B,* The urethral tube closed; the skin margins are widely undermined and elevated. *C,* The penis is sutured to the scrotum in two layers. *D,* Cross section of this approximation. Subcutaneous tissues of the scrotum attached to the tunica of the corpora, skin of penis to skin of scrotum. *E,* Following a sufficient length of time for healing and resolution of reaction, an incision is made to free the penis from the scrotum, allowing sufficient attachment of scrotal skin. *F,* The penis may be resurfaced without tension. The defect in the scrotum is closed.

stage of surgery when the chordee was corrected. At the second stage, reconstruction of the urethra was completed with a Thiersch-Duplay tube; the raw ventral surface of the penis was resurfaced by cutting loose the inferior end of the scrotal tube, opening the tube, and covering the defect with the skin flap (Fig. 95–6).

Multiple-staged hypospadias repairs have always been popular. The medical literature is replete with diagrams and descriptions of surgical maneuvers which have been proposed at one time or another for the repair of this difficult problem.

**One-Stage Repairs.** The first one-stage repair of hypospadias found in a search of the literature was that of Beck (1917), who felt the urethra could be mobilized and stretched to reach to the distal end of the penis in minor degrees of hypospadias. He reported a small series of one-stage repairs in 1922. The authors began their one-stage hypospadias repair in 1955 and first reported their results in 1961 (Devine and Horton, 1961), although they had described their use of the free full-thickness skin graft tube in hypospadias repair in a film produced in 1958 (Horton and Devine, 1958). Various other surgeons also reported a series of one-stage hypospadias operations about this time.

DesPrez, Persky, and Kiehn (1961) and Broadbent, Woolf, and Toksu (1961) used a lateral flap of ventral penile skin which may extend onto the prepuce to construct the urethra; the former base their flap on the meatus, while the latter leave a subcutaneous mesentery to vascularize the flap. Hinderer (1968) also utilized a lateral penile skin flap in a one-stage repair but buried the flap in a tunnel made beneath the tunica albuginea of the corpora. For distal hypospadias Mustardé (1971) used a flap based on the urethral meatus.

Toksu (1970) and Hodgson (1970) independently reported similar techniques for the repair of distal hypospadias (Fig. 95–7). The central area of the inner layer of the prepuce is formed into a tube, leaving the inner preputial skin tube attached to the dorsal skin by subcutaneous attachments. A buttonhole flap is then made in the prepuce; the prepuce, along with the tubed skin, is transferred to the ventral surface of the penis, where it is used to reconstruct the urethra proximal to the tip of the penis. Toksu used the V-shaped glanular flap described by the authors of this chapter to bring the urethral meatus to the tip of the glans. Hodgson, who later modified this technique to make it more useful for proximal lesions, incised triangles of glanular epithelium to locate the meatus in the glans.

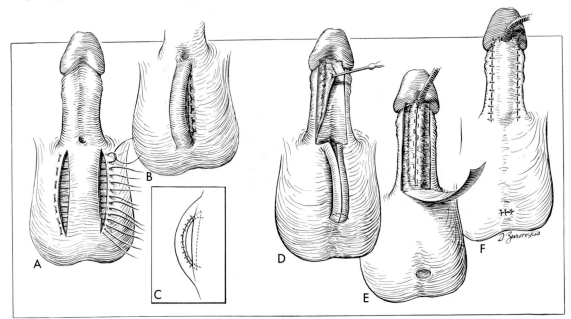

**FIGURE 95–6.** Wehrbein-Smith procedure. *A,* At the time of release of chordee, a tubed flap is formed of scrotal skin with its base at the penoscrotal junction. *B,* Closure of the tube. *C,* Closure of the scrotal skin beneath the tube. It is important that the tube be made very large. *D,* The Thiersch-Duplay urethroplasty incision surrounding the urethral meatus is continued down the midline of the tube, which is then disconnected from the scrotum at the proximal end. *E,* When the urethra has been formed, the opened tube is advanced forward. *F,* The defect on the ventral surface of the penis is covered by the opened tube.

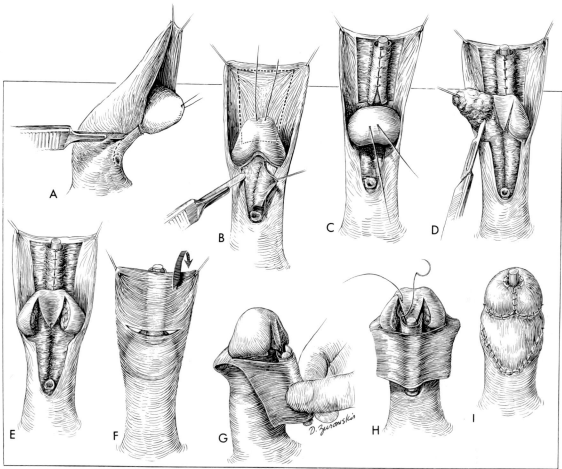

**FIGURE 95–7.** Hodgson-Toksu "tumble flap" repair. *A*, An incision is made releasing the chordee. *B*, The ventral skin distal to the meatus is excised. Dotted line outlines the portion of the inner leaf of the prepuce which will form the tube for urethroplasty. *C*, Tube formed with care taken not to damage its vascular attachments. *D*, Glanular V-flap incised; the lateral wing of the glans tissue is being mobilized by sharp dissection. *E*, Glanular V-flap sutured to the tunica of the corpora. *F*, Incision through the preputial hood which is rotated in the direction of the arrow, placing the new urethral tube in position for anastomosis. *G*, Anastomosis of the tube. *H*, The V-flap tacked high in the distal end of the tube. *I*, Completed repair.

## SURGICAL TREATMENT OF HYPOSPADIAS

Repair should be accomplished prior to school age. The penis is generally large enough by age 1½ to 2 years, and psychologic problems are mitigated if surgery is done at this age and the mother is allowed to remain in the hospital with the patient.

The type of surgical treatment is determined by the severity of the lesion. Prior to urethroplasty, it is necessary to remove all tissue causing the chordee. When the abnormal fibrous tissue is removed, the tunica albuginea of the corpora cavernosa will be completely denuded. Chordee will not recur if adequate resection has been done. Epinephrine

1:100,000 injected sparingly (1 ml) into the area of dissection and traction on a suture placed in the glans, with dorsal finger pressure on the penis, are aids which help to control bleeding. Hemostasis is best obtained by electrocoagulation applied with fine smooth-tipped forceps to each discrete bleeding point. Various incisions allow adequate exposure on the ventral surface of the penis. The area is opened widely, confident that, after the chordee is released, ventral resurfacing of the penis will not prove difficult.

Urinary diversion for distal hypospadias repairs is achieved by a small Foley catheter or preferably a No. 8 plastic feeding tube left in the bladder traversing the repair for three to four days. A perineal urethrostomy for penile hypospadias is preferred; however, if there is only a short urethra proximal to the repair, scrotal or perineal hypospadias cases are probably best diverted by suprapubic drainage.

When the meatus is in the glans but not in its normal position, chordee may be evident only in the flattened shape of the glans. Surgical correction is not necessary unless there is meatal stenosis. It has long been recognized that a meatotomy should be done in a fashion which will not increase the defect. A modification of the glanular V-flap is employed for this condition. The V-flap is outlined with the apex at the urethral meatus and the base at the tip of the glans. The flap is elevated and advanced to be inserted into an incision made in the dorsum of the urethra. The dorsal hood of the prepuce is then removed (circumcision) (Fig. 95–8) (Horton and Devine, 1971).

When chordee is a factor in the repair, three methods have been employed to reconstruct the urethra. Basic to each of these is the flap of glans tissue to place the completed meatus at the tip of the glans (Horton and Devine, 1973).

**The Authors' Technique for Distal Shaft Hypospadias.** For repair of distal shaft hypospadias, if the V-flap of glans tissue will reach the normal urethra after correction of chordee, a new urethra is constructed from a "flip-flap" of skin which is based distally on the meatus (Fig. 95–9). This flap forms the ventral and lateral sides of the urethra and is sutured to a V-shaped flap of glans tissue, which completes the roof and the sides of the new urethra. Several sutures are placed beneath the V-flap to fasten it to the tunica of the corpora, preventing its retraction out of the meatus. The tip of the glanular V-flap is inset into an incision in the dorsal surface of the urethra to open the original meatus. The lateral wings of the glans tissue are brought ventrally and approximated in the midline, changing the spatulate glans to a normal conical shape. The ventral surface of the penis is covered with a preputial buttonhole hood or preferably by split preputial flaps. The ends of the flaps are usually redundant and must be trimmed. It is desirable to use one flap to resurface past the midline and to denude the epidermis from the opposite flap so that the subcutaneous vascular tissue can be interposed as a supporting layer beneath the opposite cover.

**The Authors' Technique for Proximal Shaft Hypospadias.** When the glanular flap does not reach the existing urethra, a full-thickness skin graft is tubed and used to elongate the urethra. Generally this technique is useful in proximal and midshaft hypospadias (Fig. 95–10).

The normal urethra is first calibrated to determine the size (usually 12 French in a 2 year old child). The distance between the existing meatus and the glans is measured, and a skin segment of suitable size is taken from the distal end of the unfolded prepuce. Preputial skin is thin and is an ideal replacement for the normal urethral lining, as this skin will retain its dimensions and grow. The graft is thinned, being careful not to remove dermis but to remove all excess subcutaneous tissue. The graft is then sutured, with the raw surface outward, over a red rubber catheter. The tube is constructed with a tongue at the proximal end to fit into a slit in the urethra at the old meatus, and the seam is left incomplete at the distal end so that the flap of glans tissue can be inset (Fig. 95–10, *D, H, I*). The tubed skin graft is joined to the urethra and the glanular flap with interrupted sutures of 6–0 chromic gut, inverting all epithelial edges into the lumen (Everingham, Horton, and Devine, 1973). The lateral wings of glanular tissue are mobilized distally to cover the urethral tube and to reshape the glans over the new urethra which emerges at the glans tip (Fig. 95–10, *G to J*). Ventral coverage is obtained either by the use of the preputial hood or by the split prepuce technique. Occasionally rotation of the shaft skin held in torsion will provide ventral coverage (Fig. 95–11). The prepuce has always been adequate to cover the base of the penis, and occasionally excess prepuce must be excised. In distal lesions, when using the perforated hood technique, the ventral penile skin is incised proximally from the meatus toward the base of the penis to allow a smoother fit and to ensure that the urethral graft anastomosis is covered by well-vascularized skin. To obtain a reinforcing layer of vascularized subcutaneous tissue in proximal lesions, especially those at the penoscrotal junction, the scrotal skin is undermined, and a long flap of subcutaneous fatty vascular tissue is mobilized and interposed over the urethroplasty. Skin closure is accomplished with 6–0 chromic gut.

**The Authors' Technique for Perineal Hypospadias.** There will usually be a bifid scrotum with a central area of hairless smooth skin extending distally from the meatus to the shaft of the penis when scrotal or perineal hypospadias is present. At that point the skin becomes thin, and abnormal fibrous tissue appears to penetrate the subcutaneous layers. In order to

*Text continued on page 3859*

**FIGURE 95–8.** Authors' procedure employed when chordee is not a factor and urethral meatotomy is necessary. *A*, The skin incisions are outlined by the dotted line. The V-shaped flap of glans is incised and elevated. *B*, The flap has been elevated and an incision made on the dorsal surface of the urethra. Circumcision has been accomplished, removing the excess preputial hood. *C*, The flap of glans has been advanced into the urethra. The circumcision is then closed.

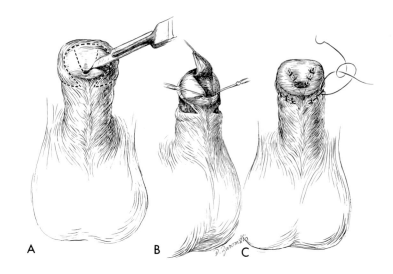

**FIGURE 95–9.** Authors' flip-flap repair is used when chordee is a factor and when the V-flap of glans will reach the urethral meatus after the tissue causing the chordee has been resected. *A*, Incisions marked (1) for the flip-flap and (2) around the penis proximal to the corona. *B*, Dissection completed. The chordee has been released. The glanular V-flap is sewn to the tunica of the corpora and an incision outlined in the midline of the prepuce. *C*, The V-flap is sutured to the incision in the dorsal surface of the urethra. *D*, The flip-flap completes the ventral surface of the urethra. *E*, The wings of glans tissue have been approximated in the midline ventral to the urethral meatus, and the skin has been closed.

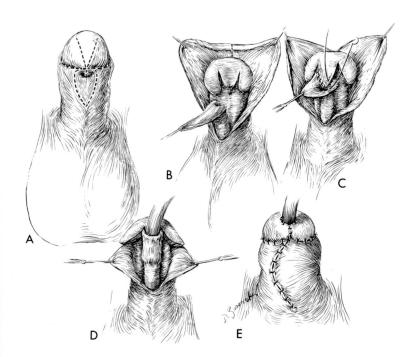

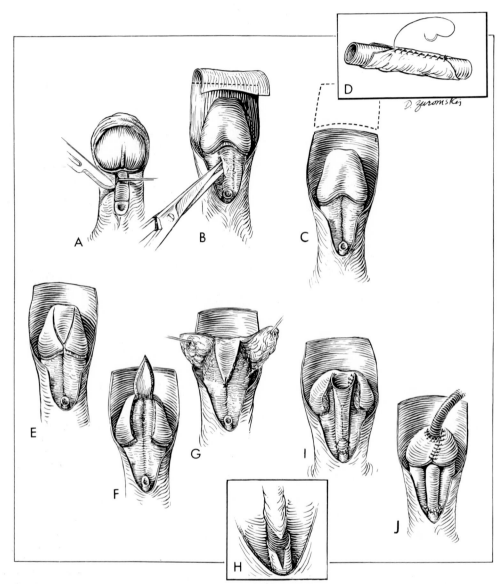

**FIGURE 95–10.** Authors' repair when the urethral meatus is proximal, the glanular V-flap will not reach, and a tubed skin graft is necessary to bridge the gap. *A*, Incisions are made circumcising the urethral meatus and extending out to the corona where they are continued around the penis. *B*, The subcutaneous tissue is excised. *C*, Cleaning the tunica albuginea of the corpora cavernosa and the urethra. The prepuce is unfolded and the distal end is excised. *D*, After subcutaneous tissue is removed from the full-thickness skin graft, a tube is constructed. A tongue is left at the proximal end opposite the seam, and the seam is not extended to the distal end, leaving a V-shaped defect. *E*, After dissecting between the glans and the corpora cavernosa, a distally based V-shaped glanular skin flap is incised. *F*, The glanular flap is elevated and thinned. *G*, The glanular flap is sutured to the tunica albuginea of the corpora cavernosa. The lateral wings of glanular tissue are mobilized. *H*, Anastomosis between the tubed skin graft and the urethra. The tongue of the graft fits in an incision in the urethra, creating a long, elliptical anastomosis. Sutures are interrupted 6–0 chromic with the knots outside the lumen. *I*, The distal end of the skin graft is anastomosed to the V-shaped glanular flap with the knots tied inside the lumen. *J*, The wings of glanular tissue have been brought ventral to the urethral meatus by a deep 5–0 chromic suture and 6–0 chromic sutures in the epithelial surface.

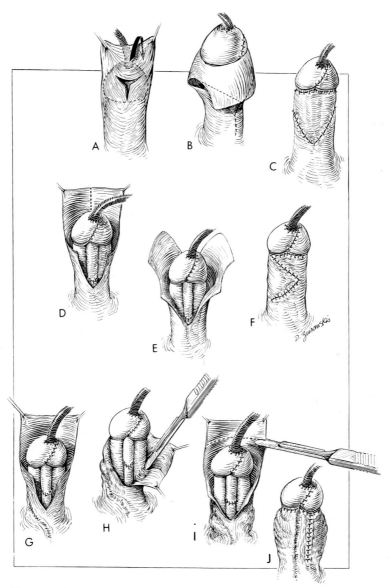

**FIGURE 95–11.** Three techniques for resurfacing the ventral portion of the penis. *A,* The perforated preputial hood is prepared. The incision through which the glans will be brought is Y-shaped. *B,* The glans has been brought through the hole. *C,* The anastomosis is completed. An incision can be made in the midline of the ventral surface of the penis and the corners of the hood trimmed for a smoother fit. *D, E,* At present, the authors prefer to make a midline incision in the prepuce, avoiding the blood vessels and rotating the flaps to the ventral surface. *F,* The flaps are closed in Z-plasty fashion. *G,* When there is torsion of the penis, the raphé will swing laterally. *H,* The skin of the penis can be freed up completely. *I,* Excess prepuce is excised. *J,* The skin is rotated to cover the ventral surface of the penis and to correct the torsion.

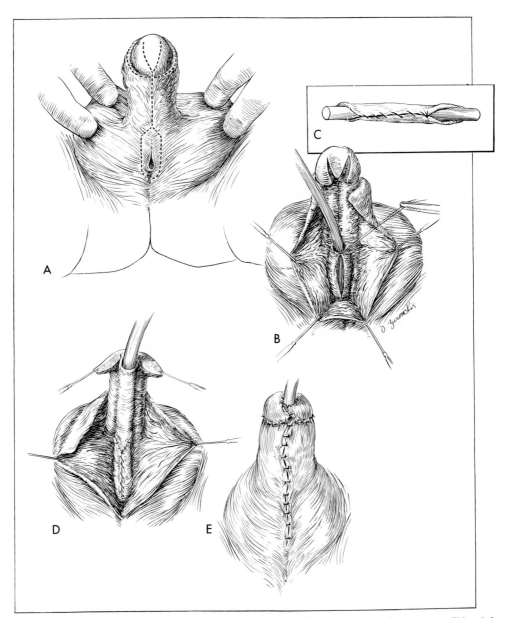

**FIGURE 95–12.**   Authors' repair when the urethral meatus is located in the perineum; the scrotum will be cleft and the meatus surrounded by an area of hairless skin. *A,* An incision is made around the area of hairless skin, extending to the midline of the penis and to the corona where it is continued around the penis. The midline glanular flap is diagrammed also. *B,* Dissection complete, the hairless skin surrounding the urethral meatus has been formed into a tube. *C,* A tube of full-thickness skin graft has been formed from preputial skin. *D,* The skin graft tube has been anastomosed to the Thiersch-Duplay type of tube at the penoscrotal junction and to the V-shaped flap of glans tissue at the new meatus. *E,* The wings of glans have been approximated ventral to the urethral meatus, and the skin on the shaft of the penis has been closed.

convert the scrotal or proximal hypospadias to a penile shaft hypospadias, a Thiersch-Duplay tube of the midline strip of hairless skin is made and used to extend the urethra distally onto the penile shaft as far as possible. All abnormal fibrous tissue is resected from beneath the tube, which is based on the meatus. Once the severe hypospadias has been converted to a proximal shaft hypospadias, a repair using a tubed full-thickness skin graft can be completed (Fig. 95–12).

## POSTOPERATIVE CARE

A light, four-tailed elastic pressure bandage is employed to give postoperative compression to the hypospadias repair, to control edema, and to prevent postoperative bleeding. The dressing should be removed immediately if there is excess bruising around the area, and any hematoma should be evacuated. The tissue flaps are fragile, and the vascular supply to the tips of the glans is precarious. Consequently, any extra pressure imposed by a hematoma could cause necrosis. Because of the effect of pressure on healing, catheters traversing the repair should be small; either a small, sterile, plastic feeding tube or a soft red rubber catheter is used.

Bladder spasm, which can cause excruciating pain and may be difficult to control, is probably the result of irritation of the trigone by the tip of the catheter. To prevent bladder spasm, the catheter used to divert the urine is inserted into the bladder until urine flows freely; the catheter is then withdrawn until the urine flow stops, after which the catheter is reinserted 2 cm further so that only the tip projects into the bladder. This maneuver avoids excess irritation of the trigone area. If bladder spasm still occurs, the patient should be given tincture of belladonna, belladonna and opium rectal suppositories, narcotics, hot tub baths, or tranquilizers as indicated. Early removal of the catheter is advised.

Postoperative erection can be troublesome in older patients, resulting in traction on the suture line, dehiscence of the wound, and bleeding. Nocturnal erections occur without the willful control of the patient, but all erotic stimulation must be avoided. Pearls of amyl nitrite are left at the patient's bedside to be broken and the fumes inhaled when an erection is first suspected. Their quick use will prevent daytime erection; however, if erections continue to be a problem, ethyl chloride can be tried. There is no systemic medication to prevent nocturnal erections, but sedation may be helpful. Routine prophylactic antibiotics are not used, but the patient is given a urinary antibacterial while the indwelling catheter is in place. The urine is observed carefully, and should an infection occur, specific antibiotic therapy is started.

In the event wound dehiscence occurs as a result of wound edema, erection, or hematoma, no attempt is made to resuture the separated edges. The friable and thin tissue becomes easily infected because of organisms present in the perineum. The area should be compressed with warm, sterile saline pads and urinary diversion continued until the injured area heals. When the tissues have healed, the resultant problems can be repaired at a secondary operation 6 to 12 months later.

Gentle technique in removing dressings is important in all cases of hypospadias repair, regardless of the technique. Tissue healing progresses slowly in this area, with little strength noted in the early phase. Injudicious and rough pulling on bandages may result in separation of suture lines. The use of a water-soluble material between the skin and dressing, tubbing the patient three times a day, and letting the bandages fall away from the wound rather than removing them manually are helpful adjuncts. A crust should not be allowed to form in the new meatus, as it could plug the urethra and cause a proximal blowout leak when the patient starts to void. Crusting can be prevented by tub baths and antibiotic ointment applied into the new meatus with an ophthalmic tipped tube.

## COMPLICATIONS

The most frequent complications of hypospadias repair are fistula, diverticulum, urethral stricture, and meatal stenosis (Ombrédanne, 1913). The rate of complications seems to be approximately the same for multistage and one-stage repairs.

The most common cause of fistulas is necrosis of a flap due to a small collection of blood under the flap, but they may also result from formation of epithelized tracts around retained sutures. Fistulas should be allowed to heal spontaneously with secondary repair six months later. A catheter can be used to divert urine for two weeks after a fistula has appeared, in the hope that the edges will reapproximate; however, it is useless to continue diversion longer than two weeks.

When a diverticulum or fistula occurs, the urethra should be checked for distal stenosis.

Since continued softening of the scarring can be expected postoperatively for two or three months, meatal stenosis may often be handled by simple dilatation. Surgery, if necessary, is best done by incising the dorsal roof of the meatus and elevating a V-shaped flap from the glans penis to be advanced into the dorsal meatotomy incision. Meatal stenosis has not been a problem since the V-shaped glanular flap has been used in primary hypospadias repair.

Strictures of the urethra pose particular problems. If a stricture is short and not dense, dilatation of the urethra may be effective. In severe strictures, secondary surgery is indicated. Internal urethrotomy may suffice in short strictures. However, in long strictures the urethra should be opened along the area of stricture and a full-thickness skin graft patch used to reconstitute the caliber of the urethra (Devine, Sakati, Poutasse and Devine, 1968). An indwelling catheter can be used to support the skin graft patch, with the outer skin closed in layers over the repair. The repair of urethral strictures is discussed in Chapter 97.

To repair a diverticulum, it is necessary to incise over the area and isolate and dissect free the diverticulum. The neck should be opened and divided so that the urothelium can be closed at the same level as the adjacent urethral walls. The overlying skin is then closed in layers and the urine diverted by an indwelling catheter.

## REFERENCES

Anger, T.: Quoted by Duplay, S.: De l'hypospadias périnéo-scrotal et de son traitement chirurgical. Presentation at the Société de Chirurgie, Paris, 1874.

Beck, C.: Hypospadias and its treatment. Surg. Gynecol. Obstet., *24*:511, 1917.

Bevan, A. D.: A new operation for hypospadias. J.A.M.A., *68*:1032, 1917.

Blair, V. P., and Brown, J. B.: The correction of the scrotal hypospadias and of epispadias. Surg. Gynecol. Obstet., *57*:646, 1933.

Broadbent, T. R., Woolf, R., and Toksu, E.: Hypospadias: One-stage repair. Plast. Reconstr. Surg., *27*:154, 1961.

Browne, D.: Hypospadias. J. Postgrad. Med., *25*:367, 1949.

Browne, D.: A comparison of the Duplay and Denis Browne techniques for hypospadias operation. Surgery, *34*:787, 1953.

Bucknall, R. T. H.: A new operation for penile hypospadias. Lancet, *2*:887, 1907.

Byars, L. T.: A technique for consistently satisfactory repair of hypospadias. Surg. Gynecol. Obstet., *92*:149, 1951.

Cecil, A. B.: Symposium on pediatric urology. Hypospadias and epispadias: Diagnosis and treatment. Pediatr. Clin. North Am., *2*:711, 1955.

Culp, O. S.: Experiences with 200 hypospadias: Evolution of a therapeutic plan. Surg. Clin. North Am., *39*:1007, 1959.

Davis, J. S.: Plastic Surgery. Philadelphia, P. Blakiston Son & Company, 1919.

DesPrez, J. D., Persky, L., and Kiehn, E. L.: One-stage repair of hypospadias by island flap technique. Plast. Reconstr. Surg., *28*:405, 1961.

Devine, C. J., Jr.: Motion picture: Embryology of the Male External Genitalia. Trans. Am. Assoc. Genitourin. Surg., *62*:123, 1970.

Devine, C. J., Jr., and Horton, C. E.: A one stage hypospadias repair. J. Urol., *85*:166, 1961.

Devine, C. J., Jr., and Horton, C. E.: Hypospadias. *In* Goldwyn, M. (Ed.): The Unfavorable Result in Plastic Surgery: Avoidance and Treatment. Boston, Little, Brown and Company, 1972.

Devine, C. J., Jr., and Horton, C. E.: Chordee without hypospadias. J. Urol., *110*:264, 1973.

Devine, P. C., Sakati, I. A., Poutasse, E. F., and Devine, C. J., Jr.: One stage urethroplasty: Repair of urethral stricture with a free full thickness patch of skin. J. Urol., *99*:191, 1968.

Dieffenbach, J. F.: Guérison des fentes congénitales de la verge, de l'hypospadias. Gaz. Hebd. Méd., *5*:156, 1837.

Duplay, S.: De l'hypospadias périnéo-scrotal et de son traitement chirurgical. Arch. Gén. Méd., *23*:513, 1874.

Duplay, S.: Sur le traitement chirurgical de l'hypospadias et l'épispadias. Arch. Gén. Méd., *5*:257, 1880.

Edmunds, A.: An operation for hypospadias. Lancet, *1*:447, 1913.

Everingham, W. J., Horton, C. E., and Devine, C. J., Jr.: Studies of urethral healing in dogs. Plast. Reconstr. Surg., *51*:312, 1973.

Gross, S. D.: A System of Surgery: Pathological, Diagnostic, Therapeutic, and Operative. 3rd Ed. Philadelphia, Blanchard and Lea, 1864.

Hinderer, U.: Hypospadias. Rev. Esp. Cirug. Plast., *1*:53, 1968.

Hodgson, N. B.: A one-stage hypospadias repair. J. Urol., *104*:281, 1970.

Horton, C. E., and Devine, C. J., Jr.: Details of this are illustrated in an animated film: Embryology of the Male External Genitalia. Eaton Medical Film Library, Norwich, New York, 1958.

Horton, C. E., and Devine, C. J., Jr.: Hypospadias. *In* Mustardé, J. C. (Ed.): Plastic Surgery in Infancy and Childhood. Philadelphia, W. B. Saunders Company, 1971.

Horton, C. E., and Devine, C. J., Jr.: Hypospadias and epispadias. Ciba Clinical Symposia, Vol. 24, No. 3, 1972.

Horton, C. E., and Devine, C. J., Jr.: Hypospadias. *In* Horton, C. E. (Ed.): Plastic Surgery of the Genital Area. Boston, Little, Brown and Company, 1973.

Humby, G.: One-stage operation for hypospadias. Br. J. Surg., *29*:84, 1941.

McCormack, R. M.: Simultaneous chordee repair and urethral reconstruction for hypospadias. Plast. Reconstr. Surg., *13*:257, 1954.

Mayo, C. H.: Hypospadias. J.A.M.A., *36*:1157, 1901.

Mettauer, J. P.: Practical observations on those malformations of the male urethra and penis, termed hypospadias and epispadias with an anomalous case. Am. J. Med. Sci., *4*:43, 1836.

Mustardé, J. C.: Reconstruction of anterior urethra in hypospadias by buried skin strip method. Br. J. Plast. Surg., *7*:166, 1954.

Mustardé, J. C. (Ed.): Plastic Surgery in Infancy and Childhood. Philadelphia, W. B. Saunders Company, 1971.

Nesbit, R. M.: Plastic procedure for correction of hypospadias. J. Urol., *45*:699, 1941.

Nové-Josserand, G.: Traitement de l'hypospadias; nouvelle méthode. Lyon Méd., *85*:198, 1897.

Ombrédanne, L.: Précis Clinique et Opération de Chirurgie Infantile. Paris, Masson et Cie, 1923, p. 851.

Rogers, B. O.: History. *In* Horton, C. E. (Ed.): Plastic Surgery of the Genital Area. Boston, Little, Brown and Company, 1973.

Rosenberger, P.: Ueber Operative Behandlung der männlichen Epispadie. Dtsch. Med. Wochenschr., *17*:1250, 1891.

Smith, D. R.: Surgical treatment of hypospadias. J. Urol., *73*:329, 1955.

Thiersch, K.: Ueber die Enstehungsweise und Operative Behandlung der Epispadie. Arch. Heilk., *10*:20, 1869.

Toksu, E.: Hypospadias: A one-stage repair. Plast. Reconstr. Surg., *45*:365, 1970.

Van Hook, W.: A new operation for hypospadias. Ann. Surg., *23*:378, 1896.

Wehrbein, H. L.: Hypospadias. J. Urol., *50*:335, 1943.

Young, H. H.: Genital Abnormalities, Hermaphroditism and Related Adrenal Disease. Baltimore, The Williams & Wilkins Company, 1937.

Young, F., and Benjamin, J. A.: Preschool age repair of hypospadias with free inlay skin graft. Surgery, *26*:384, 1949.

# CHAPTER 96

# EPISPADIAS AND EXSTROPHY OF THE BLADDER

CLIFFORD C. SNYDER, M.D.,
AND EARL Z. BROWNE, JR., M.D.

In his paper on bladder exstrophy published in 1916, Battle Malone wrote: "The pathology is as vague and indefinite as the remedies are numerous and worthless." Having been closely involved with the surgical correction of 62 epispadiac and ectopic urinary bladders, our enthusiasm is somewhat greater than Malone's, although his discouraging remark demands respect. Moreover, the physician should constantly remember that every parent of a child with epispadias regards him as a source of help.

Sorrentino and Leonetti (1958) called attention to an Assyrian tablet, dated 2000 B.C. and now located in the British Museum, which describes a case of epispadias and exstrophy of the bladder. They also cited an article written in 1595 accounting for this anomaly. From other Assyrian tablets dated about 700 B.C., it is known that these deformities existed (Thompson, 1930; Camac, 1931; Bettman, 1956). Aristotle (334 B.C.), the father of teratology, never accepted the theories that congenital anomalies were due to astral configurations in the heavens or to sexual relations between animals and man; he believed that congenital anomalies were the result of de-fective growth. The ancient Hebrews, because their religious laws required examining the meat of deformed animals, observed and recorded congenital anomalies in the 370 A.D. Talmud (Preuss, 1923). Ambroise Paré (1579), addressing a group at the Sorbonne, remarked that mystical reasons must not be discarded as causes of malformations. This Renaissance surgeon considered the Devil and witches responsible for some of the pranks encountered by mothers of deformed siblings. Fortunately, the sixteenth century anatomical studies of Andreas Vesalius (Burggraeve, 1841) and the works of Leonardo da Vinci (1492) proved some of the superstitious ideas erroneous. Harvey (1685) researched the chick embryo with a magnifying lens and reported his observations of developmental growth which were not readily accepted by many of his colleagues. There were many other early medical contributions dealing with these challenging and intriguing anomalies, but, consistent with early writings, they were vague, unfinished, and indefinite as to therapy and results (Lloyd, 1851; Simon, 1852; Roux, 1853; Wood, 1869; Smith, 1879; Maydl, 1894). Over 625 manuscripts dealing with bladder exstrophy in the medical literature in the past 115 years have been researched by the authors.

## EPISPADIAS

**Etiology and Incidence.** The anomalies of the genitourinary tract known as epispadias and exstrophy of the bladder are more frequently coexistent entities, and a synchronized description of these is appropriate (Hejtmancik, King and Magid, 1954; Kittredge and Bradburn, 1954; Uson and Roberts, 1958). Epispadias is a rare congenital deformity for which there is no etiologic explanation that has as yet received a general acceptance among embryologists (Pohlman, 1911; Fraser and Fainstat, 1951; Patten, 1954; Muecke, 1964; Arey, 1966). The theoretical divergence of opinion ranges from inborn errors of metabolism to environmental predispositions (Wyburn, 1937; Douglas, 1958; Arnesen, 1958). Patten and Barry (1952) suggested that the departure from normal development occurs early when the genital tubercle primordia are yet in their original paired position (see Chapter 93). If at this time, which is recognized as four to six weeks of embryonic life, the primordia are displaced caudally and coalesce in this position with the urogenital sinus remaining open cephalically rather than caudally as is normal, the urethral groove develops without a closing of the superior surface of the genital tubercle, and an epispadias is produced (Fig. 96–1). When this occurs, the thin cloacal membrane has a tendency to rupture, and the deformity extends in a cephalad direction, creating the commonly associated anomaly of bladder exstrophy.

Epispadias is relatively uncommon (Dees, 1949; Flocks and Culp, 1959; Marshall and Muecke, 1962), even though numerous papers have been written on the subject. For each 500 cases of hypospadias, there is only one of simple epispadias. Campbell (1951) found only three cases of epispadias in 10,712 autopsies and compared this to the discovery of one case of bladder exstrophy in 936 autopsies. The sex incidence is about three males to one female (Campbell, 1952).

The condition is defined as a groove or cleft without a covering on the upper surface of the penis and it is seen in various degrees of severity (Arey, 1954). The urethral canal is short, and there is usually a fibrous contracture or chordee drawing the spatulous penis upward (Williams, 1968). The types of epi-

spadias in the male may be divided into balanic, penile, and penopubic (Brachet, 1947).

The balanic or glanular form of epispadias is the simplest and least involved but is the least common of the three types (see Fig. 96–1, *A* to *E*). The deformity is limited to the glans and ends proximally at the coronary sulcus. The prepuce is not present on the cleft side, and the patient is continent of urine.

The penile variety is also uncommon and usually involves the penis from the glans to the symphysis pubis (see Fig. 96–1, *F* to *H*). The corpora cavernosa musculature is spread apart, and the corpus spongiosum is absent or deficient; these anomalous conditions are responsible for the flat or spatulous contour of the penis. The prostate gland is usually absent. Depending on the severity of the deformity, the patient may or may not be continent.

The penopubic type is complex and is usually associated with exstrophy of the bladder. It is the commonest form of the disease and the most difficult to treat. The penis is very short, spatulated, and curved cephalically against the pubis (see Fig. 96–1, *I* to *K*). The urethra remains unroofed in its entirety and opens into the exstrophied bladder. Because the bladder sphincter has not completely formed, the patient is incontinent of urine. While the bony pelvis is usually normal in the first two types, it is commonly separated at the pubis in the third form. Infertility may or may not be present in the male, but this is not a complication in the female (Campbell, 1957).

**Treatment.** Probably the first successful closure of epispadias was achieved by Liston (1838), a British surgeon, who reported that by paring the margins of the anterior cleft he was able to close the deformity. Mettauer (1842), an American surgeon, described epispadial repair by first using multiple incisions to release the curvature (chordee) and then inhibiting recurrence by splinting the penile shaft with a tube. He remarked that cures were complete within three weeks. The therapeutic approach to epispadias is directed toward constructing a urethral tunnel which will function as a conduit for genitourinary excretions. Sphincter competence is the ultimate goal, and every effort should be made to restore this function. This goal is not difficult in the glanular and penile forms of the anomaly, but complications may ensue when the pubic variety is encountered. When the detrusor muscle is functionally defective, the chances of achieving urinary continence are slim (Williams, 1968).

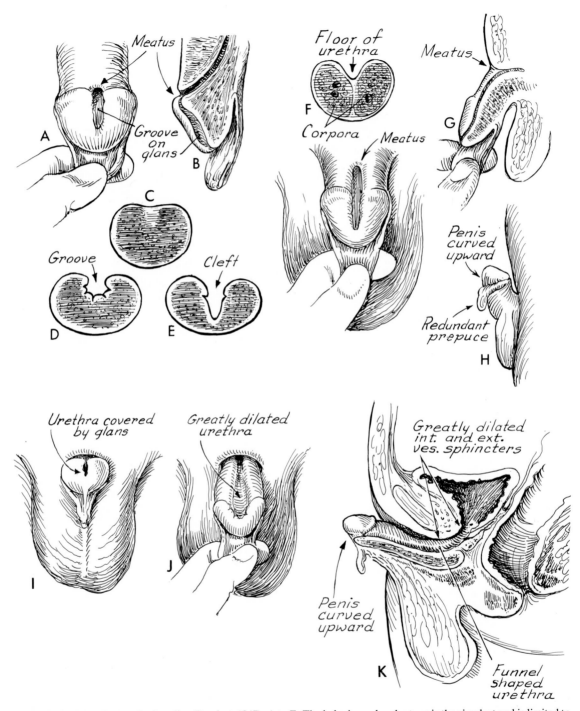

**FIGURE 96–1.** Types of epispadias (Brachet, 1947). *A* to *E,* The balanic or glanular type is the simplest and is limited to the glans and coronal eminence. There is no prepuce on the cleft side, and there is urinary continence. *F* to *H,* The penile form involves the phallic shaft, and there is continence of urine. *I* to *K,* The penopubic type is the most severe, and because the bladder sphincter is incompletely developed, there is urinary incontinence.

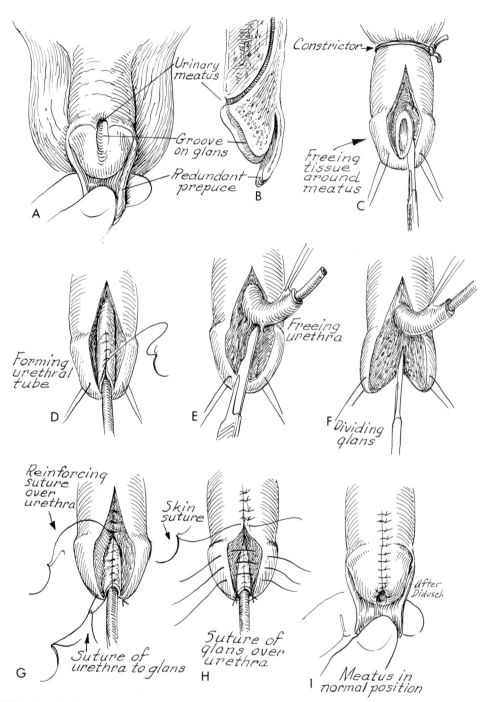

**FIGURE 96–2.** Surgical correction of the balanic type of epispadias by the technique of Lowsley and Kirwin. *A* to *C,* A tourniquet may be used. The urethral orifice and groove are dissected free. *D* to *F,* Over a catheter, the urethra is dissected proximally and the glans sectioned. *G* to *I,* After the urethra is buried deep in the glans, affording a natural position for the orifice, the wound is closed in two layers with nylon sutures.

There is a difference of opinion as to the optimum age at which to repair the deformity (Lowsley and Johnson, 1955). While some surgeons advocate allowing the full growth of the genital and urinary tissues, others consider the prepubertal age as the ideal period for surgical repair, because the patient by this time realizes the severity of his disease and is psychologically prepared for the operation. The complete form of epispadias should be surgically corrected when the newborn is stabilized in his new external environment and is free of disease which may complicate the operative procedure. Although the infant may be considered in a satisfactory surgical status before his first birthday, the authors prefer this age for the surgical repair. The organ size at 1 year is favorable, and body resistance to injury is optimum. The reparative bladder procedure should certainly be finished before the age of puberty to prevent ascending lesions of the upper urinary tract and to avoid intervening sociologic and psychologic complications, such as urinary excoriation of the skin of the abdomen and perineum and the accompanying unpleasant uriniferous odors. Affected adults find sexual intercourse a problem owing to the short, curved, penile shaft, and insemination may not take place because of diverted seminal ejection from the penopubic area.

**Repair of the Simple Type of Epispadias.** Reconstructive surgery for the simple types of epispadias in the male consists of constructing a urethral canal to the penile tip. The urine flow is first diverted by a suprapubic cystostomy. Among the more popular methods of repair are those described by Young (1918), Campbell (1952), Lowsley and Kirwin (1956), and Gross and Cresson (1958). The technique of Lowsley and Kirwin (1956) is shown in Figure 96–2. It consists of freeing the cleft urethra in an

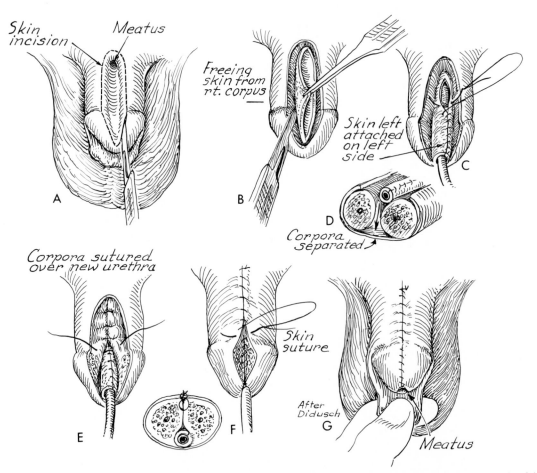

**FIGURE 96–3.** Technique of Young. *A*, Parallel incisions are made along the urethral groove. *B to D*, One margin of the urethra is dissected deeply, but the opposite edge is only slightly undermined to ensure an adequate blood supply. The urethra is tubed and buried deeply between the bulbocavernosae. *E to G*, The bulbocavernosae are closed over the urethra. The deep layer is closed with interrupted fine clear nylon sutures and the skin with a continuous nylon suture.

elliptical fashion and replanting it deep in the soft tissue of the glans. The procedure of Young (1918), as demonstrated in Figure 96–3, is used for the penile type of epispadias with continence. Parallel incisions on each side of the dorsal groove are joined proximally where the urethral orifice opens. The dissection on one side is carried deep to free the urethra, whereas the parallel incision on the opposite side is made shallow, leaving the wall attached to the corpus cavernosum to ensure an adequate blood supply. The tubed urethra is rolled between the divided corpora, and the latter are approximated with sutures over the reconstructed urethra. The skin is approximated to finish the procedure. Campbell (1952) has adapted the Denis Browne

(1953) hypospadias operation for surgical repair of epispadias (see Chapter 95), and it is the technique preferred by the authors for the correction of the simple type of epispadias (Fig. 96–4).

Occasionally, unsatisfactory results are observed following the repair of the simple glanular type of epispadias. Consequently, careful evaluation of the patient, including consultation in some cases, is suggested before considering any type of surgical approach. Even if the condition is a minor dorsal slit in the glans and there is no existent bladder or upper urinary tract disease, the parents of the patient should be informed of the possible complications that may follow an operative procedure. Surgery may not improve the original deformity and, in fact, may result in

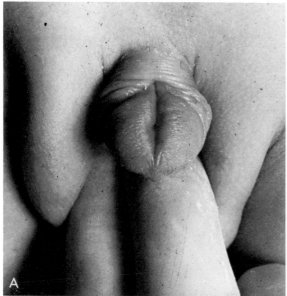

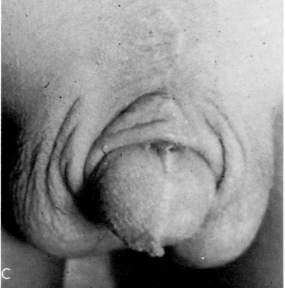

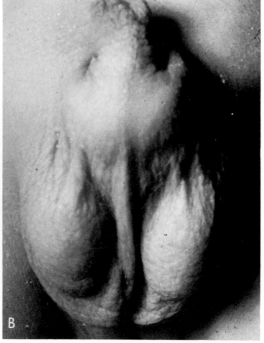

**FIGURE 96–4.** Authors' repair of penopubic epispadias. *A,* Preoperative view of the cleft involving the glans and extending into the bladder neck. Patient is incontinent at age 10 years. *B,* The prepuce on the uncleft underside of the glans. *C,* The ligaments between the pubic crests and rami and the rudimentary bladder neck musculature have been incised, crossed anteriorly, and sutured to construct a sphincter. The patient can urinate through the glanular tip and is continent.

scarring, fistulas, stenosis, and atresia. If the parents insist on correction of the minor variant of the anomaly, diversion of the urinary stream should be considered prior to surgical correction of the defect. Wound dehiscence is all too common, especially if the operative site is continually bathed in urine.

**Repair of the Complete Type of Epispadias.** The treatment of the complete or penopubic form of epispadias, in which there is incontinence of urine, should be directed toward constructing a sphincter for control of the urine (White and Dennison, 1958). The sphincter can be obtained by constructing a bladder neck. If this procedure is not feasible due to associated genital, urinary, or abdominal anomalies or if sphincter reconstruction fails, the urinary stream can be diverted into the intestinal tract, where the anal sphincter is utilized for urinary control.

If the decision is made to construct a bladder neck, the procedure must include closure of the bladder wall, with special care taken to use all of the available tissue at the bladder neck and interpubic area in order to form a vesical sphincter. This approach is conventional, and modifications are abundant with variable results (Lattimer, Dean and Furey, 1957a, b; Sweetser, 1960). Remnants of the arcuate ligament, which normally connects one pubic bone to the other at the symphysis in front of the urethra, should be utilized. The transverse pelvic ligament, which lies posterior to the urethra between the pubic rami, should also be conserved. A portion of either of these ligaments may be used, as well as a portion of the superficial triangular ligament, to construct a bladder sphincter for urinary continence.

The authors employ a two-stage procedure in correcting the incontinent penopubic types of male epispadias (Fig. 96–5), but only one stage is required for the repair of female epispadias. In the male, the first stage is done at the age of 1 year, at which time the cicatricial chordee is corrected and the prepuce is buttonholed and transferred from the underside of the penile shaft to the upper aspect. Sufficient tissue is gained for second stage urethral construction, and also additional length is obtained for the short, curved, penile body. A waiting period of three months is sufficient in order to complete the repair. The canal must be made sufficiently large at the corona and within the glans, areas which have a tendency toward scar contraction. The incisions are extended proximally to correct the defect in the inferior

portion of the bladder and to locate the transverse ligamentous and muscle attachments to the symphysis pubis. The insertions of the abdominal recti muscles are in part severed at their pubic attachments, decussated anteriorly, and reattached with steel wire to the opposite pubic bone. This maneuver corrects the diastasis of the rectus abdominis muscles and prevents direct hernias. The ligamentous structures are dissected from their lateral attachments and folded medially over the urethra, forming a sphincterlike structure. The tissues are sutured over a catheter placed in the bladder. The soft tissues are closed using mattress sutures of either nylon or stainless steel wire. If there is difficulty in bringing the tissues into approximation, the iliac bones are divided lateral to the sacroiliac joint; the pubes are advanced medially and sutured in juxtaposition with stainless steel wires. There are various techniques described regarding ileostomy (Trendelenburg, 1906; Schultz, 1959; Lattimer and associates, 1960; Marshall and Muecke, 1962). The skin edges are approximated with deep sutures of stainless steel wire which are removed after 10 to 12 days. A suprapubic cystostomy is used in males, but only an indwelling catheter is required to divert the stream in females. Because the clitoris is bifid and the anterior vaginal vault is absent, both of these structures must be repaired. They are surgically pared and approximated in the one-step procedure. The dressing is positioned with only a moderate amount of pressure and is removed on the fourth postoperative day. The wound is left open thereafter but cleansed daily. The suprapubic cystostomy catheter is removed on the twelfth day after operation. If a decision is initially made to shunt the urinary stream, there are a variety of techniques available for diverting the urine into various portions of the intestinal tract, abdominal wall, or perineum (Connelly, 1901; Burns, 1924; Brickel, 1926; Cecil, 1932; Allison, 1933; Cabot, 1937; Blair and Byars, 1938).

Fracture of the pelvic bones in order to approximate the pubes at the symphysis is performed only in females. The techniques are numerous (Trendelenburg, 1906; Shultz, 1959; Lattimer and associates, 1960). There are many gradients of female epispadias, but to simplify the classification, three are demonstrated in Figure 96–6. Female epispadias is not as difficult to correct as that in the male. However, it is necessary to divert the urinary stream for a few days by catheter. In constructing a snug vesical sphincter, the operation is similar to that in the

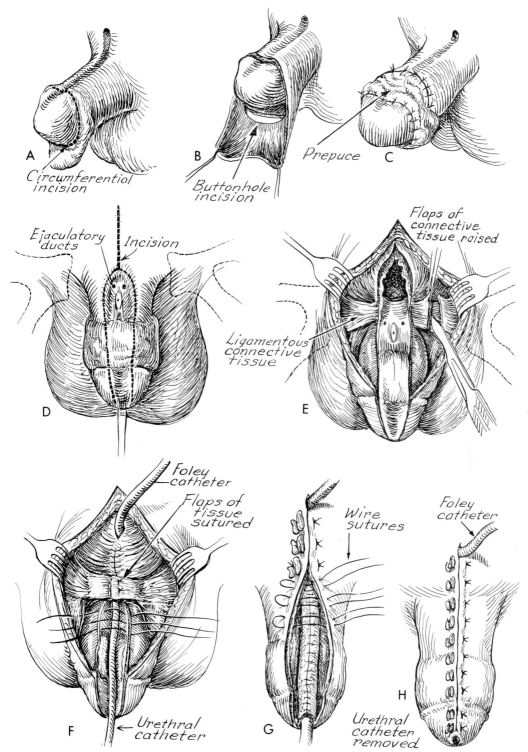

**FIGURE 96–5.** Authors' repair of penopubic epispadias. *A* to *C,* In a first stage the preputial hood is transposed from the undersurface to the top surface of the penile shaft through a buttonhole incision. *D* to *H,* The second stage is performed three months later. Two parallel incisions will construct the urethra and accommodate the ejaculatory ducts. Interpubic ligamentous tissue and the remnants of the bladder neck muscle are used to construct a sphincter over a temporary catheter conformer. Urinary diversion is necessary until the wound heals. Nylon sutures are used to approximate the deep tissues, and stainless steel wires are tied over cotton bolsters in mattress fashion to coapt the skin.

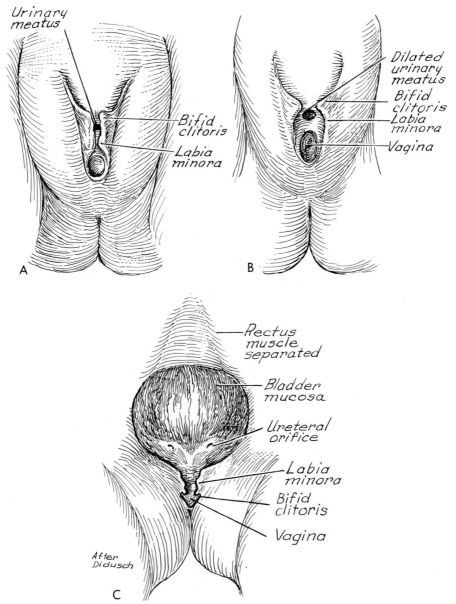

**FIGURE 96–6.** Female epispadias may exist in many gradients, three of which are shown. *A,* The first type exhibits a short urethra, positioned abnormally cephalad, and is associated with a cleft clitoris and labia. *B,* The second type is more pronounced, and the patient is incontinent of urine. *C,* The most severe type is associated with exstrophy of the bladder.

male, with the exception that the bifid clitoris and the anterior wall of the vagina must be constructed as mentioned above.

## EXSTROPHY OF THE BLADDER

This congenital cleft of the midline ventral body wall, which usually extends from the umbilicus to the perineum, is also known as ectopia vesicae, ectopic bladder, cloacal exstrophy (Tank and Lindenauer, 1970), and superior vesical fistula (Wainstein and Persky, 1968). The deformity does not represent an absence of tissue but is secondary to a failure of anterior midline convergence (see Chapter 93). The exposed, everted, red and redundant bladder mucosa is exquisitely tender, is irritated by even a diaper, and bleeds easily. The umbilicus is shallow or absent (Fig. 96–7).

Bladder exstrophy is associated with diastasis of the rectus abdominis muscles, nonunion of the bony pelvis at the symphysis pubis, and usually a cleft of the penile shaft and glans (epispadias). In the female a bifid or cleft clitoris is commonly present, and there is an absence of the anterior vaginal vault with widely separated labia (Higgins, 1959). The anterior and posterior rectus sheaths, as well as the peritoneum and skin, extend to the periphery of the exposed bladder mucosa. The margin of the bladder mucosa is sharply demarcated as a fixed, indurated, and fibrous rim. The ureteral orifices are usually located on elevated villi in their normal position and excrete urine externally. The penile shaft is short and spatulous. While there is an absence of the prepuce on the anterior aspect, a redundancy is noted on the posterior surface. The bladder sphincters do not function, since they are also cleft. The verumontanum and occasionally the prostate gland, if present, may be visible. The pubic bones are usually widely separated, a finding which may be demonstrated by manual palpation and roentgenographic study (Fig. 96–8). The pubic bones, however, remain connected by fibrous tissue. There are many references in the literature to children showing a duck-waddle gait, but this has not been a consistent finding in the 62 patients in the authors' series. In 11 of these patients, the right rectus was dissected and found to be present in its entirety. Its origin is from the pubococcygeus and pubovesicalis muscles in the perineal area.

In the child with bladder exstrophy, other genitourinary as well as nongenitourinary anomalies are commonly found. Among the former

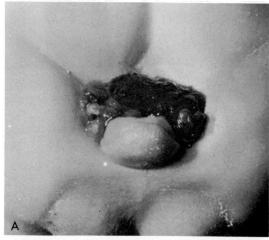

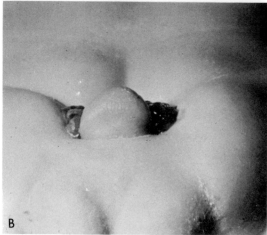

**FIGURE 96–7.** Bladder exstrophy represents a cleft of the midline ventral body wall. *A,* The exposed mucosa is red, redundant, edematous, and tender. The penis is cleft and short. *B,* Although hernias may be present, the pubic eminences are usually fat pads. The scrotum is small, sometimes cleft, but usually contains testes. Note the pyramidal defect of the diastatic rectus muscles.

are cryptorchidism, megaloureter, ureteral aplasia, ureteral stricture, vesicorectal fistulas, omphalocele (Fig. 96–9), and renal developmental disorders (Simon, 1852; Ladd and Lanman, 1940; Engle, 1948; McIndoe, 1948; Eagle and Barrett, 1950; Higgins, 1950; Overstreet and Hinman, 1954; Riparetti and Charnock, 1954; Powell, 1955; Paul and Kanagasuntheram, 1956; van der Vuurst de Vries, 1960; Lock, Gatling and Wells, 1961). Nongenitourinary anomalies that have been observed are imperforate anus (Bill, Johnson and Foster, 1958), anal and rectal prolapse (Fig. 96–10), ear malformations (Vincent, Ryan and Longnecker, 1961), cloacal exstrophy (Von Geldern, 1959), cleft lip, cleft palate, spina bifida, clubfoot, hernia,

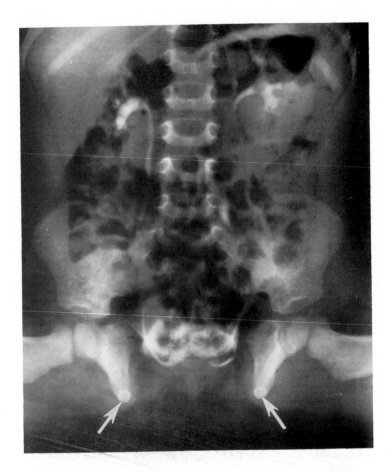

**FIGURE 96–8.** Roentgenogram of a complete bladder exstrophy. The arrows show widely separated pubic bones. The dye outlines of the renal pelves, ureters, and bladder remnants can also be seen.

**FIGURE 96–9.** Primordial cleft of the entire abdominal wall musculature and the skin. The omphalocele is associated with bladder ectopia and vaginal dysgenesis.

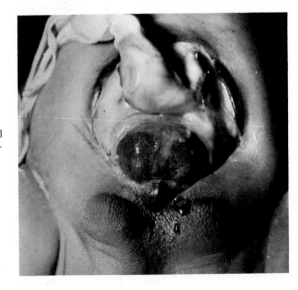

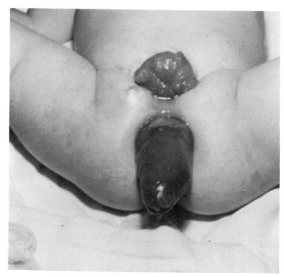

**FIGURE 96–10.** Exstrophy of the bladder associated with a complete rectoanal prolapse.

viduals reach maturity and that two-thirds of these are crippled with such diseases as pyelonephritis, hydronephrosis, and megaloureter (Harvard and Thompson, 1951; Cross and Barber, 1959). There have been 39 cases of bladder malignancy diagnosed pathologically in the exposed bladder mucous membrane, and 82.6 per cent of the malignancies were in patients under the age of 30 years (Abeshouse, 1943; Davidson, 1950; Goyanna, Emmett and McDonald, 1951; Staubitz, Oberkircher and Lent, 1956; Wattenbert, Beare and Tormey, 1956). However, some patients live to be elderly (Fisher, 1938; Burns, Kittredge and Hyman, 1947; Dixon and Weissmann, 1948; McEachern, 1950; Boyce and Vest, 1951; Jacobs and Stirling, 1952; Garrett and Mertz, 1954; Clinton-Thomas, 1955; Jonas, 1959), and one patient who had vesical exstrophy with a transitional cell carcinoma of the mucosa was alive at age 66 years (Cordonnier and Spjut, 1957).

hydrocephalus, and others (Wyburn, 1937; White and Dennison, 1958; Lapides, 1962; Culp, 1964).

**Etiology and Incidence.** Though many theories have been proposed, the cause of bladder exstrophy remains unknown (Ballentyne, 1904; Von Geldern, 1924; Muecke, 1964). Patten and Barry (1952) proposed an embryologic explanation for the various accompanying defects characteristic of the complete syndrome. According to these authors, the paired primordia of the genital tubercle are situated more caudally than normal, and the mesodermal ingrowth is tardy in its coverage, thus leading to the exstrophied state. Connelly (1901) divided the theories of causation into three categories: mechanical, pathologic, and arrested development. He listed many causes in his paper, but none of these has ever been confirmed (see Chapter 93).

Fortunately the incidence of bladder exstrophy is low, for it remains one of the few congenital abnormalities for which the problems of surgical treatment have not been completely solved (McIntosh, 1954). From statistics available in the literature, it appears that at least 100 children are born each year in the United States with bladder exstrophy. Campbell (1952) reported that the number of newborns yearly afflicted with this condition was approximately 75 in the United States. The anomaly is universally more prevalent in the male infant. In the authors' series of 62 patients, only 11 were female. It has been reported (Mayo and Hendricks, 1926) that only 10 per cent of these indi-

**Treatment.** In the historical development of the surgical therapy for exstrophy of the bladder, attention was focused on closing the bladder wall and covering it with abdominal skin, because the exposed bladder mucosa and ureteral orifices were a focus for upper urinary tract infection. In 1844, Pancoast demonstrated the closure of an ectopic bladder by using adjacent skin flaps, but the flap edges sloughed and a fistula resulted. The chief source of complaint of exstrophied patients is incontinence of urine. The latter persisted following the early operations because they failed to construct a functioning urinary sphincter. The surgical trend, therefore, gradually changed to diversion of the urinary stream. Sir John Simon (1852) is given credit for the first procedure of this type, although it was not successful when he established a urinary-colic fistula in 1851. Later, the technique was modified by excision of the bladder and transplantation of the ureters to the skin, into the alimentary tract, or even into the penis. Various types of bags were used as urine receptacles, but these were soon discarded. Thiersch (1869) apparently initiated the construction of the urethral canal with buried skin islands, a popular method today. He made two parallel skin incisions to form an island of skin on the penile shaft of an epispadiac patient; the skin island was tubed and covered with adjacent skin. The technique is identical to Denis Browne's method of urethral construction (see Chapter 95). Maydl (1894) reported an improved technique of diversion, in which the bladder trigone and attached ureters were coapted into the anterior rectosigmoid wall and the anal sphincters used for urinary control. However, 25 per cent of his patients died. Peters (1901) implanted the ureters separately into the rectum extraperitoneally by using a small section of trigone around each ureter. A flux of unusual procedures thereafter followed, such as ureteroileal (Merricks, Gilchrist, Hamlin and Rieger, 1951), ureterocecal (Malone, 1916), ureterosigmoid, and ureterorectal fistulas (Moynihan, 1906; Foulds, 1933; Goodwin and Hudson, 1951; Kiefer and Linke, 1958; Wilkins and Wills, 1959).

Coffey (1932) published a method of transplanting the ureters between the layers of the colonic wall to achieve a valvelike function. He further elaborated upon his technique, and these modifications became known as the Coffey No. 1, No. 2, and No. 3 techniques. Harvard and Thompson (1951) summarized the results of 144 patients who had undergone the Coffey type of ureteroenteric anastomosis. There were 18 deaths during the initial hospitalization. At the end of the first ten years, 88 of the patients were still alive; 11 lived throughout the twentieth postoperative year, but only 2 were alive 30 years later. These poor survival rates were due to progressive renal insufficiency secondary to pyelonephritis, hydronephrosis, renal calculi, and cicatrical obstruction at the site of ureteral anastomosis. Autopsy of several patients showed necrosis and slough at the ureteroenteric junction, with resultant urinary peritonitis. In addition, four deaths were attributed to bladder cancer.

It became apparent that an advance in surgical technique must be sought, and different methods were proposed (Cabot, 1931; Estes, 1934; Walters and Braasch, 1934; Ferris, 1948; Flocks, 1949; Boyce and Vest, 1952; Hinman, 1958). Colostomies were recommended to shunt the fecal stream in order to reduce ascending urinary infection (Harlin and Hamm, 1953). Gross and Cresson (1952) were of the belief that urinary incontinence should be managed by constructing an autogenous receptacle to receive and discharge urine, that the bladder should be removed, and that the existing deformities should be corrected by plastic surgical procedures. Loops of small bowel and segments of colon were used as urinary receptacles and exteriorized on the abdominal wall or the perineum. Hepburn (1951) curetted the redundant bladder mucosa and closed the abdominal wall over it without complications. Swenson (1957) published data on simple closure of the abdominal wall defect, with emphasis placed on close approximation of tissues at the bladder neck, simulating the procedure of Young (1942).

More recently, another surgical approach has been to separate the iliac bones by posterior osteotomy (Shultz, 1960; Chisholm, 1961) in order to bring the pubes together anteriorly (Fig. 96–11). The pubic rami are approximated with wire. The pelvis is held in the desired position with a brace or cast. The results are excellent in female patients, but such a procedure in the male shortens the penis, a goal which is not desirable.

The definition of a "good" result in the treatment of bladder exstrophy requires interpretation. The parents of a child born with this appalling congenital affliction anxiously accept any advice and type of therapy offered by their

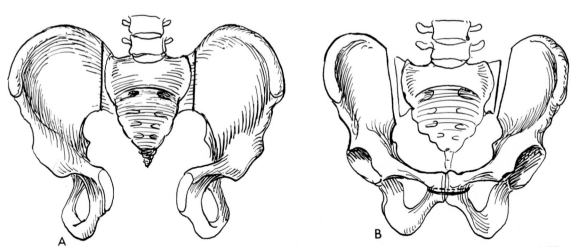

**FIGURE 96–11.** Bilateral iliac osteotomy allows anterior pelvic rotation so that the pubes may be approximated. The technique is of help in repairing female exstrophy, but in the male it shortens the length of the penile shaft.

physician. The mere closure of the abdominal wall is comforting to them, but this initial reaction is only temporary. They soon come to realize their child will be a social outcast because of urinary incontinence and the offensive odor which accompanies it. They also become discouraged with the child's repeated bouts of elevated temperature, dysuria, and abdominal pain secondary to cystitis and nephritis. A bladder that cannot retain urine, even one which "dribbles just a little bit," does not represent a surgical triumph. The thought that time will cure the dribble is one of futility. Therefore, the ideal therapeutic goals are (1) to correct the urinary incontinence, (2) to preserve renal-ureteral function, (3) to reconstruct a functional penis or vagina, and (4) to reconstruct the abdominal wall.

TECHNIQUE. Although there is no recognizable standard procedure acceptable to all surgeons, there are currently two popular approaches: functional reconstruction and urinary diversion. Swenson (1957) and Marshall and Muecke (1962) have reported similar results in repairing bladder exstrophy by functional reconstruction; about 25 per cent of the treated patients are placed in the category of fair to good. Those surgeons who are attracted to the urinary diversion technique usually choose one of three procedures: urinary-intestinal anastomoses, ileal conduits, or cystectomy. Those patients who have undergone urinary-intestinal anastomoses and remain satisfied are the exception rather than the rule; the operating physician is in constant fear of chronic cystitis, pyelonephritis, and pyonephrosis. Ileal conduits, favored by many surgeons, are not without complications, such as a lack of volume control, leakage at anastomotic junctions, malfunctioning stenotic orifices, reflux problems, and the continued use of an uncomfortable external receptacle. When a cystectomy is the procedure of choice, all of the "bridges are burned," and any future hope to be "normal again" is lost. With the advances in electronics and in engineering on the horizon of medicine, it can be speculated that functionless bladders may once again become organs of health. Because the various maneuvers described, including primary closure of the bladder sphincter, have not proved completely successful, other procedures warrant testing. Construction of a urinary receptacle with a functioning sphincter, completely divorced from the alimentary tract (which also must maintain a controllable sphincter), should achieve the surgical goal of a normal life expectancy without intercurrent urinary complications. The technique of the authors is described below (Snyder,

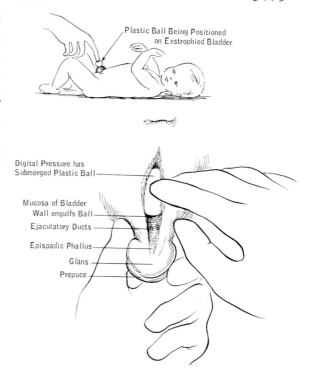

Plastic Ball Being Positioned on Exstrophied Bladder

Digital Pressure has Submerged Plastic Ball

Mucosa of Bladder Wall engulfs Ball
Ejaculatory Ducts
Epispadic Phallus
Glans
Prepuce

**FIGURE 96–12.** The edematous, redundant, protruding bladder mucosa may be flattened by pressure using a plastic globe or Ping-Pong ball for 48 hours prior to surgery.

1958). A requisite of the procedure is a functioning anal sphincter.

Preoperative laboratory studies include a hemogram, ureteral urinalysis, pyelograms, and pelvic roentgenograms. The intestinal tract is prepared preoperatively with enemas and a combined sulfa-neomycin medication. The redundant bladder mucosa may be flattened by pressure using a plastic ball or similar object for 48 hours prior to surgery (Fig. 96–12).

Under general endotracheal anesthesia, the abdomen, perineum, buttocks, and thighs are surgically prepared and draped. Ureteral catheters are inserted. The circumferential fibrous band at the junction of the bladder mucosa and the abdominal skin is excised. The bladder is dissected from the abdominal wall and adjacent soft tissues, isolating the ureters and preserving the vesical blood vessels (Fig. 96–13). The incisions may be made longitudinally or transversely, care being taken to preserve the ejaculatory ducts in the urethral trough exterior to the dissected bladder wall. The rectum is elevated from the pelvic floor and transected 5 cm above the anal outlet. A fenestration is made in the posterior bladder wall between and slightly above the ureters. The distal rectal segment is approximated to it with a double layer of surgical catgut sutures. The ureteral catheters are intro-

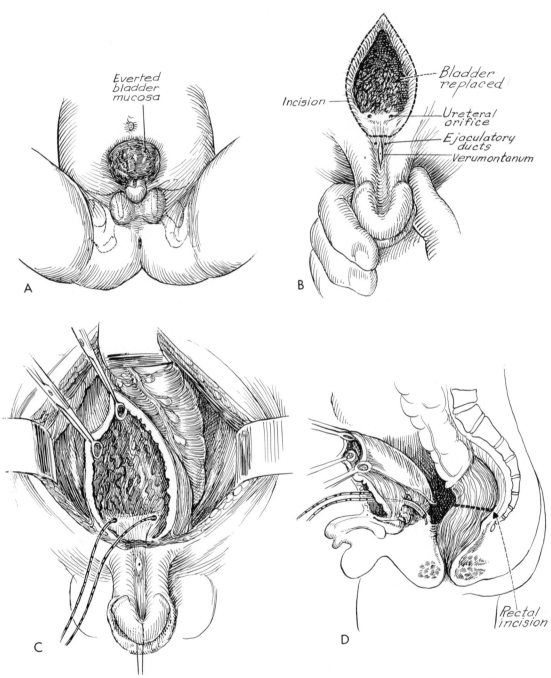

**FIGURE 96–13.** Authors' technique of repair of bladder exstrophy. *A*, Complete exstrophy of the bladder associated with epispadias. *B*, The circumferential rim of scar is excised. The ureteral orifices are contained within the bladder mucosa, but the ejaculatory ducts are left in the urethral cleft external to the bladder incision. *C*, With ureteral catheters in position, the bladder is dissected from the surrounding soft tissues. *D*, The rectum is divided 5 cm above the anal outlet.

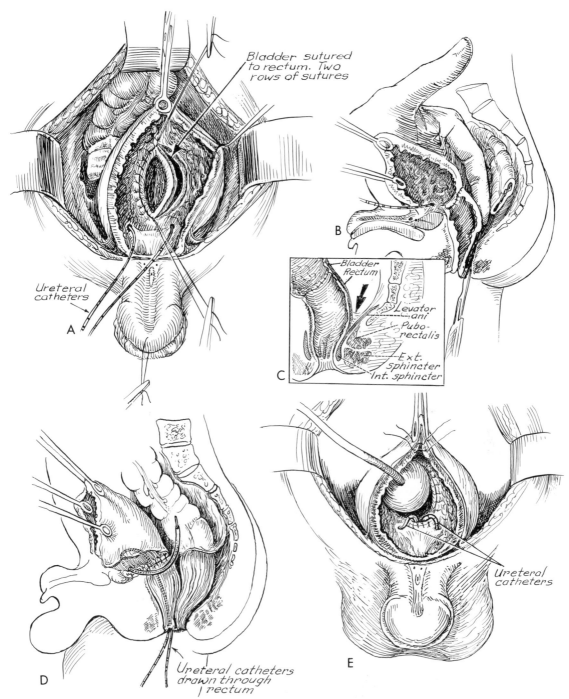

**FIGURE 96–14.** Repair of exstrophy of the bladder (continued). *A*, The posterior wall of the bladder is fenestrated above and between the ureteral orifices, and the distal end of the divided rectum is sutured to the bladder. *B*, The proximal end of the bowel is advanced caudally. *C*, The dissection must be carefully done and should be in a plane between the muscular wall of the remaining rectum and the levator ani musculature. The nerve supply to the sphincter muscles must not be disturbed. *D*, The newly constructed anal outlet is made by an incision in the skin, and the alimentary tract is completely separate from the urinary tract. *E*, A Foley catheter is inflated within the bladder, and the bladder is closed over it in two layers.

duced through the fenestration and to the exterior via the new urinary receptacle (Fig. 96–14).

The operative field is transferred to the perineum, and an incision is made posterior to the anal outlet but within the anal sphincters. The sphincteric musculature is not incised with a scalpel, but the muscle fibers are spread apart with a hemostat. The proximal rectal segment is grasped gently with an Allis forceps and brought through the levator ani sling and within the anal muscle sphincters. Meticulous care is taken to preserve the nerve and blood supply to the area. The distal end of the bowel segment is sutured to the perianal integument with surgical catgut sutures, leaving 1.5 cm of exterior bowel redundancy. The excess will contract to the level of the skin. A small finger flap is brought between the anus and bladder outlet. The surgical site is transferred back to the bladder region. The bladder is closed in two layers over an inflated balloon catheter, which functions as a conformer until the bladder is closed. After the catheter is removed, the rectus abdominis muscles are detached from the pelvic rim, decussated, and sutured to the opposite pubic crests. This maneuver corrects the diastatic muscles and prevents the development of a midline hernia. The abdominal wall is closed in layers with steel or nylon sutures (Fig. 96–15).

There are many methods of closing the abdominal wall (Baret, Demuth, Murphy, and Muir, 1953; Steffensen, Ryan and Sinclair, 1956; Spencer, 1957; Longacre and coworkers, 1958, 1959; Thompson, 1961), and each may be adapted to the individual case. The epispadias may or may not be repaired during the first operation. The ureteral catheters are of little use after 48 hours and are removed. Early and long-term follow-up studies of renal function, cystograms, intravenous roentgenograms, sphincter control, and social relations are necessary.

The complete separation of the urinary tract from the fecal stream adds a definite advantage, as this eliminates ascending renal infection, which is a common postoperative complication. There is no problem of ureteral obstruction at the site of anastomosis, because the ureters are left intact to empty their contents as they should into the bladder. The patient is no longer a social outcast because of soiled clothes or uriniferous odors, since the anal sphincters serve a dual purpose in retaining both urine and feces (Fig. 96–16). Plaster casts or long periods of bed rest are not necessary in the male patients, because the pelvic bones are not fractured. The ilia are osteotomized in all female subjects.

The operative technique described above has been used in 51 males. There have been

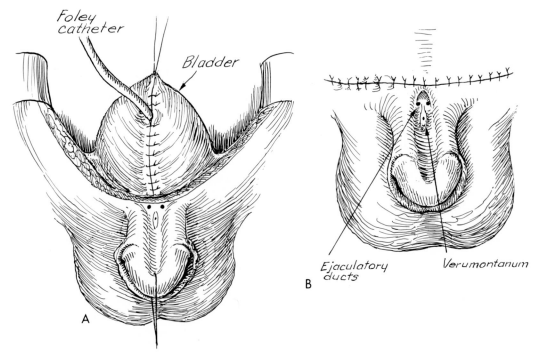

**FIGURE 96–15.** Repair of exstrophy of the bladder (continued). *A,* After the bladder is constructed, the Foley catheter is deflated and removed. *B,* The abdominal wall is closed in layers using stainless steel sutures.

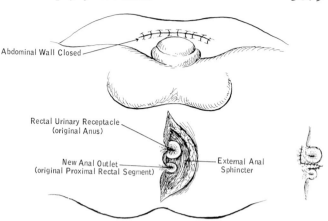

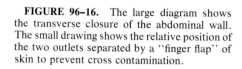

**FIGURE 96–16.** The large diagram shows the transverse closure of the abdominal wall. The small drawing shows the relative position of the two outlets separated by a "finger flap" of skin to prevent cross contamination.

four complete failures, all occurring in patients who had been previously treated by other methods. The patient group does not include 28 other exstrophied bladders treated by other techniques. Three patients have been lost to follow-up. The postoperative studies included questioning about incontinency, and degree if present, diarrhea, bouts of chills and fever, perianal rash, penile length, and activities (swimming, contact sports, and so forth), and roentgenographic examination for ureteral size, renal anatomy, and pathology. Of the remaining 44 patients, five are yet under the age of 7, but the remainder are of an age which permits clinical evaluation. Twenty-six of these patients are satisfied with their continency and do not wear any type of protective gear (diapers, urinal, and so forth). Intermittent diarrhea was a complaint of three, but the reasons were not fully established. Eleven have experienced serious bouts of chills and fever, and diagnoses of acute and chronic pyelonephritis, hydronephrosis, and cystitis have been established. Four patients have been plagued with intervals of anal rash, but this condition has cleared with topical medications. Thirty-one adolescent patients desire penile lengthening. All of the patients enjoy sports activities, and most participate in sunbathing, swimming, and other athletic activities.

PRESENT ATTITUDES TOWARD TREATMENT. Though the final answer for the ideal treatment of bladder exstrophy is still wanting, there definitely exists a universally accepted belief that this condition can be surgically treated. The pendulum of operative therapy has oscillated from one extreme to the other, and at present there remains a divergence of opinion as to whether the urinary stream should be guided through the penile shaft or diverted to other means of excretion. It was Hugh Young (1942)

who reported the correction of bladder exstrophy with resultant normal bladder sphincter control and who inspired contemporary surgeons to utilize again the method of primary bladder closure and urethral construction for micturition. Later, the patient who underwent this type of repair was found to be incontinent. The time factor in all corrective surgery is paramount, and even though the immediate postoperative results are important, only the judgment of time permits the final evaluation of a technique.

It is also unwise to be prejudiced against those operative procedures that advocate transplantation of the ureters into a conduit or the distal bowel. Such operations represent the labors of surgeons who have obtained numerous good results (Allison, 1933). Some surgeons who use this type of operation have reported problems with electrolyte imbalance, but Falk and Benjamin (1951) have found little effect on electrolyte balance, if the urine is directed into the bowel at the age of 1 year. In order to prevent ureteral necrosis and dehiscence as well as cicatricial and obstructive changes when the transplantation procedure is used, Boyce and Vest (1952) devised a procedure to connect the bladder to the rectum and to perform a colostomy that functioned only once daily. The results were exceptionally good. Many surgeons have corrected bladder exstrophy in staged operations, but Ferris (1948) has been ingenious in achieving this treatment in one operation. He performed a cystectomy, ureterosigmoidostomy, and abdominal closure in one stage.

Many methods have been offered to treat this anomaly, and improved methods should be forthcoming. Reconstructive surgeons should combine their efforts in the years ahead to conquer this malady.

# REFERENCES

Abeshouse, B. S.: Exstrophy of the bladder complicated by adenocarcinoma of the bladder and renal calculi. J. Urol., 49:259, 1943.

Allison, P. R.: Result of transplantation of ureters more than a quarter of a century after operation. Brit. J. Surg., 20:529, 1933.

Arey, L. B.: Developmental Anatomy. 6th Ed. Philadelphia, W. B. Saunders Company, 1954, p. 302.

Arey, L. B.: Developmental Anatomy. 7th Ed. Philadelphia, W. B. Saunders Company, 1966, p. 295.

Aristotle: De Partibus Animalium. Translated into English by A. Platt. Oxford, Clarendon Press, 1910.

Arnesen, K.: Exogenous causes for malformations. Tidsskr. Nor. Laegeforen., 78:935, 1958.

Ballentyne, J. W.: Manual of Antenatal Pathology and Hygiene. The Embryo. Edinburgh, W. Greene & Son, Ltd., 1904, p. 539.

Baret, A., Demuth, W. E., Jr., Murphy, J. J., and Muir, M. W.: Experimental repair of exstrophy of the bladder by using a free fascial graft. Surg. Gynecol. Obstet., 97:633, 1953.

Bettman, O. L.: A Pictorial History of Medicine. Springfield, Ill., Charles C Thomas, Publisher, 1956, p. 8.

Bill, A. H., Jr., Johnson, R. J., and Foster, R. A.: Anteriorly placed rectal opening in the perineum. Ectopic anus. A report of 30 cases. Ann. Surg., 147:173, 1958.

Blair, V. P., and Byars, L. T.: Hypospadias and epispadias. J. Urol., 40:814, 1938.

Boyce, W. H., and Vest, S. A.: Rehabilitation of genitourinary malformations. Va. Med. Monthly, 78:176, 1951.

Boyce, W. H., and Vest, S. A.: A new concept concerning treatment of exstrophy of the bladder. J. Urol., 67:503, 1952.

Brachet, J.: Embryologie Chimique. Paris, Masson & Cie, 1947.

Braithwaite, F., and Wilson, J. S. P.: Some observations on the deformity of ectopia vesicae. Br. J. Plast. Surg., 15:1, 1962.

Brickel, A. C. J.: Ectopia vesicae. Anat. Rec., 34:1, 1926.

Browne, D.: A comparison of the Duplay and Denis Browne techniques for hypospadias operations. Surgery, 34:787, 1953.

Burggraeve, A. P.: Studies of Andre Vesale. In C. Annoot-Braeckman, Gaud, 1841.

Burns, E., Kittredge, W. E., and Hyman, J.: Bilateral cutaneous ureterostomy eighteen years after ureterosigmoidostomy for exstrophy of the bladder. Ann. Surg., 125:788, 1947.

Burns, J. E.: A new operation for exstrophy of the bladder. Preliminary report. J.A.M.A., 82:1587, 1924.

Cabot, H.: The treatment of exstrophy of the bladder by ureteral transplantation. New Engl. J. Med., 205:706, 1931.

Cabot, H.: Treatment of epispadias in the male. Br. J. Urol., 9:793, 1937.

Camac, C. N. B.: Imhotep to Harvey. New York, P. B. Hoeber, 1931.

Campbell, M. F.: Clinical Pediatric Urology. Philadelphia, W. B. Saunders Company, 1951.

Campbell, M. F.: Epispadias; a report of fifteen cases. J. Urol., 67:988, 1952.

Campbell, M. F.: Principles of Urology. Philadelphia, W. B. Saunders Company, 1957.

Campbell, M. F.: Urology. 2nd Ed. Philadelphia, W. B. Saunders Company, 1962.

Cecil, A. B.: Surgery of hypospadias and epispadias in the male. J. Urol., 27:507, 1932.

Chisholm, T. C.: Exstrophy of the urinary bladder. Am. J. Surg., 101:649, 1961.

Clinton-Thomas, C. L.: A case of ectopic vesicae in an elderly woman. Br. J. Urol., 27:232, 1955.

Coffey, R. C.: Transplantation of ureters into large intestine by submucous implantation. J.A.M.A., 99:1320, 1932.

Connelly, F. G.: Exstrophy of the bladder. J.A.M.A., 36:637, 1901.

Cordonnier, J. J., and Spjut, H. J.: Vesical exstrophy and transitional cell carcinoma: Unusual longevity following ureterosigmoidostomy. J. Urol., 78:242, 1957.

Cross, R. R., Jr., and Barber, K. E.: Exstrophy of the bladder: Follow-up of survivors. J. Urol., 82:333, 1959.

Culp, D. A.: The histology of the exstrophied bladder. J. Urol., 91:536, 1964.

Davidson, J. A.: Report of three cases of carcinoma occurring in exstrophy of the bladder. Urol. Cutan. Rev., 54:206, 1950.

da Vinci, L.: On the Human Body. New York, H. Schuman, 1953.

Dees, J. E.: Congenital epispadias with incontinence. J. Urol., 62:513, 1949.

Dixon, C. F., and Weissmann, R. E.: Polyps of the sigmoid occurring 30 years after bilateral ureterosigmoidostomy for exstrophy of the bladder. Surgery, 24:1026, 1948.

Douglas, B.: The role of environmental factors in the so-called congenital malformations. Plast. Reconstr. Surg., 22:204, 1958.

Eagle, J. F., Jr., and Barrett, G. S.: Congenital deficiency of abdominal musculature with associated genitourinary abnormalities: A syndrome. Pediatrics, 6:721, 1950.

Engle, W. J.: Ureteral ectopic opening into the seminal vesicle. J. Urol., 60:46, 1948.

Estes, W. L.: Exstrophy of the urinary bladder. Ann. Surg., 99:223, 1934.

Falk, G., and Benjamin, J. A.: Observations on water diuresis and on ureteral peristalsis in an infant with exstrophy of the bladder. Surg. Gynecol. Obstet., 93:159, 1951.

Ferris, D. O.: Simultaneous multiple surgical procedures for correction of exstrophy of the bladder: Report of case. Proc. Staff Meet. Mayo Clin., 23:430, 1948.

Fisher, J. H.: A case of ureteral transplantation surviving twenty-two years. Br. J. Urol., 10:241, 1938.

Flocks, R. H.: Management of patients undergoing ureterointestinal anastomosis. Preoperative, operative, and postoperative measures. J.A.M.A., 139:626, 1949.

Flocks, R. H., and Culp, D. A.: The perineum in epispadias. J. Urol., 81:443, 1959.

Fonseca Ely, J.: Plastic surgery in vesical exstrophy. Rev. Lat. Am. Cirug. Plast., 5:102, 1961.

Foulds, G. S.: Historical data on ureteral transplantation. Am. J. Surg., 23:217, 1933.

Fraser, F. C., and Fainstat, T. D.: The causes of congenital defects. Am. J. Dis. Child., 82:593, 1951.

Garrett, R. A., and Mertz, J. H. O.: Follow-up studies of bladder exstrophy with ureterosigmoidostomy. J. Urol., 71:299, 1954.

Geldern, C. E. Von: Etiology of exstrophy of the bladder. Arch. Surg., 8:61, 1924.

Geldern, C. E. Von: The etiology of cloacal exstrophy and allied malformations. J. Urol., 82:134, 1959.

Goodwin, W. E., and Hudson, P. B.: Exstrophy of bladder treated by rectal transplantation of divided trigone. Modification of the Maydl-Bergenheim operation. Surg. Gynecol. Obstet., 93:331, 1951.

Goyanna, R., Emmett, J. L., and McDonald, J. R.: Exstrophy of the bladder complicated by adenocarcinoma. J. Urol., 65:391, 1951.

Gross, R. E., and Cresson, S. L.: Exstrophy of the bladder: Observations from 80 cases. J.A.M.A., *149*:1640, 1958.

Harlin, H. C., and Hamm, F. C.: Exstrophy of the urinary bladder. N.Y. State J. Med., *53*:289, 1953.

Harvard, M. B., and Thompson, G. J.: Congenital exstrophy of the urinary bladder: Late results of treatment by the Coffey-Mayo method of ureterointestinal anastomosis. J. Urol., *65*:223, 1951.

Harvey, W.: Exercitationes de generatione animalium. *In* LeClerc, D.: Bibliotheca Anatomica. Geneva, J. A. Chovet, 1685.

Hejtmancik, H. J., King, W. B., and Magid, M. A.: Pseudo-exstrophy of the bladder. J. Urol., *72*:829, 1954.

Hepburn, T. N.: Repair of exstrophy of the bladder. J. Urol., *65*:389, 1951.

Higgins, C. C.: Exstrophy of the bladder: Review of 70 cases. J. Urol., *63*:852, 1950.

Higgins, C. C.: Exstrophy of the bladder: Review of one hundred fifty-six cases. J.A.M.A., *171*:1922, 1959.

Higgins, C. C.: Exstrophy of the bladder: Report of 158 cases. Am. Surg., *28*:99, 1962.

Hinman, F., Jr.: A method of lengthening and repairing the penis in exstrophy of the bladder. J. Urol., *79*:237, 1958.

Jacobs, A., and Stirling, W. B.: The late results of uretero-colic anastomosis. Br. J. Urol., *24*:259, 1952.

Jonas, K. C.: Results of surgical reconstruction in exstrophy of the bladder. Arch. Surg., *78*:146, 1959.

Kiefer, J. H., and Linke, C.: Ureterorectostomy and pre-anal colostomy for bladder exstrophy. J. Urol., *79*:242, 1958.

Kittredge, W. E., and Bradburn, C.: Incomplete exstrophy of the bladder. J. Urol., *72*:38, 1954.

Ladd, W. E., and Lanman, T. H.: Exstrophy of the bladder and epispadias. New Engl. J. Med., *222*:130, 1940.

Lapides, J.: Urinary incontinence in the male. South. Med. J., *25*:965, 1962.

Lattimer, J. K., Dean, A. L., Jr., Furey, C. H., and Ballantyne, L.: Reconstruction of the urinary bladder in children with exstrophy. N.Y. State J. Med., *57*:746, 1957a.

Lattimer, J. K., Dean, A. L., Jr., Furey, C. H., and Ballantyne, L.: Reconstruction of urinary bladder in children with exstrophy. J. Urol., *77*:424, 1957b.

Lattimer, J. K., Dean, A. L., Jr., Dougherty, L. J., Ju, D., Ryder, C., and Uson, A.: Functional closure of the bladder in children with exstrophy: A report of twenty-eight cases. J. Urol., *33*:647, 1960.

Liston, R.: Practical Surgery: With One Hundred and Thirty Engravings on Wood. Philadelphia, Thomas and Cowperthwait, 1838, p. 367.

Lloyd, M. R.: Ectopia vesicae. Lancet, *2*:370, 1851.

Lock, F. R., Gatling, H. B., and Wells, H. B.: Difficulty in the diagnosis of congenital abnormalities. J.A.M.A., *178*:711, 1961.

Longacre, J. J., deStefano, G. A., and Davidson, D. A.: Congenital medial defects of the central body. Plast. Reconstr., *22*:458, 1958.

Longacre, J. J., deStefano, G. A., and Davidson, D. A.: Plastic repair of congenital defects of the ventral body wall with particular reference to exstrophy of the bladder. Plast. Reconstr. Surg., *23*:260, 1959.

Lowsley, O. S., and Johnson, T. H.: A new operation for creation of an artificial bladder with voluntary control of urine and feces. J. Urol., *73*:83, 1955.

Lowsley, O. S., and Kirwin, T. J.: Clinical Urology. 3rd Ed. Baltimore, The Williams & Wilkins Company, 1956, p. 113.

McEachern, A. C.: Ectopia vesicae in an adult woman. Br. J. Surg., *37*:471, 1950.

McIndoe, A. H.: Deformities of the male urethra. Br. J. Plast. Surg., *1*:29, 1948.

McIntosh, R.: Incidence of congenital malformations: Study of 5,964 pregnancies. Pediatrics, *14*:505, 1954.

Mackay, J., and Syme, J.: Monthly J. Med. Sci., *9*:934, 1849.

Malone, B.: A discussion of the different methods of exclusion in the treatment of exstrophy of the bladder with case report. Trans. South. Surg. Assoc., *29*:240, 1916.

Marshall, B. F., and Muecke, E. C.: Variations in exstrophy of the bladder. J. Urol., *88*:766, 1962.

Mathews, D. N.: Ectopia vesicae. Br. J. Plast. Surg., *11*:118, 1958.

Maydl, K.: Ueber die Radikaltherapie der Blasenektopie. Wien. Med. Wochenschr., *44*:25, 1894.

Mayo, C. H., and Hendricks, W. A.: Exstrophy of the bladder. Surg. Gynecol. Obstet., *43*:129, 1926.

Merricks, J. W., Gilchrist, R. K., Hamlin, H., and Rieger, J. T.: A substitute bladder and urethra, using cecum as bladder and ileum as urethra. J. Urol., *65*:581, 1951.

Mettauer, J. P.: Practical observations on those malformations of the male urethra and penis, termed hypospadias and epispadias, with an anomalous case. Am. J. Med. Sci., *4*:43, 1842.

Moynihan, B. G. A.: Extroversion of the bladder. Relief by transplantation of the bladder into the rectum. Ann. Surg., *43*:237, 1906.

Muecke, E. C.: The role of the cloacal membrane in exstrophy. The first successful experimental study. J. Urol., *92*:659, 1964.

Overstreet, E. W., and Hinman, F., Jr.: Some gynecologic aspects of bladder exstrophy with report of an illustrative case. West. J. Surg., *64*:131, 1954.

Pancoast, J.: A Treatise on Operative Surgery. Philadelphia, Carey and Hart, 1844, p. 317.

Paré, A.: Chysurgery. Paris, J. leRoyer, 1579.

Patten, B. M.: Human Embryology. 2nd Ed. New York, McGraw-Hill Book Company, 1953, p. 607.

Patten, B. M.: Mechanisms of Congenital Malformation. New York, John B. Watkins, 1954.

Patten, B. M., and Barry, A.: A genesis of exstrophy of the bladder and epispadias. Am. J. Anat., *90*:35, 1952.

Paul, M., and Kanagasuntheram, R.: The congenital anomalies of the lower urinary tract. Br. J. Urol., *28*:64, 1956.

Peters, G. A.: Transplantation of ureters into rectum by an extraperitoneal method for exstrophy of bladder. Br. Med. J., *1*:1538, 1901.

Pickerill, H. P., and Pickerill, C. M.: Ectopia vesicae. Aust. N. Z. J. Surg., *15*:91, 1945.

Pohlman, A. G.: The development of the cloaca in human embryos. Am. J. Anat., *12*:1, 1911.

Powell, T. O.: Certain anomalies of the genitourinary tract in children. South. Med. J., *48*:68, 1955.

Preuss, J.: Biblisch-talmudische Medizin. Basel, S. Karger, 1923.

Rickham, P. P.: The treatment of ectopia vesicae. Br. J. Plast. Surg., *10*:300, 1958.

Riparetti, P. P., and Charnock, D. A.: Urological problems in the agenesis of the abdominal wall musculature. J. Urol., *72*:541, 1954.

Roux, W.: Gesammelte Abhandlungen uber Entwicklung der Organismen. Leipzig, Engelman, 1853.

Shultz, W. G.: An ideal surgical correction of ectopia vesicae. J. Int. Coll. Surg., *31*:674, 1959.

Shultz, W. G.: Plastic repair of exstrophy of the bladder combined with bilateral osteotomy of the ilia: Progress report. Am. Surg., *26*:158, 1960.

Simon, J.: Ectopia vesicae. Lancet, *2*:568, 1852.

Smith, T.: Account of an unsuccessful attempt to treat bladder extroversion. St. Bart. Hosp. Rep., *15*:29, 1879.

Snyder, C. C.: A new therapeutic concept of the exstrophied bladder. Plast. Reconstr. Surg., *22*:1, 1958.

Sorrentino, F., and Leonetti, P.: Terapia della Estrofia Vesicale. Naples, Edizioni Scientifiche Italiane, 1958, p. 13.

Spencer, H. M.: A simplified technique for cystectomy and repair of the abdominal defect in exstrophy of the bladder. J. Urol., *77*:428, 1957.

Staubitz, W. J., Oberkircher, O. J., and Lent, M. H.: Carcinoma in exstrophy of the bladder. N.Y. State J. Med., *56*:386, 1956.

Steffensen, W. H., Ryan, J. A., and Sinclair, E. A.: A method of closure of the abdominal wall defect in exstrophy of the bladder. Am. J. Surg., *92*:9, 1956.

Sweetser, T. H.: Plastic reconstruction for exstrophy of the urinary bladder. South. Med. J., *53*:1519, 1960.

Swenson, O.: Changing trends in management of exstrophy of the bladder. Surgery, *42*:61, 1957.

Tank, E. S., and Lindenauer, S. M.: Principles of management of exstrophy of the cloaca. Am. J. Surg., *119*:95, 1970.

Thiersch, K.: The cause, surgical correction and rehabilitation of epispadias. Arch. Heilk., *10*:20, 1869.

Thompson, C. J. S.: The Mystery and Lore of Monsters with Accounts of Some Giants, Dwarfs and Prodigies. London, Williams and Norgate, 1930.

Thompson, I. M.: Management of exstrophy of the urinary bladder by primary closure. South. Med. J., *54*:1069, 1961.

Trendelenburg, F.: The treatment of ectopia vesicae. Ann. Surg., *44*:281, 1906.

Uson, A. C., and Roberts, M. S.: Incomplete exstrophy of the urinary bladder: A report of two cases. J. Urol., *79*:57, 1958.

Vincent, R. W., Ryan, R. F., and Longnecker, C. G.: Malformation of the ear associated with urogenital anomalies. Plast. Reconstr. Surg., *28*:214, 1961.

Vuurst de Vries, J. H., van der: Exstrophy of the bladder. Arch. Chir. Neerl., *12*:169, 1960.

Wainstein, M. L., and Persky, L.: Superior vesical fistula. Am. J. Surg., *115*:397, 1968.

Walters, W., and Braasch, W. F.: Ureteral transplantation to the rectosigmoid. Am. J. Surg., *23*:255, 1934.

Wattenbert, C. A., Beare, J. B., and Tormey, A. R.: Exstrophy of the urinary bladder complicated by adenocarcinoma. J. Urol., *76*:583, 1956.

White, M., and Dennison, W. M.: Surgery in Infancy and Childhood. Edinburgh, E & S Livingstone, 1958, p. 276.

Wilkins, S. A., Jr., and Wills, S. A.: The rectal bladder for urinary diversion. Surg. Gynecol. Obstet., *109*:1, 1959.

Williams, R. H.: Textbook of Endocrinology. Philadelphia, W. B. Saunders Company, 1968, p. 451.

Wood, J.: Fission and extroversion of bladder and epispadias. Med.-Chir. Trans., London, *52*:85, 1869.

Wyburn, G. M.: The development of the infra-umbilical portion of the abdominal wall with remarks on the etiology of ectopic vesicae. J. Anat., *71*:201, 1937.

Young, H. H.: A new operation for epispadias. J. Urol., *2*:237, 1918.

Young, H. H.: Exstrophy of the bladder—The first case in which a normal bladder and urinary control have been obtained by plastic operations. Surg. Gynecol. Obstet., *74*:729, 1942.

# CHAPTER 97

# STRICTURES OF THE MALE URETHRA

PATRICK C. DEVINE, M.D.,
AND CHARLES E. HORTON, M.D.

---

Peyronie's Disease
*Charles E. Horton, M.D.,
and Charles J. Devine, Jr., M.D.*

## Anatomy

The male urethra can be divided into five segments. These anatomical divisions are useful in considering the pathology and treatment of strictures of the urethra.

1. *Prostatic urethra.* The prostatic urethra is lined with transitional epithelium (Fig. 97–1) and extends from the triangular ligament to the vesical neck (Fig. 97–2).

2. *Membranous urethra.* The membranous urethra is also lined with transitional epithelium and extends from the inferior to the superior leaf of the triangular ligament (see Fig. 97–2).

3. *Bulbous urethra.* The bulbous urethra is lined with squamous epithelium distally, with a gradual change to delicate transitional epithelium proximally (Fig. 97–3). The bulbous urethra extends from the suspensory ligament of the penis to the triangular ligament (see Fig. 97–2).

4. *Pendulous urethra.* The epithelium of the pendulous urethra is squamous (Fig. 97–4) and extends from the fossa navicularis to the level of the suspensory ligament of the penis (see Fig. 97–2).

5. *Glanular urethra.* The glanular urethra, which traverses the glans penis, is lined with stratified squamous epithelium (Fig. 97–5) and extends from the external urethral meatus to the fossa navicularis (see Fig. 97–2).

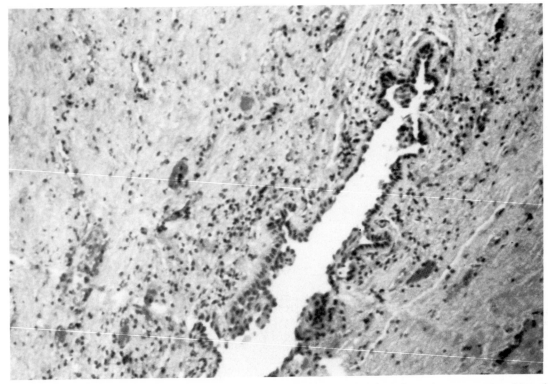

**FIGURE 97-1.** Photomicrograph of the urethra at the junction of the prostatic and membranous urethra. Note the lining of transitional epithelium. × 63.

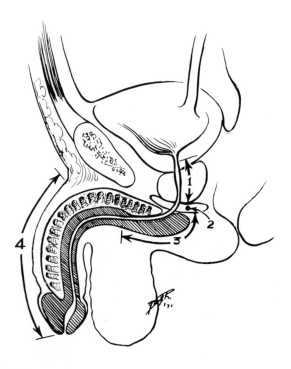

**FIGURE 97-2.** Sagittal section of urethra: (1) prostatic urethra; (2) membranous urethra; (3) bulbous urethra; (4) pendulous urethra.

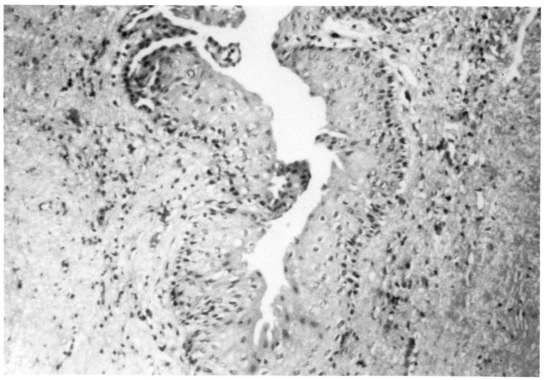

**FIGURE 97–3.** Photomicrograph of the mid-bulbous urethra. Note the lining of squamous epithelium. × 63.

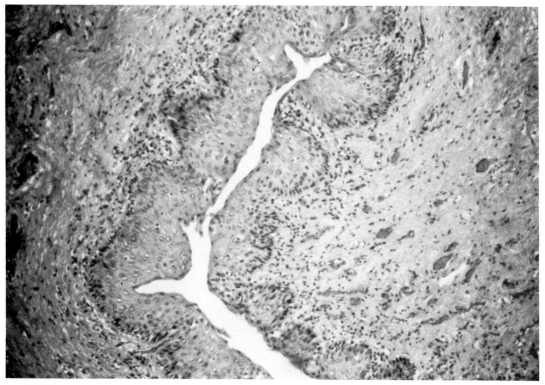

**FIGURE 97–4.** Photomicrograph of the pendulous urethra. Note the lining of squamous epithelium. × 10.

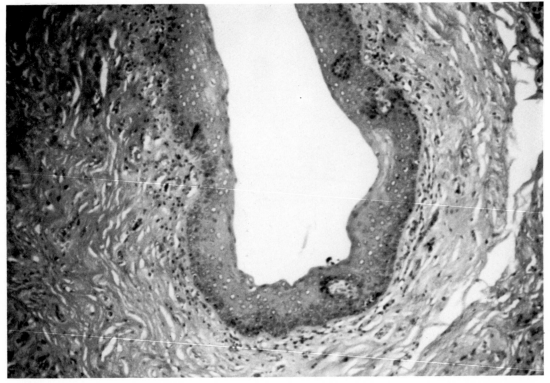

**FIGURE 97–5.**   Photomicrograph of the urethra at the fossa navicularis lined with squamous epithelium. × 10.

## Pathology

Traumatic urethral strictures may involve only the epithelial lining of the urethra or the epithelium and supporting structures of the urethra. More commonly, inflammatory strictures involve the entire thickness of the urethra and the surrounding tissues, including the corpus spongiosum and overlying skin (Fig. 97–6) (Beard and Goodyear, 1948).

## Diagnosis

The diagnosis of urethral stricture is suspected in the patient who has a decrease in the size and force of his urinary stream. Diagnosis is confirmed by a urethrogram, which shows the presence, length, and number of strictures (but not the caliber of the stricture). The latter information must be obtained by gentle calibration of the urethra with a bougie à boule. The retrograde urethrogram is made while the urethra is filled with contrast medium. The material used for injection of the urethra should be suitable for intravenous use, because of the possibility of intravascular intravasation of the material when

the urethra is distended sufficiently to demonstrate the stricture (Fig. 97–7).

The technique of retrograde injection can be facilitated either by wrapping a strip of sterile gauze around the coronal sulcus to allow traction to be placed on the urethra while the injection is being made or by use of the Brodny (1941) urethrographic clamp (Beard, Goodyear and Weens, 1952).

## Treatment

Treatment can vary from simple urethral dilatation to total excision and replacement of the urethra. Several factors must be considered in selecting treatment for any patient. Among these are the length and severity of the stricture; the general state of health of the patient; the presence of urethritis and periurethritis, including possible abscess formation; the degree of urinary continence; and osseous distortion secondary to pelvic fracture, which might complicate the operative exposure of the strictured urethra.

Urinary continence in the normal male is primarily controlled by the internal urethral sphincter and prostatic urethra. The internal urethral

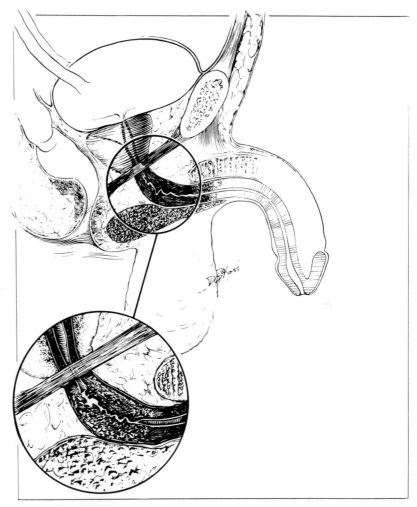

**FIGURE 97–6.** Sagittal section of a stricture of the bulbous urethra showing involvement of the corpus spongiosum.

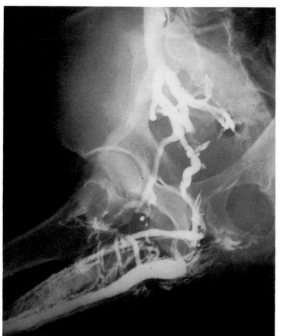

**FIGURE 97–7.** Venogram of the penis, pelvis, and inferior vena cava following injection of the urethra.

sphincter is a circular band of smooth muscle located at the vesical neck. Urinary continence is secondarily controlled by the external urethral sphincter, which is composed of striated muscle fibers surrounding the membranous urethra and terminal prostatic urethra at the triangular ligament. Either of the sphincters can be damaged without loss of urinary continence if the other is intact. One must be cautious, however, in the surgical approach to the external sphincter if the internal sphincter has been removed at prostatectomy. Similarly, if the external urethral sphincter has been damaged or bypassed by trauma or surgery, simple prostatectomy may result in urinary incontinence.

Urethral stricture is commonly accompanied by urinary infection. The causative organisms should be identified and appropriate antibacterial therapy started prior to any instrumentation of the urinary tract. When a periurethral abscess develops secondary to the stricture with extravasation of urine into the scrotum and perineum, emergency drainage and urinary diversion are required. Secondary surgical correction of the strictured urethra must be deferred until the local tissue reaction has subsided and all secondary abscesses have been drained and healed. Multiple periurethral abscesses and urethrocutaneous fistulas in the perineum often develop in the patient with a long-term untreated stricture. The fistulous tracts should be excised and abscesses drained while the urine is diverted proximally; the strictured urethra can be secondarily repaired.

When urinary diversion is required prior to repair of a urethral stricture because of extravasation or abscess formation, suprapubic cystostomy is usually the method of choice. This can be accomplished either by exposure of the bladder and intubation under direct vision or by trocar insertion of a catheter. Suprapubic cystostomy affords excellent vesical drainage and diverts the urine away from the diseased urethra. Direct antegrade urethrography before and after surgical repair of the stricture is facilitated by the diversion.

Surgical treatment of strictures of the urethra usually consists of one or more of the procedures listed below:

1. Dilatation
2. Internal urethrotomy
3. Excision
4. External urethrotomy
5. Marsupialization and secondary reconstruction
6. Incision or excision and skin graft

**Dilatation.** Prior to instrumentation, the urethral meatus and surrounding tissues are carefully prepared with a suitable detergent and 1:750 aqueous benzalkonium (Zephiran chloride) solution. The urethra and all instruments are lubricated with a sterile anesthetic lubricating jelly, such as Anestacon (lidocaine). The urethra is then gently calibrated with a soft catheter to locate the distal limit of the stricture. Dilatation must be done without force, because trauma results in further scarring and subsequent increase in both the length and density of the stricture. The properly sterilized filiform and Phillips woven urethral bougies are the most satisfactory instruments for safe, gentle dilatation of the urethra. The spiral-tipped filiform is passed into the bladder and is then used to guide firmly attached bougies through the urethra. Dilatation should be gradual and should be done at intervals over a period of several weeks, if necessary, until adequate dilatation can be obtained. Dilatation beyond 24 French in the adult male is seldom indicated. After dilatation, 15 ml of nitrofurazone (Furacin) solution diluted 1:10 is instilled into the bladder. When the urinary tract is infected, appropriate antibacterial therapy should be started prior to the introduction of instruments, thus reducing the risk of bacteremia. Urethral strictures, unless they can be surgically corrected, usually require periodic dilatation for the remainder of the patient's life.

**Internal Urethrotomy.** Internal urethrotomy should be carried out with the use of a suitable urethrotome, such as the Maisonneuve or Otis model (Fig. 97-8). The urethrotome is gently passed through the urethra, and the stricture is incised by multiple cuts in one plane until the entire thickness of the stricture has been incised. Internal urethrotomy is generally more applicable to traumatic strictures than to inflammatory strictures, because of the relative thickness of the wall of an inflammatory stricture.

**Excision.** Dugas in 1836 reported the first use of this technique, in which a short stricture was excised and allowed to heal across an indwelling catheter. Subsequently, many techniques have been reported for excision of the strictured urethra, with the defect bridged by a flap of proximal urethra which was then allowed to regenerate into a tube (Watson, 1935; Wells, 1941). A method of excision of the diseased posterior urethra, involving mobilization of the normal posterior urethra with a pull-through of the normal urethra into the prostatic urethra,

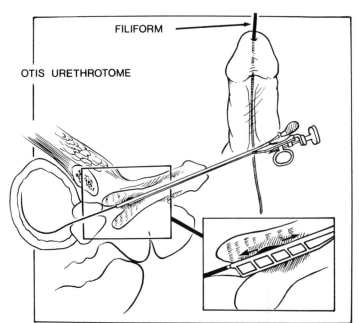

**FIGURE 97–8.** Otis urethrotome incising the urethral stricture with the bladder elevated.

was described by Badenoch in 1950 (Fig. 97–9). Waterhouse modified this procedure and, by removing the pubis and transporting the proximal urethra anterior to the triangular ligament, was able to bypass a longer segment of strictured urethra with less tension on the unaffected urethra (Figs. 97–10 and 97–11) (Waterhouse, Abrahams and Gruber, 1972).

**External Urethrotomy.** The early attempts at external urethrotomy were simple incisions of the urethra guided by a grooved director, as performed by Wheelhouse, Syme, and Freyer before the turn of the century.

In 1926, this technique was improved by Young and Davis, who removed the entire inflammatory wall of the stricture and allowed the stricture to regenerate from a bridge of the anterior urethral wall.

**Marsupialization.** Marsupialization procedures were first suggested by Stewart in 1948, when he described marsupialization of the strictured urethra and subsequent urethroplasty by the Ombrédanne (1923) method of hypospadias repair. Following this, Johanson in 1953 reported techniques of marsupialization of strictures with secondary reconstruction by the Denis Browne (1949) method of hypospadias repair. The technique of marsupialization followed by reconstruction has been subsequently modified by Turner-Warwick (1960), Leadbetter (1960), and Gil-Vernet (1966).

**Incision and Graft.** Incision or excision of the stricture with replacement by grafts has included the implantation of a silicone tube (De Nicola, 1950), grafting bladder mucosa which reportedly failed (Stevenson and Mackey, 1951), a cadaver urethral transplant (Bourque, 1952), a split-thickness skin graft (Peyton and Headstream, 1956), and a full-thickness skin graft (Devine and coworkers, 1963, 1968).

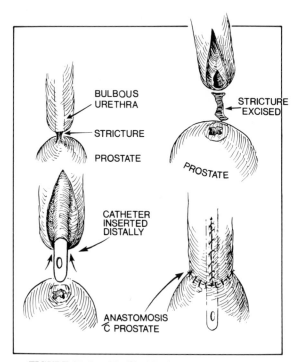

**FIGURE 97–9.** Modified Badenoch urethroplasty.

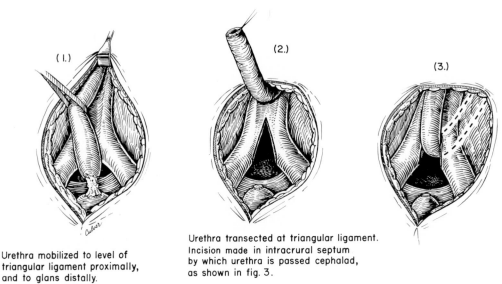

Urethra mobilized to level of
triangular ligament proximally,
and to glans distally.

Urethra transected at triangular ligament.
Incision made in intracrural septum
by which urethra is passed cephalad,
as shown in fig. 3.

**FIGURE 97–10.** Waterhouse urethroplasty, perineal view. (From Transactions of the American Association of Genito-Urinary Surgeons. Vol. 64, p. 20. Copyright 1972, The Williams and Wilkins Company, Baltimore.)

## Surgical Techniques

The techniques of surgery which the authors recommend vary somewhat, depending on the location of the stricture.

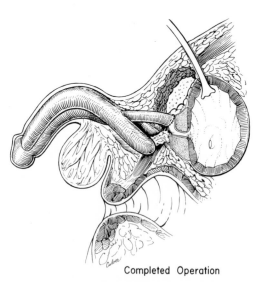

Completed Operation

Note: I. Urethra passes between crura.
    2. Scar tissue remains in place.
    3. Anastomosis is anterior to scar tissue.

**FIGURE 97–11.** Waterhouse urethroplasty, sagittal section. (From Transactions of the American Association of Genito-Urinary Surgeons. Vol. 64, p. 19. Copyright 1972, The Williams and Wilkins Company, Baltimore.)

**Urethral Meatus.** A simple meatotomy is recommended for a stricture at the urethral meatus. The ventral margin of the urethral meatus is infiltrated with 1 per cent Xylocaine anesthetic solution and clamped with a straight clamp, which is allowed to remain attached for a five-minute period. Following this, an incision is made in the center in the midportion of the crushed tissue to open the urethral meatus. The meatotomy is gently opened daily, by the patient or his family, until it is completely healed in order to maintain patency. The anterior meatotomy which Horton and Devine (1972) described for repair of the distal type of hypospadias with meatal stenosis can be used for meatal stricture. A V-shaped flap is outlined with the apex at the urethral meatus and is extended forward with its base at the most distal end of the glans. The flap is then elevated, and an incision is made through the dorsal portion of the urethra, opening the urethra widely. The tip of the flap is then sutured into the urethra as far proximally as possible using 6–0 chromic sutures, and the edges are approximated with the same material. A catheter can be left indwelling to allow the flap to seal.

**Pendulous Urethra.** The authors treat most strictures of the pendulous urethra by circumcising the skin of the penis at the coronal sulcus, retracting the penile skin to expose the strictured urethra, and incising the strictured urethra with extensions into the unaffected urethra proximally and distally for a distance of at least 1 cm. Methylene blue, 5 ml of 1 per cent solution, is instilled in the urethra prior to the incision, staining the urethral mucosa and making it more easily identified during the procedure. The mucosa of the strictured urethra is selectively stained to a greater degree so that the stricture is easily identified (Fig. 97–12). A patch graft of full-thickness skin from the prepuce or from some other hairless area is sutured over the defect with the epithelial surface toward the urethral lumen (Fig. 97–13). The skin of the penis is resutured at the coronal sulcus, and a urethral stent catheter (24 French in the adult) is allowed to remain in the urethra for ten days. A moderate amount of pressure is placed around the urethra with a dressing that is allowed to remain for a four-day period. The authors employ a marsupialization procedure in those strictures of the pendulous urethra complicated by fistulas or periurethral abscesses, in which it is necessary to remove the fistulous tract and drain the abscess prior to reconstruction of the urethra. The method described by Johanson (1953) is used except that the second stage is modified, when enough skin is available, to close the urethra as a complete tube rather than simply as a buried strip.

**Bulbous Urethra.** For strictures of the bulbous urethra, the patient is placed in the lithotomy position, and methylene blue is instilled in

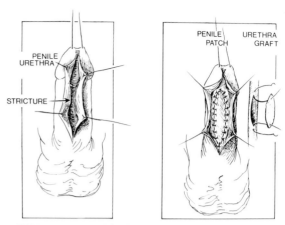

**FIGURE 97–13.** Distal urethral stricture incised and repaired by a patch graft of full-thickness skin.

the urethra for identification of the stricture. A Y-type incision is made in the perineum; the anterior compartment of the perineum is exposed; the bulbocavernous muscles are separated in the midline; and the urethra along with the corpus spongiosum is incised (see Fig. 97–12). The incision is extended for at least 1 cm into the normal urethra proximal and distal to the stricture. At this point one of three modifications of the technique is used. If the stricture is less than 1 cm in length, the entire stricture is excised; the urethra is mobilized and reapproximated with interrupted sutures of 4–0 chromic catgut (Fig. 97–14). When the stricture is more than 1 cm in length, after incision of the stricture and extension of the incision into the normal urethra, a full-thickness patch graft of hairless skin is placed over the defect and approximated with interrupted and continuous sutures of 4–0 chromic catgut (Fig. 97–15). When the stric-

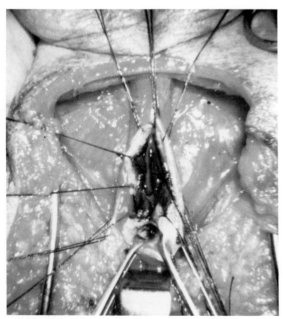

**FIGURE 97–12.** Urethra incised exposing the stricture deeply stained with methylene blue.

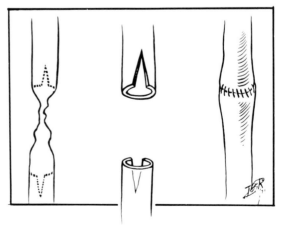

**FIGURE 97–14.** Stricture excised, urethra opened ventrally and dorsally, and the urethra anastomosed.

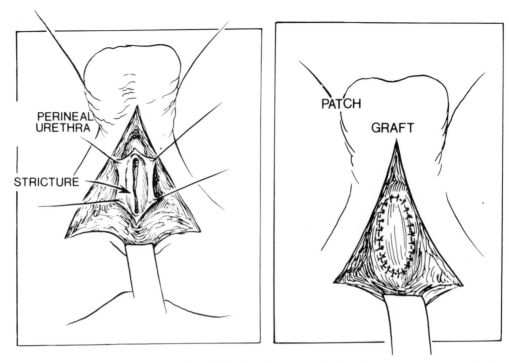

**FIGURE 97–15.** Perineal urethral stricture incised and a patch graft of full-thickness skin sutured in place.

ture is longer than 1 cm and the lumen is so distorted or destroyed that it is not suitable for reconstruction by the patch graft technique, the entire strictured area of urethra is excised and the resultant defect replaced by a tube of full-thickness graft of hairless skin with the epithelial surface toward the lumen of the urethra (Fig. 97–16).

When strictures of the bulbous urethra are complicated by fistulous tracts or abscesses, adequate drainage is necessary prior to urethroplasty. The urethra is therefore marsupialized at

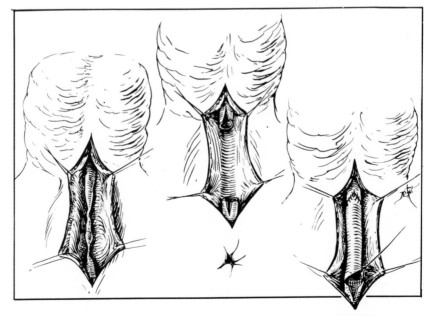

**FIGURE 97–16.** Perineal urethral stricture exposed, excised, and replaced with a full-thickness (tubed) skin graft.

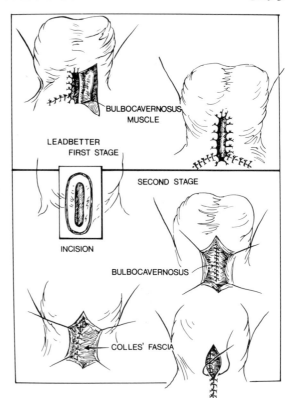

**FIGURE 97–17.** Leadbetter urethroplasty: marsupialization stage and secondary closure.

the time of excision and drainage, using the technique described by either Turner-Warwick (1960) or Leadbetter (1960) (Fig. 97–17). The urethra is closed in the second stage as a tube rather than as a buried strip in all cases.

**Membranous Urethra.** Strictures of the membranous urethra are usually traumatic in origin and are not associated with abscesses or fistulous tracts. The patient is placed in the exaggerated lithotomy position. An inverted V-incision is made in the perineum; dissection in the ischiorectal fossa is developed, and the rectum is stripped free from the posterior surface of the prostate gland, exposing the apex of the prostate gland. The bulbous urethra is then identified; the bulbocavernous muscles are separated in the midline, and the urethra with its surrounding corpus spongiosum is freed proximally to the inferior surface of the triangular ligament and distally 3 to 4 cm beyond the stricture. The stricture, if short, can be excised and the normal bulbous urethra passed through the incised triangular ligament with reapproximation to the prostatic urethra after the method of Badenoch (1950), except that it is preferable to approximate the bulbous urethra to the prostatic urethra under direct vision (see Fig. 97–9). If

the stricture is long, it can be completely excised; a full-thickness graft of hairless skin, which is tubed, is placed between the apex of the prostate gland and the normal bulbous urethra (Figs. 97–18 and 97–19). The graft is placed over a catheter with the epithelial surface toward the lumen and is approximated with interrupted sutures of 4–0 chromic catgut. The urethral catheter, used for drainage of urine and for stenting, should be left in place for 10 to 14 days.

A novel approach to urethroplasty for traumatic strictures of the membranous urethra was described by Waterhouse in 1972. The patient is placed in the Trendelenburg position with his legs in the frog position to expose simultaneously the suprapubic area and the perineum. The pubic bone is removed through a lower abdominal incision; the bulbous urethra is exposed through a perineal incision, divided at the membranous urethra, and freed distally for at least 5 to 6 cm. The intracrural septum is then divided, exposing the retropubic space of Retzius. The urethra is moved dorsally over the triangular ligament and reapproximated to the anterior surface of the prostatic urethra immediately proximal to the stricture (see Figs. 97–10 and 97–11). The authors feel, however, that most

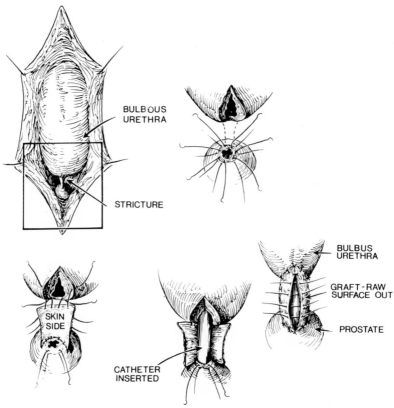

**FIGURE 97–18.** Patch graft urethroplasty: membranous urethral stricture exposed, excised, and replaced with a full-thickness skin graft which is wrapped around a catheter.

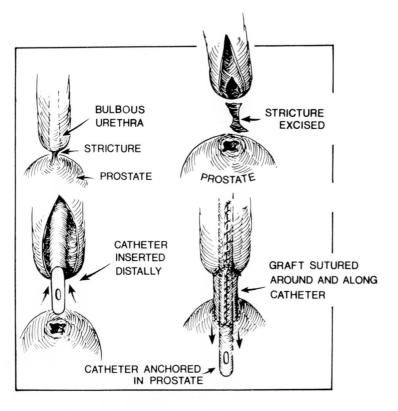

**FIGURE 97–19.** Membranous urethral stricture excised and replaced with a full-thickness skin graft which is sutured around a catheter.

patients with membranous urethral strictures can be treated by perineal exposure of the bulbous, membranous, and prostatic urethra without removal of the pubic bone.

The surgeon should select certain procedures with which he is most adept as his primary oper-ation for strictures in each urethral location. It is imperative, however, that each surgeon be familiar with alternative procedures for use in situations in which his primary operations are not applicable.

# Peyronie's Disease

## Charles E. Horton, M.D., and Charles J. Devine, M.D.

Peyronie's disease, first described by François de la Peyronie (1819), physician to Louis XIV, has been called by many names, such as plastic induration of the penis, fibrositis, fibrous caver-nositis, fibrous plaque of the penis, and fibrous sclerosis of the penis. Because of the unknown etiology of the condition, the eponym Peyronie's disease is likely to persist.

## Etiology

The cause of Peyronie's disease is unknown. Sexual excess, phlebitis, and sexual abstinence have all been described as possible contribu-tors. Dupuytren's palmar contracture or plantar fibromatosis occurs in 10 per cent of patients with Peyronie's disease, and 3 per cent of pa-tients with Peyronie's disease have Dupuy-tren's contracture. There is also an apparent association with fibrosis of the male breast and a rare association with fibrosis of the ears. Smith (1966) demonstrated a loss of the normal space between the tunica albuginea of the corpora and the intercorporal vascular erectile tissues in Peyronie's disease. He postulated that this may be caused by a vasculitis with fibrosis and that an inflammatory process is the cause of Peyronie's disease.

## Signs and Symptoms

Peyronie's disease is characterized by a plaque in the tunica albuginea of the corpus caverno-sum, usually located on the dorsum. The plaque may vary in length and thickness or exist as a chord or nodules, often involving the septum. The plaque is irregular, firm to hard, and may contain cartilage or bone. The patient gives a typical history of slow, limited growth of the nodule, with a severe curvature of the erect penis that produces extreme discomfort with erection but is painless when the penis is flaccid. The disease is most frequently seen in patients between the ages of 40 and 60, although the authors have observed it in younger and in older patients.

## Diagnosis

Peyronie's disease is suspected when a patient reports a painful curvature of the erect penis without previous trauma or infection of the area. A dense, fibrous, or ossified plaque may be palpated in many cases. If the patient is asked to photograph the erect penis, a distinct curvature can be noted. A simple office test, which is of assistance in the diagnosis, consists of placing a tourniquet around the base of the penis and injecting 50 ml of sterile saline into the corpora to produce erection of the penis (Gittes and McLaughlin, 1974) (Fig. 97–20). The inter-corporal septum is a lattice-like partition which allows transmission of fluid from one corporal body to the other, and distention can be accom-plished with a single needle. An adequate pre-operative appraisal of the true curvature of the penis can be obtained in all cases with this tech-

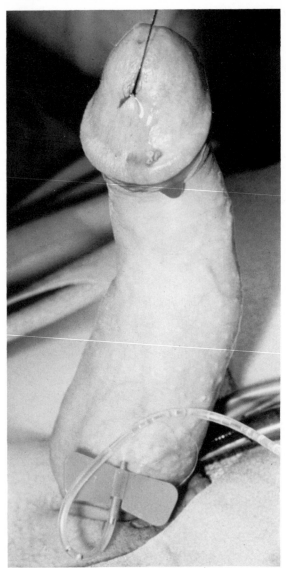

**FIGURE 97–20.** Preoperative filling of the penis with saline to demonstrate the penile defect. The tourniquet at the base is secured with a clamp. Note that the saline injected into the corpora leaks from the suture punctures in the glans.

nique. Preoperative X-ray studies will often show ossification or calcification in the suspected plaque area. A corpus cavernosogram may show lesions located in the septum (Byström, Johansson, Edgren, Alfthan and Kohler, 1974).

## Pathologic Physiology

The tunica albuginea is a distensible and expansible covering of the vascular tissue of the corpora. When the corpora enlarge, the tunica albuginea allows expansion of the penis; if the tunica is equally expansible in all areas, a straight and turgid penis results during erection. If one portion of the expansible tunica albuginea becomes scarred, as in Peyronie's disease, this portion of the tunica will not expand, and the penis will be shortened on this side, causing a curvature. Location of the curvature is important to diagnose the exact site of the plaque and to determine the amount of pathologic involvement of the tunica albuginea.

## Treatment

Systemic treatment with potassium para-amino-benzoate (Potaba), potassium iodide, dimethyl sulfoxide, and steroids has been disappointing. While a high rate of spontaneous remission has been observed, symptoms are usually progressive, and the phallus becomes increasingly angulated and painful. Vitamin E (100 mg three times a day) is the only systemic medicine which has given relief of pain. Although the response to vitamin E is not consistent, the authors recommend it in all patients prior to surgery.

Surgical removal of small plaques may be successful without any type of reconstruction; however, if a large area of tunica is excised, postexcision scar tissue in the area of resection will cause a recurrence of the penile curvature. Poutasse (1971, 1973) has reported success with multiple incisions of the plaque to release the acute angulation, but he allows the diseased tunica albuginea to remain. Lowsley advocated excision of the diseased tunica and insertion of a fat graft into the defect (Lowsley, 1943; Lowsley and Boyce, 1950). X-ray, radium, physiotherapy, and ultraviolet light have all been advocated for the treatment of Peyronie's disease. In our experience, the patients who have had radiation therapy or injections with steroids and who require surgery are the most difficult to manage because of increased fibrosis in the area of dissection.

Since 1970 the authors have advocated surgery for Peyronie's disease. The technique consists of total excision of the diseased tunica albuginea and replacement of the tunica albuginea with a dermal graft to restore continuity of the covering of the vascular spaces of the corpora (Horton and Devine, 1973; Devine and Horton, 1974). The dermal graft does not have the same elastic expansibility as the normal adjacent tunica albuginea but in time recovers most of the characteristics. A firm envelope to surround the vascular spaces is restored, a property which allows normal erection and correction of the curvature in most cases.

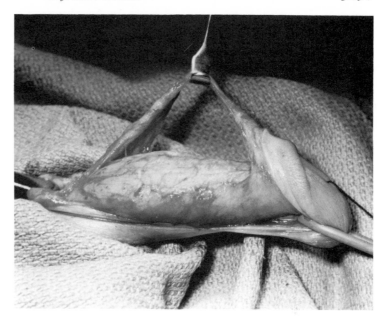

**FIGURE 97-21.** Buck's fascia and the dartos fascia have been dissected, with preservation of the blood supply and innervation to the glans. Retraction is by means of a red rubber catheter at the frenulum and a retractor at the base of the penis.

## Surgical Technique

An incomplete circumcising incision is made just proximal to the coronal sulcus, and the skin of the penile shaft is retracted to the base of the penis, thereby exposing the corpora. The skin in the region of the frenulum is left intact. An incision is made in the dartos and Buck's fascia; the tissue containing the paired dorsal artery, vein, and nerves is dissected from the tunica. Incisions are made on each side of the penis, and dissection is extended to the midline, raising the artery, veins, and nerves as a single bundle (Fig. 97–21). Careful attention should be paid to the dissection so that the innervation to the glans is not impaired. When the subcutaneous tissue containing the vascular and nerve structures is elevated, the diseased plaque of the penis can be identified by visual inspection and by palpation. There is always reaction between the fascia and the plaque, making the dissection tedious. However, as the margins of the plaque are passed, the two tissue layers are easily separated. The plaque is generally discrete but often merges into the surrounding normal tunica albuginea. If neces-

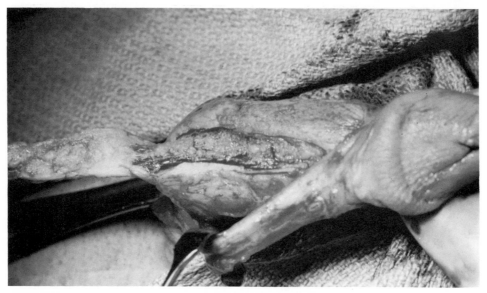

**FIGURE 97-22.** Plaque being excised. Note the minimal bleeding and retraction of the neurovascular bundle.

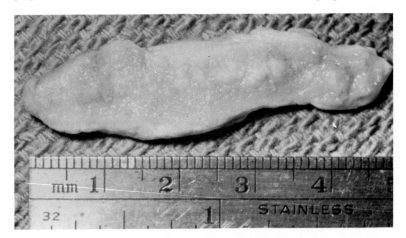

**FIGURE 97-23.** Deep surface of the excised plaque. Note the points of attachment of the strands of septum; the hyalinization process extends into the septum.

sary, a tourniquet at the base of the penis and distention of the penis with saline at this stage are helpful to define the limits of the plaque. An incision is made around the plaque, which is dissected free by sharp and blunt dissection (Fig. 97-22). The plaque is adherent to the vascular tissue of the corpora, but less bleeding is encountered than might be expected. After removal of the tunica, the vascular spaces do not bleed and remain contained within the depth of the defect. The edges of the excised area should be carefully palpated; a gritty sensation may reveal thickened tunica not visible to the naked eye. All abnormal tunica should be excised (Fig. 97-23). In many cases the defect may measure 3 to 4 cm in width and 6 to 8 cm in length. The edge of the excised area should be incised at several points, providing darts which prevent a straight line closure with the dermal graft (Fig. 97-24).

The dermal graft is obtained from a relatively hairless area of the body, usually the groin or lower abdomen. It is not necessary that the area be totally hairless, since the dermal graft hair follicles will gradually atrophy when used in a buried graft (Fig. 97-25). The graft is tailored to

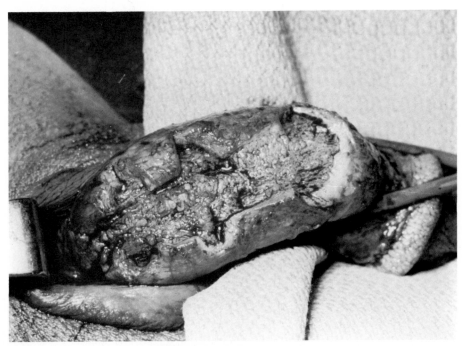

**FIGURE 97-24.** The plaque has been resected, and multiple dartlike incisions have been extended into the unaffected tunica surrounding the lesion. Note the erectile tissue in the defect.

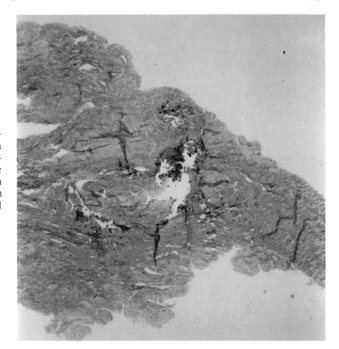

**FIGURE 97–25.** Photomicrograph of the portion of the dermal graft removed for biopsy in a patient who had a subsequent penile implant because of impotence secondary to diabetes. The dark area in the center is the result of a reaction around a nylon suture. The tunica albuginea is on the right and the dermal graft on the left. All skin appendages are atrophic.

fit the defect of the tunica albuginea and is sutured with multiple interrupted sutures of nonabsorbable material, such as braided nylon sutures (Fig. 97–26). The defect in the abdomen can be closed primarily. The dermal graft should be inserted into the defect with the dermal side toward the vascular space. After the graft is securely sutured, the penis can be engorged with further injections of saline to confirm that all of the curvature is corrected.

The subcutaneous tissue is returned to its original position (Fig. 97–27); the sleeve of penile skin is replaced; and the circumcising incision is closed with 5–0 chromic catgut interrupted sutures. An elastic pressure bandage is applied to the penis. A catheter is usually not used, as the patient can ordinarily void through the pressure bandage without difficulty. Sexual intercourse is banned for at least six weeks after surgery. To prevent erec-

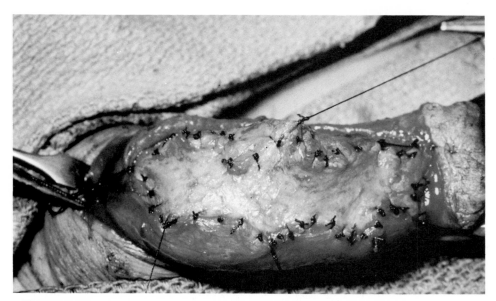

**FIGURE 97–26.** Dermal graft in situ secured with multiple nonabsorbable sutures.

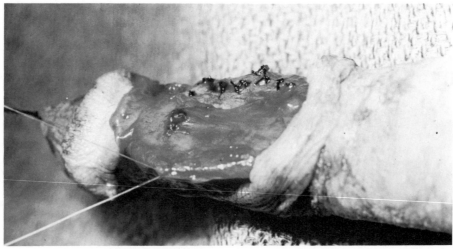

**FIGURE 97-27.**   The layer of dartos and Buck's fascia being reapproximated to cover the dermis graft. A sleeve type of penile incision will then be approximated.

tions the patient is heavily sedated and given amyl nitrite pearls to be broken and inhaled when an erection is impending.

### Results

In the approximately 40 patients operated on with this technique, the results have been generally satisfactory. One case required a penile implant because of impotence secondary to diabetes and lack of ability to obtain an erection. Some patients have had difficulty in initiating erections or in obtaining a full erection. Filling the penis with saline has demonstrated that the defect has been corrected, and this encouragement has helped in later physiologic erections. All of the remaining patients report improvement in sexual function, and most have a straight penis. The curvature is not totally corrected in some because the degree of distention and elasticity of the dermal graft is not exactly the same as that of the normal tunica albuginea. However, curvature has been adequately corrected in all cases, allowing intercourse. The painful erection problem has been eradicated in all patients. There has been no recurrence or extension of the disease, although the primary excision was inadequate in one patient, and a secondary excision of diseased tissue in the septum was required. Since dermal grafts soften over a period of six months, early results may seem disappointing until adequate softening of the grafts has occurred.

It is important to construct the patch to the exact size of the defect to prevent constriction

of the phallus or ballooning of the tunica at the site of a graft that is too large.

Victims of Peyronie's disease universally express a strong desire to continue sexual intercourse. However, unless the disease is corrected, they experience increasingly limited sexual activity which finally becomes difficult or even impossible. Vitamin E is the initial treatment; if this results in regression of symptoms and relief of discomfort, surgery is not recommended. If, however, the patient is incapacitated by progressive disease, excision of the diseased plaque and replacement with a dermal graft are advised.

A dermal graft has also been used to correct chordee in a patient who had had multiple operations for what was originally chordee without hypospadias. The residual chordee was due to iatrogenic scar in the tunica albuginea. The tissue was resected and replaced with a dermal graft. Subsequent urethroplasty has resulted in a satisfactory reconstruction (Devine and Horton, 1975).

### REFERENCES

Badenoch, A. W.: A pull-through operation for impassable traumatic stricture of the urethra. Br. J. Urol., *22*:404, 1950.

Beard, D. E., and Goodyear, W. E.: Urethral stricture: A pathological study. J. Urol., *59*:619, 1948.

Beard, D. E., Goodyear, W. E., and Weens, H. T. S.: Radiologic Diagnosis of the Lower Urinary Tract. Springfield, Ill., Charles C Thomas, Publisher, 1952.

Bourque, J. P.: New surgical procedure for cure of scrotal hypospadias: Grafting of a male human urethra taken from a fresh cadaver. J. Urol., *67*:698, 1952.

Brodny, M. L.: A new instrument for urethrography in the male. J. Urol., *46*:350, 1941.

Browne, D.: An operation for hypospadias. Proc. R. Soc. Med., *42*:466, 1949.

Byström, J., Johansson, B., Edgren, J., Alfthan, J., and Kohler, R.: Induratio penis plastica. Scand. J. Urol. Nephrol., *8*:155, 1974.

De Nicola, R.: Permanent artificial (silicone) urethra. J. Urol., *63*:168, 1950.

Devine, C. J., Jr., and Horton, C. E.: Surgical treatment of Peyronie's disease with a dermal graft. J. Urol., *111*:44, 1974.

Devine, C. J., Jr., and Horton, C. E.: Use of dermal graft to correct chordee. J. Urol., *113*:56, 1975.

Devine, P. C., Horton, C. E., Devine, C. J., Sr., Devine, C. J., Jr., Crawford, H. H., and Adamson, J. E.: Use of full-thickness skin grafts in repair of urethral strictures. J. Urol., *90*:67, 1963.

Devine, P. C., Sakati, I. A., Poutasse, E. F., and Devine, C. J., Jr.: One stage urethroplasty: Repair of urethral strictures with a free full-thickness patch of skin. J. Urol., *99*:191, 1968.

Dugas, L. A.: Stricture of the urethra successfully treated by excision of the indurated portion of the canal. South. Med. Surg. J., *1*:293, 1836.

Gil-Vernet, J. M.: Un traitement des sténoses traumatiques et inflammatoires de l'urètre postérieur. Nouvelle methode d'uretroplastie. J. Urol. Nephrol., *72*:97, 1966.

Gittes, R. F., and McLaughlin, A. P.: Injection technique to induce penile erection. Urology, *4*:473, 1974.

Horton, C. E., and Devine, C. J., Jr.: Clinical Symposia: Hypospadias and Epispadias. Vol. 24, No. 3. Summit, New Jersey, Ciba Pharmaceutical Company, 1972.

Horton, C. E., and Devine, C. J., Jr.: Peyronie's disease. Plast. Reconstr. Surg., *52*:503, 1973.

Johanson, B.: Reconstruction of the male urethra in strictures, Acta Chir. Scand. Suppl. 176, 1953.

Leadbetter, G. W., Jr.: A simplified urethroplasty for strictures of the bulbous urethra. J. Urol., *83*:54, 1960.

Lowsley, O. S.: Surgical treatment of plastic induration of the penis (Peyronie's disease). N. Y. J. Med., *43*:2273, 1943.

Lowsley, O. S., and Boyce, W. H.: Further experience with an operation for the cure of Peyronie's disease. J. Urol., *63*:888, 1950.

Ombrédanne, L.: Precis clinique et operatoire de chirurgie infantile. Paris, Masson & Cie, 1923.

Peyronie, F. de la: Sur quelques obstacles qui s'opposent à l'ejaculation naturelle de la semence. Mém. Acad. Chir. (New Ed.). 1819, pp. 316–323, 425–434.

Peyton, A. B., and Headstream, J. W.: Construction of perineal urethra by split thickness skin graft. J. Urol., *76*:90, 1956.

Poutasse, E. F.: Peyronie's disease. Trans. Am. Assoc. Genitourinary Surg., *63*:97, 1971.

Poutasse, E. F.: Peyronie's disease. *In* Horton, C. E. (Ed.): Plastic and Reconstructive Surgery of the Genital Area. Boston, Little, Brown and Company, 1973.

Pressman, D., and Greenfield, L.: Reconstruction of the perineal urethra with a free full-thickness skin graft from the prepuce. J. Urol., *69*:677, 1953.

Smith, B. H.: Peyronie's disease. Am. J. Clin. Pathol., *45*:670, 1966.

Stevenson, A. J., and Mackey, J. F.: Urethroplasty: Use of bladder mucosa. J. Missouri State Med. Assoc., *48*:990, 1951.

Stewart, H. H.: Discussion on the surgery of urethral stricture. Proc. R. Soc. Med., *41*:843, 1948.

Turner-Warwick, R. T.: A technique for posterior urethroplasty. J. Urol., *83*:416, 1960.

Waterhouse, K., Abrahams, J. I., and Gruber, H.: The transpubic approach to the lower urinary tract. Trans. Am. Assoc. Genitourinary Surg., *64*:18, 1972.

Watson, E. M.: Complete rupture of the urethra: A method of repair in delayed cases. J. Urol., *33*:64, 1935.

Wells, C. A.: Ruptured urethra: A technique for secondary repair. Br. J. Urol., *13*:8, 1941.

Young, H. H., and Davis, D. M.: Young's Practice of Urology. Vols. 1 and 2. Philadelphia, W. B. Saunders Company, 1926, pp. 565–596.

# CHAPTER 98

# RECONSTRUCTION OF THE MALE GENITALIA

## VINKO ARNERI, M.D.

### INJURIES TO THE MALE GENITALIA

Injuries to the external male genitalia are not infrequent because of the widespread use of high-speed machinery in industry and agriculture and because of the constantly rising number of traffic accidents. The incidence of these injuries in modern warfare is also increasing; during the conflict in Vietnam, for example, because of frequent use of land mines, such injuries accounted for 41.6 per cent of all urogenital trauma (Salvatierra, Bucklew and Morrow, 1969).

The great majority of these injuries are of the avulsive type, with considerable loss of skin, and therefore require plastic surgical methods of repair. They must be treated as emergency cases in order to prevent infection and the attending complications. Treatment of the latter poses serious difficulties for the surgeon and further frustrates the patient who, due to prolonged and ineffective treatment, is often emotionally depressed.

**Mechanism and Etiology.** The mechanism of the injuries is typical and is similar to a traumatic avulsion of the scalp. The hairs or clothes are caught in a rotating machine or driving wheel, and the skin is torn off by traction and twisting.

Blood loss is rarely a problem because the avulsion occurs in the relatively bloodless plane superficial to Buck's fascia, just beneath the dartos layer. In the scrotum, the plane of cleavage is superficial to the cremaster. In this layer of loose areolar tissue and as a result of the cremasteric reflex, the skin is easily torn off (Fig. 98–1). Consequently, the deep structures of the penis and testes are usually intact. According to the force and duration of traction, different degrees of skin avulsion may result.

Partial avulsion of the skin of the penis is the injury most often observed; combined avulsion of the penoscrotal skin or isolated avulsion of the scrotal skin is less frequent, while associated perineal and perianal injuries are even less frequently seen.

Wartime wounds of the external genitalia are more extensive and involve the urethra with partial or even total loss of the penis and testicles.

Apart from the injuries described above, unusual cases of direct scrotal avulsion caused by a bull's horn during bullfights have also been reported (Gonzalez-Ulloa, 1963).

Causes other than mechanical factors are less common and may include thermal burns (Julian, Klein and Hubbord, 1969), electrical burns, and chemical burns; gangrene of the skin may occur after urinary infections or Fournier's disease (Moustafa, 1967). The skin defect in this group of cases is the result of skin necrosis and should be treated by secondary skin grafting procedures, in contradistinction to

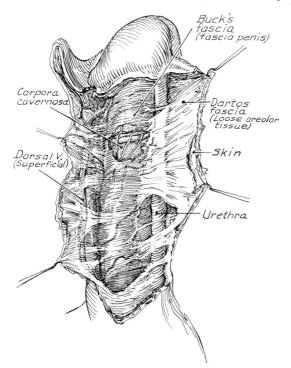

Buck's
fascia
(fascia penis)

Corpora
cavernosa

Dartos
fascia
(Loose areolar
tissue)

Dorsal V.
(Superficial)

Skin

Urethra

**FIGURE 98–1.** The skin is avulsed in a plane just beneath the dartos layer in the loose areolar tissue.

skin defects caused by mechanical factors, which must always be primarily repaired.

Penile skin loss may also result from the treatment of squamous cell carcinoma of the shaft by irradiation. The treatment of this type of condition poses special problems because of the poor blood supply resulting from the widespread vascular destruction caused by the irradiation (Casson, Bonnano and Converse, 1971).

In traffic accidents, the lesions of the external genitalia may often be associated with other injuries. In one of the author's cases, a totally denuded penis and partial avulsion of the scrotum were associated with a fracture of the pelvis, subluxation of the left femur, and extensive injuries of the soft tissues of the thighs. This type of trauma is usually accompanied by severe physiologic alterations, and complex resuscitative efforts are indicated (Fig. 98–2, *A*, *B*).

**Historical Aspects.** Before the present century, only two reports on these injuries were recorded in the medical literature. Credit must be given to Gibbs (1855) for being the first surgeon to report on penile and scrotal repair in a patient with traumatic avulsion of the skin. Twenty-six years later, a second report on the same subject appeared. At the turn of the century, the incidence of these injuries increased with the development of technology and industry.

The present number of reported cases in the literature varies according to different authors. Up to 1942, Owens had collected 13 cases of penoscrotal avulsion described in the literature. Gonzalez-Ulloa (1963) found 28 such cases; Kubaček (1957) cited 60 cases, of which 22 were combined penoscrotal skin avulsion; Santoni-Rugiu (1966) mentioned reports of 30 cases of similar injuries.

Although all authors agreed on the need for primary repair, their surgical techniques differed widely. Cottle (1924) buried the denuded testicles in skin pockets on the thighs between the fascia and subcutaneous tissue, while he inserted the penis through a skin tunnel in the inguinal region. Owens (1942) in a similar case

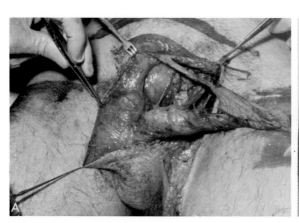
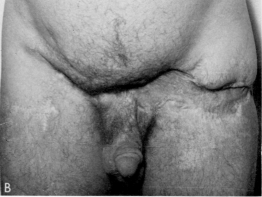

**FIGURE 98–2.** *A*, Totally degloved penis and partial loss of the scrotum combined with massive injuries of the skin and muscles of the thighs, fracture of the pelvis, subluxation of the femur, and shock. The wound surface on the penis was covered by replanting the avulsed skin as a full-thickness skin graft. The defect on the scrotum was closed by direct approximation. *B*, Appearance 11 years later.

applied Cottle's technique to the testes and covered the penis with a skin graft. Whelan (1944), in a patient with a loss of scrotum and intact penis, first buried the testes in a pocket under the skin of the thighs and later, by a three-stage procedure, formed the scrotal sac by means of previously planned skin flaps over the pockets.

In order to avoid multistage operations in reconstructing the scrotum, some authors reported successful results by raising skin flaps from the thigh (Douglas, 1951) or pubic region (Kubaček, 1957) in one stage.

Others published satisfactory results in covering the denuded testes and penis by skin grafts (Balakrishnan, 1956; Campbell, 1957; Alton, 1963; Manchanda, Singh, Keswani and Sharma, 1967).

The avulsed skin has also been reapplied as a full-thickness skin graft for covering the denuded scrotum with only variable results (Gibson, 1954; Alton, 1963).

The skin of the scrotum has also been used for resurfacing the shaft of the penis (Banham, 1948; Casson and coworkers, 1971). Regardless of differences in techniques, all authors are unanimous that these injuries require immediate treatment to prevent infection, subsequent deformities, and impairment of testicular function.

**Diagnosis.** A detailed examination of the wound is essential, and the following points should be carefully evaluated: first, the extent of skin loss on the penis and scrotum; second, the viability of the avulsed skin; third, possible lesions of the corpora cavernosa or urethra; and fourth, the severity of the combined lesions and general condition of the patient in cases of multisystem injury.

The exact assessment of the extent of skin loss is essential in deciding the method of treatment. This is particularly important in covering the defect on the scrotum, the elastic skin of which often permits the covering of even large defects by direct approximation. Therefore, the curled and retracted skin should be stretched with skin hooks in order to evaluate the possibility of direct closure of the wound without undue tension.

Proper assessment of the viability of the skin is of no less importance. The contused or excoriated skin with impaired vascularity should be excised primarily and the wound covered by using one of the transplantation techniques. This is also important in deciding whether the avulsed skin can be replanted as a full-thickness skin graft (see Fig. 98–2).

**Treatment.** Primary treatment includes sedation by opiates or their substitutes when the patient is restless, and the application of a well-fixed dressing. The wound should not be subjected to washing with disinfectants. The patient should be immediately transported to a hospital that can provide the necessary specialized treatment.

Upon admission to the hospital, the patient should be given tetanus antitoxin and/or a booster and antibiotics. Blood transfusions are rarely indicated in cases of simple avulsion, in which the loss of blood is usually moderate, but are frequently required in combined injuries.

The actual treatment, which is performed in the operating room, is as follows: the wounded area is first covered with sterile gauze, and the surrounding intact skin around the wound and on the thighs and pubis is prepared with soap and water, and an antiseptic solution. Thereafter the gauze is removed from the wound, and the denuded area is meticulously cleansed and all nonviable tissue carefully excised. Subfascial hematomas should be incised and blood clots evacuated. As to the treatment of isolated avulsion of the skin of the penis, all authors today agree that the split-thickness skin graft is the method of choice. Skin flaps from the abdomen or thighs should be mentioned only to be condemned, as the resulting penis is overly large, ungainly, and hairy and subsequent excision of the flap and application of a split-thickness skin graft is necessary.

In cases of combined injuries, when the general condition of the patient does not permit a protracted operation, or when the surgeon is not familiar with skin grafting techniques, the denuded penis may be temporarily buried in a subcutaneous tunnel in the pubic or inguinal region, or under the scrotum if the latter is not damaged, allowing the glans to protrude through a buttonhole incision. A Foley catheter is inserted. After approximately one week, during which time the general condition of the patient has improved, the penis is retrieved from the tunnel and definitive grafting is completed. As a rule, however, primary grafting is usually possible, and the surgeon should grasp this opportunity, as the penis in most instances is in erection during the first few hours after the accident, thus allowing the surgeon to establish the size of the skin graft necessary to cover the defect and enabling the graft to be fixed more firmly. An indwelling urethral catheter is inserted before the application of the skin graft.

If the patient is not admitted to the hospital immediately after the injury, the primary grafting may be undertaken 24 or even 48 hours after injury, provided that the wound is dry and free of infection. This, of course, is an exception, and the decision is left to the assessment and experience of the surgeon.

If the wound is infected, it must be treated as any other infected wound followed by delayed skin grafting techniques.

In cases of partial avulsion of the skin of the penis, the length of the unfolded preputial skin which is left undamaged may on rare occasions be sufficient to cover the whole denuded shaft. It cannot be sutured to the base of the penis if this involves any tension. An extensive persisting edema, which subsides after a variable length of time, is the usual complication.

In all other circumstances, the preputial remnants should be excised and only a small cuff left around the corona, to the edges of which the graft is sutured (Ferris, 1949; Huffman and coworkers, 1956).

Most often the avulsed skin is damaged and should be discarded, and the wounded surface should be immediately covered with a split-thickness skin graft. In unusual circumstances, the totally avulsed skin can be replanted as a full-thickness graft (see Fig. 98–2).

The optimum thickness of the graft in primary repair is that of a split-thickness skin graft of intermediate thickness. In the secondary repair of a relatively infected surface, a thinner graft may be indicated.

The denuded penis should be covered by a single piece of skin graft in order to avoid the scars and constrictions which could result when multiple grafts are used. Therefore, the surgeon who performs such operations should be completely familiar with skin graft removal techniques (see Chapter 6).

SKIN GRAFTING. The donor site that will yield a skin graft of sufficient size (10 × 20 cm) must be healthy and hairless. The most common donor sites are the medial aspects of the arms and thighs. The graft should preferably be taken by a separate operating team. This shortens the time of the operation and minimizes the risk of infection of the donor site. Before the graft is applied, an assistant stretches the penis to its full length in order to assess the required length of the graft. This is particularly important in patients in whom the penis is not in full erection. The graft is first fixed in position by means of pilot sutures at the base of the penis. The distal edge of the graft is stretched by mosquito forceps or skin hooks over the penis (Fig. 98–3, *A*). The edges of the graft are then cut with pointed

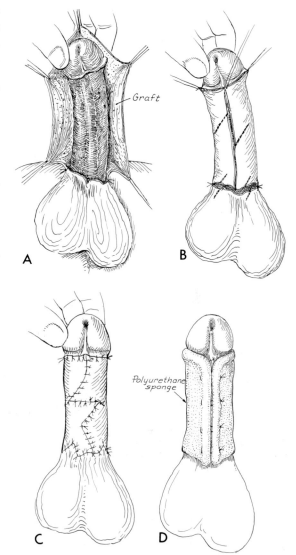

**FIGURE 98–3.** Skin grafting the shaft of the penis following skin avulsion. *A,* Split-thickness graft being placed over the defect. Note that the penis is stretched. *B,* After the graft has been sutured to the proximal and distal ends of the raw area, oblique cuts are made with scissors through the graft in order to interrupt the straight line of suture between the two edges of the graft. *C,* The graft is sutured in place. Note the broken suture line on the ventral aspect of the shaft of the penis and also at the junction line between the graft and the skin at the proximal portion of the penis. *D,* A polyurethane sponge has been sutured over the graft.

scissors in such a way as to produce a zigzag suture line on the ventral aspect of the shaft of the penis. The same procedure is done at the proximal end of the graft in order to interrupt the circular suture line (Fig. 98–3, *B, C*). At the base of the penis and around the corona, the graft is fixed to the underlying tissue by a few additional interrupted sutures. The graft is definitively fixed in position by encircling gauze sponges or by cotton wool dressings reinforced by tie-over pressure sutures. The author has observed that the best results were obtained by using a polyurethane sponge. A sheet of sponge of matching size is carefully molded around the penis and fixed by sutures at moderate pressure (Fig. 98–3, *D*). The glans is left free so that its color may be observed. The sponge is not toxic; it allows evaporation, ensures more balanced pressure, and is also simpler than the clumsy bolus dressing technique which is most often used.

POSTOPERATIVE TREATMENT. The patient is kept in bed for 10 to 14 days, until the catheter is removed. The bladder is washed several times a day through a closed drainage system with sterile saline or 3 per cent boric acid. This technique ensures the free drainage of urine, which may be blocked by mucoid or crystalline deposits. Occasional bladder spasms, which may be provoked by the tip of the catheter, are controlled by antispasmodic therapy. Prophylactic antibiotic treatment is continued for seven to ten days. Possible erections will not disturb the healing of the graft if it is properly fixed.

The sponge is removed on the tenth day, and the catheter is left in place for another two days. Vascularization of the graft is usually 100 per cent successful.

Within three to four weeks the graft has become well established. In some cases in which the preputial skin was not sufficiently excised, edema may appear around the corona, and this usually takes longer to subside.

The patient is cautioned to avoid sexual intercourse for approximately six weeks after complete healing. Erection of the penis is moderately painful in some patients in the first few months, but later sexual function becomes unremarkable.

RESURFACING THE SHAFT OF THE PENIS WITH SCROTAL SKIN. When the scrotal skin is intact and when conditions may be unfavorable for skin grafting, the penis is buried in a bed under the scrotal skin; the glans is extruded through an incision placed in the dependent portion of the sac (Fig. 98–4, *A, B*). Four weeks later, bilateral incisions 8 cm in length diverging from the base of the glans (Fig. 98–4, *C*) are made through the skin and dartos, and the scrotal skin is undermined laterally. Closure of the flaps is partially completed along the ventral aspect of the shaft, and a Z-plasty is done to interrupt the linear closure (Figs. 98–4, *D, E* and 98–5).

COMBINED AVULSION OF PENOSCROTAL SKIN. While the primary repair of isolated avulsion of the penis by split-thickness skin grafts has become a routine technique, the management of degloved testes is more complicated, and a definitive technique has not been developed. It is essential to cover the denuded testes primarily in order to avoid infection and thrombosis of the spermatic vessels. Any remnants of the scrotal skin should be spared, as scrotal skin, due to its elasticity and healing capacity, can often be used for covering the defect. In fact, this should be the method of choice because of its simplicity and associated rapid recovery.

Huffman, Culp, Greenleaf, Flocks, and Brintnall (1956) recommended suturing the remaining scrotal skin, even under considerable tension, emphasizing that within a few months the scrotum expands almost to normal size and permits free testicular mobility. However, the well-known dangers of suturing a wound under tension should not be forgotten. In addition to necrosis of the skin and infection, tension, particularly in this area, can be fatal for the normal function of the testes. Therefore, in cases in which the skin defect cannot be closed except under tension, other surgical methods should be considered. At this point it is important to call attention to the fact that there is no universal method which can be applied in all cases of avulsion of the scrotum.

Among the more commonly used methods, the following should be mentioned: burying the testes in skin pockets in the thigh or inguinal area, covering the testes by skin grafts, and reconstruction of the scrotum by local flaps. All of the above mentioned methods can be successful if correctly indicated and properly performed.

In principle, if the testes have been totally denuded of their tissue or damaged, the techniques of burying the testes in thigh pockets or covering them by skin flaps are indicated. If, however, the testes are covered by their own tissue and undamaged, the application of skin grafts is the preferable method of treatment.

Technically, the method of burying the testes in an upper thigh pocket is quite simple: through an oblique incision in the upper thigh, the testes and spermatic cord are buried in a pocket formed just under the skin; the pocket should be large enough to allow free mobility of the testes and avoid pressure. The testes should also be placed posteriorly in the thigh to prevent the stretching of the spermatic cord when the thighs are abducted. This method, however, may have serious physiologic consequences for normal

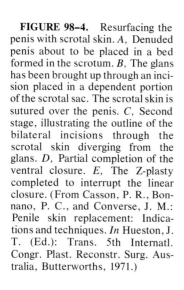

**FIGURE 98–4.** Resurfacing the penis with scrotal skin. *A,* Denuded penis about to be placed in a bed formed in the scrotum. *B,* The glans has been brought up through an incision placed in a dependent portion of the scrotal sac. The scrotal skin is sutured over the penis. *C,* Second stage, illustrating the outline of the bilateral incisions through the scrotal skin diverging from the glans. *D,* Partial completion of the ventral closure. *E,* The Z-plasty completed to interrupt the linear closure. (From Casson, P. R., Bonnano, P. C., and Converse, J. M.: Penile skin replacement: Indications and techniques. *In* Hueston, J. T. (Ed.): Trans. 5th Internatl. Congr. Plast. Reconstr. Surg. Australia, Butterworths, 1971.)

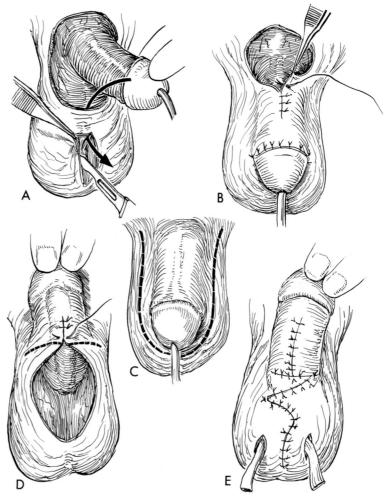

spermatogenesis if the testes are buried deep under the subcutaneous tissue. In studying the environmental temperature in the thighs and comparing it with that in the abdominal cavity, Huffman, Culp, Greenleaf, Flocks, and Brintnall (1956) demonstrated that the deep thigh and intra-abdominal temperatures were the same, while the superficial thigh temperature was similar to that of the normal scrotum. Consequently, they suggested that the testes should be buried in a plane superficial to the subcutaneous tissue, that is, just beneath the skin.

In forming the superficial skin pocket, it is of prime importance to undermine the skin in the proper subcutaneous plane and to make sure that the flap is of uniform thickness. This precaution is essential to avoid impairment of the vascularity of the skin and resulting necrosis.

In burying the testes, even minimal torsion of the spermatic cord should be avoided.

In view of its simplicity, this method, as an emergency procedure, can be performed by most surgeons. In many instances it is also a definitive operation, as the patients are usually satisfied with the result and request no further reconstruction of the scrotal sac. Huffman found that several patients so treated had normal sperm counts in terms of number, motility, and viability.

In cases of total avulsion of the skin of the scrotum and totally denuded testes, the design and transfer of skin flaps from the pubic region (Kubaček, 1957) or from the thigh (Douglas, 1951) are more complicated and are tedious procedures which should be performed only by experienced plastic surgeons.

Reconstruction of the scrotum by skin flaps as a secondary procedure, after the testes have been primarily buried in skin pockets (Whelan, 1944; Baxter, Hoffman, Smith and Stern,

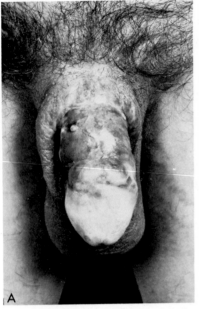
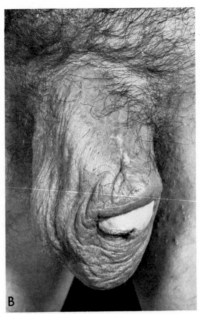
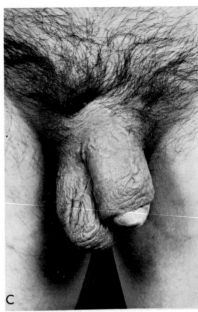

**FIGURE 98–5.** Scrotal resurfacing of the penis. *A,* Appearance of penis five years after radiotherapy for squamous cell epithelioma. *B,* Appearance of the penis in the scrotal tunnel four weeks after the first operation. *C,* Final appearance three months after the second stage. (From Casson, P. R., Bonnano, P. C., and Converse, J. M.: Penile skin replacement: Indications and techniques. *In* Hueston, J. T. (Ed.): Trans. 5th Internatl. Congr. Plast. Reconstr. Surg. Australia, Butterworths, 1971.)

1949; May, 1950; Gonzalez-Ulloa, 1963), requires multistaged operations and is justified only if the patient insists on a new scrotum.

Scrotal reconstruction by split-thickness skin grafts was first successfully performed by Balakrishnan (1956). This method should be used in cases in which there has been total avulsion of the scrotal skin but not of the enveloping tissues of the testes. Each testis with its spermatic funiculus may be covered separately with a one-piece split-thickness skin graft. The resulting bifid scrotum can later be joined by an operation performed under local anesthesia (Alton, 1963). The grafts are fixed by one of the techniques described above, and they are usually successful. Occasional small nonepithelized areas are treated by routine lavage with saline solution and dressed with Vaseline gauze. The initial contraction of the graft gradually loosens as it becomes smooth and elastic.

This method of treatment is especially suitable in cases in which the skin of the scrotum has been totally avulsed while the penis is undamaged, because the fixation of the grafts is then much simpler.

In a five-year follow-up of patients, Manchanda and coworkers (1967) and Balakrishnan (1956), who have so far treated the largest number of cases, found that spermatogenesis was normal in most patients. Possible sterility in some patients may be attributed to primary damage of the spermatic vessels with subsequent atrophy of the testes. In such cases, atrophy is inevitable irrespective of the surgical method used to resurface the testes.

**Complications.** In split-thickness skin grafting techniques, the most common complication is hematoma. In such cases, the affected section of the graft should be excised, the hematoma evacuated, and the raw surface regrafted within three to five days. For this purpose it is advisable to remove extra skin grafts and preserve them in an ordinary refrigerator, so that they may be applied should secondary grafting be necessary. When infection is present at the primary operation, a most infrequent occurrence (except when the patient's treatment has been delayed), the principles of delayed skin grafting should be applied (see Chapter 6).

Among late complications are persistent lymphedema and scar contracture. Lymphedema should be treated by excision of a rim of hypertrophic skin around the corona. Contractures of the graft occur most often in children, and in some cases regrafting of the penis is required at a later date. For this reason, the method of flaps or skin pockets may be preferable for covering the testes when the patients are children.

In the skin flap techniques, hematoma or partial necrosis may occur. In such instances, the necrotic skin should be excised and the remaining defect covered by a thin split-thickness skin graft.

In the skin pocket technique, severe compression of the testes may develop as a result of a collection of blood or serum. The early discovery of this complication and immediate evacuation of blood clots or serum are essential in order to prevent irreparable damage to the testes. Suction drainage will help to avoid this complication.

## RECONSTRUCTION OF THE PENIS

**Etiology.** Total loss of the penis is frequently of traumatic origin. Frumkin (1944) reported a number of wartime casualties during World War II in which loss of the penis was caused by gunshot or explosive wounds. Best, Angelo, and Mulligan (1962) reported a case of self-amputation in a mental patient. Julian, Klein, and Hubbord (1969) recorded loss of the penis due to severe thermal injury. Tagirov (1959) described three cases of loss of the penis in children, two of which were caused by pig bites; the third case was that of a boy whose penis had been cut off by another boy while playing games. Loss of the penis may also result from gangrene (Barclay and Hendrick, 1948; Hamm and Kanthor, 1949). However, most cases in which reconstruction of the penis is indicated involve patients who have undergone radical surgery for cancer (Gelb, Malament, and Loverme, 1959). Many of the patients are relatively young and do not, as a rule, develop metastases. Hence, reconstructive phalloplasty in these cases should certainly be considered on a much wider scale than has been the practice to date.

Of the twelve patients the author has treated, loss of the penis was due to sexual crime in five, to radical excision for cancer in six, and to gunshot wound in one.

The loss of the penis may be partial or total. Partial losses are mostly traumatic in origin and are often associated with scrotal and penile skin avulsion. In partial losses of the shaft, the reconstruction of a new penis is rarely indicated, as remnants of penile copora cavernosa may assure satisfactory coitus and micturition.

**History.** The first basic article on total reconstruction of the penis was published by Bogoraz (1936) and has since been repeatedly cited in the literature. Originally, Bogoraz unsuccessfully attempted to construct a penis by forming two tube skin flaps on the abdominal wall, one for the shaft and the other for the urethra. Later, he employed scrotal skin to construct the urethra. However, in reporting 16 cases of total reconstruction of the penis at the All-Soviet Congress (1938), he stated that he had constructed the urethra in only 10 cases.

In reconstructing the penis, most authors prefer to use an abdominal tube flap (Bogoraz, 1936; Frumkin, 1944; Maltz, 1946; Gillies, 1948; McIndoe, 1948; Majal, 1947; Thorek and Egel, 1949; Tagirov, 1959; Morgan, 1963; Arneri, 1959). Some authors favor tube flaps from the thighs (Cowan, 1944; Julian, Klein and Hubbord, 1969) or the scrotum (Goodwin and Scott, 1952; Morales, O'Connor and Hotchkiss, 1956).

The abdominal tube flap is best suited for construction of the penis, because it affords the best possibility of obtaining an acceptable appearance and of incorporating material for rigidity and a new urethra. If the abdominal skin is not available, the thigh is the next choice as a donor site for the tube flap; the scrotum is the least suitable donor site.

To achieve rigidity of the reconstructed penis, various materials have been used. Autogenous cartilage is most often reported in the literature (Bogoraz, 1936; Frumkin, 1944; Gillies, 1948; Chappell, 1953; Morgan, 1963), and some authors have used acrylic implants (Goodwin and Scott, 1952; Morales, O'Connor and Hotchkiss, 1956). Munawar (1957) incorporated a tibial periosteal bone graft, and Lash, Zimmerman, and Loeffler (1964) used silicone implants. Some authors did not implant any material (Majal, 1947; McIndoe, 1948; Farina and Freirre, 1954), claiming that fibrosis in the tube is sufficient to ensure a rigid penis. As may be concluded from a review of the literature, the best results were achieved with an autogenous cartilage graft. In most of the reported cases, acrylic implants were eventually rejected.

Orticochea (1972) has described a method for muscular control of the penis. This technique employs the gracilis muscle, whose neurovascular supply remains intact, to achieve erection.

In reconstruction of the penis, the formation of a new urethra is the most difficult aspect. Because of poor results, a number of surgeons did not attempt to construct a new urethral canal, being satisfied with a urethral orifice at the penoscrotal junction (Chappell, 1953; Munawar, 1957).

Various techniques have been used to construct an artificial urethral canal. The inlay skin graft technique suggested by McIndoe (1948) was used by Cowan (1944) on a mold and by Julian, Klein, and Hubbord (1969) on a silastic tube. Morales, O'Connor, and Hotchkiss (1956) employed a bladder mucosal graft, which resulted in failure, as did most of the inlay skin grafts; Best, Angelo, and Mulligan (1962) preferred a full-thickness skin graft inlay.

The use of scrotal skin for constructing an artificial urethra has also been reported by Frumkin (1944), Bergman, Howard, and Barnes (1948), and Goodwin and Scott (1952). The difficulties involved, however, were such as to make Frumkin state that no urethra could be successfully incorporated in the tube flap (quoted by Gillies, 1948). The idea of incorporating a skin canal in a tube flap to form the urethra was suggested for the first time by Maltz (1946) and successfully achieved by Gillies in 1948, who formed a "composite" tube flap which included a skin canal and a cartilage graft. This technique was favored by many authors (Huffman and coworkers, 1956; Morgan, 1963; Bishop and Villiers, 1967). Most of the authors claim good results in using the Gillies technique, although some failures have also been reported, such as the sloughing of the skin urethra (Evans, 1963, 1973), skin necrosis of the tube flap due to pressure of the incorporated cartilage (Morgan, 1963), and strictures. The Gillies technique does not place the meatal opening at the distal end of the reconstructed penis; instead, the urinary flow is from a meatus located on the ventral aspect of the glans. With the exception of the Gillies method, most of the reported procedures in producing an artificial urethra were complicated by fistulas, necrosis, and strictures, all of which greatly delayed the entire treatment.

The ability of self-conversion of a buried strip of skin into a skin canal is well known. In view of the results obtained with this technique in the construction of the urethra in the hypospadiac penis (Duplay, 1874; Marion and Pérard, 1942; Browne, 1949) and in view of the author's experience with the buried strip of skin in the construction of an artificial urethra and in the reconstruction of the skin-lined esophagus (Arneri, 1964), this method was applied for the construction of the urethra in the total or subtotal reconstruction of the penis.

**Total Reconstruction of the Penis: The Author's Technique.** Before undertaking the operation, certain conditions must be satisfied. *First,* the psychologic condition of the patient must be stabilized. Through an initial interview, the patient should be encouraged to cooperate during the whole period of treatment in order to establish confidence. He should be informed of the length of treatment and the multiple procedures involved. *Second,* the remaining external orifice of the urethra must allow free passage of the urine, which is a condition sine qua non for successful phalloplasty. Any preexisting strictures of the urethra must be relieved by surgical means. *Third,* remnant stumps of the corpora cavernosa must be present if a functional result is to be expected. In traumatic loss of the penis, the remaining corpora cavernosa are often buried among heavily scarred tissues, and in dissecting the scars, care must be taken to spare these structures. After radical surgery for cancer, only a static penis can be obtained. *Fourth,* the abdominal skin should be pliable and of good quality. Thick, rigid, and hairy skin is not suitable for reconstructive phalloplasty.

FIRST STAGE. By means of two parallel incisions made along previously marked lines on the hairless surface of the thoracoabdominal wall, a strip of skin 18 cm long and 3 cm wide is outlined (Fig. 98–6, *A*). When making the incisions, the mobile abdominal skin must be held firmly in place by the assistants.

The edges of the outlined strip are undermined over a few mm (Fig. 98–6, *B*). When the skin is being incised, the edges of the outlined strip should be slightly outwardly inclined in order to provide a wider base for the strip and thus ensure a better blood supply (Fig. 98–6, *C*). The next step is to raise two advancement flaps on both sides of the original skin strip. The undermining must be extensive in order to secure maximum mobility of the flaps. It is important to find the proper plane of cleavage so as to minimize bleeding. All bleeding points must be carefully controlled by electrocoagulation. The flaps are sutured together over the buried strip of skin in two layers by catgut (subcutaneous) sutures and by nylon (cutaneous) sutures (Fig. 98–6, *D*). The sutures of the flaps at the proximal and distal ends must include the subdermal edges of the skin strip (Fig. 98–6, *E*). In this way, a raw surface is avoided, and the edges of the skin strip tend to curl inward spontaneously.

The first stage of the reconstructive phalloplasty is completed by the application of a specially constructed apparatus at some distance from the suture lines. This apparatus (Fig. 98–6, *F*) reduces the tension on the suture lines, prevents the collection of blood and serum

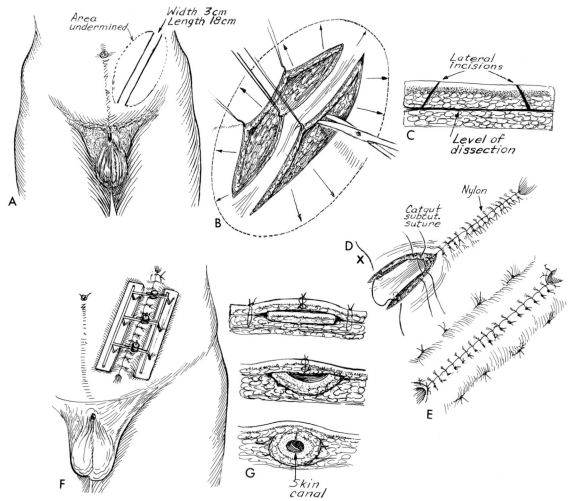

**FIGURE 98–6.** Reconstruction of the penis (first stage). *A*, A strip of skin 3 cm in width and 18 cm in length is outlined, and the skin lateral to the incisions is widely undermined. *B*, The edges of the outlined strip are undermined over a few millimeters to facilitate the curling of the strip upon itself. *C*, When the incisions outlining the buried strip are being made, the edges of the strip should be beveled outward in order to provide a wider base for the strip and thus ensure a better blood supply. *D*, The lateral advancement flaps are sutured together over the buried strip of skin. *E*, The sutures at the proximal and distal ends must include the subdermal edges of the buried skin strip, thus avoiding a raw area. *F*, A specially constructed apparatus is used to reduce tension. *G*, Diagrammatic illustration of the curling of the new skin canal.

under the flaps, and encourages the curling of the strip of skin and the epithelization of the new skin canal (Fig. 98–6, *G*). The apparatus consists of two metal bars which are connected by an articulator. It is fixed to the skin by adhesive tape, and the articulator is fastened by screws.

SECOND STAGE. The second stage is undertaken four to five weeks later. Within this time, the buried strip of skin has been fully converted into a skin canal, through which a Nélaton catheter (No. 24) is easily introduced (Fig. 98–7, *A*). The formation of the composite tube flap starts with an 18- to 20-cm incision on each side of the new skin canal. The distance between the two incisions should be approximately 10 to 12 cm.

In raising the bipedicle flap from the abdominal fascia, particular attention must be paid to the skin canal, which must be raised intact with the flap (Fig. 98–7, *B, C*). A cartilage graft is taken from the eighth and ninth ribs, on the right side of the thorax. The cartilage is carved in the shape of a pencil and fixed with chromic catgut along the length of the skin canal (Fig. 98–7, *B, C*).

The tube which is now formed represents the future penis, incorporating the skin canal for the urethra and the cartilage graft for rigidity (Fig. 98–7, *D, E*). It should be emphasized that the tube must be free of all tension; thus, in the initial planning, correct estimation of its size is of utmost importance. The secondary defect on the

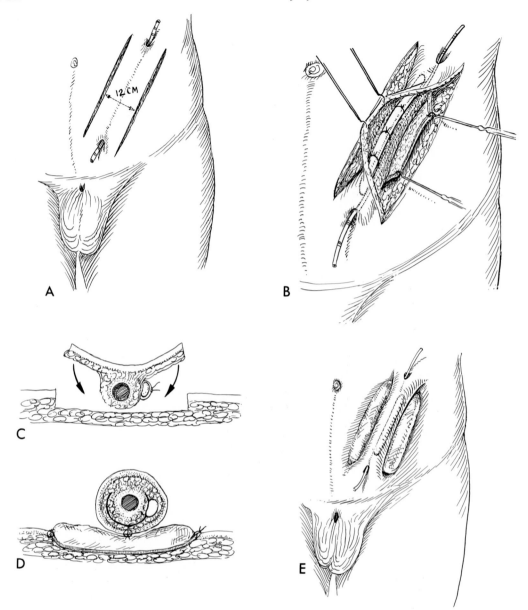

**FIGURE 98–7.** Reconstruction of the penis (second stage). *A*, Formation of the tube flap is initiated by parallel incisions 12 cm apart and 18 to 20 cm in length on each side of the new urethra. *B*, The flap is raised from the abdominal wall; the new urethra must be raised with the flap. The illustration shows a cartilage graft sutured along the length of the new urethra. *C*, Diagrammatic section showing the urethra raised with the skin flaps and the cartilage graft prior to tubing. *D*, Cross section illustrating the completed tubing. A split-thickness skin graft covers the resulting raw area and is maintained by a pressure dressing. *E*, The completed tube flap containing the new urethra and the cartilage graft.

abdominal wall is covered by a split-thickness skin graft (Fig. 98–7, *D*, *E*).

The sutures from the tube flap are removed between the tenth and twelfth days.

THIRD STAGE. The third stage requires attention to delicate surgical technique and should therefore not be undertaken before five to six weeks after the second stage in order to allow the tube to become fully stabilized. This operative stage starts with a perineal urethrotomy for the temporary diversion of the urine. The transposition of the tube to the stump of the penis is done by severing the upper end of the tube and joining it directly to the stump of the penis (Fig. 98–8, *A*). This is the usual procedure in most cases. However, if the tube is not sufficiently flexible, transfer is performed using the wrist as a carrier. The scars which usually cover the area of the amputated penis are excised, and the corpora cavernosa are meticulously dissected from the fibrous tissue (Fig. 98–8, *B*). The distal end of the original urethra

is freed from scars and mobilized to facilitate an end-to-end anastomosis with the skin urethra within the tube. The two corpora cavernosa are separated within the interseptum in order to avoid bleeding and obtain a suitable bed for the cartilage graft (Fig. 98–8, *C*). A similar procedure is performed on the divided end of the tube. The skin urethra within the tube is dis-

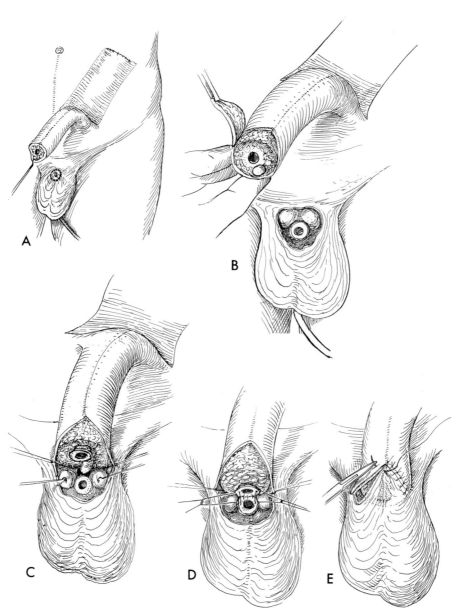

**FIGURE 98–8.** Reconstruction of the penis (third stage). *A,* Division and transfer of the tube flap to the penile stump. *B,* Removal of some skin from the surface of the tube flap. The corpora cavernosa and the urethra are skeletonized. *C,* Insertion of the cartilage graft between the separated corpora cavernosa. *D,* Anastomosis of the urethra and skin tube. *E,* Approximation of the skin edges.

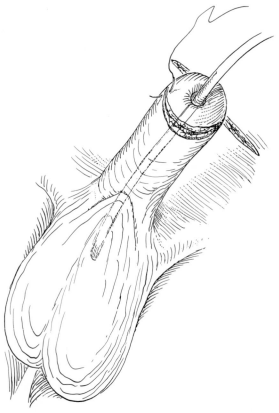

**FIGURE 98–9.** Reconstruction of the penis (fourth stage). Terminal end of the skin urethra is sutured to the edges of the tube flap. A glans is also fashioned from the distal end of the flap.

sected up to 1 cm, while the cartilage is freed for 2 cm in anticipation of final insertion into the composite tube. The end of the cartilage graft is first embedded between the separated corpora cavernosa and sutured into the interseptum with 4–0 chromic catgut (Fig. 98–8, *C*). This is followed by direct end-to-end anastomosis between the skin urethra and the original urethra (Fig. 98–8, *D*). Sutures of 4–0 chromic catgut are used for this purpose. The operation is completed by approximating the edges of the tube to the skin edges around the corpora cavernosa (Fig. 98–8, *E*). Subcutaneous suction drainage is employed for 24 hours. The sutures are removed after eight to ten days.

FOURTH STAGE. The last stage, which is also the simplest from a technical standpoint, is done four to five weeks later under local anesthesia. The abdominal or wrist end of the tube is divided. The edges of the terminal end of the skin urethra are sutured to the edges of the skin of the tube. The distal end of the new penis can be further shaped by excising redundant skin from the end of the tube (Fig. 98–9). The sutures are removed after eight days and the catheter from the perineal urethrotomy after 14 days.

RESULTS. In the evaluation of the functional results of the operative technique, it was found that erection occurred in four patients in whom remnants of corpora cavernosa had been preserved. The patients were able

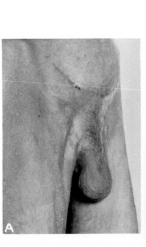

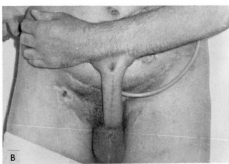

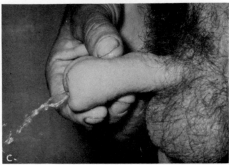

**FIGURE 98–10.** Reconstruction of the penis following radical excision for carcinoma. *A*, Appearance of patient following the radical excision. *B*, The tube containing the newly formed skin-lined urethra has been transported via the wrist. The wrist was used as a carrier because of the poor flexibility of the tube due to prior radiation treatment. *C*, Static penis obtained. Rigidity is provided by the cartilage graft. Photograph was taken ten years after reconstruction of the penis. Note the voiding of urine from the distal end of the reconstructed penis. As the corpora cavernosa had been excised, coitus was possible only by manual introduction of the penis.

to effect normal coitus penetration, and one reported having become a father. With respect to ejaculation, the patients reported that digital pressure was needed to void the sperm content. In cases in which remnants of the corpora cavernosa had not been preserved, as after radical excision for cancer, a static penis was obtained (Fig. 98–10, *A, B*). The psychologic effect, however, was satisfactory. The six patients who had penile reconstruction following ablative surgery for cancer were able to effect coitus by introducing the penis manually and to urinate in a normal way (Fig. 98–11, *C*).

Stimulation within the first two years derives principally from the remnants of the corpora cavernosa or the pubic area. In a follow-up of the patients for a period of up to 12 years, it was found that the sensibility of the terminal end of the new phallus, although not complete, was quite satisfactory.

The stream of urine through the new urethra, which is a little thinner in the first few months, gradually becomes thicker and is normal within one year. No dilation procedures were necessary in any of the author's twelve cases (Fig. 98–11).

In certain instances it may be necessary to

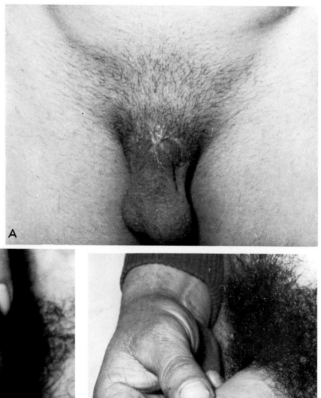

**FIGURE 98–11.** Reconstruction of the penis following amputation. *A,* Total loss of the penis as the result of a sexual crime. The corpora cavernosa were enmeshed in scarred tissue. There is an almost complete stricture of the external urethral orifice. *B,* Appearance of the reconstructed penis 14 years after reconstruction. Note the erection of the penis. *C,* The urine flows from the urethral opening situated at the distal end of the penis. Two years after the operation, the patient became the father of a male child.

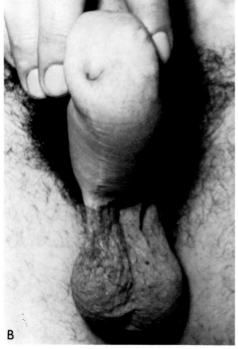

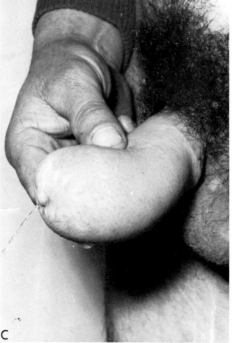

reconstruct the entire urethra as well as the penis. This is usually necessary only after the penis has been completely ablated for extensive invasive carcinoma. Bonanno and Converse (1975) reconstructed the penis in a 40 year old male who had extensive squamous cell carcinoma, which was treated by total resection of the penis and staged bilateral radical groin dissection. The patient was left with a perineal urethrostomy. The reconstruction, based upon the Arneri technique, was employed, with the addition of a midline scrotal tube to bridge the perineal orifice to the new urethra in the penis (Fig. 98–12).

**Replantation.** In special cases replantation of a cleanly divided penis should be attempted because of the well-known regenerative capacity of the corpora cavernosa.

The author has treated a patient in whom the amputated penis had been replanted one hour after the injury by a general surgeon, who had sutured the corpora cavernosa and the skin and had also anastomosed the blood vessels. Although the skin and the distal end of the urethra had sloughed (Fig. 98–13, *A, B*), the corpora cavernosa survived completely. The remaining granulating surface over the corpora cavernosa was successfully covered by a split-thickness

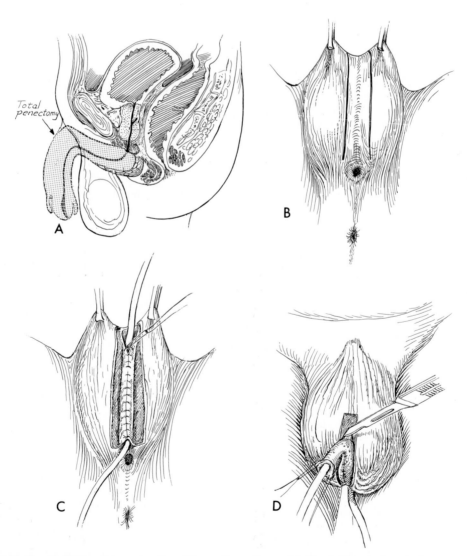

**FIGURE 98–12.**    Technique of reconstruction of the urethra using scrotal skin. *A,* Proposed urethral reconstruction in a patient who had undergone a total amputation of the penis and a perineal urethrostomy. *B,* Outline of the midline scrotal tube. *C,* Formation of the scrotal tube. *D,* One end of the tube is detached, and the tube is raised.

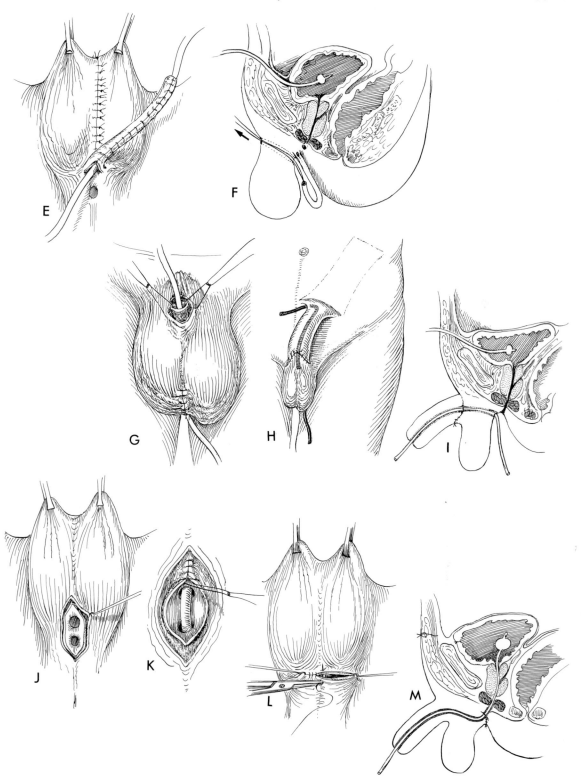

**FIGURE 98–12** *Continued.* *E,* The tube has been raised, being left attached at one end. *F,* Sectional view showing the introduction of the tube into the scrotum. *G,* After its passage through the scrotum, the skin of the new skin-lined urethra is anastomosed to the skin of the scrotum. *H,* The anastomosis of the scrotal tube with the penile urethra formed according to the Arneri technique. *I,* Sectional diagram illustrating partial restoration of the urinary tract. *J, K,* Anastomosis of the scrotal and perineal urethras. *L,* Skin closure. *M,* Sagittal view. (From Bonnano and Converse, 1975.)

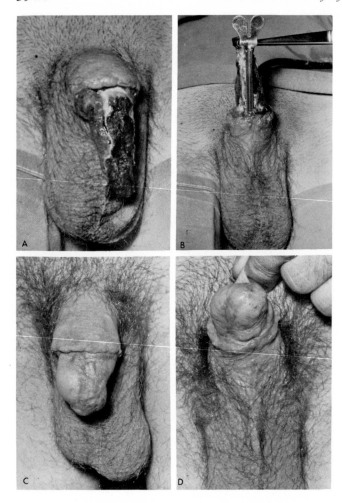

**FIGURE 98–13.** Replantation of the penis. *A*, Appearance following replantation. Note the sloughing of skin but preservation of the corpora cavernosa. *B*, Sloughing of the distal urethra. *C*, *D*, Result following resurfacing with a split-thickness skin graft.

skin graft, and a satisfactory functional penis was obtained (Fig. 98–13, *C, D*).

A similar case was reported by Best, Angelo and Mulligan (1962), who obtained the same result by simply suturing first the corpora cavernosa and then the skin, without attempting the anastomosis of the blood vessels.

Undoubtedly recent advances in microsurgical techniques should ensure total survival of the amputated penis. The successful clinical replantation of an amputated penis by microneurovascular repair has recently been reported (Cohen and associates, 1977). The midline superficial dorsal vein, the paired dorsal arteries, and two dorsal nerves were repaired.

**Complications.** Most of the complications reported in the literature are related to the construction of the artificial urethra, and the majority of cases involve sloughing, strictures, and fistulas. Consequently, many authors were discouraged from further attempts at making a new urethra.

In the author's series, the only complications were fistulas, which occurred in two of the twelve cases. Both fistulas were localized at the anastomosis between the artificial urethra and the original urethral stump. In one patient, a punctate fistula appeared on the seventh postoperative day but healed spontaneously within four weeks. In the second case, the fistula which appeared on the eighth day became well established, and a reanastomosis was necessary. This was successfully performed on the sixteenth day after the operation. During the entire period of treatment, the catheter was not removed from the urethrotomy.

No strictures were noted in any of the twelve cases of reconstructive phalloplasty, and hence no dilatation procedures were required. In none of our cases did rejection of cartilage occur, as has been reported in other techniques in which various implants were used.

Among other possible complications, disruptions of the wound or skin necrosis may occur; these are not specific for phalloplasty and are treated in the usual way.

## REFERENCES

Alton, J. D. McG.: Complete avulsion of the scrotum. *In* Broadbent, T. R. (Ed.): Transactions of the Third International Congress of Plastic Surgery, Oct. 13–18. Amsterdam, Excerpta Medica Foundation, 1963.

Arneri, V.: Phalloplasty (film). Presented at the Second International Society of Plastic Surgeons, London, 1959.

Arneri, V.: Reconstruction of skin oesophagus—A new method. Br. J. Plast. Surg., *17*:413, 1964.

Arneri, V.: Reconstruction of the Penis. II. *In* Horton, C. E. (Ed.): Plastic and Reconstructive Surgery of the Genital Area. Boston, Little, Brown & Company, 1973.

Arneri, V.: Reconstruction of the penis after loss of various etiology. Round Table, Sixth International Congress, Paris, 1975.

Balakrishnan, C.: Scrotal avulsion: A new technique of reconstruction by split-skin graft. Br. J. Plast. Surg., *9*:38, 1956.

Banham, A. R.: Total denudation of the penis. Br. J. Surg., *36*:268, 1948.

Barclay, L. T., and Hendrick, E. B.: Spontaneous gangrene of the scrotum, Fournier's gangrene. Plast. Reconstr. Surg., *3*:56, 1948.

Baxter, H., Hoffman, M., Smith, E., and Stern, K.: Complete avulsion of the skin of the penis and scrotum: Surgical, endocrinological, and psychological treatment. Plast. Reconstr. Surg., *4*:508, 1949.

Bergman, R. T., Howard, A. H., and Barnes, R. W.: Plastic reconstruction of the penis. J. Urol., *59*:1174, 1948.

Best, J. W., Angelo, J. J., and Mulligan, B.: Complete traumatic amputation of penis. J. Urol., *87*:134, 1962.

Bishop, B. W., and Villiers, W.: Report on a case of reconstruction of the penis. S. Afr. Med. J., *41*:750, 1967.

Bogoraz, N. A.: Ueber die volle plastische Wiedenherstellung eines zum Koitus fähigen Penis (from Russia). Zentralbl. Chir., *63*:1271, 1936.

Bonnano, P. C., and Converse, J. M.: Unpublished case report, 1975.

Browne, D.: An operation for hypospadias. Proc. R. Soc. Med., *42*:466, 1949.

Campbell, R. M.: Dermatome grafting of the totally denuded penis. Plast. Reconstr. Surg., *19*:509, 1957.

Casson, P. R., Bonnano, P. C., and Converse, J. M.: Penile skin replacement: Indications and techniques. *In* Hueston, J. T. (Ed.): Transactions of the Fifth International Congress of Plastic and Reconstructive Surgery, Feb. 22–26. Australia, Butterworths, 1971.

Chappell, B. S.: Utilization of the scrotum in reconstruction of the penis. J. Urol., *69*:703, 1953.

Cohen, B. E., May, J. W., Jr., Daly, J. S. F., and Young, H. H.: Successful clinical replantation of an amputated penis by microneurovascular repair. Plast. Reconstr. Surg., *59*:276, 1977.

Cottle, G. F.: Avulsion of scrotum, left testicle and sheath of penis. U. S. Naval Med Bull., *20*:457, 1924.

Cowan, R. J.: Total reconstruction of the penile urethra following a gunshot wound. Br. J. Plast. Surg., *17*:66, 1964.

Douglas, B.: One-stage reconstruction for traumatic denudation of the male external genitalia. Ann. Surg., *133*:889, 1951.

Duplay, S.: De l'hypospadias périnéo-scrotal et de son traitement chirurgical. Arch. Gén. Méd., *133*:657, 1874.

Evans, A. J.: Buried skin-strip urethra in a tube pedicle-phalloplasty. Br. J. Plast. Surg., *16*:280, 1963.

Evans, A. J.: Reconstruction of the penis. *In* Horton, C. E.: Plastic and Reconstructive Surgery of the Genital Area. Boston, Little, Brown and Company, 1973.

Farina, R., and Freire, G. de C.: Total reconstruction of the penis. Plast. Reconstr. Surg., *14*:351, 1954.

Ferris, D. O.: Traumatic avulsion of the skin of penis and scrotum. J. Urol., *62*:523, 1949.

Frumkin, A. P.: Reconstruction of the male genitalia. Ann. Rev. Soviet Med., *2*:14, 1944.

Gelb, J., Malament, M., and LoVerme, S.: Total reconstruction of the penis. Plast. Reconstr. Surg., *24*:62, 1959.

Gibbs, R. W.: A case where the entire scrotum and perineum together with one testicle and its cord attached and nearly all the integument of the penis were torn off. Recovery with preservation of sexual powers. Charleston Med. J. Rev., *10*:145, 1855.

Gibson, T.: Traumatic avulsion of the skin of the scrotum and penis: Use of the avulsed skin as a free graft. Br. J. Plast. Surg., *6*:283, 1954.

Gillies, H., and Harrison, R. J.: Congenital absence of the penis, with embryological considerations. Br. J. Plast. Surg., *1*:8, 1948.

Gonzalez-Ulloa, M.: Severe avulsion of the scrotum in a bullfighter: Reconstructive procedure. Br. J. Plast Surg., *16*:154, 1963.

Goodwin, W. E., and Scott, W. W.: Phalloplasty. J. Urol., *68*:903, 1952.

Hamm, W. G., and Kanthor, F. F.: Gangrene of the penis following circumcision with high frequency current. Plastic reconstruction of the penis. South. Med. J., *1*:1531, 1949.

Huffman, W. C., Culp, D. A., Greenleaf, J. S., Flocks, R. H., and Brintnall, E. S.: Injuries to the male genitalia. Plast. Reconstr. Surg., *18*:344, 1956.

Julian, R., Klein, M., and Hubbord, H.: Management of the thermal burn with amputation and reconstruction of the penis. J. Urol., *101*:580, 1969.

Kubaček, V.: Complete avulsion of skin of penis and scrotum. Br. J. Plast. Surg., *10*:25, 1957.

Lash, H., Zimmerman, D. C., and Loeffler, R. A.: Silicone implantation: Inlay method. Plast. Reconstr. Surg., *34*:75, 1964.

Majal, V. S.: New method for restoration of the penis. Khirurgia (Bucur), *2*:85, 1947.

Maltz, M.: Evolution of Plastic Surgery. New York, Frobin Press, 1946, p. 278.

Manchanda, R. L., Singh, R., Keswani, R. K., and Sharma, C. G.: Traumatic avulsion of scrotum and penile skin. Br. J. Plast. Surg., *20*:97, 1967.

McIndoe, A.: Deformities of the male urethra. Br. J. Plast. Surg., *1*:34, 1948.

Marion, G., and Pérard, J.: Technique des Opérations Plastiques sur la Vessie et sur L'Uretre. Paris, Masson et Cie, 1942.

May, H.: Reconstruction of scrotum and skin of the penis. Plast. Reconstr. Surg., *6*:134, 1950.

Morales, P. A., O'Connor, J. J., and Hotchkiss, R. S.: Plastic reconstructive surgery after total loss of the penis. Am. J. Surg., *92*:403, 1956.

Morgan, B. L.: Total reconstruction of the penis in an eleven year old boy. Plast. Reconstr. Surg., *4*:467, 1963.

Moustafa, M. F. H.: Gangrene of the scrotum: An analysis of ten cases. Br. J. Plast. Surg., *20*:90, 1967.

Munawar, A.: Surgical treatment of the male genitalia. J. Int. Coll. Surg., *27*:352, 1957.

Orticochea, M.: A new method of total reconstruction of the penis. Br. J. Plast. Surg., *25*:347, 1972.

Owens, N.: Reconstruction for traumatic denudation of the penis and scrotum. Surgery, *12*:88, 1942.

Salvatierra, O., Bucklew, W. B., and Morrow, J. W.:

Penetrating ureteral injuries. Surg. Gynecol. Obstet., *128*:591, 1969.

Santoni-Rugiu, P.: Possilita della chirurgia ricostructiva nei traumi peno-scrotum. Minerva Chir., *21*:20, 1966.

Tagirov, K. K.: Plastic operation connected with the loss of the penis. Khirurgiya, 7:122, 1958; *13*:4150, 1959.

Thorek, P., and Egel, P.: Reconstruction of the penis with a split-thickness skin graft. Plast. Reconstr. Surg., *4*:469, 1949.

Whelan, E.: Repair of the avulsed scrotum. Surg. Gynecol. Obstet., *78*:649, 1944.

## ADDITIONAL REFERENCES

Agostinelli, E.: Note di falloplastica. A proposito di un caso di strappamento della cute del pene a dello scroto. II Policlinico (Sez. Pratica), *46*:1303, 1939.

Ahmad, S.: Cut penis: A short case of reconstruction. Br. J. Plast. Surg., *14*:59, 1961.

Bagozzi, I. C.: Reconstruction du scrotum et des téguments du pénis avulsé par lésion traumatique. Minerva Chir., *14*:1133, 1959.

Bean, L. I.: Skin grafted penis. U.S. Naval Med. Bull., *47*:715, 1947.

Bessel-Hagen: Ueber plastische Operationen bei volhommenen Verluste der Hautbeckungen am Penis and Scrotum. Verh. Dtsch. Ges. Chir., 733, 1901.

Blum, V.: A case of plastic restoration of the penis. J. Mt. Sinai Hosp., *4*:506, 1938.

Borges, A.: Reconstruccion del pene con piel de escroto. Rev. Lat. Am. Cir. Plast., *1*:43, 1953.

Bramann, F., and Ramnsted, C.: Lesioni traumatiche del pene. *In* German, E.: Trattato di chirurgia plastica. Soc. Ed. Libraria Milano, *4*:602, 1909.

Brown, J. B., and Fryer, M. P.: Surgical reconstruction of the penis. G. P., *17*:104, 1958.

Bruner, J.: Traumatic avulsion of the skin of the external male genitalia. Plast. Reconstr. Surg., *6*:334, 1950.

Byars, L. T.: Avulsion of the scrotum and skin of the penis. Technique of delayed and immediate repair. Surg. Gynecol. Obstet., *77*:326, 1943.

Cafer Tayyar Kankat: Traumatic total loss of the penis; Plastic reconstruction by the author's method. Turk Tip Cemiy. Mecm., *8*:549, 1954.

Clarkson, P.: Problems in penile reconstruction. Guy's Hosp. Rep., *9*:2750, 1955.

Colmer, F.: Ueber Plastische Operationen am Penis nach Zerstorungen seiner Hautbedeckunge. Arch. Klin. Chir., 65, 1901.

Conley, J. J.: One-stage operation for the repair of the denuded penis and testicles. New York J. Med., *56*:3014, 1956.

Cullen, T. H.: Avulsion of the skin of the penis and scrotum. Br. J. Urol., *38*:99, 1966.

Culp, D. A., and Huffman, W. C.: Temperature determination in the thigh with regard to burying the traumatically exposed testis. J. Urol., *76*:436, 1956.

Davis, A. D., and Berner, R. E.: Primary repair of total avulsion of the skin from the penis and scrotum. Plast. Reconstr. Surg., *3*:417, 1948.

Derdoy, J. B.: Traumatic avulsion of the skin of the penis and scrotum. Rev. Argent. Urol., *30*:133, 1961.

Dexelmann, F.: Ueber einen Fall von Isolierter Skalpierung des Penis und Scrotum. Zentralbl. Chir., *2*:760, 1932.

Diffenbach, J. F.: Die operative Chirurgie. Leipzig, 1845.

El-Masri, D.: Polyethylene prosthesis of the corpora cavernosa of the penis. J. Med. Liban, 5:365, 1965.

Esser, J. F.: Use of preputial skin in "structive" surgery. J. Int. Coll. Surg., 7:469, 1944.

Ewell, G. H.: Avulsion traumatique de la peau du pénis et du scrotum. J. Int. Coll. Surg., *19*:207, 1953.

Frocks, R. H., and Culp, D. A.: Surgical Urology. Chicago, Year Book Medical Publishers, 1954.

Gaisford, J. C., and Hanna, D. C.: Reconstruction of the penis. Plast. Reconstr. Surg., *3*:277, 1965.

Gelbke, H.: Penishautplastiken. Zentralbl. Chir., *79*:935, 1954.

George, P.: Un cas d'avulsion traumatic complète de la peau du pénis et du scrotum. Presse Med., *53*:2581, 1962.

Henninger, H.: Erfolge und Misserfolge plastischer Operationen bei Totalverlust des Penis. Z. Urol., *44*:146, 1951.

Hiklova-Sera, D., and Wondrak,: Contributions au traitement primaire de la perte traumatique de la peau des organes genitaux chez l'homme. Zentralbl. Chir., *84*:1127, 1939.

Ilyinsky, V.: Zur Frage der plastischen Operationen, am mannlichen Gliede. Chirurgya, 1937, 142; rip. Im. Z. O. f. D. Gesamte Chir., Vol. 86,583.

Jacobs, F. M., and Berry, J. L.: Reconstruction of the scrotum, a new use for the prepuce. J. Urol., *61*:956, 1949.

Joseph, K. C.: Skin graft for the scrotum—Antiseptic. Madras, *46*:55, 1949.

Judd, E., and Havens, E.: Traumatic avulsion of skin of penis and scrotum. Am. J. Surg., *62*:246, 1945.

Kearns, W.: Testicular transplantation. Ann. Surg., *114*:886, 1941.

Kendall, A. R., and Karafin, L.: Repair of the denuded penis. J. Urol., *98*:653, 1967.

Kenny, T. B., and Morello, M.: Asportazioni traumatiche delle cute del pene e dello scroto. Prensa Med. Argent., *15*:1549, 1929.

Loeffler, R. A., and Soyegh, E. S.: Perforated acrylic implants in the management of organic impotence. J. Urol., *84*:559, 1960.

Malbec, E. F., and Quaife, J. V.: Avulsion of the scrotum and skin of the penis. Plast. Reconstr. Surg., *22*:535, 1958.

Mamanov, G. L.: Une méthode pour la conservation du testicule dans le cas de perte complète du scrotum, d'origine traumatique. Khirurgiia (Mosk.), *35*:127, 1959.

Marberger, H., and Wilflingseder, P.: Plastische Eingriffe bei Verletzungen des ausseren Genitales. Klin. Med. (Wien), *21*:373, 1966.

Meyer, I. I.: Phalloplastik nach schindung. Arch. Orthop. Chir., *27*:437, 1929.

Millard, D. R.: Scrotal construction and reconstruction. Plast. Reconstr. Surg., *38*:10, 1966.

Moore, C. R.: Physiology of the testis. J.A.M.A., *116*:1638, 1941.

Mukin, M. V.: Total plastic reconstruction of the penis and urethra. Vestn. Khir. Grekov. (Mosk.), 5:5888, 1951.

Mukin, M. V.: Total phalloplasty. Kirov Milit. Med. Acad. Leningrad. Chir. Plast., *2*:130, 1968.

Neumann, A.: Sulla plastica del pene. Rev. Med del Rosario, *22*:292, 1949.

Patania, A.: Les opérationes plastiques dans les pertes de revètement cutane du pénis et du scrotum. Minerva Chir., *4*:391, 1949.

Penn, J.: Penile reform. Br. J. Plast. Surg., *16*:3, 1963.

Pfeiffer, D., and Miller, D.: Traumatic avulsion of the

skin of the penis and scrotum. Plast. Reconstr. Surg., 5:520, 1950.

Prokhorov, J. M.: Remote results of plastic surgery of skin avulsion of the penis and scrotum. Urologiia (Mosk.), 27:63, 1962.

Robertson, J.: Avulsion and reconstruction of scrotum and penis. South. Med. Surg., 93:527, 1931.

Robinson, D., Stephenson, K., and Padgett, E.: Loss of coverage of the penis, scrotum and urethra. Plast. Reconstr. Surg., 1:58, 1946.

Robinson, D., Stephenson, K., and Padgett, E.: Surface losses of the scrotum, penis and urethra. Plast. Reconstr. Surg., 2:378, 1947.

Roth, R. B., and Warren, K. W.: Traumatic avulsion of skin of penis and scrotum. J. Urol., 52:162, 1944.

Rowan, R. L.: Etheron sponge dressing for skin grafting penis. J. Urol., 93:709, 1965.

Russe, O.: Plastie cutanée de l'appareil génital masculin. Chirurgie, 23:270, 1952.

Saravia, C. E.: Operazioni plastiche sulla copertura del pene e dello scroto, specialmente nelle lesioni traumatiche. Rev. Chir. (Buenos Aires), 6:662, 1927.

Sawhney, C. P.: Management of the urethra following total amputation of the penis. Br. J. Urol., 39:405, 1967.

Silveira, L. M.: Total avulsion of the skin of the penis and scrotum. Rev. Paul. Med., 62:313, 1963.

Snyder, C. C.: Restoration of the skin of the male external genitalia following trauma. Am. Surg., 18:806, 1952.

Sung, R. Y.: Reconstruction of the genitalia. Chin. Med. J., 6:446, 1954.

Sutton, L. E.: Reconstruction following complete avulsion of the skin of penis and scrotum (case). N. Y. State J. Med., 43:2279, 1943.

Takashima, R., and Kusano, M.: Ueber einen Fall von totalem defekt der Penishaut durch Machine. Zentralbl. Chir., 1:84, 1936.

Thierry, W.: Ein Fall von Totalgangran des scrotum und der Penishaut. Munch. Klin. Wochenschr., 66:937, 1919.

Torres, G. A., and Osacar, E. M.: Avulsion of the skin of the penis and scrotum: Reparative genitoplasty. Bol. Trab. Soc. Cir. Cordoba, 7:225, 1946.

Veseen, L. L., and O'Neill, C. E.: Plastic operation on the penis. J. Urol., 30:375, 1933.

Watson, J.: Skin loss on scrotum: Repair by skin grafts. Br. J. Plast. Surg., 8:33, 1956.

Wetherell, F.: Loss of scrotum integument: Simple method of repair. Surgery, 18:525, 1945.

# CHAPTER 99

# ABNORMALITIES OF THE EXTERNAL FEMALE GENITALIA

### RICHARD BOIES STARK, M.D.

Vaginal Reconstruction Following
Ablative Surgery by Gracilis
Myocutaneous Flaps
*John B. McCraw, M.D.,*
*and Fred M. Massey, M.D.*

Congenital absence of the vagina was found by Counseller (1948) to account for 1:4000 female admissions to the Mayo Clinic. Of the 41 cases which he evaluated, only 20 had normal urinary tracts. The other 21 patients had a variety of anomalies, including absence of one kidney, ectopia of a solitary kidney, horseshoe kidney, and duplication of the ureter.

In addition, the uterus may be atrophic, infantile, or bicornuate, and there may be associated rectovesical or rectoperineal fistula. The ovaries are ordinarily unaffected, so that the secondary sexual characteristics—libido, breast development, vaginal introitus, and triangular pubic hair pattern—are normal. TeLinde (1962) has stated, "In our personal experience we have never seen a woman with a congenital absence of the vagina who was not typically feminine physically."

### HISTORICAL ASPECTS

The first report of vaginal agenesis was by Realdus Columbus, successor to Vesalius, in

1573. Skin flaps from the labia or inner thigh have been used by Heppner (1872), Abbé (1898), Beck (1900), and Graves (1908), all of whom had indifferent success, and by Frank and Geist (1927), whose "satchelhandle" tube flap proved to be too complicated.

Segments of the gastrointestinal tract have also been utilized. Sneguireff (1904), Popow (1910), Schubert (1914), and Conway and Stark (1953) all used the rectum, while Baldwin (1904) employed a loop of ileum. These procedures were associated with significant morbidity and mortality and were complicated by prolapse and/or disagreeable mucosal secretions.

Frank and Geist (1927) attempted to produce a lined vaginal cavity using graduated test tube conformers with a pulsion force exerted against the perineum. Wharton (1938) dissected a vaginal canal and attempted to maintain its patency with an obturator while it became spontaneously epithelialized. Counseller (1948) used this technique in 14 cases.

In a married patient with absence of the vagina, Abbé (1898) grafted the dissected neovaginal canal with "Thiersch skin grafts" placed cut surface outward over a condom stuffed with iodoform gauze. The mold was removed after ten days; Abbé reported, "The grafts had taken universally." Postoperatively, the patient continued to wear a wax candle conformer. Abbé concluded that the operation had "fulfilled at least one of its functions—giving gratification to the mated couple." McIndoe (1950) incorrectly reported that "the results were unimpressive."

A solution to the problem similar to Abbé's was popularized by McIndoe, beginning in 1937 and culminating in his report of 63 cases over the ensuing 12 years. Counseller (1948), who followed the McIndoe technique, reported the successful use of the skin graft technique in 70 patients.

## PATHOGENESIS

The female external genitalia may be said to represent those of the male with arrested development. This is true, since the genital development of both sexes is identical until the third month of intrauterine life.

In the embryologic differentiation of the external genitalia, each embryo develops with a pair of internal ducts, one of which will potentially produce male ducts (the wolffian system, developing into the epididymis, vas deferens, seminal vesicles, and ejaculatory duct) and one of which will potentially produce female ducts (the müllerian system, developing into the fallopian tubes, uterus, and vagina). With development, the ducts of the opposite sex become rudimentary. The uterus begins at the second month as paired structures—the müllerian ducts—from which the fallopian tubes and vagina also arise.

Although the double-barreled uterus rarely persists at birth, the usual, indeed the expected, development consists of polarization and death of cells of the intervening septum, thus uniting the two cavities into a single channel. The cervix and vagina, initially solid in form, become hollow by the process of polarization and cell death. As the cavity burrows toward the pubic surface, the urogenital sinus—which is well on its way toward becoming the vaginal vestibule—becomes more concave until only a cluster of cells, called the müllerian tubercle, remains to divide the two approaching tunnels. The müllerian tubercle persists after birth as the hymen, one of the few branchial membranes (like the tympanic membrane) to remain.

Abnormalities of the müllerian system include a Y-shaped fundic uterine cavity; double cavities; Y-shaped bicornuate uterus; bicornuate uterus with two cavities; a double uterus with double vagina (as is the case in marsupials); a bicornuate uterus, one horn of which is rudimentary; atresia of the fallopian tube; cervical atresia; and agenesis of the vagina.

## THERAPY

With the popularization by McIndoe (1937) of partial thickness grafts of skin for lining of the neovaginal canal, the use of other tissues which were associated with more hazard and less likelihood of success (intestinal conduit, hernia sac, peritoneum, vaginal labia, amniotic membrane) waned. McIndoe had extrapolated the principle of the Esser oral inlay graft to another structure. He recognized the need for absolute hemostasis and prolonged dilation of the graft during the period of postoperative contraction. In all of these matters, McIndoe was echoing, with an impressive series of cases, Abbé's discovery of the feasibility of using partial thickness skin for lining the vagina; if it were obturated, it would serve its connubial function. The procedure commonly employed today should be termed the Abbé-McIndoe operation.

Significantly, the widespread acceptance of this procedure coincided with the development of simplified instruments with which one could predictably obtain large sheets of partial thickness skin (dermatomes, guarded knives, and so forth).

The optimum time, indeed the only time, to perform construction of the vagina is prior to sexual initiation. Failure to obturate the neovagina first by a mold and then by intercourse will cause the cavity to shrink to obliteration.

## OPERATIVE TECHNIQUE

The operation is performed with the patient in the lithotomy position. The author prefers to use the abdomen, between the umbilicus and the pubic hair, as the donor site for the skin graft. The graft is removed with a precision drum dermatome (Reese) at a calibration of 0.014 inch. This technique provides a graft 8 by 4 inches with a dermal thickness which assures resilience. The donor site, if properly managed, will usually heal without incident.

Landmarks for dissection of the vaginal canal are flagged by placing a sound in the urethra and a doubly gloved finger in the rectum. A saline-epinephrine solution (1:100,000) is injected into the intervening space so as to promote hemostasis and vascularization of the skin transplant.

An incision in the shape of an X is made within the introitus, avoiding clitoris and urethra (Fig. 99–1, *A*). The vaginal canal is easily and safely formed by blunt scissors and finger dissection (Fig. 99–1, *B*). Any visible bleeding points are electrocoagulated. The canal is packed with a saline-epinephrine–soaked sponge.

The graft may be transplanted to the side walls of the cavity in one of two ways. The first utilizes a mold cast of the new cul-de-sac. Dental compound, a material made up of several waxes, becomes soft when heated in warm water. Several pieces of the compound are needed and, when soft, are pushed into the cavity and held until a firm mold is formed.

The mold is painted with dermatome cement. The skin graft is wrapped around the mold, the dermal surface outward. The margins of the graft are sutured with fine chromic catgut, so that the mold is completely covered with skin. The mold with graft is inserted into the cavity (Fig. 99–1, *C*), and the labia minora are sutured loosely together using horizontal mattress sutures tied over boluses to facilitate removal.

The second method of transplanting the graft to the cavity is to suture the graft together, dermal surface outward, in a form to simulate the vaginal canal. The graft is advanced over a vaginal speculum which is placed in the new channel, and the graft is meticulously filled with vaginal packing so that the graft is in intimate juxtaposition with the walls of the neovagina. The labia are sutured so as to secure the graft against the cavity walls without movement.

The patient is kept at absolute bed rest with the foot of the bed elevated to minimize premature extrusion of the mold. A constipating regimen is prescribed.

At the end of a week, the labial sutures and the mold or packing are removed. After this interval

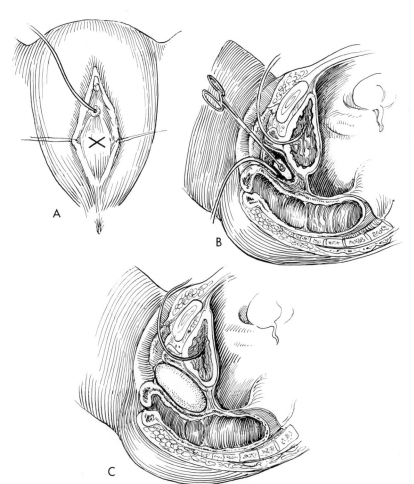

**FIGURE 99–1.** *A,* Incision in the shape of an X within the introitus, avoiding the clitoris and urethra. *B,* Vaginal canal formed by blunt dissection. *C,* Skin graft–covered mold in the vaginal canal.

of time, the graft should be adherent to the side walls of the cavity, and the mold can be removed without difficulty. The neovagina is irrigated with saline and inspected using a speculum. If small areas exist where the graft has been unsuccessful (usually over a hematoma), these will produce hillocks of granulations which must be cauterized with silver nitrate sticks to facilitate epithelization. The patient is placed on a twice-daily douche and Sitz bath regimen.

A vaginal mold must be worn constantly to prevent obliteration of the cavity. The heavier dental compound mold is replaced by a lighter one. The author favors a mold of similar size fashioned of balsa wood surfaced with a condom. This can be worn without discomfort, eliminating the danger of erosion by a heavier object through the rectovaginal septum.

Other types of molds have been used in the past: acrylic, Pyrex glass, and condoms filled with cotton. Braley (1971) advocated the use of molds made from silicone rubber mix after a prototype is cast in dental stone. The silicone rubber mold can be made in the operating room and can also be used to prevent contraction of the neovagina, even after successful vascularization of the skin grafts. Castañares (1963) felt the soft mold must be worn day and night for the first three months and only at night for an additional three months.

Shortly after epithelization is complete, coitus is permitted. Skin transplanted into the vaginal tract soon appears like mucosa, and normal cyclical changes have been reported to occur.

Steffanoff (1973) reported the development of a squamous cell carcinoma in the skin graft site 20 years following the construction of a neovaginal vault.

# RECONSTRUCTION OF THE EXTERNAL FEMALE GENITALIA

The occurrence of ambiguous external genitalia is seen in one of every 30,000 births. The condition may occur in a genetic female virilized by androgens (female pseudohermaphrodite); in a male pseudohermaphrodite; in a true hermaphrodite; or in asymmetric gonadal dysgenesis (see Chapter 100).

In the diagnosis of a female pseudohermaphrodite, the sex must first be verified. Virilization and the pathogenic factor or factors must also be considered. The timing and method of reconstruction are the last factors to be considered.

Verification of the sex involves buccal smears (presence of chromatin bodies in more than 30 per cent of cells); karyotype; gonadal biopsy; 24-hour urine specimens for 17-ketosteroids and pregnanediol; and examination of the upper and lower urinary tracts (urethroscopy, cystourethrogram, intravenous pyelogram).

The question of ongoing virilization can be answered by measuring titers of circulating androgens or their excretion products. If increased urinary levels are not present, virilization is due to exogenous androgens usually iatrogenically administered to prevent premature birth. In this situation, the source is self-limited, and the ambiguity of the external female genitalia must be corrected.

In the case of the genetic female, prevention is the crux of the matter. Progestational compounds with the basic steroid molecule containing 21 carbon atoms (C–21) will support the pregnancy without being androgenic; this is not true of C–18, C–19, or C–19 #1 compounds, which should not be used because of their ineffectiveness in treating threatened abortion and because of their virilizing effect.

While the use of exogenous androgens is the major cause of ambiguous female external genitalia, a virilizing tumor in the mother is not uncommon. If circulating androgens are present in the infant or child, they are commonly due to the adrenogenital syndrome, resulting from either a virilizing tumor or congenital hyperplasia of the adrenals. Such a cause must be corrected before genital reconstruction is undertaken.

It is necessary, if normal psychosexual behavior patterns are to be established, that complete reconstruction of the external genitalia be accomplished in the preschool period.

Treatment of female pseudohermaphroditism may consist of construction of the vagina with subtotal amputation of the clitoris, prepuce, and labia minora.

In reducing the elongated clitoris, a subtotal wedge resection of the corpus proximal to the tip will preserve sensation. An excessive prepuce should be trimmed appropriately as one would perform a circumcision. The labia minora may resemble redundant leaves; they should be marginally resected and sutured with fine catgut, leaving a normal wishbone configuration about the clitoris.

The treatment of intersex problems is also discussed in Chapter 100.

# Vaginal Reconstruction Following Ablative Surgery by Gracilis Myocutaneous Flaps

JOHN B. McCRAW, M.D.,
AND FRED M. MASSEY, M.D.

Reconstruction of a functional vagina following vaginectomy remains an unsolved surgical problem. The abdominoperineal resection and total pelvic exenteration usually leave patients with crippling defects that are associated with prolonged healing and inadequate vaginal function.

Ideally, vaginal reconstruction should provide immediate anatomical restoration and primary healing at the time of tumor resection. The neovagina must have the desirable characteristics of sensibility, softness, pliability, and durability. The biologic donor tissue should be expendable and transferrable, with minimal morbidity and without any life-threatening risk to the patient. These criteria can be satisfied by using gracilis island myocutaneous flaps.

The concept that skin is sustained, primarily, by its underlying muscle, has been applied only recently. Owens (1955) and Bakamjian (1963) pioneered the clinical application of compound myocutaneous flaps by using the sternocleidomastoid muscle and its overlying skin to repair defects of the cheek and palate, respectively. Subsequently, pectoralis (Hueston and McConchie, 1968), trapezius (Des Prez, Kiehn and Eckstein, 1971), latissimus dorsi (Orticochea, 1972) and gracilis myocutaneous flaps have been employed. All of the authors recognized the principle of a certain cutaneous dependence upon the underlying muscle. None of the authors recognized a "primary" island myocutaneous flap as an integral skin-muscle unit that is totally supported by a single muscle neurovascular pedicle. When elevated as a compound flap,

this discrete and definable area of skin and muscle will survive without any delay procedure, because its blood supply is essentially unchanged. This concept allows the surgeon to use "primary" island gracilis myocutaneous flaps for total vaginal reconstruction. The operative technique has been described by McCraw, Massey, Shanklin and Horton (1976).

Myocutaneous flaps are also discussed in Chapters 6 and 86.

## CASE REPORTS

A 54 year old Caucasian female underwent resection of a Bartholin's gland carcinoma, including two-thirds vaginectomy, radical vulvectomy, and bilateral inguinal node dissections. The vulvar defect was closed using local flaps, and the hemivaginal reconstruction was accomplished using a unilateral gracilis island myocutaneous flap (Fig. 99–2). All wounds healed primarily, and within a three-month period the patient resumed normal vaginal function (Fig. 99–3). While prolapse of the bladder is a common complication following radical ablative vaginal surgery, muscular reconstitution of the pelvic floor by the myocutaneous flap technique apparently prevented this complication.

A 46 year old Caucasian female underwent radical hysterectomy and total vaginectomy for carcinoma of the cervix following irradiation therapy. Vaginal reconstruction, using

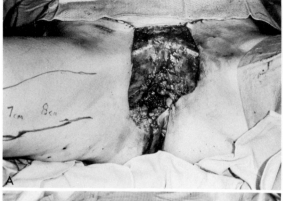

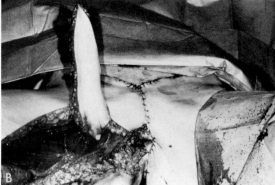

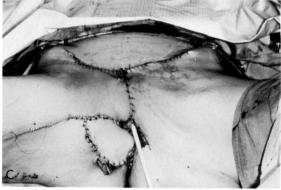

**FIGURE 99–2.** *A,* Operative defect following hemivaginectomy, radical vulvectomy, and bilateral inguinal node dissections. Note the outlined myocutaneous flap along the medial aspect of the right thigh. *B,* Unilateral gracilis island myocutaneous flap elevated. *C,* Primary closure of the perineal defects.

split-thickness skin grafts, was attempted but failed completely (Fig. 99–4, *A*). Elective total vaginal reconstruction with bilateral island gracilis myocutaneous flaps was accomplished (Fig. 99–4, *B* to *D*). A large pocket was developed between the remaining bladder and rectum, and the wounds were primarily closed (Fig. 99–4, *E*). After a four-month period, the patient experienced completely normal vaginal function (Fig. 99–4, *F, G*).

## COMPLICATIONS

The common complications of prolonged healing, pelvic abscesses, and dramatic interstitial fluid shifts (related to the pelvic burn) were not seen in any of the 26 patients who underwent partial or total vaginal reconstruction by the myocutaneous flap technique. Several significant complications did occur, and these included:

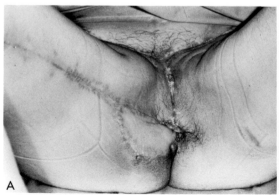

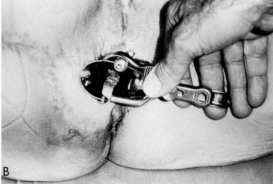

**FIGURE 99–3.** Patient shown in Figure 99–2. *A, B,* Two months postoperatively.

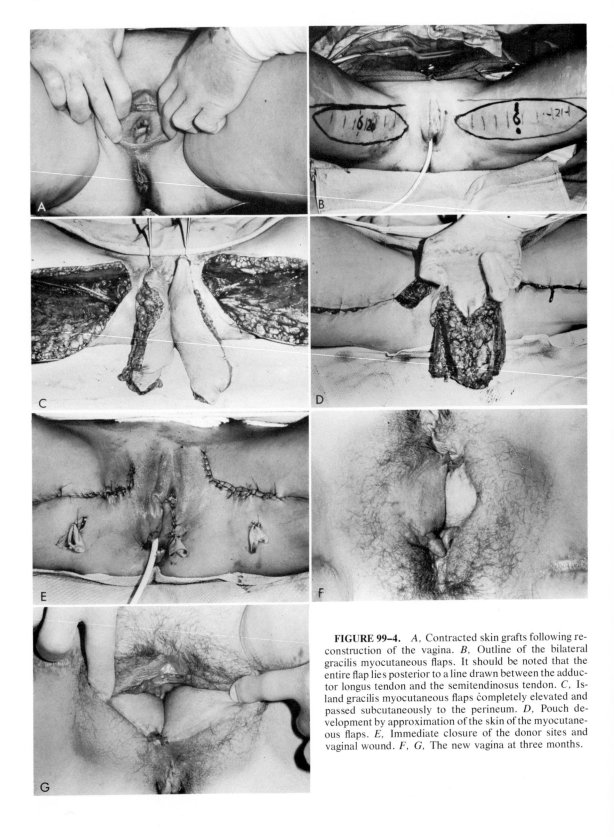

**FIGURE 99–4.** *A,* Contracted skin grafts following reconstruction of the vagina. *B,* Outline of the bilateral gracilis myocutaneous flaps. It should be noted that the entire flap lies posterior to a line drawn between the adductor longus tendon and the semitendinosus tendon. *C,* Island gracilis myocutaneous flaps completely elevated and passed subcutaneously to the perineum. *D,* Pouch development by approximation of the skin of the myocutaneous flaps. *E,* Immediate closure of the donor sites and vaginal wound. *F, G,* The new vagina at three months.

1. A pulmonary embolus was sustained by one patient who had preexisting venous hypertensive disease. This resolved without difficulty.

2. Partial necrosis of the flaps occurred in several patients, but this was related to poor flap design. When the flaps are adequately designed and viability is determined by using fluorescein, the problem of flap necrosis should be obviated.

3. Hematoma and infection were common and were related to the susceptibility of perineal fat to infection. All of the infections were low-grade and subsided with conservative therapy. In none of the cases was it necessary to open widely the leg or the pelvic wound for drainage.

4. Vault contraction occurred in one patient in whom an adequate presacral pouch was not developed. In all of the patients in whom an adequate pouch was constructed, vault contraction was not a problem. In fact, flap redundancy rather than vault contraction was the rule.

5. Sensibility of the flaps to touch is fair to good but it is never normal. Satisfactory pressure sensibility is maintained, and this is the more valuable sensory modality of the normal vagina.

## REFERENCES

Abbé, R.: New method of creating a vagina in a case of congenital absence. Med. Rec., Dec. 10, 1898.

Bakamjian, V.: A technique for primary reconstruction of the palate after radical maxillectomy for cancer. Plast. Reconstr. Surg., *31*:103, 1963.

Baldwin, J. F.: The formation of an artificial vagina by intestinal transplantation. Ann. Surg., *40*:398, 1904.

Beck, C.: A new method of colpoplasty in a case of entire absence of the vagina. Ann. Surg., *32*:572, 1900.

Braley, S. A.: Do-it-yourself vaginal molds of silicone rubber. Plast. Reconstr. Surg., *47*:192, 1971.

Castañares, S.: Plastic construction of the artificial vagina in congenital total absence. Plast. Reconstr. Surg., *32*:368, 1963.

Conway, H., and Stark, R. B.: Construction and reconstruction of the vagina. Surg. Gynecol. Obstet., *97*:573, 1953.

Counseller, V. S.: Congenital absence of the vagina. J.A.M.A., *136*:861, 1948.

DesPrez, J. B., Kiehn, C. L., and Eckstein, W.: Closure of large meningomyelocele by composite skin-muscle flaps. Plast. Reconstr. Surg., *47*:234, 1971.

Frank, R. T., and Geist, S. H.: Formation of an artificial vagina by a new plastic technique. Am. J. Obstet. Gynecol., *14*:712, 1927.

Graves, W. P.: Operative treatment of atresia of the vagina. Boston Med. Surg. J., *163*:753, 1908.

Heppner (1872): Cited by Paunz, A.: Formation of an artificial vagina to remedy a congenital defect. Zentralbl. Gynak., *47*:833, 1923.

Hueston, J. J., and McConchie, I. H.: A compound pectoral flap. Aust. N.Z. J. Surg., *38*:61, 1968.

McCraw, J., Massey, F., Shanklin, K., and Horton, C.: Vaginal reconstruction using gracilis myocutaneous flaps. Plast. Reconstr. Surg., *58*:176, 1976.

McIndoe, A.: The application of cavity grafting. Surgery, *1*:535, 1937.

McIndoe, A.: The treatment of congenital absence and obliterative conditions of the vagina. Br. J. Plast. Surg., *2*:254, 1950.

Orticochea, M.: A new method of total reconstruction of the penis. Br. J. Plast. Surg., *25*:347, 1972.

Owens, N.: A compound neck pedicle designed for the repair of massive facial defects. Plast. Reconstr. Surg., *15*:369, 1955.

Popow, D. D. (1910): Cited by Meyer, H. W.: Kolpoplastik. Zentralbl. Gynak., *37*:639, 1918.

Schubert, G.: Concerning the formation of a new vagina in the case of congenital malformation. Surg. Gynecol. Obstet., *193*:376, 1914.

Sneguireff, W. F.: Zwei neu Fälle von Restitutio Vaginiae per Transplantationen Ani et Recti. Zentralbl. Gynak., *28*:772, 1904.

Steffanoff, D. N.: Late development of squamous cell carcinoma in a split-skin graft lining a vagina. Plast. Reconstr. Surg., *51*:454, 1973.

TeLinde, R. W.: Operative Gynecology. Philadelphia, J. B. Lippincott Company, 1962, p. 716.

Wharton, L. R.: A simple method of constructing a vagina: Report of four cases. Ann. Surg., *107*:842, 1938.

# CHAPTER 100

# INTERSEX PROBLEMS AND HERMAPHRODITISM

## CLIFFORD C. SNYDER, M.D., AND EARL Z. BROWNE, JR., M.D.

Sex is no longer a word to eschew; it has been accepted in the literature as a quality of the individual, whether it be anatomical, physiologic, psychiatric, or social. From a medical standpoint, it is a complex mosaic which needs constant investigation, as evidenced by developments in the past 25 years. Research has converted many previous "confirmed sex facts" into unrealities. These scientific investigations of a fascinating array of sex anomalies have afforded the surgical profession a better understanding of the ambiguities involved and have provided methods of precise therapeutic reasoning. Diagnosis of sex variants can now be definitely established, and treatment can be instituted early.

For the physician to detect specific gender as well as to diagnose individual sex characteristics, it is helpful to review a few elementary biological principles (see also Chapter 4). Chromosomes are the vehicles for transmission of genetic matter, and they provide for genetic segregations and breeding behaviors. Human chromosomes are found in the nuclei of cells in pairs, and when cell mitoses begin, the chromosomes split at the same instant and distribute genetic material equally into the two newly formed cells. Interest in human nuclear cytology began to gain momentum at the turn of the present century.

At first, the cytogeneticists found the new science confusing because there were so many chromosomes, they were so small, and the methods of preparing them for observation were inadequate. The genesis of significant advances in the study of sex was not initiated until 1949, when two Canadian scientists (Barr and Bertram, 1949) discovered there was a difference in the chromatin morphology between the nuclei of men and women. The nuclear chromatin in the female cell was found to stain very deeply, and this characteristic was absent in the male cell nucleus. Today, chromatin cell staining is as routine a test as a physical examination of the external genitalia of the newborn, and it has been adapted for the diagnosis of sex anomalies.

The next advance was reported three years later when Hsu (1952) exposed chromosomes to hypotonic solution and observed them swelling and dispersing individually. This technique afforded an easy means of analyzing and counting the chromosomes.

A series of technical developments ensued, such as changing the sectioned slides to squash or smear slides to enable the flattening of individual cells for inspection in more detail, a technique which in turn provided the opportunity to examine biopsies from any organ or tissue. By changing the culture medium, cytologists were able to grow cells indefinitely and abundantly with chromosomal organization never before realized (Tjio and Levan, 1956). As a result of the achievements, Tjio and Levan (1956) demonstrated that the previously accepted number of 48 chromosomes was an error, and that the human cell contained a diploid number of 46. Lejeune, Turpin, and Gautier (1959) identified an extra chromosome in mongolism, an important finding which stimulated others (Jacobs and Strong, 1959; Hayward, 1960; Sandberg, Koepfe, Crosswhite and Hauschke, 1960; Ford, 1961) to find chromosomal abnormalities in the Sturge-Weber syndrome, Gaucher's disease, and neurofibromatosis.

With the advent of isotopes as tracers to mark chromosome deformities and the utilization of the electron microscope, the means for studying the chromosome have been simplified (Hsu, Hooks and Pomerat, 1953; Young and Corner, 1961; Barlow and Vosa, 1970; Caspersson, Zech and Johannsson, 1970; Pearson, Bobrow and Vosa, 1970; Lamborot-Manzur, Tishler and Atkins, 1971; Hale, Vaughn and Engel, 1973).

It still remained difficult to isolate the cell nucleus during equatorial division and maturation in order to be able to examine the chromosome at the time of metaphase. This problem was solved when it was discovered that the drug colchicine added to the cell medium arrested mitoses during the metaphase stage (Ohno and Makino, 1961). Following the metaphase, each chromosome divides longitudinally into chromatids at opposite poles. The splitting polar movement is called disjunction, and it is at this time that potential errors can occur. However, peripheral blood was the common substance used in examining chromosomes, and the nuclei of white blood cells did not divide frequently. In 1960, Nowell and Hungerford discovered that a kidney bean extract, phytohemagglutinin, accelerated the division of white blood cells to less than 72 hours.

The normal chromosomal complement in man is 22 paired autosomes associated with two sex chromosomes. The basic difference in gender is seen in the sex chromosome pattern, which is XX in the female and XY in the male (Bankoff, 1956). There is definite confirmation that an ovum harbors two X chromosomes and a spermatozoon carries an X chromosome and a smaller Y chromosome (Cabot, 1946). Sex is initiated at fertilization when the ovum is impregnated with a sperm cell containing an X or a Y chromosome, though sexual differentiation is not evident until the seventh or eighth week of gestation (Campbell, 1937). The combination of XX chromosomes develops into a female and of XY chromosomes into a male (Frazer, 1931; Goldschmidt, 1938).

In the past, these chromosomal configurations have been of only casual interest to most clinicians. With the advent of new concepts in cellular structure, they have become most helpful in distinguishing and treating sex anomalies. Studies have shown that genotypes of ovarian agenesis (Turner's syndrome) have an XO chromosomal make-up (only one sex chromosome and a total of 45 chromosomes) (Bergada, Cleveland, Jones and Wilkins, 1962), whereas those of testicular dysgenesis (Klinefelter's syndrome) have an XXY chromosomal pattern (with a total of 47 chromosomes) (Grumbach, Van Wyk and Wilkins, 1955; Ford and coworkers, 1959; Richart and Benirschke, 1960). Jacobs and associates (1959) reported the "super female" with a chromosome plan of XXX plus 22 pairs of autosomes. A YO prototype has never been observed and is considered incompatible with survival. These atypical forms of chromosome patterns are caused by irregular mitosis, but the precise mechanism is not known (Sinnott, 1958). When these patterns contradict the normal in sex chromosome studies, various sexual anomalies result.

It is thus apparent that any single characteristic intended to distinguish a male from a female must undergo careful study before it can be regarded as established. In fact, it has become rather difficult to define accurately the simple terms "man" and "woman."

## VERIFICATION OF SEX IDENTIFICATION

The physician may be called upon to examine an infant of doubtful sex and may find it difficult to obtain help in assigning the youngster to the correct sex. Far too often the clinician postpones making a decision, and this is responsible for future psychiatric, endocrinologic, and surgical problems. The parents, who have come for help and expect a prompt decision, remain confused; the children, who are regarded as atypical of either sex, must be assigned to one or the other in order to fit into social patterns. The physician who examines the infant or child with the puzzling sex should include in his physical survey the following criteria: the size and contour of the phallus or clitoris (by word description and photographs), the position of the urethral orifice; the scrotal or labial contour and contents; and the presence or absence of a vaginal introitus and vault. Other physical findings which should be noted are the facies, neck contour, possible hernias, and any other body abnormality. Suspected mental retardation is also a noteworthy finding which should be thoroughly investigated. Certain laboratory tests must confirm the chromatin sex pattern, the chromosome karyotype, the ketosteroids, gonadotropins, estrogens, and electrolytes. As the child grows older, continued assessment of the contours of the limbs and trunk, the development of the breasts and genitalia, hair distribution, fat apportionment, voice changes, and menstrual and sperm data should be made.

**The Sex Chromatin Mass.** One helpful guide to the clinician in making a diagnosis is to utilize information regarding the sex chromatin mass. In 1949 Barr, an anatomist, in collaboration with his colleague Bertram described a small, dark area at the inner periphery of the nucleus in the brain cells of cats. The uniqueness of this discovery was that it could be seen only in the nuclear chromatin of *female* cats. It was soon recognized as a notable contribution. The accumulation of a sizable body of literature was prompted by this original discovery of sex distinction at the cell level (Howard, 1951; Hsu, 1952; Moore, Graham and Barr, 1953; Davidson and Smith, 1954; Marberger, Bocabella and Nelson, 1955; Bunge and Bradbury, 1957; Huffman, 1958; Haddad and Wilkins, 1959; Ford, 1960). The sex chromatin mass (Fig. 100–1) is referred to as the "Barr body." It is also known as the "chromatin sex body" or "mass." If the chromatin sex mass is present, the nuclear sex is female; if it is absent, the nuclear sex is male. Chromatin sex bodies have now been identified in the female monkey, ferret, cat, dog, coyote, wolf, fox, deer, goat, bear, mink, skunk, raccoon, opossum, pig, cow, horse, and marten (Moore, 1960). The body is not easily visible in rodents, because they naturally have large, dark chromatin particles dispersed throughout their nuclei, and these are indistinguishable from sex chromatin masses.

Innumerable studies have substantiated the validity of the sex chromatin in humans. It is thought that the sex chromatin is derived from sex chromosomes, although direct proof is lacking (Young and Corner, 1961). The sex chromosomes tend to be stabilized into a compact mass and stain heavily with basic dyes (Allen, Danforth and Doisy, 1939), whereas the autosomes or somatic chromosomes are diffuse and stain lightly. It is therefore considered that the apposition of two X chromosomes produces the typical deep pyknotic appearance; the mass is sufficiently large to be readily visible under the oil immersion lens of

the microscope. The small size of the Y chromosome could explain the fact that it is not visible in the cells of males.

The sex chromatin unit measures about 1 micron in diameter (Kiefer, McGrew, Rosenthal and Bronstein, 1957), is planoconvex, contains nucleic acid, mainly of the deoxyribose type (Shettles, 1956), and is usually found adjacent to the inner surface of the nuclear cell membrane (see Fig. 100–1). It is sex-specific, and cells harboring sex chromosomes are called chromatin-positive, whereas those that lack it are known as chromatin-negative. Though cells of all body tissues may contain the structure (Briggs and Kupperman, 1956) and it has been demonstrated in embryos, infants, adolescents, the aged, and cadavers (Pratt, 1958), only certain tissue cells are employed for the test because they are readily accessible. The cells commonly used for rapid sex determination are those from the skin (Moore, Graham and Barr, 1953; Barr, 1954), blood (Davidson and Smith, 1954; Briggs and Kupperman, 1956), mucous membrane (Moore and coworkers, 1953; Rathbun, Plunkett and Barr, 1958), and amniotic fluid (Eastman, 1960). Scrapings from the epidermis and the oral mucosa or smears from the vagina may be prepared and read within three hours (Naib, 1961). In blood smears it is customary to observe at least 500 to 1000 cells before a diagnosis is made. A drop or two of peripheral blood is thickly smeared on a slide to ensure that a large number of polymorphonuclear leukocytes is available for examination. The sex chromatin drumstick appendage is apparent in only about 1 per cent of the leukocytes. The slide is dried and stained by the May-Giemsa-Grünwald method. One must be able to differentiate irregular nuclei, minor lobulations, and sessile mounds from the true pedunculated sex body. The normal female will show at least five or six drumsticks when counting 500 white blood cells. When there are less than five typical sex masses per 500 cells, correct interpretation is in doubt, and additional slide smears are indicated. The chromatin sex pattern should always be compared to the chromosomal analysis and the hormonal and the gonadal sex patterns.

Sex differences are also seen in the circulating polymorphonuclear leukocytes, such as accessory nuclear lobules or drumstick appendages (see Fig. 100–1, *B*). The drumstick is characteristic of mature neutrophils. It is only rarely seen in nonsegmented forms and is never observed in the precursor cells of leukocytes. A patient

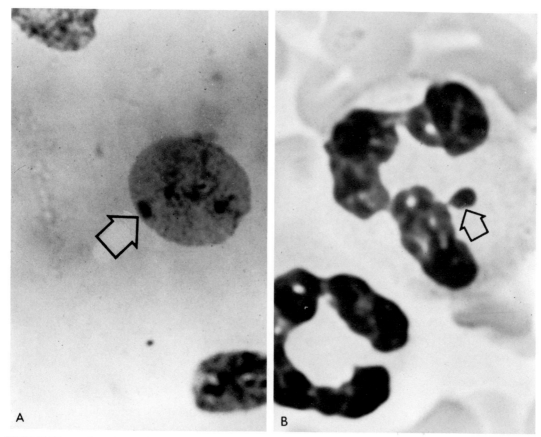

**FIGURE 100–1.** Sex chromatin mass. *A,* Chromatin mass silhouette (arrow) poised on the inner periphery of the nuclear membrane is the sentinel of the female gender. These masses may be found in the cells of all body tissues of embryos, infants, adolescents, adults, and cadavers. This cell was scraped from oral mucosa. *B,* Drumstick appendages on the nuclei of leukocytes are also sex-specific for the female gender. These accessory nuclear lobules are named after their discoverer and are called Barr bodies.

with an acute severe infection, displaying a toxic shift to the left, may fail, therefore, to show the characteristic drumstick. A blood smear from a female presenting a shift to the right will be laden with the diagnostic chromatin patterns.

It is also possible to determine sex by prenatal examination (Blakely, 1937; Dewhurst, 1956; Fuchs and Riis, 1956; James, 1956). This may be done between the fourth and seventh months of pregnancy by aspirating and examining the cells of the amniotic fluid (Serr, Sachs and Dannon, 1957). Though this may be of significant benefit in horses, cows, and other domestic animals, there is a divergence of opinion as to its merits in man.

The importance of the sex chromatin mass is demonstrated in differentiating hermaphrodites or individuals who are phenotypical deviates from those of the normal sex type (Bergemann, 1961). A review of the literature suggests that

there are approximately 90 hermaphroditic phenotypes. Overzier (1955) reviewed 74 of these phenotypes. It would be difficult to obtain a figure regarding the number of so-called pseudohermaphrodites. New genotypes are currently being described as investigative procedures become more diagnostic. As has been previously mentioned, some hermaphrodites have an XO (Turner's syndrome) or an XXY (Klinefelter's syndrome) chromosomal pattern (Turner, 1938; Klinefelter, Reifenstein and Albright, 1942). The gonadal dysgeneses are now recognized (Richart and Benirschke, 1960; Bergada, Cleveland, Jones and Wilkins, 1962), and this adds to the growing problems of identifying the genotypes. These unusual patterns result from the abnormal behavior of the chromosomes during the mitotic phases of the maturing germ cell (Fig. 100–2).

The complexity of chromosomal gains and losses is a stimulus in the search for other means

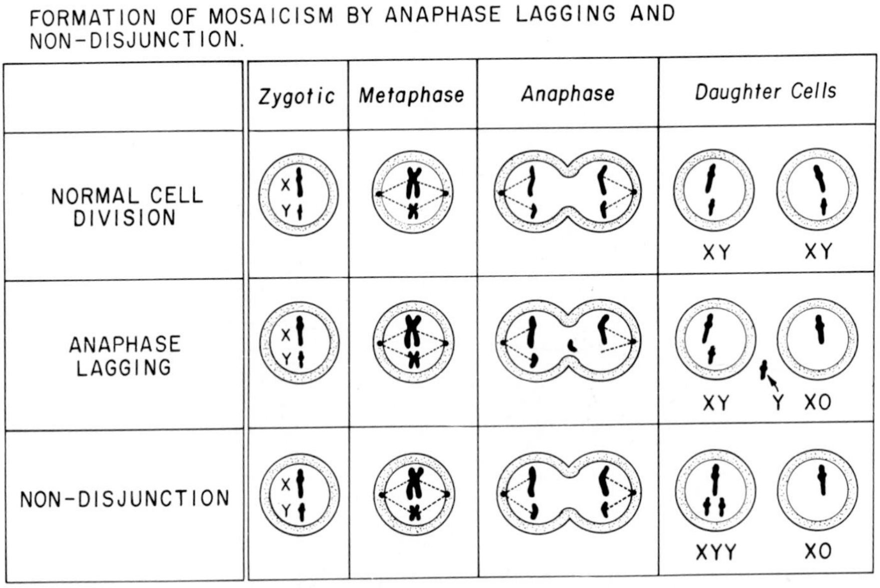
FORMATION OF MOSAICISM BY ANAPHASE LAGGING AND NON-DISJUNCTION.
Zygotic
Metaphase
Anaphase
Daughter Cells
NORMAL CELL DIVISION
XY
XY
ANAPHASE LAGGING
XY
Y
XO
NON-DISJUNCTION
XYY
XO

**FIGURE 100–2.** From a single fertilized ovum, thousands of body cells develop, and each cell comprises the identical genetic endowment of the original zygote. If an error develops during cell division, the altered chromosome will initiate an entire new lineage, each of the cells incorporating the aberrant complement.

and methods of describing the intersex problem. The assignment of sex requires verification beyond the finding of chromatin masses within cells; this test alone is not dependable.

**The Chromosome Karyotype.** Chromosome analyses should be referred to geneticists, cytologists, or those who make these determinations on a regular basis. The test may be accomplished by using cultures of skin, mucous membrane, or bone marrow, but peripheral blood is less painful and less difficult to obtain. The peripheral blood sample is heparinized and treated with phytohemagglutinin, a French bean extract which promotes growth of the leukocytes and precipitates the hemoglobin. The white blood cells are segregated and incubated in a commercial tissue culture medium for three days, at which time mitoses become accelerated. Colchicine is then used to halt mitoses in the metaphase stage. A hypotonic solution is added to swell the cells and disperse the chromosomes. Careful digital manipulation and squashing of the cells on a slide with a coverslip will flatten them for easier identification. Cytogeneticists describe this conglomeration as ''lobster pincers'' or ''rabbit feet markings on the snow'' (Fig. 100–3). Chromosomes present specific characteristics which identify them into patterns. They have large and small bodies, long or short arms and legs, a narrow waist or isthmus called the centromere, and sometimes satellites. The chromosomes are microphotographed and enlarged on white prints so that they can be cut out, counted, and arranged in alphabetical groups based on surface contour (Fig. 100–4). The chromosomes are then rearranged into homologous pairs according to the Denver classification (Fig. 100–5). In 1960, cytogeneticists established an orderly classification and nomenclature for human chromosomes. There are seven major groups of chromosomes, of which the X chromosome belongs to the larger one, and the Y chromosome is a small, single acrocentric type without satellite bodies. The latter is not present in the normal female. To ensure accuracy in karyotyping, large numbers should be counted. If a chromosome has been lost, the karyotype is called a monosomy, and an example would be Turner's syndrome (XO). A karyotype with an extra chromosome is a trisomy, and this is exemplified by Klinefelter's syndrome (XXY). Chromosomal determinations yield valuable data in genital ambiguities.

**The Gonadal Sex.** The obstetrician usually assigns the newborn infant to its specific sex on the basis of an initial glance and casual examination of its external genitalia. Though it has been proved by experience that this conventional criterion may be misleading (Bunge and Bradbury, 1956; Hamblen, 1957), it is still by far the most common method of sex assignment util-

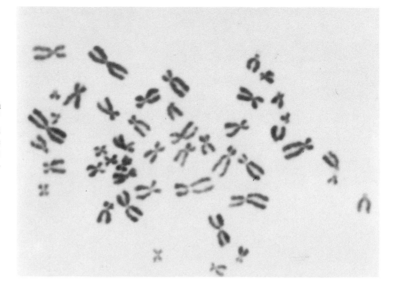

**FIGURE 100-3.** Microphotograph of chromosomal "lobster pincers" from a peripheral blood sample which has been prepared. They are ready to be segregated by cutting with scissors like paper dolls into individual chromosomes and grouped.

ized. The need for closer examination of the child is demonstrated by recent statistics showing that sexual anomalies are more common than suspected. One authority states that there is at least one intersex in every thousand births (Wilkins, 1957), a statistic which places this congenital deformity close to the same incidence as cleft lip and palate. Hermaphroditism or intersex has been reported in ten sets of twins (Col-

lier, 1948) and in brothers and sisters (Cavellero and Zanardi, 1953) and may be a family trait through many generations (Campbell, 1951, 1954). Four cases of female hermaphroditism have been reported in one family (Phillips, 1886). Deming, Goettsch and Humm (1949) reported a family of four sisters all of whom had sexual ambiguities of the same type. Snyder and Cleveland (1975) treated three sisters who were fe-

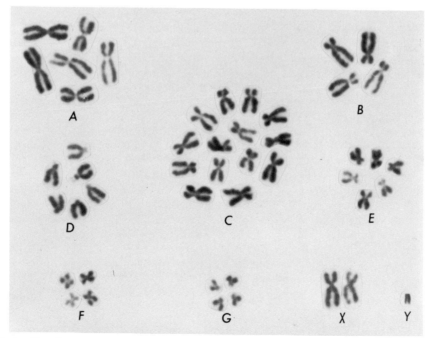

**FIGURE 100-4.** The chromosome pairs are arranged into seven groupings according to their size, shape, arm and leg lengths, centromeres, and satellites. The initial pieces of the karyotypic mosaic are ready to be aligned into a sex assignment.

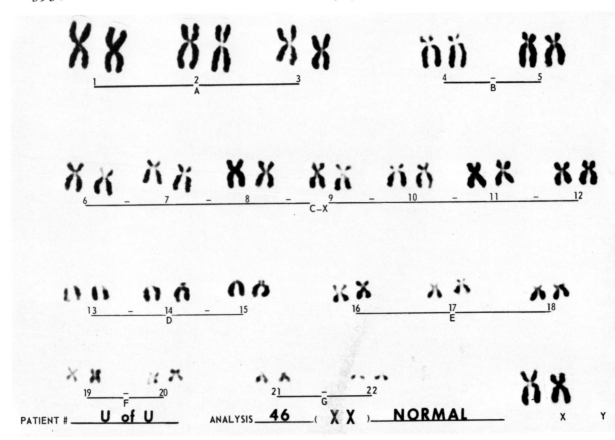

**FIGURE 100–5.** The karyotype segregated into seven (A to G) groupings of 22 homologous paired autosomes and two sex chromosomes representative of both the Denver and Patau methods. This idiogram is that of a normal female.

male hermaphrodites with congenital adrenal cortical hyperplasia (Fig. 100–6). Blocker, Lewis, and Snyder (1953) reported 13 cases of hermaphroditism, including one set of twins. Many patients reported as having an absence of the vagina may be hermaphrodites (Bryan, Nigro and Counseller, 1949).

Although legal authorities and social traditionalists acknowledge only two sexes, medical authorities, geneticists, biologists, zoologists, and botanists recognize at least three sexes with many aberrations. The assignment of the newborn to the sex seemingly indicated by its external genitalia may be the causative factor of mental and physical imbalance throughout life. The decision, therefore, should take into account the knowledge of the normal as well as of the various abnormal embryologic and anatomical developments.

**Developmental Anatomy of the Genitalia.** The earliest visible sexual primordium in the human embryo is the gonadal anlage, which remains undifferentiated until the fetus is about 5 cm in length (Jordan and Kindred, 1942; Murphy, 1947; Hamilton, Boyd and Mossman, 1962). This is followed by the development of the genital tract, which consists of the genital tubercle or phallus, the urethral groove, and the labioscrotal eminences. Even at this stage, the gonadal or genetic sex is unknown (Glenister, 1954). The urethral groove becomes continuous with the urogenital sinus, and soon the coronary sulcus and the prepuce take form. When the fetus is about seven or eight weeks of age, sexual differentiation is definite (Spaulding, 1921; Warkany, 1947). The urethral groove remains open to form the vulva in the female, but it closes to form the penile urethra in the male. The fusion of the urethral folds in the male is seen as the perineal raphé, whereas the nonfused urethral folds in the female become the labia minora. The genital eminences are called scrotal swellings in the male and labial swellings in the female (Arey, 1954; Dmowski and Greenblatt, 1971).

During the seventh month the testes complete their migration into the scrotum. Removal of the female fetal ovaries does not modify femininity, but castration of the male testes does change masculinity. In other words, the male fetal testes produce male characteristics of wolffian origin and inhibit female characteristics of müllerian origin. If there is a deficiency of testicular function, depending on the time this occurs, various masculine characteristics are inhibited (Jost, 1953). There is a critical stage in the developing fetus during which testicular bombardment and organ formation take place. If any interference with this progress is introduced at this time, abnormalities may ensue. Because the gross examination of external genitalia may be deceiving, sex identification is necessary by means of microscopic studies of sections of tissue from the gonads. Such identification is the basis of Klebs' classification (1876).

The development of the internal genitalia is of little significance in the assignment of sex but influences the function of the genitals. Panhysterectomies are done in females without any change in their sex assignment, but resultant hormonal symptoms may require therapy.

The embryology of the genitourinary system is discussed in more detail in Chapter 93.

**The Hormonal Sex.** Most of the knowledge concerning hormonal influence on sex is based upon experiments conducted with freemartins (Lillie, 1916, 1917; Buyse, 1935). Cattle breeders have been acquainted with this animal for many years. The freemartin is an intersex anomaly, being a sterile female calf twinborn to a normal male calf. It has typically female external genitals and udder but is usually bisexual and well developed, although all variants are possible. This syndrome is very constant, and it has been concluded that the abnormal development of the female twin is due to a hormone produced by the male twin. This in turn suggests that the testicular hormone is activated before the ovarian hormone (Bascom, 1923). These studies prompted further investigation with parabiosis (Burns, 1925), gonadal grafting, injection of pure hormones (Kozelka and Gallagher, 1934), castration, and the transformation of testes by administration of estrogenic substances (Jones, 1958).

The hormonal influence on the human external genitalia is observed in such entities as hyperadrenocorticogenitalism (Young, 1937; Wilkins and coworkers, 1952), hypoadrenocorticogenitalism (Moore, 1947; Wilkins and coworkers, 1958), gonadal dysgenesis (Ehrenfeld and Brom-

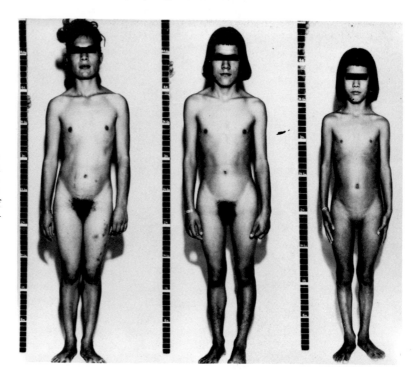

**FIGURE 100-6.** Female hermaphroditism is the most common type of intersex and is occasionally a familial trait. These three sisters show the typical virilism of congenital adrenocortical hyperplasia.

berg, 1958; Hamblen, Palma and Poshyachinda, 1960), and feminizing testicularism (Berthrong, Goodwin and Scott, 1949; Morris, 1953). In the hyperadrenocortical type of hormonal disorder, the adrenal glands secrete a virilizing hormone, producing the hermaphroditic condition. In the feminizing testicularism form, the testes are estrogen-producing in nature. The hormonal factor is responsible for body contour, epiphyseal fusion, hirsutism, acne formation, and fat habitus, as well as genital morphology. Early diagnosis of the hormonal sex is paramount for therapy, which occasionally may be lifesaving. The easiest and most rapid method of determining the hormonal status is the collection and examination of 24-hour urine specimens for 17-ketosteroid levels (Mason and Engstrom, 1950; Young and Corner, 1961).

## THE PROBLEM OF SEX ASSIGNMENT

The importance of sex assignment or rearing in bisexual individuals has frequently been emphasized (Money, Hampson and Hampson, 1955; Hamblen, 1957). There is no disagreement about the concept that all humans have varying amounts of masculinity and femininity in their make-up. However, it is necessary to adhere to the universal designation of humans as either male or female and to assign one of these sexes to those who are unfortunate enough to be born into the category of the intersex.

Hermaphroditism should not be confused with homosexuality. The hermaphrodite does not share the sexual desires of the homosexual (Witschi and Mengert, 1942). The homosexual's chromatin status is as consistent with his sex as that of a normal individual. The transsexual, however, often convinces himself that his genitals have been erroneously given to him and frequently insists on surgical removal and reconstruction of the type he prefers. Surgical and hormonal therapy in the transvestite should be discouraged, whereas in the hermaphrodite it should be encouraged. The transsexual will be discussed later in the chapter.

Occasionally, it is impossible to assign sex, such as in the premature infant born before sex differentiation can be made or in newborns before sex chromatin studies are interpretable. When sex assignment is not possible immediately after birth, the parents should be informed that, as soon as tests are feasible, a definite sexual assignment will be made. At times, this may be difficult because of religious objections, legal interference, or possibly because the parents already have several children of one sex and desire the newborn to be of the opposite sex.

When the patient has been erroneously assigned a definite sex and the decision is later made by the physician that the sex should be changed, the parents should consent before the child is 2 years of age. The gender role is not fixed at this early age, and it is not too late to change previously assigned sex. The gender role and orientation are described by Hampson (1955) as "those things that a person says or does to disclose himself or herself as having the status of a male or female." The gender role is established while the person is maturing chronologically and is concerned with such factors as hair style, dress, and mannerism. If sex assignment is changed after childhood, serious mental sequelae may ensue.

## CLASSIFICATION OF INTERSEXUALITY

Contrary to previously held opinion, it is now acknowledged that hermaphroditism is a design of variables ranging from the typical female gender to the typical male gender. These variables may be confusing at first glance. The variable known as female hermaphroditism has male-type external genitals. The male hermaphrodite's external genitalia are female-appearing. Individuals with Klinefelter's syndrome possess male external genitalia but are gonadal females. Those with Turner's syndrome have female external sex organs but are gonadal males. The so-called true hermaphrodite may resemble either sex. There is no controversy over the existence of these variables, but there remains a lack of conformity in terms of their classification. Hooks (1949) has suggested that a "Genitourinary Intersexuality Register" be organized to collect and analyze all data on these variables and that this register be used to evaluate, classify, and formulate standard methods of therapy.

Since antiquity, both lay persons and physicians have relied upon the appearance of the external gonads to designate sex. Later this method was found to be unreliable, and the next approach was to remove a section from the external gonads for microscopic study. To this method was added the comparative examination of the external and internal gonads. These concepts are the basis of a popular classification of hermaphrodites (Klebs, 1876). Examination of Klebs' classification (Table 100–1) indicates

TABLE 100–1. *Classification of Klebs (1876)*

HERMAPHRODITISMUS VERUS
Bilateralis—ambisexual gonadal tissue on both sides.
Unilateralis—ambisexual gonadal tissue on one side.
Lateralis—alternating gonadal tissue (male one side, female other side).
Completus—gonadal tissue present on both sides.
Incompletus—gonadal tissue present on only one side.
MALE PSEUDOHERMAPHRODITISM (ambisexuals with entirely male gonads)
Completus—testes present but feminine internal and external genitalia.
Internus—testes present but well-developed uterus, tubes, and maybe vagina.
Externus—testes present but feminine external genitalia.
FEMALE PSEUDOHERMAPHRODITISM (ambisexuals with entirely female gonads)
Completus—female with ovaries but male internal and external genitalia.
Internus—female with ovaries but vestigial Gartner's duct, prostate, and vas.
Externus—female internal genitalia but external male genitalia.

that it is too complex and obviously incomplete in view of current knowledge. It is included only for historical interest.

Wilkins (1957) used the pathogenetic features in hermaphroditism for his classification, with emphasis on corticomedullary antagonism and dominance. He categorized the intersex abnormalities into defective development of the gonads, abnormal secretion of male hormone by fetal testes, masculinization of the fetus by extragonadal male hormone, and postnatal virilization of females. Under these four headings he described the degrees of hermaphroditism.

Money, Hampson, and Hampson (1955) organized eight different variables of the intersex problem and then explained how each may contradict the others. They emphasized the variable of sex assignment and sex rearing as being the most important in the prognosis of the gender role. The variables were arranged systematically and included sex assignment and sex rearing, external genital morphology, internal accessory reproductive structures, hormonal sex and secondary sexual characteristics, gonadal sex, chromosomal sex, gender role and orientation established during growth and development, and gonadal agenesis or dysgenesis.

Hamblen (1957) classified and described the ambiguities of sex (Table 100–2) and prognosticated the sex assignments.

Jones and Scott (1971) grouped the hermaphrodites according to etiology and then classified them into the various patterns which they fitted (Table 100–3).

Intersex or hermaphroditism has thus been divided and subdivided into unwieldy numbers of categories, and it is because of this incongruity that the authors' classification has been devised for purposes of simplicity (Table 100–4).

In summary, it may be said that sex is variable, limited not merely to two distinct types but extending into a variety of entities. Among the variables are patterns of chromosomal (genetic), hormonal (endocrine), and gonadal (morphologic) sex design. If the individual is past infancy, a fourth factor must be considered—that is, sex rearing and gender. Final

TABLE 100–2. *Classification of Hamblen (1957)*

FEMALE PSEUDOHERMAPHRODITISM DUE TO CONGENITAL ADRENAL HYPERPLASIA
Chromatin-positive.
External genitalia android completely or incompletely.
Internal genitalia gynecoid.
Precocious android pubescence.
FEMALE PSEUDOHERMAPHRODITISM NOT DUE TO CONGENITAL ADRENAL HYPERPLASIA
Chromatin-positive.
External genitalia android.
Internal genitalia gynecoid.
MALE PSEUDOHERMAPHRODITISM
Chromatin-negative.
External genitalia android or ambiguous.
Internal genitalia gynecoid, maybe android vestiges.
Usually android pubescence.
MALE PSEUDOHERMAPHRODITISM
Chromatin-negative.
External genitalia android or ambiguous.
Internal genitalia android, maybe gynecoid vestiges.
Android or gynecoid pubescence.
MALE PSEUDOHERMAPHRODITISM
Chromatin-negative.
External genitalia gynecoid.
Internal genitalia gynecoid, maybe uterus absent.
Gynecoid pubescence.
TRUE HERMAPHRODITISM
Chromatin-positive 75%.
External genitalia android and gynecoid.
Internal genitalia android and gynecoid.
Android or gynecoid pubescence.
MORPHOLOGIC GYNECOID EXTERNAL AND INTERNAL GENITALS (MOST OF TURNER'S SYNDROME AND "OVARIAN AGENESIS")
Chromatin-negative.
External genitalia gynecoid ⎤ rudimentary
Internal genitalia gynecoid ⎦ or absent.
Absent pubescence.
MORPHOLOGIC ANDROID EXTERNAL AND INTERNAL GENITALS EXCEPT PUBESCENT GYNECOMASTIO–CHROMATIN-POSITIVES
Chromatin-negative.
External genitalia android with normal Leydig but degenerated seminiferous cells.
Internal genitalia android.
Absent pubescence.

TABLE 100–3.　Classification of Jones and Scott (1971)*

| ETIOLOGY | GROUP | CRITERIA OF SEX | | | | | | | | |
|---|---|---|---|---|---|---|---|---|---|---|
| | | Chromosomal Arrangement | Sex Chromatin | Gonadal Structure | Morphology of External Genitalia | Morphology of Internal Genitalia | Hormonal Dominance | Sex of Rearing | | Gender Role |
| | | | | | | | | Actual | Preferred | |
| Chromosomal aberration in most cases | Gonadal aplasia and dysplasia | XO, XO/XX, etc. | Negative or positive | None | Feminine | Feminine | None | As women | As women | As women |
| Unknown (probably genetic) | Male intersexuality (masculinizing) | XY, etc. | Negative | Testis | Mixed | Mixed | Masculine | Either, but mostly as women | Either, but mostly as women | Either, but mostly as women |
| Genetic | Male intersexuality (feminizing) | XY | Negative | Testis | Feminine | None | Feminine | As women | As women | As women |
| Chromosomal aberration | Klinefelter's syndrome | XXY, etc. | Positive or negative | Testis | Masculine | Masculine | Masculine | As men | As men | As men |
| Unknown | Other syndromes of male intersexuality | XX, etc. | Positive or negative | Testis | Masculine | Masculine | Masculine | As men | As men | As men |
| Congenital adrenal hyperplasia (genetic) | Female intersexuality with adrenal hyperplasia | XX | Positive | Ovary | Mixed | Feminine | Masculine | Either, but mostly as women | As women | Either, but mostly as women |
| Maternal androgen in some cases | Female intersexuality not due to adrenal hyperplasia | XX | Positive | Ovary | Mixed | Feminine | Feminine | Either, but mostly as women | As women | Either, but mostly as women |
| Chromosomal aberration | Other syndromes of female intersexuality | XXX, etc. | Double positive, etc. | Ovary | Feminine | Feminine | Feminine | As women | As women | As women |
| Unknown | True hermaphroditism | XX, etc. | Positive or negative | Testis and ovary | Mixed | Mixed | Mixed | Either | Either | Either |

*From Jones, H. W., Jr., and Scott, W. W.: Hermaphroditism, Genital Anomalies and Related Endocrine Disorders. Copyright 1971, The Williams & Wilkins Company, Baltimore.

TABLE 100–4. *Degrees of Hermaphroditism*

| | TRUE HERMAPHRODITISM | FEMALE HERMAPHRODITISM | MALE HERMAPHRODITISM | FEMINIZING TESTICULARISM |
|---|---|---|---|---|
| CHROMOSOMAL SEX PATTERN | | SEX CHROMATIN POSITIVE | | |
| HORMONAL SEX PATTERN 17 KETOSTEROIDS | **17** NORMAL TO DECREASED | **17** USUALLY ELEVATED | **17** NORMAL | **17** NORMAL |
| GONADAL SEX PATTERN | | UTERUS OVARIES MEGALOCLITORIS | USUALLY GYNECO-MASTIA USUALLY SMALL PHALLUS AND ECTOPIC TESTES | USUALLY FEMALE BREASTS SHALLOW VAGINA NORMAL CLITORIS IMMATURE TESTES |
| SEX ASSIGNMENT | | | | |

judgment should not be based upon any specific one of the above four sex criteria; instead, a thorough investigation of all of the criteria should be instituted.

## TREATMENT OF INTERSEX PROBLEMS

### True Hermaphroditism

If there actually existed an individual of *pure* hermaphroditic design, a more appropriate name for this sexual ambiguity would be "andro-gyne," which signifies, from its Greek deriva-tion, one-half man and one-half woman. A true hermaphrodite would possess internal and ex-ternal gonads of both sexes and would be able to function as either a male or a female; such a pattern has not been demonstrated. The term "true hermaphroditism" is accepted, therefore,

as one of relative value in classifying intersex designs.

**Diagnosis.** The diagnosis of true hermaphro-ditism is strictly dependent upon the gonadal sex pattern. Both testicular and ovarian tissue must be present, whether in one or both gonads. When one gonad contains both types of tissue, it is known as an ovotestis, and all of our patients were of this type. The gonad may be abdominal, inguinal, or labioscrotal in position; there may be a uterus; the phallus may be penile or clitoral; the labia may be bifid, as in the female, or fused, resembling the scrotum of the male.

Pubertal development may be android, gyne-coid, or ambiguous. Many true hermaphrodites develop female-like breasts, and some have been reported to menstruate. The chromosomal sex pattern differed in our patients, but six were XX and two XY; all were chromatin-positive. The hormonal sex pattern is of little diagnostic value, as the estrogens or androgens are normal or minimally decreased. There are less than 100 cases of true hermaphroditism reported in the literature, and the diagnosis in many of these is questionable (Gudernatsch, 1911, 1945; Photakis, 1916; Stojalowski and Debski, 1933; Raynaud, Marill and Xicluna, 1939; Cecil, 1940; Lattimer, Engle and Yeaw, 1943; Brachetto-Braun, Grimaldi and Rochello Costa, 1943; McKenna and Kiefer, 1944; Engle, Yeaw and Lattimer, 1946; Davis and Scheffey, 1946; Sterling, 1946; Demoura and Pinto Basto, 1946; Greene and coworkers, 1952; Fischer, Lischer and Byars, 1952; Zondek, Unger and Leszynsky, 1953; Delore and coworkers, 1953; Charlewood and Friedberg, 1955; Lauterwein and Kladetzky, 1955; Minervini, Schwarzenberg, Canibus and Natoli, 1969).

The treatment of these problem patients is controversial, but it would not be if each individual problem were understood. Young patients should be assigned to the sex which their patterns resemble, and the reconstructive procedure that is easier, usually female, should be performed. In older patients consideration should be given to their established gender role and the sex to which they have been oriented. It is evident that the hermaphrodite is destined to the role of either a male or a female. This can be achieved only if careful scientific investigation is undertaken. The assigned sex in the adult is not necessarily the one that is in agreement with the sex patterns, that is, chromosomal, hormonal, or gonadal. If such a plan is instituted, the patient may encounter difficulties in later life and require psychiatric treatment.

The parents must be cognizant of the situation and agreeable to the sex assigned their sibling. Legal documents must be in order, including correction of the birth certificate and name substitution.

**Surgical Procedures.** The surgery should be designed after a mutual decision is reached by the parents and the physician concerned and should be followed later by appropriate endocrine and, if necessary, psychiatric therapy. If possible, the operation should be performed when the patient is young, preferably before the age of 3, in order that memory of the incident be minimized (Fig. 100–7). Surgical feminization should be decided upon in all true hermaphrodites whenever possible and especially in those under 5 years of age, because a serviceable vaginal vault can be constructed without difficulty. Late adolescents and early adult-aged true hermaphrodites who have been reared as males should be given the privilege of choosing their sex preference. If they elect to undergo the necessary surgical procedures to achieve the physical attributes of masculinity, they should be informed that the procedures are time-consuming, staged operations. They should also be advised as to the future consequences which are encountered functionally after inadequate phallic reconstruction.

**Construction of the Vagina.** The surgical approach is through a paramedian incision with a catheter in the bladder. The lower abdominal cavity is explored and the anatomical structures

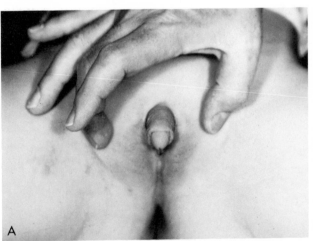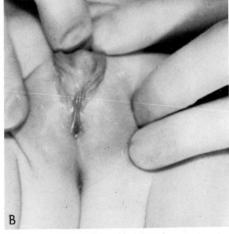

**FIGURE 100–7.** True hermaphroditism is a complex entity which presents difficult decisions in assigning the correct sex. *A,* Young patient demonstrating ambiguous external genitalia in the form of an android phallus but also having gynecoid bifid labia. *B,* Elevation of the masculine phallic structure exposes a hypospadiac urethra, a deep median raphé, and lateral eminences devoid of contents, all of which are characteristics of femininity.

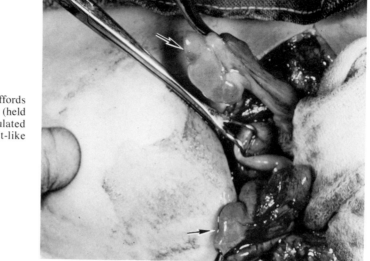

**FIGURE 100–8.** Pelvic exploration affords gross identification of an infantile uterus (held by Babcock forceps) and bilateral lobulated gonads (arrows) suspended by oviduct-like structures.

identified (Fig. 100–8). The gonads are brought into sight, and elliptical specimens are removed from each for biopsy purposes (Fig. 100–9). These are carefully labeled "right gonad" and "left gonad" and given to the pathologist for microscopic study (Figs. 100–10 and 100–11). During the microscopic examination, the gonadal incisions are closed with either an interrupted or a running catgut suture. Additional examination of the pelvis determines whether the uterus has a palpable cervix, whether the inguinal canals are normal, and whether any other abnormalities are present. A rapid examination of other peritoneal viscera should elicit any other anomalies.

If the pathologist reports that each gonad consists of both ovarian and testicular tissue and that a uterus is present, the patient should be surgically "feminized." The ovotestes are left in position because the testicular portion of a mixed gonad does not function when left in this environment. Furthermore, the testicular portion becomes atrophic. If masculinizing signs begin to appear, such as beard growth, masculine distribution of hair, and changes in body proportion, the ovotestes should be removed and estrogen therapy instituted (Cooper, 1929).

The abdominal wound is closed, and the surgical field is transferred to the pubic and perineal area. An incision is made between the phallic structure and the anal outlet. Using blunt or digital dissection, a vaginal vault is constructed, and the presence or absence of a cervix is established (Fig. 100–12). The phallic structure (or megaloclitoris) is sacrificed, but the integumental cloak, which is used to line the constructed vagina, is salvaged. If a cervix is present, it should be left exposed. The phallic integumental flap remains innervated and thus preserves erotic sensation when transposed into

**FIGURE 100–9.** True hermaphroditic gonads must be investigated, and it is necessary to obtain ample tissue by longitudinal excision. The gonadal wound is closed with catgut sutures.

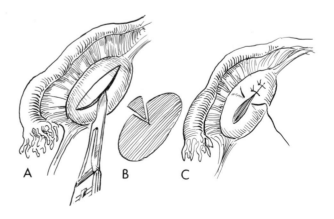

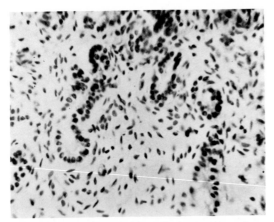

**FIGURE 100–10.** Microscopic inspection of true hermaphroditic gonads may disclose a mixture of testicular and ovarian stroma (ova-testis). Photomicrograph of a histologic section of a gonad shows a typical fetal testis with immature tubular formation.

the vaginal vault. Labioscrotal folds which are fused may now be separated to resemble female labia. A catheter is placed in the bladder to prevent wound soiling. The results of surgical feminization are rewarding as the child learns to cuddle, as well as to walk, talk, and act in a feminine fashion (Fig. 100–13). If one gonad is purely ovarian and the other is strictly testicular, a decision must be made to remove one and feminize or masculinize accordingly. The authors prefer to resect the testicular component and feminize the patient.

**Construction of the Male Genitalia.** Construction of the male external genitalia is done in multiple stages, and this type of surgery is best adapted to the patient who has ample penile and

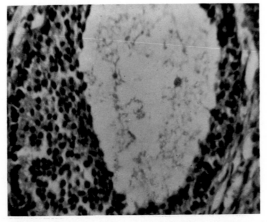

**FIGURE 100–11.** Photomicrograph of another area of the gonad pictured in Figure 100–10 showing a graafian follicle in ovarian parenchymal architecture.

testicular tissue and a prostate gland, and who is personally convinced of his choice of male sex assignment. The masculinizing procedures are initiated by designing a penile shaft which houses an integument-lined urethra (Figs. 100–14, 100–15, and 100–16). The ideal donor site is the linea alba of the abdominal wall, because it is nearly devoid of hair. Other sites beside the abdomen for penile construction are the inguinal region and the thigh. The scrotum is constructed in two stages from the skin of the thighs and perineum (Figs. 100–17 and 100–18). Silicone prostheses are placed within the fabricated scrotal sac to resemble testes. The constructed penile urethra must be joined with the perineal urethra, and this is achieved by making two parallel incisions between the two urethras, tubing the skin island, and covering it with the adjacent skin (Fig. 100–19). The newly made penile shaft functions satisfactorily as a guide for micturition, but erectile function and integumental sensation are absent (Fig. 100–20). The reader is also referred to Chapter 98 for additional details of penile construction.

### Female Hermaphroditism

Though this type of intersexuality is known by various names, probably the most popular is female pseudohermaphroditism associated with adrenal cortical hyperplasia. The adrenal cortex and the gonads synthesize compound F (hydrocortisone), androgens (17-ketosteroids), and other related steroids. The synthesis is accelerated by the action of adrenocorticotropin (ACTH) of the pituitary. If the adrenal cortex is not producing the hormones in the needed quantities, there is a compensatory increased perfusion of ACTH into the adrenal gland, and the cortical portion eventually becomes hyperplastic (Sydnor and coworkers, 1953). This endocrine situation leads to an increased secretion of adrenal androgens and hydrocortisone. If this cycle of events occurs in utero, it may produce the congenital anomaly designated as adrenocortical hyperplasia or female hermaphroditism.

One of the precursors of hydrocortisone production in the reticularis portion of the adrenal cortex is 17-hydroxyprogesterone. An excretion product of 17-hydroxyprogesterone is pregnanetriol (Jones, 1958). Laboratory analyses show an increase in the urinary 17-ketosteroids and pregnanetriol, and the 17-hydroxysteroids are low or not even measurable in congenital adrenocortical hyperplasia (virilizing adrenal

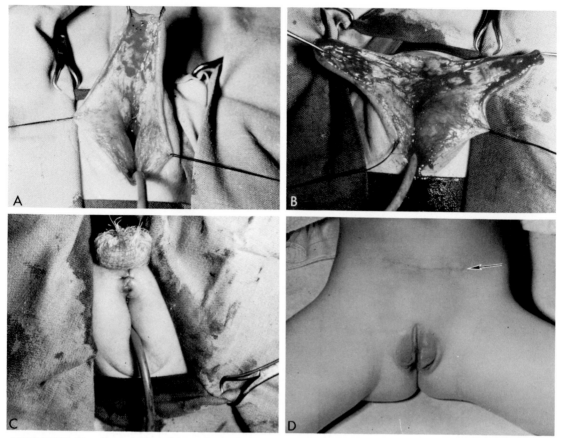

**FIGURE 100–12.** Construction of the vaginal vault. *A*, The phallic musculature is sacrificed, but the integumental hood is preserved to surface the newly constructed vaginal vault. *B*, The hood may be split and each half used to line the walls of the vagina. *C*, The flaps are inverted and the apices held in position by a mattress suture of steel wire tied over a gauze bolster. The catheter is in the bladder. *D*, The pelvic scar (arrow) and the reconstructed gynecoid external gonads six months following surgery.

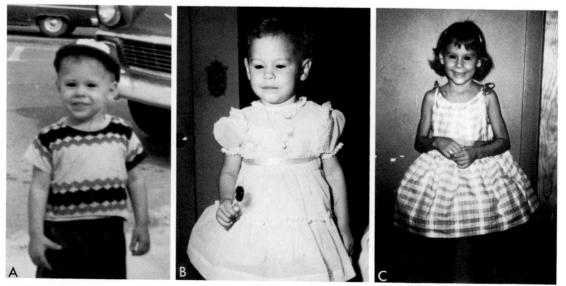

**FIGURE 100–13.** True hermaphrodite. *A*, At 18 months of age being reared as a boy. *B*, Six months following surgical sex assignment. *C*, Several years later. The patient has the characteristics and mental attitude of the female sex.

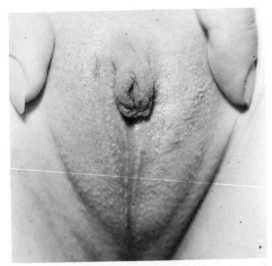

**FIGURE 100-14.** External genitalia of a true hermaphrodite who is 19 years of age and was reared as a male. A structure resembling a clitoris with redundant skin similar to a penile shaft is present. The deep median raphé separates the lateral labia-like enlargements which are without contents.

hyperplasia). If cortisone products are administered to the patient with congenital hyperadrenocorticogenitalism, the levels of steroids in the urine will approach normal values (Ely, Kelley and Raile, 1953; Wilkins, 1957). This is a diagnostic point of considerable importance. It is probable that the administered cortisone product suppresses the excess ACTH action on the adrenal reticularis and interrupts secretion of the virilizing hormone.

Female hermaphroditism is the most common of all the intersexual anomalies (Williams, 1952). The condition may be familial, as seen in Figure 100-6. It is to be suspected in any newborn with abnormal external genitalia. A study of the embryology (Greene, Matthews, Hughesdon and Howard, 1952; Gruenwald, 1947; Greenfelder and Lasch, 1949) is suggestive of wolffian duct atrophy. Derivatives of the urogenital sinus, such as the genital tubercle that forms the clitoris, the cephalic portion of the urogenital sinus that forms the urethra, and the caudal portion that results in the vagina and the labia, do not grow normally (Lattimer and coworkers, 1943; Campbell, 1963).

The patient with this intersexual abnormality has an enlarged clitoris which may resemble a hypospadiac penis (Fig. 100-21). The clitoris has two corpora cavernosa, but the urethra is absent and is found at the base of the clitoris or in the urogenital sinus. The glans penis is small, and the prepuce is usually redundant. The labia are fused in the midline, simulating a male scrotum with a median raphé; they do not contain gonads. It is common to locate a vaginal meatus, which is very small, by digital lateral traction of the labia. An opaque material can be instilled into the vaginal meatus and will show by roentgenography a vagina and possibly a uterus with oviducts (Fig. 100-22). Various modifications of the external genitalia are found. The internal genitals, including the ovarian structures, are gynecoid because the müllerian duct is normal.

**Diagnosis.** Early diagnosis of congenital adrenal cortical hyperplasia is sometimes necessary as a life-saving procedure. Because of the increased secretion of steroids by the adrenals, severe electrolyte disturbances may ensue. Persistent vomiting, dehydration, and malnutrition may lead to an erroneous diagnosis of congenital pyloric stenosis, a complicated electrolyte disorder, or some disease of inanition. The infant becomes moribund unless an accurate diagnosis is established early and cortisone products with sodium are administered.

These children grow much faster than normal, but the epiphyses of the bones close earlier; thus, when the child nears pubescence, she is shorter and heavier than other children of her age (Fig. 100-23). Full anatomical growth may be attained before the age of 12 years. Owing to an abnormal secretion of virilizing steroids, hair growth is also precocious. Mature growth of pubic and axillary hair appears early, followed by beard hair that may necessitate regular shaving. Skin blemishes, acne, and sebaceous cyst formation are common (Fig. 100-24).

In contrast to these various premature findings, the adult with congenital hyperadrenocorticogenitalism usually does not menstruate. The ovarian parenchymal structure is normal during infancy and childhood, but as age progresses there is minimum follicular maturation and an absence of ovulation and menstruation. Theoretically, the excess adrenal androgen and estrogen secretion inhibits pituitary gonadotropin production, with resultant ovarian quiescence (Jones, 1958). The breast tissues rarely develop to resemble those of the adult female mammary gland.

This anomaly is also observed in the male and is known as macrogenitosomia precox. The symptoms and physical findings simulate those of the female type, with adult dimensions of the external genitalia in childhood, stocky and muscular body build, and sterility.

*Text continued on page 3951*

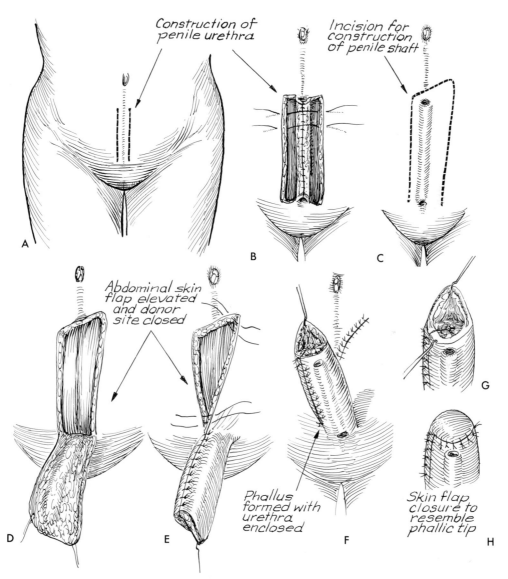

**FIGURE 100–15.** Construction of male genitalia. *A,* The linea alba is nearly hairless and is an ideal site for penile construction. *B,* Two parallel incisions are tubed to form the urethra. *C,* Six weeks later a skin flap is outlined by incisions only. *D,* The skin flap is delayed a second time and tubed with the urethral canal within it. *E,* The donor site is closed primarily. *F, G, H,* The tip of the skin flap is folded loosely to simulate a penis. The urethra does not extend through the folded flap end.

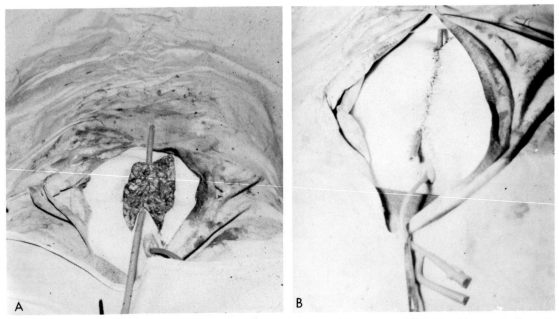

**FIGURE 100–16.** Construction of male genitalia. *A,* The urethral canal is constructed from the skin over the linea alba which is devoid of hair. Previous exploration revealed a complete absence of internal gonads and uterus. A catheter is used as a conformer. *B,* The new urethra is covered by abdominal skin, leaving the urethral conformer in place until healing is complete. The other catheter is placed in the bladder.

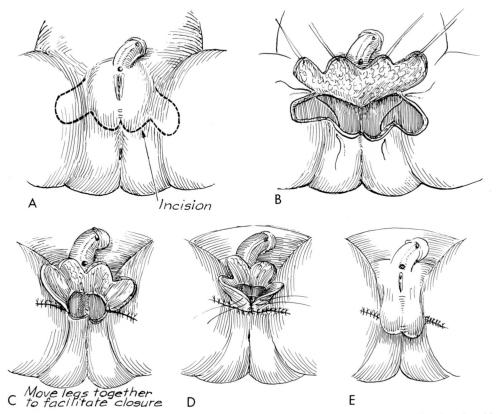

**FIGURE 100–17.** Construction of the scrotum. *A, B,* The scrotum is constructed in two stages by elevating skin flaps from the medial aspects of the thighs and perineum. *C,* The legs are moved closer together to facilitate primary approximation of the donor sites. *D,* The scrotal sac is sutured without tension. *E,* Two silicone prostheses are placed within the sac for cosmesis.

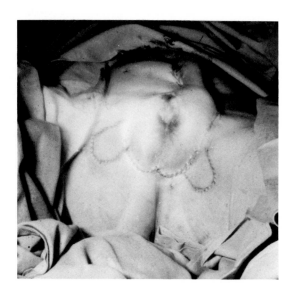

**FIGURE 100–18.** Photograph illustrating the first-stage delay of the outlined scrotal construction. One side is purposefully made lower than the other to conform with ideal masculinization.

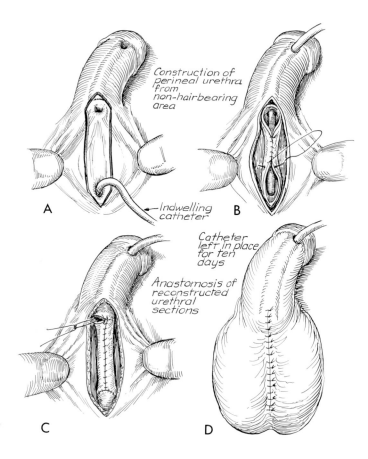

**FIGURE 100–19.** Union of the perineal and reconstructed urethras. *A*, The perineal urethra is completed by two parallel incisions joining the remaining orifices. *B*, The canal must be sufficiently large to avoid stricture formation. *C*, Absorbable sutures are used to close the urethra. *D*, Closure of the skin with interrupted nylon or wire sutures.

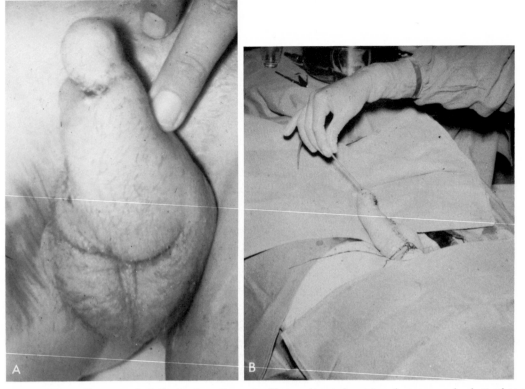

**FIGURE 100–20.** Constructed phallus and scrotum. *A*, The constructed scrotum becomes redundant when the phallic shaft is surgically thinned as in *B*. *B*, The phallus simulates a true penis and acts as a guide for the urinary stream; it has no erectile properties, and the skin is devoid of sensation.

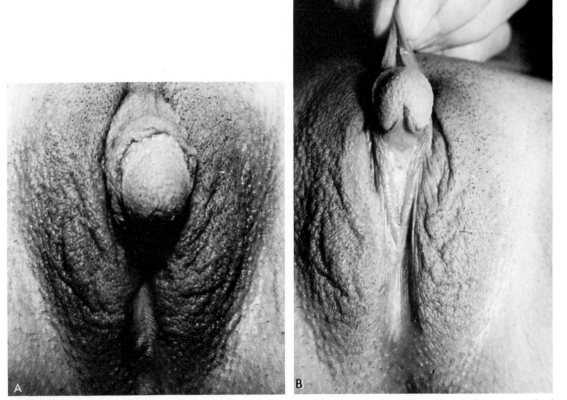

**FIGURE 100–21.** Female hermaphroditism (adrenal cortical hyperplasia) in a 10 year old child. *A*, The megaloclitoris had erroneously been circumcised. The labia, though bifid, are enlarged and redundant. Hirsutism is present (hair has been shaved). *B*, Digital elevation of the hypertrophied clitoris reveals no phallic urethra. The urogenital sinus houses the urethral orifice and conceals the vaginal vault, which can be probed.

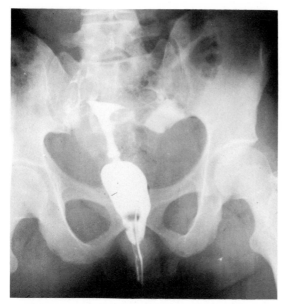

**FIGURE 100–22.** Abdominal exploration is not necessary in adrenal cortical hyperplasia, because an opaque medium inserted into the small vaginal orifice demonstrates a vagina, cervix, uterus, and patent oviducts.

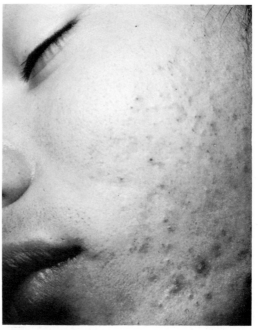

**FIGURE 100–24.** A form of hermaphroditism is also exemplified by lip hair, acne, comedo plugging, sebaceous cyst formation, and early facial scarring and pitting.

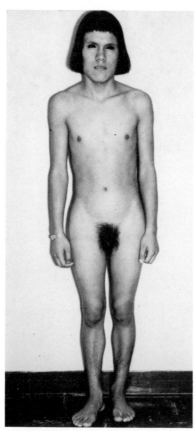

**FIGURE 100–23.** A 10 year old female hermaphrodite typically shows android characteristics, with wide shoulders, flat chest, narrow pelvis, muscular development, hirsutism, and short stature due to early epiphyseal closure.

Any patient who exhibits uncertain or undifferentiated external sex organs should be subjected to chromosomal examination. The smears from the buccal mucosa, vagina, blood, or skin will show a positive chromosomal sex mass within the cell if the patient is a female hermaphrodite.

**Differential Diagnosis.** The congenital type of adrenocorticohyperplasia must be differentiated from the acquired form of the disease, which is caused by either a masculinizing adrenal tumor (Meyer, 1925; Wilkins, 1948), idiopathic oversecretion of adrenocorticotropin (DeVaal, 1949), or exogenous administration of an androgenic or progestogenic substance to the gravid mother (Jones, 1958; Wilkins and coworkers, 1958; Nellhaus, 1958; Black and Bentley, 1959). The acquired prototype of the congenital form which is due to a masculinizing tumor occurs after birth, and therefore the genetic sex is never in doubt. The levels of 17-ketosteroids are elevated, but the concentrations of 17-hydroxysteroids and pregnanetriol are normal. Administration of cortisone products does not change the 17-ketosteroid excretion, and the anatomical configuration of the sex organs remains stationary. Diagnostic laparotomy is not necessary, as once believed. The subtypes of acquired adrenocortical hyperplasia, caused by an idiopathic oversecretion of adrenocorticotropin or exogenous administration of androgenic or progestogenic substances to the pregnant mother, may be identified by a history of medicinal therapy during pregnancy. The urinary 17-ketosteroid determinations are normal, and there is no progressive virilization. One consolation is that such subtypes are rare (Hamblen, 1957).

**Treatment.**    The sex assignment of congenital adrenocorticohyperplasia is female. Therapy is specifically endocrinologic, with possible surgical correction of the external genitalia. The therapeutic approach should be delegated to a pediatric endocrinologist because of the various complications involving electrolyte imbalance, bone growth, and maintenance doses of hormone treatment for lengthy periods of time. Relatively large doses of the corticoid are given to suppress adrenal activity, especially if surgery is anticipated in the near future. When the urinary 17-ketosteroids are reduced to the de-

sired level, a maintenance suppressive dosage schedule is formulated, and this is regulated by serial urinary determinations. If therapy is begun before 2 years of age, normal development is observed and precocious virilization remedied. If epiphyseal fusion has not occurred (under 7 years of age), cortisone therapy will prolong this natural process, and the child will continue to grow. If bone growth has reached the stage of epiphyseal closure, therapy will not be of assistance in this regard. Though hair growth and skin blemishes may have already appeared, treatment usually inhibits further manifestations of these symptoms. At the same time puberty may arrive normally, the breasts begin to enlarge, and the patient begins to menstruate.

SURGICAL TREATMENT    The types and methods of corrective surgery depend upon the judgment of the surgeon. The technique em-

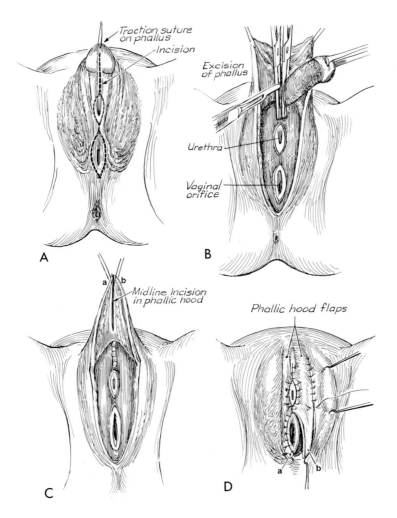

**FIGURE 100–25.** Surgical correction of female hermaphroditism is directed toward feminization. *A,* A midline incision is directed through the anterior wall of the urogenital sinus, and a catheter is placed in the urethra. *B,* The megaloclitoris is sacrificed. *C,* The stumps of the bulbocavernosus muscles are closed with sutures for purposes of hemostasis. The clitoral skin hood is also divided. *D,* Each half of the flap is used to cover the raw surfaces and to outline the vaginal and urethral orifices with formation of a fourchette.

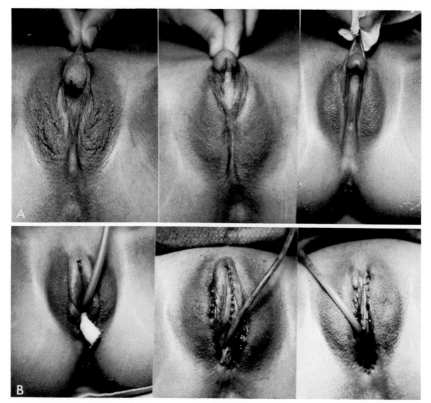

**FIGURE 100–26.** Three sisters with female hermaphroditism. *A*, Preoperative android features with differences in urogenital sinus development and positions of the urethral orifices. *B*, Postoperative appearance following construction of the vaginal vaults and labia minora.

ployed by the authors follows. A suture is placed through the glans for retraction, and a catheter is placed through the urethral meatus into the bladder. If the urethral orifice is concealed by a urogenital sinus, an incision is made from the opening at the base of the phallus, through the urogenital sinus, until the urethral orifice is found (Fig. 100–25). A Foley catheter is then introduced into the bladder and inflated. The megaloclitoris is removed, leaving the integumental covering as a skin flap. The stump of the corpora cavernosa is sutured for hemostatic purposes (Gardner, 1969). The remaining clitoral skin flap is then divided into equal halves and tailored to fit the surgical defect, i.e., to form the external limits of the vaginal vault, labia majora, and labia minora. The inferior portion of the vaginal mucosa is sutured to the integument. All suture material is of the absorbable type. A small lubricated tampon is inserted into the vagina, and the catheter is left in position. Figure 100–26 shows the manifestations of the syndrome in three sisters before and after surgery.

## Male Hermaphroditism

Synonymous terms used to designate this type of intersexuality include male pseudohermaphroditism (Hinman, 1953), hypoadrenocorticogenitalism, and gonadal dysgenesis. Three subtypes of this anomaly are usually described. The first is the combination of android or ambiguous external genitalia and gynecoid (or vestigial android) internal genitalia. The second type combines android or ambiguous external genitalia and android (or vestigial gynecoid) internal genitalia. In the third form the patient has gynecoid external genitalia and ectopic testes (inguinal or abdominal).

Regardless of the subtype, all of these types of male hermaphroditism are chromatin-negative. Adrenal gland function is normal, and the urinary 17-ketosteroids are neither elevated nor decreased. Though there are records of patients with a familial history, this is not the usual finding.

Because the patient with male hermaphroditism harbors ectopic testes, the scrotum is empty of contents and may appear gynecoid. The child may be mistaken for a female because the phallus is usually short and may show hypospadias, and the glans is very small (Fig. 100–27). On occasion there is a separate vaginal opening. As the individual reaches adulthood, android characteristics may develop, or, on the contrary, gynecoid characteristics may appear in the form of enlarged breasts (gynecomastia), resembling those of a woman. Some of these individuals marry and adjust successfully. The vaginal opening may be deep enough to permit coitus. There is an absence of menstruation, and shaving of facial hair may be necessary.

**Treatment.** The problem must be approached by the endocrinologist, the psychiatrist, and the surgeon. There is no known method of producing activity in testes that are aspermatogenic. Estrogen administration will sometimes enlarge the breasts, inhibit androidal growth of hair, and assist in keeping the voice alto or soprano. The endocrinologist utilizes these properties of estrogenic compounds. The psychiatrist directs his therapy toward achieving an emotionally adjusted patient, and

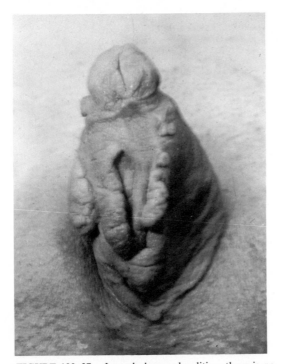

**FIGURE 100–27.** In male hermaphroditism there is no typical configuration but rather a variety of gradients. The patient, who has a short phallic structure with an abnormally small glans, was previously diagnosed as a female. Attempts to construct a vagina were unsuccessful. Though scrotal eminences are present, there are no contents.

this has proved to be of unequivocal assistance.

Inguinal hernias are common in this type of intersex, and it is often after a hernioplasty that the true sex of the patient is discovered.

The surgical procedure required in this type of hermaphrodite, after other determinations fail to supply sex assignment, includes exploration of the pelvis. The findings in the pelvis, in addition to the chromosomal and the external gonadal patterns, supply the evidence for further surgical intervention. If the decision is made to masculinize the patient, an orchiopexy is accomplished, if possible (Fig. 100–28). The testes are brought through the inguinal canals into the scrotum, with care taken to avoid injury to the testicular blood supply by excessive stretching of the testicular pedicles (Browne, 1949). The hypospadias is repaired and the vaginal vault obliterated at subsequent operations. If a decision is made to feminize the patient, the surgeon must either leave the internal gonads or remove them. It has been suggested that the gonads should be removed because of possible android secretions and carcinogenic properties. Neither of these possibilities has been confirmed. The external genitalia are treated by removing all android characteristics and improving gynecoid structures.

### Feminizing Testicularism

This interesting type of bisexuality is usually diagnosed after pubescence. The patient becomes cognizant that she is lacking the normal female function of menstruation or, later when she is married, that she is unable to satisfy her mate as she lacks a vaginal vault. The condition is strongly familial, and one set of twins with this type of bisexuality has been described (Blocker, Lewis and Snyder, 1953).

The usual distribution of female adiposity, as well as normally developed female breasts, is noted on physical examination. The voice is high-pitched and feminine. The scalp is usually well covered with hair, and there is an absence of facial hair. The axillary areas may be either scantily supplied or entirely devoid of hair, and the pubic hair, when present, is feminine in distribution. There are no aberrations of mental or physical sex status; the patient usually demonstrates attraction toward the male. Examination of the external genitalia shows average sized labia and clitoris; the vaginal vault is absent or shallow. A visible uterine cervix cannot be detected, and occasionally there is a

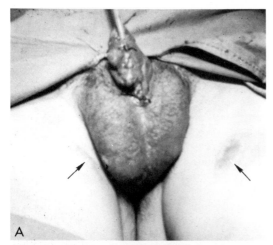

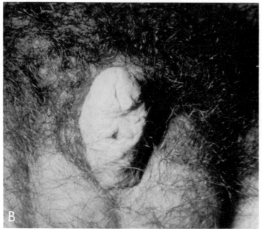

**FIGURE 100–28.** Surgical reconstruction in male hermaphroditism. *A*, First-stage reconstruction to retrieve the undescended testes and anchor them in their natural scrotal habitat by wire-elastic fixation to the thighs (arrows). A urethral canal with the meatus at the corona is also constructed. A scrotal diversion of the urinary stream protects the urethroplasty during healing. *B*, Appearance following reconstruction. The patient is married and the germinal father of two normal siblings.

bicornuate uterus (Fig. 100–29). The hormonal sex pattern is normal, and the chromosomal sex pattern is of the male type. One type of Turner's syndrome of ovarian dysgenesis blends into this category.

Diagnosis is aided by surgical exploration of the pelvis, which usually reveals an infantile or anomalous uterus and normal sized gonads which grossly simulate ovaries. However, microscopic examination of the gonads demonstrates immature seminiferous tubules without spermatogenesis. A preponderance of Sertoli and interstitial cells, instead of secreting male sex hormone, secrete female hormone.

The sex assignment of these patients should

definitely be female. Some endocrinologists believe the gonads should be removed because they are estrogen-producing. As previously stated, others who have studied this condition are concerned with the possibility of malignant degeneration of the abnormal gonads and recommend their removal. If the latter procedure is undertaken, exogenous estrogenic supplementation is administered (Freeman and Miller, 1969), because the patient develops a surgical menopause syndrome, with hot flashes, nervousness, and the usual concomitant manifestations.

The blind vaginal vault should be deepened by surgery (McIndoe, 1950; May, 1955), and a split-thickness skin graft should be inserted to serve as a lining (Fig. 100–30). A conformer made of plastic or a filled condom (Fig. 100–31) ensures successful vascularization of the graft and keeps the vault from shrinking in size (Owens, 1946). The conformer must re-

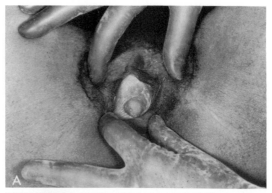

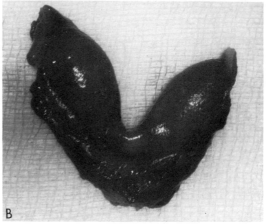

**FIGURE 100–29.** Feminizing testicularism. *A*, Patient with feminizing testicularism (testicular feminization) who is 19 years old and has a normal vaginal introitus but no vault. The clitoris, labia, and urethra and the distribution of pubic hair are normally gynecoid. The patient had never menstruated. *B*, On pelvic exploration, a uterus bicornis without cervix was found and removed.

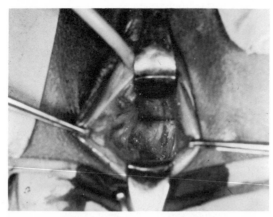

**FIGURE 100–30.** Following pelvic closure, the vaginal introitus is opened and a vault is made by digital dissection. The dissecting plane is nearly bloodless and should be of adequate dimension in depth and circumference.

main in place for three months and is removed only for cleansing and sexual intercourse. There are other methods of vaginal construction (Baldwin, 1907; Grad, 1932; Frank, 1940), and the subject is also discussed in Chapter 99.

### Turner's Syndrome

The original syndrome described by Turner in 1938 is more of historical than definitive interest, because many ovarian agenesis and dysgenesis conditions that have been discovered are much different from those discovered by Turner. The classic syndrome of Turner is designated gonadal agenesis and is represented by a short female with a thick webbed neck, cubitus valgus, retarded growth, primary amenorrhea, and infertility—the syndrome of infantilism (Fig. 100–32). It was soon discovered that most patients with Turner's syndrome are chromatin-negative with an XO karyotype and only 45 chromosomes (Fig. 100–33). Subsequent studies showed that other patients with similar features were found to have mosaics such as XO/XX, XO/XXX, XO/XX/XXX, and even an XY karyotype. Additional somatic differences have been noted, including lymphedema of the legs, cleft lip, cleft palate, hypertrophic scarring, congenital bands, ear deformities, micrognathia, deafness, epicanthal folds, and mental retardation (Fig. 100–34). Today, Turner's syndrome is considered a constellation of anomalies involving males as well as females. In fact, there are even individuals with features actually resembling those of the original Turner's syndrome, but in whom no intrinsic or extrinsic abnormali-

ties can be determined. Jones (1958) believed that it is inconsequential to resolve the nomenclature puzzle of this eponym, but one should realize that the syndrome comprises sexual infantilism due to streaks, short stature, and two or more of the mentioned somatic anomalies. Absent or undeveloped ovaries are characterized by thin streaks of white, firm, fibrous tissue (Fig. 100–35), which are microscopically indistinguishable from ovarian parenchyma.

**Treatment.** Both the sexual and somatic differences merit surveying. There is no known endocrine or chemical therapy that may rejuvenate a streak gonad, but such treatment is used, however, as replacement therapy following surgery. Surgical removal of the streaks is debatable, because neoplastic development is rare or nonexistent in XO patients. Less than 15 gonadoblastomas have been reported in XY karyotypes (Freeman and Miller, 1969). Because these children are sterile and there is a remote possibility of a neoplasm developing under endocrine therapy, the authors routinely ablate the streaks.

Following routine laboratory and clinical tests (cystoscopic, endoscopic, sigmoidoscopic), a laparotomy is performed, the pelvic organiture is examined, and a bilateral salpingogonadectomy is performed. The specimens are sent to the pathologist for histologic review. Surgical exploration has uncovered typical juvenile oviducts and an abundance of lutein and Leydig-like cells in the streaks with numerous immature tubules. No additional surgical sacrifice is necessary. The patients are placed on estrogen-progesterone therapy indefinitely, and the dosage is regulated according to the symptoms of a surgical climacteric. The authors administer 125 mg of Premarin (estrogen) for 21 days and 10 mg of Provera (progesterone) for seven days following surgery and continue this therapy indefinitely on a monthly basis.

Somatic anomalies are treated only when the patient and surgeon are in agreement. Congenital bands are released by Z-plasties (Fig. 100–36). Nuchal webs are also corrected by Z-plasties (see also Chapter 34). Cleft lips and cleft palates are repaired, and misplaced ears are repositioned.

### Klinefelter's Syndrome

Although the syndrome of gynecomastia, small testes, azoospermia, and increased urinary

*Text continued on page 3960*

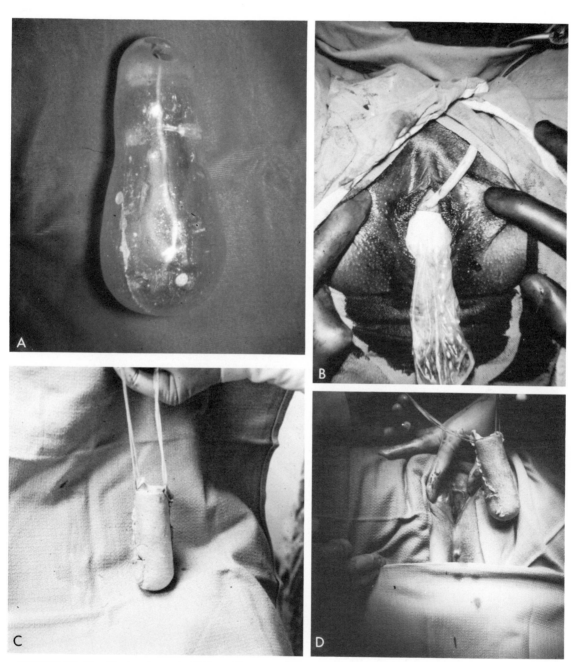

**FIGURE 100–31.** Vaginoplasty. *A*, Hollow silicone conformer. *B*, Condom filled with gauze or cotton. *C*, The skin graft is glued to the conformer with the raw surface exposed. *D*, The conformer with skin graft is inserted into the vaginal canal where it remains for seven days before removal. After the conformer and the vault are cleansed, the conformer is replaced; it remains there for three months and is removed only for cleansing or coitus.

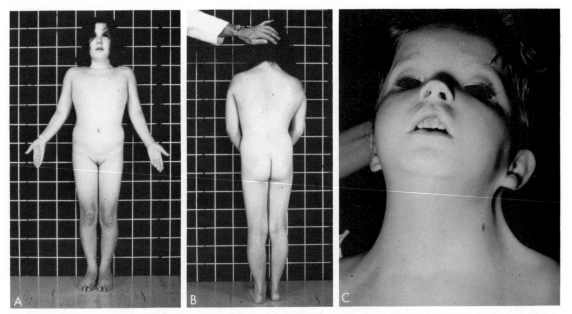

**FIGURE 100–32.** Turner's syndrome. Young female representing one gradient of Turner's syndrome, exemplified by a short stature, thickness and webbing of the neck, primary amenorrhea, and infertility.

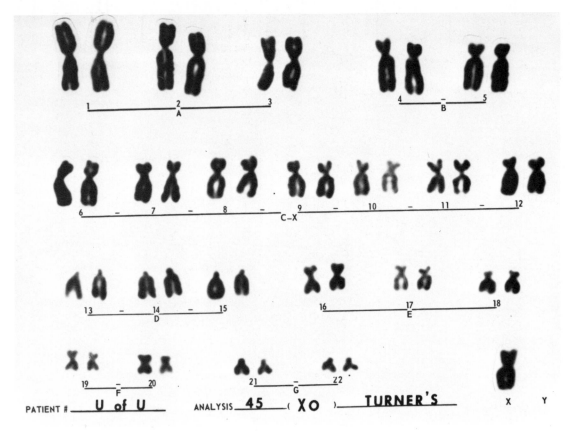

**FIGURE 100–33.** Karyotype of patient with Turner's syndrome. Note XO karyotype and the fact that there are only 45 chromosomes in the diagram.

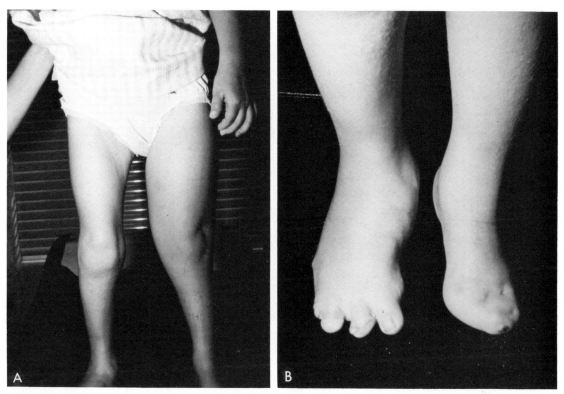

**FIGURE 100–34.** Turner's syndrome. Additional somatic differences include leg lymphedema, limb contractures, congenital bands, and talipes valgus.

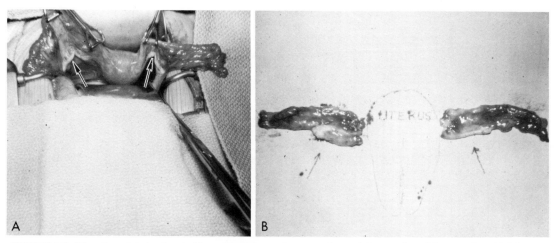

**FIGURE 100–35.** Gonadal streaks. *A,* Turner's syndrome is a type of gonadal agenesis and dysgenesis, which is represented by gonadal streaks (arrows) in the pelvic organiture. *B,* Appearance after they have been removed.

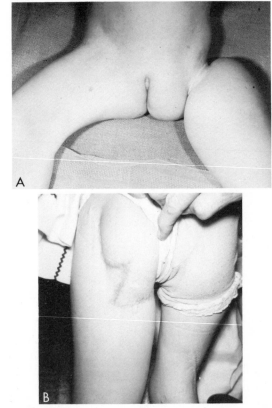

A

B

**FIGURE 100–36.** Congenital band in Turner's syndrome. *A,* A severe circumferential congenital band of the buttock and thigh. *B,* Completely relieved by multiple Z-plasties extended to the bone in depth.

gonadotropins was described in 1942 by Klinefelter, Reifenstein, and Albright, there were others who had previously published reports (Lereboullet, 1877; Meige, 1895). The typical patient is tall, with long limbs, narrow shoulders, broad hips, scanty body hair, enlarged breasts, and small and tender testes; he also tends to answer questions slowly and unintelligently (Fig. 100–37, *A, B*). Another common phenotype is a short, fat individual with the same secondary characteristics (Fig. 100–37, *C, D*). Many patients are chromatin-positive, although chromatin-negative individuals are not uncommon. The genotype is usually XXY with 47 chromosomes (Fig. 100–38). Although the testes may be normal in size and the patient may enjoy penile erection and sexual relations, his semen contains no sperm, and a testicular biopsy shows tubular hyalinization and fibrosis. The patients are infertile; the urinary 17-ketosteroids are diminished, but the follicle-stimulating hormone is increased.

Klinefelter's syndrome is common, and there are many persons with the condition who are actually unaware of their anomaly. These people usually become embarrassed and seek aid for their large, bilateral breasts or seek an explanation for their inability to have children. There is no presently known drug which will reduce the mammary hypertrophy, increase the intelligence quotient, or produce fertility through gametogenesis. Considerable improvement is gained by reduction mammaplasty (Fig. 100–39) and substitutional androgen therapy. Removal of the large breasts helps the patient gain confidence, and his mental status usually improves. The best results are achieved with intramuscular or oral administration of testosterone in doses of 1000 mg administered every two weeks. If the patient shows improvement with a noticeable increase in masculine characteristics, the testosterone dosage is decreased to 500 mg bimonthly and less, if feasible. Often the body fat deposits are replaced by muscle tissue. A decrease in eunuchoid proportions occurs, as well as an increase in masculine distribution of body hair. Changes in personality characterized by lessened' irritability and increased aggressiveness, self-confidence, and ambition are seen following therapy.

### Transsexualism

A preferable term for transsexualism may be psychopathia transsexualis, because the individual is dominated by a fantasy preferring the opposite gender role to the one endowed him. Cauldwell (1949) is credited with being the first person to use the word "transsexualism." The desire for some males to assume feminine roles is primeval. The male transsexual is disgusted with his normal male phenotype and genotype and is anxious to shed his male characteristics by surgical and hormonal feminization. There are examples of self-inflicted genital mutilation to satisfy this desire. The transsexual male states that he prefers heterosexual companions and disapproves of sex relations with homosexual males. The desire for the male transsexual to adopt female mannerisms begins early in childhood and progresses convincingly as the youngster develops secondary sex characteristics. The cross-gender behavior consists of wearing dresses, lace panties, and high heeled shoes, of playing and associating strictly with females, and of participating in all daily activities as a woman. The female transsexual, who wishes to be a male, similarly abhors her body contour and dreams of being a male and participating in masculine activities.

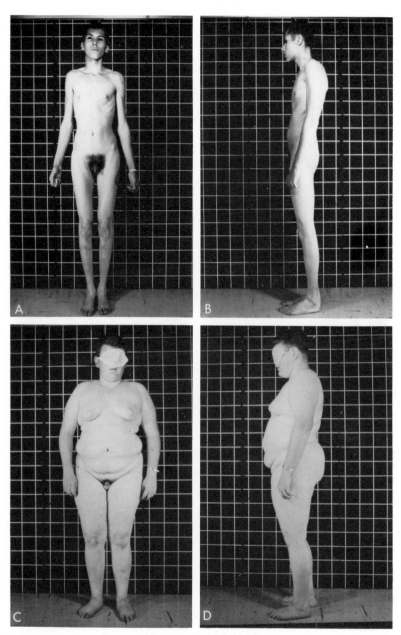

**FIGURE 100–37.** Klinefelter's syndrome. *A, B,* Klinefelter's syndrome may be represented by a tall stature, long arms, narrow shoulders, broad hips, scanty body hair, enlarged breasts, and small tender testes. *C, D,* The patient may also be adipose and short in stature.

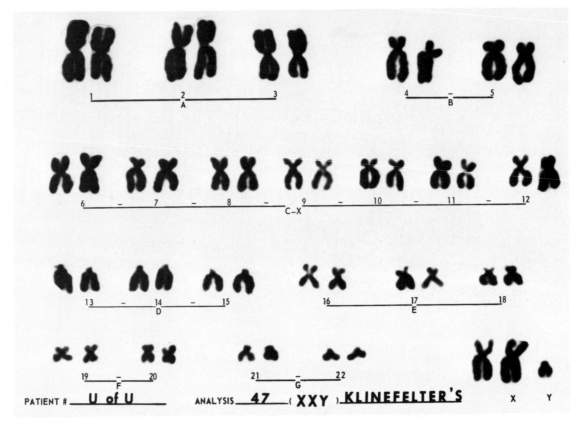

**FIGURE 100–38.** Klinefelter's syndrome. The genotype is usually expressed by an additional chromosome (47) and by a karyotype of XXY.

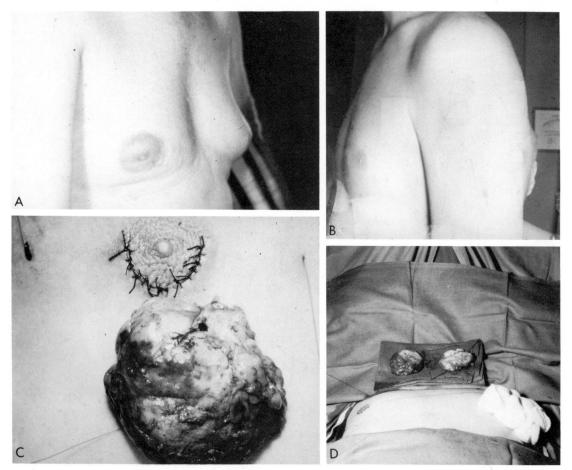

**FIGURE 100–39.** Gynecomastia associated with Klinefelter's syndrome. *A*, Three-quarter view before surgery. *B*, Profile view after surgery. *C*, Specimen following reduction mammaplasty. *D*, Bilateral specimens superimposed on the chest.

Many gender teams prefer to separate the transsexual from the transvestite and homosexual by distinguishing between their sexual and gender motives. They report that the true transsexual presents a persistent contragender role as a child, long before homosexuality or genital sexuality is known by the child. The transsexual hates his genitals and will sacrifice them any time; the homosexual enjoys the use of his genitals and will not tolerate their removal. The transsexual is considered to have a weak sexual drive or libido and will avoid genital relations to keep his sex identity hidden, whereas the transvestite makes considerable efforts to have genital contact. There are many authors who feel that the number of transsexuals is woefully underestimated (Pauly, 1969; Fogh-Andersen, 1969; Walinder, 1967; Benjamin, 1967) and that the incidence is increasing. Pauly (1969) believed that there is one male transsexual

to every 100,000 men and one female transsexual to every 400,000 women. Walinder (1967) in Sweden estimated incidences of 1:37,000 and 1:103,000, respectively. The reported age distributions vary; our youngest patient was 26 years of age and the oldest 53. The results of sex reassignment surgery are difficult to evaluate, because many of the patients are transient and answers to questionnaires are sporadic. Our estimate of satisfied postsurgical patients is about 65 per cent, but it can be said that improvement in terms of emotional and social adjustment is very good in the majority of patients.

When the psychiatrist feels he has reached his limits of therapy and the desired results have not yet been achieved, hormonal and surgical therapy is considered. The gender clinic physicians make the final decision regarding conversion surgery, and this usually requires three to six months of preliminary studies and tests. Parents and guardians are thoroughly familiarized with every facet, and their permission, along with the decision of the patient, is considered reason for conversion of sex. Surgical intervention in transsexualism without psychiatric approval is detrimental and may possibly terminate in suicide (Hoopes, Knorr and Wolf, 1969). Laub and Fisk (1974) require that the patient live and function in the gender of his choice for several years before reconstructive surgery is recommended.

Surgery for the male transsexual is a one-stage procedure involving the genitals and the breasts. Two operating teams work concomitantly, one augmenting the breasts with silicone prostheses while the other team is converting the male genitals to resemble those of a female. Outlines of incisions are made with a marking pen on the penile shaft and scrotum (Fig. 100–40, *A*). The corpora cavernosa as well as the gonads are removed, and the remaining integumental cloaks are sewn together to be used in forming the anterior and posterior walls of the vaginal vault and the labia (Fig. 100–40, *B*). The urethra is brought through a buttonhole in the skin flap and sutured in the natural position. At times a portion of the male glans penis is converted to mimic a clitoris. A planned silicone conformer (or cotton-filled condom) is employed to hold the skin flaps in position within the vagina (Fig. 100–40, *C*).

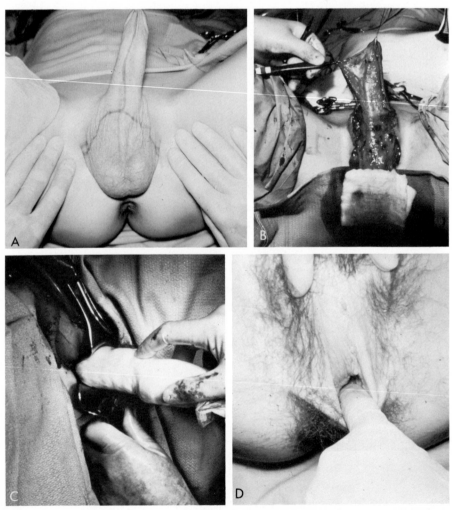

**FIGURE 100–40.**   Genital reconstruction in the transsexual. *A,* The initial incision is extended from the prepuce to the base of the shaft, where it is made to diverge to the scrotal-inguinal junction. The penile skin is separated from the corpus cavernosum muscles and the urethra, and the scrotal skin is dissected from its contents. The remaining genital tissues except the urethra are sacrificed. *B,* The penile and scrotal integumental cloaks are sutured at their distal ends and inverted into the new vaginal vault. *C,* The skin flap lining is maintained in position with a stent made of plastic or a condom filled with soft material. *D,* The vaginal canal must be large enough for coital relations, and the introitus must be soft and pliable.

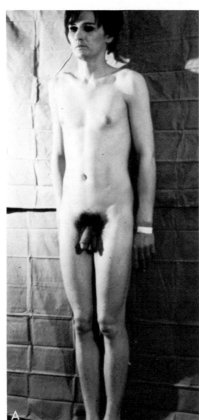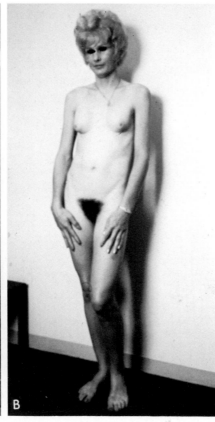

**FIGURE 100–41.** Surgical reconstruction in the transsexual. *A,* Preoperative photograph of a transsexual with normal masculine phenotype and genotype. *B,* Postsurgical appearance.

The transformation is a reasonable facsimile of female genitalia (Fig. 100–40, *D*), and the change in torso structure is quite noticeable (Fig. 100–41).

A modification of the Baldwin (1907) technique to construct a vaginal vault has also been employed. The low abdominal approach affords excellent exposure to the distal ileum, where a segment measuring approximately 14 cm is isolated on its neurovascular pedicle (Fig. 100–42, *A*) and transferred to the opening in the perineum to form the vaginal vault (Fig. 100–42, *B*). Initially, there is a minimal amount of mucosal excretion, but this decreases with vaginal douches and conscientious hygiene.

The female transsexual who wishes to be masculinized must endure five to six stages of surgical procedures similar to those described earlier in the chapter for the true hermaphrodite. A skin flap is devised from either the abdominal wall, the inguinal region, or the thigh, with skin innervation remaining intact. The scrotal skin is sometimes used as a covering, including its sensory innervation. The urethra is fabricated from a segment of ileum, with its neurovascular supply attached. The bowel segment is rotated into a canal made specifically for it in the penile shaft. Thus, urethral sensation as well as external skin sensation is provided. The pectineus muscle is transposed to act as a suspensory ligament and penile shaft elevator. Orticochea (1972) reconstructed the penile shaft and the urethra from innervated inguinal and thigh skin flaps, which included the gracilis muscle and a silicone rod for erectile purposes. Noe, Birdsell, and Laub (1974) marsupialized an external skin tube on the penile shaft. A plastic implant was inserted for erection purposes and removed at the patient's will for cleansing. The authors have used this procedure for treatment of impotence due to various spinal injuries among other causes (Fig. 100–43).

In summary, the gender clinic staff should conduct all examinations and extend requests for consultations. For sex reassignment surgery, the patient must be a true transsexual. A legal change of sex should be established and psychotherapy instituted postoperatively.

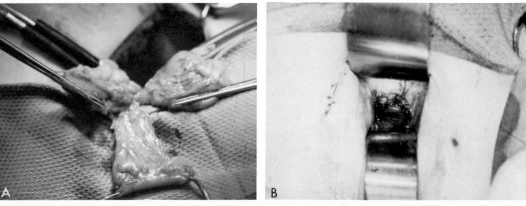

**FIGURE 100–42.** An alternate method of vaginal construction is to utilize a segment of ileum or sigmoid with preservation of the neurovascular pedicle. *A,* Exteriorized intestinal segment. *B,* The bowel segment is brought into the dissected area between the bladder and rectum, sutured to the introital inlet, and the deep end closed to form the vault.

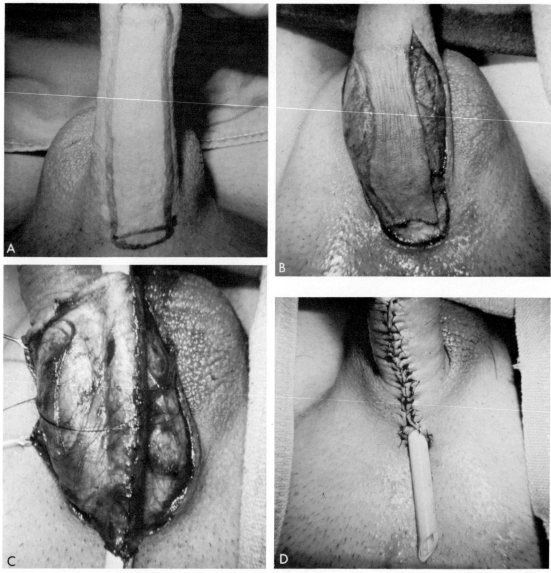

**FIGURE 100–43.** Construction of a penile rod for impotence. *A,* For erection purposes, two parallel lines are drawn on the penile shaft. *B,* Incisions are made. *C,* A skin-lined tube is constructed which will later be the site for a Teflon or silicone ramrod. *D,* The tube is constructed over a catheter conformer, which is left in place until the wound edges are healed.

# REFERENCES

Allen, E., Danforth, C. H., and Doisy, E. A.: Sex and Internal Secretions. 2nd Ed. Baltimore, The Williams & Wilkins Company, 1939.

Arey, L. B.: Developmental Anatomy. 6th Ed. Philadelphia, W. B. Saunders Company, 1954.

Baldwin, J. F.: Formation of an artificial vagina by intestinal transplantation. Am. J. Obstet. Gynecol., 56:636, 1907.

Bankoff, G. A.: Plastic Repair of Genito-urinary Defects. New York, Philosophical Library, 1956.

Barlow, P., and Vosa, C. G.: The Y chromosome in human spermatozoa. Nature (Lond.), 226:961, 1970.

Barr, M. L.: An interim note on the application of the skin biopsy test of chromosomal sex to hermaphrodites. Surg. Gynecol. Obstet., 99:184, 1954.

Barr, M. L., and Bertram, E. G.: A morphological distinction between neurones of the male and female, and the behavior of the nucleolar satellite during accelerated nucleoprotein synthesis. Nature, 163:676, 1949.

Bascom, K. F.: The interstitial cells of the gonads of cattle, with especial reference to their embryonic development and significance. Am. J. Anat., 31:223, 1923.

Benjamin, H.: Transvestism and transsexualism in the male and female. J. Sex Res., 3:107, 1967.

Bergada, C., Cleveland, W. W., Jones, H. W., Jr., and Wilkins, L.: Gonadal histology in patients with male pseudohermaphroditism and atypical gonadal dysgenesis: Relation to theories of sex differentiation. Acta Endocr., 40:493, 1962.

Bergemann, E.: Sex determination in newborn infants. Schweiz. Med. Wochenschr., 91:292, 1961.

Berthrong, M., Goodwin, W. E., and Scott, W. W.: Estrogen production by the testis. J. Clin. Endocr., 9:579, 1949.

Black, J. A., and Bentley, J. F. R.: Effect on the fetus of androgens given during pregnancy. Lancet, 1:21, 1959.

Blakely, S. B.: The diagnosis of the sex of the human fetus in utero. Am. J. Obstet. Gynecol., 34:322, 1937.

Blocker, T. G., Lewis, S. R., and Snyder, C. C.: Plastic construction of an artificial vagina. Plast. Reconstr. Surg., 11:177, 1953.

Brachetto-Braun, D., Grimaldi, F., and Rochello Costa, A. O.: Hermaphroditismus verus lateralis. Rev. Assoc. Méd. Argent., 57:900, 1943.

Briggs, D. K., and Kupperman, H. S. L.: Sex differentiation by leukocyte morphology. J. Clin. Endocr., 15:1163, 1956.

Browne, D.: Treatment of undescended testicle. Proc. R. Soc. Med., 42:643, 1949.

Bryan, A. L., Nigro, J. A., and Counseller, V. S.: One hundred cases of congenital absence of the vagina. Surg. Gynecol. Obstet., 88:79, 1949.

Bunge, R. G., and Bradbury, J. T.: Genetic sex; chromatin test versus gonadal histology. J. Clin. Endocr., 16:1117, 1956.

Bunge, R. G., and Bradbury, J. T.: The sex chromatin test in clinical practice. J. Urol., 77:759, 1957.

Burns, R. K., Jr.: The sex of parabiotic twins in amphibia. J. Exp. Zool., 42:31, 1925.

Buyse, A.: A case of extreme sex modification in an adult bovine freemartin. Anat. Rec., 66:43, 1935.

Cabot, H.: Modern Urology. Vol. 5. Philadelphia, Lea & Febiger, 1946.

Campbell, M. F.: Pediatric Urology. Vol. 2. New York, The Macmillan Company, 1937.

Campbell, M. F.: Clinical Pediatric Urology. Philadelphia, W. B. Saunders Company, 1951.

Campbell, M. F.: Urology. Vol. 1. Philadelphia, W. B. Saunders Company, 1954.

Campbell, M. F.: Urology. 2nd Ed. Philadelphia, W. B. Saunders Company, 1963.

Carpentier, P. J., Stolte, L. A. M., and Visschers, G. P.: Gonadal dysgenesis and testicular tumors. Lancet, 1:386, 1956.

Caspersson, T., Zech, L., and Johansson, C.: Differential binding of alkylating fluorochromes in human chromosomes. Exp. Cell Res., 60:315, 1970.

Cauldwell, D. O.: Psychopathia transsexualis. Sexology, 16:274, 1949.

Cavallero, C., and Zanardi, F.: Male pseudohermaphroditism in three siblings. A.M.A. Arch. Pathol., 55:142, 1953.

Cecil, A. B.: A true hermaphrodite. S. Afr. Med. J., 29:238, 1955.

Collier, T. W.: Pseudohermaphroditism in twins: Report of tenth case. Am. J. Dis. Child., 76:208, 1948.

Cooper, E. R. A.: Histology of the retained testis in human subject at different ages and its comparison with scrotal testis. J. Anat., 64:5, 1929.

Davidson, W. M., and Smith, D. R.: A morphological sex difference in the polymorphonuclear neutrophil leukocytes. Br. Med. J., 2:6, 1954.

Davis, D. M., and Scheffey, L. C.: A case of true hermaphroditism. J. Urol., 56:715, 1946.

Delore, P., Noel, R., Perrin, J., Guinet, P., and Blanc, J.: A case of true hermaphroditism with a histological study of the testicle and ovary. Pédiatrie, 8:458, 1953.

Deming, C. L., Goettsch, J. B., and Humm, F. D.: Clinical and hormonal studies in familial pseudohermaphroditism. J. Urol., 61:144, 1949.

DeMoura, A. C., and Pinto Basto, L.: True hermaphroditism. J. Urol., 56:725, 1946.

DeVaal, O. M.: Gonads, adrenals and intersexuality. Gynaecologia (Basel), 128:205, 1949.

Dewhurst, C. J.: Diagnosis of sex before birth. Lancet, 1:471, 1956.

Dmowski, W. P., and Greenblatt, R. B.: Abnormal sexual differentiation. Am. Fam. Physician, 3:1, 1971.

Eastman, N. J.: Prenatal determination of sex. Obstet. Gynecol. Surv., 15:636, 1960.

Ehrenfeld, E. N., and Bromberg, Y. M.: Syndrome of gonadal dysgenesis with enlarged clitoris in chromosomal males. Acta Endocr., 28:540, 1958.

Ely, R. S., Kelley, V. C., and Raile, R. B.: Studies of 17-hydroxycorticosteroids in children; peripheral blood levels in health and disease. J. Pediatr., 42:38, 1953.

Engle, E. T., Yeaw, R. C., and Lattimer, J. K.: True hermaphroditism: Supplementary report of a case. J. Urol., 56:931, 1946.

Fischer, H. W., Lischer, C. E., and Byars, L. T.: True hermaphroditism. Ann. Surg., 136:864, 1952.

Fogh-Andersen, P.: Transsexualism, an attempt at surgical management. Scand. J. Plast. Reconstr. Surg., 3:61, 1969.

Ford, C. E.: Human cytogenetics: Its present place and future possibilites. Am. J. Hum. Genet., 12:104, 1960.

Ford, C. E.: The cytogenetic analysis of some disorders of sex development. Am. J. Obstet. Gynecol., 82:1154, 1961.

Ford, C. E., Jones, K. W., Palami, P. E., deAlmeida, J. C., and Briggs, J. H.: A sex chromosome anomaly in a case of gonadal dysgenesis (Turner's syndrome). Lancet, 1:711, 1959.

Frank, R. T.: The formation of an artificial vagina without operation (intubation method). N.Y. J. Med., 40:1669, 1940.

Frazer, J. E.: A Manual of Embryology. The Development of the Human Body. London, Tindall and Cox, 1931.

Freeman, M. V. R., and Miller, O. J.: XY gonadal dysgenesis and gonadoblastoma. Obstet. Gynecol., 34:478, 1969.

Fuchs, F., and Riis, P.: Antenatal sex determination. Nature (Lond.), *177*:330, 1956.

Gardner, L. J.: Endocrine and Genetic Diseases of Childhood. Philadelphia, W. B. Saunders Company, 1969, p. 422.

Glenister, T. W.: The origin and fate of the urethral plate in man. J. Anat., *88*:413, 1954.

Goldschmidt, R.: Physiological Genetics. New York, McGraw-Hill Book Company, 1938.

Grad, H.: The technique of formation of an artificial vagina. Surg. Gynecol. Obstet., *54*:200, 1932.

Greene, R. R.: Embryology of sexual structure and hermaphroditism. J. Clin. Endocr., *4*:335, 1944.

Greene, R. R., Matthews, D., Hughesdon, P. E., and Howard, A.: A case of true hermaphroditism. Br. J. Surg., *40*:263, 1952.

Greenfelder, B., and Lasch, W.: Anomalies. Ann. Paediatr., *173*:388, 1949.

Gruenwald, P.: Mechanisms of abnormal development. Arch. Pathol., *44*:398, 1947.

Grumbach, M. M., Van Wyk, J. J., and Wilkins, L.: Chromosomal sex in gonadal dysgenesis (ovarian agenesis); relationship to male pseudohermaphroditism and theories of human sex differentiation. J. Clin. Endocr., *15*:1161, 1955.

Gudernatsch, F.: True hermaphroditism: Concerning the 37 cases reported. J. Urol., *52*:620, 1945.

Gudernatsch, J. T.: Hermaphroditismus verus in man. Am. J. Anat., *11*:267, 1911.

Haddad, H. M., and Wilkins, L.: Congenital anomalies associated with gonadal aplasia. Pediatrics, *23*:885, 1959.

Hale, M. T., Vaughn, W. K., and Engel, E.: Fluorescent male sex chromatin in white blood cells. South. Med. J., *66*:340, 1973.

Hamblen, E. C.: The assignment of sex to an individual: Some enigmas and some practical clinical criteria. Am. J. Obstet. Gynecol., *74*:1228, 1957.

Hamblen, E. C., Palma, E., and Poshyachinda, D.: The congenital rudimentary gonad syndrome. Clin. Obstet. Gynecol., *3*:207, 1960.

Hamilton, W. J., Boyd, J. D., and Mossman, H. W.: Human Embryology. 3rd Ed. Baltimore, The Williams & Wilkins Company, 1962.

Hampson, J. G.: Hermaphroditic genital appearance, rearing and eroticism in hyperadrenocorticism. Bull. Johns Hopkins Hosp., *96*:265, 1955.

Hayword, M.: Chromosomal trisomy associated with Sturge-Weber syndrome. Lancet, *2*:844, 1960.

Hinman, F.: The Principles & Practice of Urology. Philadelphia, W. B. Saunders Company, 1935.

Hooks, C. A.: Clinical aspects of intersexuality. J. Urol., *62*:528, 1949.

Hoopes, J. E., Knorr, C. P., and Wolf, F. S.: Transsexualism: Considerations regarding sexual reassignment. J. Nerv. Ment. Dis., *147*:510, 1969.

Howard, F. S.: Mammalian chromosomes in vitro. 1. The karyotype of men. J. Hered., *43*:167, 1952.

Hsu, T. C., Hooks, C. A., and Pomerat, C. M.: Opportunities for determining sex in human tissues. Texas Rep. Biol. Med., *11*:585, 1953.

Huffman, J. W.: Disorders of the external genitalia and vagina during childhood. Pediatr. Clin. North Am., *5*:35, 1958.

Jacobs, P. A., Baikie, A. G., Court Brown, W. M., MacGregor, T. N., Maclean, N., and Harnden, D. G.: Evidence for the existence of the human "super female." Lancet, *2*:423, 1959.

Jacobs, P. A., and Strong, J. A.: A case of human intersexuality having a possible XXY sex determining mechanism. Nature, *183*:302, 1959.

James, F.: Sexing foetuses by examination of amniotic fluid. Lancet, *1*:202, 1956.

Jones, H. W., Jr.: Masculinization of the female fetus. The role of exogenous progestogens during pregnancy. Curr. Med. Dig., *25*:53, 1958.

Jones, H. W., Jr., and Jones, G. E. S.: The gynecological aspects of adrenal hyperplasia and allied disorders. Am. J. Obstet. Gynecol., *68*:1330, 1954.

Jones, H. W., Jr., and Scott, W. W.: Hermaphroditism, Genital Anomalies and Related Endocrine Disorders. Baltimore, The Williams & Wilkins Company, 1971, p. 75.

Jordan, H. E., and Kindred, J. E.: A Textbook of Embryology. 4th Ed. New York, D. Appleton-Century Company, 1942.

Jost, A.: Problems of fetal endocrinology: The gonadal and hypophyseal hormones. Rec. Prog. Horm. Res., *8*:379, 1953.

Kiefer, J. H., McGrew, E. A., Rosenthal, I., and Bronstein, I. P.: Sex chromatin determination in intersex states. J. Urol., *77*:762, 1957.

Klebs, E.: Handbuch der pathologischen Anatomie. Berlin, August Hirschwald, 1876.

Klinefelter, H. F., Jr., Reifenstein, E. C., Jr., and Albright, F.: Syndrome characterized by gynecomastia, aspermatogenesis without aleydigism, and increased excretion of follicle-stimulating hormone. J. Clin. Endocr., *2*:615, 1942.

Kozelka, A. W., and Gallagher, T. F.: Effect of male hormone extracts, theelin and theelol on the chick embryo. Proc. Soc. Exp. Biol. Med., *31*:1143, 1934.

Lamborot-Manzur, M., Tishler, P. V., and Atkins, L.: Fluorescent drumsticks in male polymorphs. Lancet, *1*:973, 1971.

Lattimer, J. K., Engle, E. T., and Yeaw, R. C.: True hermaphroditism: Case report, with interpretations. J. Urol., *50*:481, 1943.

Laub, D. R., and Fisk, N.: A rehabilitation program for gender dysphoria syndrome by surgical sex change. Plast. Reconstr. Surg., *53*:388, 1974.

Lauterwein, C., and Kladetzky, J.: Hermaphroditismus glandularis (H. verus) mit Ovotestis. Z. Geburtshilfe. Gynaekol., *143*:257, 1955.

Lejeune, J., Turpin, R., and Gautier, M.: Le mongolisme, premier exemple d'aberration autosomique humaine. Ann. Genet., *2*:41, 1959.

Lereboullet, L.: Contribution à l'étude des atrophies testiculaires et des hypertrophies mammaires observies à la suite de certaines orchites (feminisme). Gaz. Hebd. Med., *14*;533, 1877.

Lillie, F. R.: The theory of the freemartin. Science, *43*:611, 1916.

Lillie, F. R.: The freemartin: A study of the action of sex hormones in the foetal life of cattle. J. Exp. Zool., *23*:371, 1917.

Lowsley, O. S., and Kirwin, T. J.: Clinical Urology. 3rd Ed. Baltimore, The Williams & Wilkins Company, 1956, p. 182.

McIndoe, A.: Treatment of congenital absence and obliterative conditions of the vagina. Br. J. Plast. Surg., *2*:254, 1950.

McKenna, C. M., and Kiefer, J. H.: Two cases of true hermaphroditism. J. Urol., *52*:464, 1944.

Marberger, E., Boccabella, R. A., and Nelson, W. O.: Oral smear as a method of chromosomal sex detection. Proc. Soc. Exp. Biol. Med., *89*:488, 1955.

Mason, H. L., and Engstrom, W. W.: 17-Ketosteroids; their origin, determination and significance. Physiol. Rev., *30*:321, 1950.

May, H.: The metamorphosis of a male pseudohermaphrodite. Plast. Reconstr. Surg., *15*:433, 1955.

Meige, H.: Infantilism, La Feminism et L'Hermaphrodite. Paris, G. Masson, 1895.

Meyer, R.: True and false hermaphroditism and gonad tumors. Arch. Gynak., *123*:675, 1925.

Minervini, F., Schwarzenberg, T. L., Canibus, R., and Natoli, G.: The surgical therapy of intersexuals. Arch. Ital. Pediatr. Pueric., *26*:275, 1969.

Money, J., Hampson, J. G., and Hampson, J. L.: Hermaphroditism; recommendations concerning assignment of sex, change of sex and psychologic management. Bull. Johns Hopkins Hosp., *97*:284, 1955.

Moore, C. R.: Embryonic Sex Hormones and Sexual Differentiation. Springfield, Ill., Charles C Thomas, Publisher, 1947, p. 7.

Moore, K. L.: Sex, intersex and the chromatin test. Modern Med., Oct. 1, 1960, p. 235.

Moore, K. L., and Barr, M. L.: Smears from the oral mucosa in the detection of chromosomal sex. Lancet, *2*:57, 1955.

Moore, K. L., Graham, M. A., and Barr, M. L.: The detection of chromosomal sex in hermaphrodites from a skin biopsy. Surg. Gynecol. Obstet., *96*:641, 1953.

Morris, J. M.: Syndrome of testicular feminization in male pseudohermaphrodites. Am. J. Obstet. Gynecol., *65*:1192, 1953.

Murphy, D. P.: Congenital Malformations: A Study of Parental Characteristics. 2nd Ed. Philadelphia, J. B. Lippincott Company, 1947.

Naib, Z. M.: Chromosomal sex determination. Obstet. Gynecol., *18*:64, 1961.

Nellhaus, G.: Artificially induced female pseudohermaphroditism. New Engl. J. Med., *258*:935, 1958.

Noe, J. M., Birdsell, D., and Laub, D. R.: The surgical construction of male genitalia for the female-to-male transsexual. Plast. Reconstr. Surg., *53*:511, 1974.

Nowell, P. G., and Hungerford, D. A.: Chromosome studies on normal and leukemic human leukocytes. J. Natl. Cancer Inst., *25*:85, 1960.

Ohno, S., and Makino, S.: Derivation of sex chromatin. Lancet, *1*:78, 1961.

Orticochea, M.: A new method of total reconstruction of the penis. Br. J. Plast. Surg., *25*:347, 1972.

Overzier, C.: Hermaphroditismus verus. Acta Endocr., *20*:63, 1955.

Owens, N.: A suggested Pyrex form for support of skin grafts in the construction of an artificial vagina. Plast. Reconstr. Surg., *1*:350, 1946.

Pauly, I. P.: The current status of the change of sex operation. J. Nerv. Ment. Dis., *147*:460, 1969.

Pearson, P. L., Bobrow, M., and Vosa, C. G.: Technique for identifying Y chromosomes in human interphase nuclei. Nature (Lond.), *226*:78, 1970.

Phillips, J.: Four cases of spurious hermaphroditism in one family. Am. J. Obstet. Gynecol., *8*:1108, 1886.

Photakis, B.: Ueber einen Fall von Hermaphroditismus verus lateralis masculinus dexter. Arch. Pathol. Anat., *221*:107, 1916.

Pratt, J. P.: Determination of sex by sex chromosomes. Clin. Obstet. Gynecol., *1*:686, 1958.

Rathburn, J. C., Plunkett, E. R., and Barr, M. L.: Diagnosis and management of sex anomalies. Pediatr. Clin. North Am., *5*:375, 1958.

Raynaud, R., Marill, F. G., and Xicluna, R.: Hermaphrodisme vrai. Presse Med., *47*:459, 1939.

Richart, R. M., and Benirschke, K.: Diagnosis of gonadal dysgenesis in newborn infants. Obstet. Gynecol., *15*:621, 1960.

Sandberg, A. A., Koepf, G. F., Crosswhite, L. H., and Hauschke, T.: The chromosome constitution of human marrow in various development and blood disorders. Am. J. Hum. Genet., *12*:231, 1960.

Serr, D. M., Sachs, L., and Danon, M.: The diagnosis of fetal sex during pregnancy. Surg. Gynecol. Obstet., *104*:157, 1957.

Shettles, L. B.: Nuclear morphology of cells in human amniotic fluid in relation to sex of infant. Am. J. Obstet. Gynecol., *71*:834, 1956.

Sinnott, E. W.: Principles of Genetics. 5th Ed. New York, McGraw-Hill Book Company, 1958.

Snyder, C. C., and Cleveland, W. W.: Adrenocorticohyperplasia (female hermaphroditism) in 3 sisters. 1975 (in preparation).

Spaulding, N. H.: The development of the external genitalia in the human embryo. Contrib. Embryol., No. 61, *13*:69, 1921.

Sterling, W. C.: Report of a case of true hermaphroditism; a discussion of thirty two cases previously reported. J. Urol., *56*:720, 1946.

Stojalowski, K., and Debski, J.: Ein neuer Fall von Hermaphroditismus verus beim Menschen. Arch. Pathol. Anat., *290*:358, 1933.

Sydnor, K. L., Kelly, V. G., Raile, R. B., Ely, R. S., and Sayers, G.: Blood adrenocorticotropin in children with corticoadrenohyperplasia. Proc. Soc. Exp. Biol. Med., *82*:695, 1953.

Tjio, J. H., and Levan, A.: The chromosome number of men. Hereditas, *42*:1, 1956.

Tjio, J. H., and Puck, T. T.: Somatic chromosomes of men. Proc. Natl. Acad. Sci. USA, *44*:1229, 1958.

Turner, H. H.: A syndrome of infantilism, congenital webbed neck and cubitus valgus. Endocrinology, *23*:566, 1938.

Walinder, J.: Transsexualism. Goteburg, Sweden, Scandinavian University Books, 1967.

Warkany, J.: Etiology of Congenital Malformations. *In* Levine, S. E., et al. (Eds.): Advances in Pediatrics. Vol. 2. New York, Interscience Publishers, Inc., 1947.

Wilkins, L.: Feminizing and virilizing adrenal tumors. Classification of adrenal disorders. J. Clin. Endocr., *8*:122, 1948.

Wilkins, L.: The Diagnosis and Treatment of Endocrine Disorders in Childhood and Adolescence. 2nd Ed. Springfield, Ill., Charles C Thomas, Publisher, 1957, p. 287.

Wilkins, L., Gardner, L. I., Crigler, J. F., Jr., Silverman, S. H., and Mageon, C. J.: Further studies on the therapy of congenital adrenal hyperplasia with cortisone. J. Clin. Endocr., *12*:257, 1952.

Wilkins, L., Jones, H. W., Jr., Holman, G. H., and Stempfel, R. S., Jr.: Masculinization of the female fetus associated with administration of oral and intramuscular progestins during gestation: Non-adrenal female pseudohermaphrodism. J. Clin. Endocr., *18*:559, 1958.

Williams, D.: The diagnosis of intersex. Br. Med. J., *1*:1264, 1952.

Witschi, E., and Mengert, W.: Endocrine studies on human hermaphrodites and their bearing on the interpretation of homosexuality. J. Clin. Endocr., *2*:279, 1942.

Young, H. H.: Genital Abnormalities, Hermaphroditism and Related Adrenal Diseases. Baltimore, The Williams & Wilkins Company, 1937.

Young, W. C., and Corner, G. W.: Sex and Internal Secretions. 3rd Ed. Baltimore, The Williams & Wilkins Company, 1961.

Zondek, H., Unger, H., and Leszynsky, H. E.: Unilateral hermaphroditismus verus associated with ovarian endometriosis. Acta Endocr., *14*:137, 1953.

# EPILOGUE

As Evelyn Waugh said of women parking cars, we have not finished this book, we have abandoned it. The second edition of *Reconstructive Plastic Surgery* appears at a timely moment in the history of our specialty. A great leap forward has occurred in the last decade, and many advances have been incorporated even as the treatise was being written. Although additions and revisions were responsible for a delay in publication, they have greatly enhanced the value of the book as a reference text. Many of our techniques are in a constant state of change, partly under the influence of the ingenuity and imagination of the surgeon and development of new technology, and partly under the influence of new findings of biological scientists. A special (or new) concept or technique is necessarily followed by a period of time before it is finally accepted, rejected, modified or incorporated into the body of knowledge.

Although technical advances will continue to arise from clinical experience, progress in medicine has always originated from major basic science discoveries. At this time, 23 years from the twenty-first century, we can form a hypothetical image of future changes in the state of the art: our costly hospital system undergoing radical changes; blood loss during operations being reduced to a minimum; new methods of anesthesia making present ones obsolete; the incidence of congenital malformations being reduced as a result of genetic manipulation and immunogenetic research; cancer cells being destroyed by the unleashing of selective immunologic responses; esthetic surgery becoming more commonly practiced as the competition for employment becomes more acute and the desire of the aging population to remain active increases. Closer to the realm of science fiction, when the immunologic barrier responsible for the rejection of allografts is overcome, and if the problem of axonal disorientation in replantation can be solved, it is not unthinkable that the transplantation of composite tissue from cadavers will become a reality.

We confidently anticipate these future developments, but we also realize how inexact is prophesy. We inscribe this book to the plastic surgeons who will make of it a foundation for the next decade of achievements.

John Marquis Converse, M.D.
J. William Littler, M.D.
Joseph G. McCarthy, M.D.

# INDEX

*Note:* Page numbers in *italics* refer to illustrations. Page numbers followed by the letter "t" refer to tables.